Clues in the Diagnosis of Non-tumoral Testicular Pathology

Manuel Nistal
Pilar González-Peramato
Álvaro Serrano

Clues in the Diagnosis of Non-tumoral Testicular Pathology

Springer

Manuel Nistal
Universidad Autónoma de
Madrid (UAM)
School of Medicine
Madrid
Spain

Pilar González-Peramato
School of Medicine, Universidad
Autónoma de Madrid (UAM)
University Hospital La Paz
Department of Pathology
Madrid
Spain

Álvaro Serrano
University Hospital Clinico San Carlos
Department of Urology
Madrid
Spain

ISBN 978-3-319-84145-8 ISBN 978-3-319-49364-0 (eBook)
DOI 10.1007/978-3-319-49364-0

Softcover reprint of the hardcover 1st edition 2017

Printed on acid-free paper

This Springer imprint is published by Springer Nature
The registered company is Springer International Publishing AG
The registered company address is: Gewerbestrasse 11, 6330 Cham, Switzerland

To my wife, Piedad
To my children Rodrigo, Gonzalo, Beatriz, and Natalia
In memoriam, to my father Manuel

Manuel Nistal

To my husband, Alvaro
To my children Álvaro, Teresa, and Javier
In memoriam, to my parents Antonio and Pilar

Pilar González-Peramato

To my wife, Pilar
To my children Álvaro, Teresa, and Javier
In memoriam, to my father Lope

Álvaro Serrano

Preface

This book is a work based on the study and reflection of the authors about hundreds and hundreds of biopsies, surgical specimens, and autopsy material reported during more than 40 years in a university hospital, which treated testicular pathology – and precisely non-tumoral testicular and epididymal pathology – as a hobby. Therefore, this book does not pretend to be a compendium on this pathology, but a presentation of diagnostic problems that to be solved need knowledge on urology, andrology, pediatric gynecological endocrinology, and genetics apart from the usual pathological armamentarium. The success that the book *Testicular and Epididymal Pathology* by Nistal M and Paniagua R, editors, had in the 1980s has encouraged us to continue being specially interested in the non-tumoral testicular and epididymal pathology that has not raised a special interest in other pathology books.

What is the difference of this book from other books of pathology? In the majority of the treatises, the non-tumoral testicular pathology is reduced to a few items where the pathologist does not seem to play an important role. Our purpose is to present the diagnostic problems from the morphology of the lesions and build the diseases and their differential diagnosis under this perspective. Although the book is written in a schematic form, details necessary to get a deeper knowledge of this pathology and its differential diagnosis are included.

The chapters have been selected considering three reasons: first, that the different fields of non-tumoral testicular pathology – genetic, malformative, developmental, functional, vascular, or inflammatory – would be represented; second, that the topics should present problems on their differential diagnosis; and, third, that the pathologies included in this book should be uncommon enough to make this book a highly consultable text to solve certain problems in non-tumoral testicular pathology.

The chapters have been divided in eight parts: genetic and developmental pathology of the testes, infertility, vascular pathology of the testes, inflammatory pathology, pathology of the rete testis, pathology of the epididymis, pathology of the vaginal tunica and paratesticular structures, and miscellanea.

Bearing in mind that in pathology images are as important as – or even more important than – text, figures have been carefully selected in each chapter. Furthermore, in many chapters, to stand out the main characteristics of the lesions or to ease the diagnostic process, a variety of diagrams or algorithms have been included. In addition, legends are straightforward.

The authors have to thank the important contribution along many years of many pathologists in the study of the cases presented in this book, either as pathologist in training or sending cases in consultation that have been kindly and enthusiastically given up. We also have to emphasize the unconditional support of our clinicians and surgeons without whose collaboration this book of clues on non-testicular and epididymal pathology couldn't have been written.

Madrid, Spain Manuel Nistal
Madrid, Spain Pilar González-Peramato
Madrid, Spain Álvaro Serrano

Acknowledgments

First, our thanks are due to our publishers, the Springer-Verlag team, in particular, our associate editor, Inga von Behrens, for giving us the opportunity of publishing this book and our project coordinator, Palanisamy Dhanapal, for his support.

The authors would like to heartily thank the University Hospital La Paz, one of the first big hospitals in Spain, in which two of the authors have developed their professional activity for many years. Special thanks go to all staff members and residents of the Department of Pathology at University Hospital La Paz for their support and for bringing to our attention items and cases of special diagnostic and descriptive interest. We also express our appreciation and gratitude to technical staff of the Department of Pathology at University Hospital La Paz for their careful preparation of the slides shown in this book. We would also like to recognize with thanks the Universidad Autonoma de Madrid where we have carried out our teaching and research activity.

We would also like to express our deepest thanks and appreciation to a large number of colleagues, co-workers, and friends who throughout the years have generously contributed cases in consultation, many of which are very rare and hence precious materials.

Finally, we wish to acknowledge Ana Weyland for her invaluable help to improve the English grammar and syntax of our manuscripts to transform them into readable documents.

Manuel Nistal
Pilar González-Peramato
Álvaro Serrano

Contents

What Does the Presence of Seminiferous Tubules Inside the Tunica Albuginea Mean?

1

Manuel Nistal, Pilar González-Peramato, and Álvaro Serrano

1.1 Structure of the Normal Tunica Albuginea

Together with the interlobular septa, the albuginea forms the structures of the testicular parenchyma support. They divide the testis in 250 lobules with a pyramidal shape. The base, peripheral, is formed by tunica albuginea and the sidewalls by interlobular septa. The lobules, the seminiferous tubules, and the interstitium are located inside with Leydig cells outstanding in the latter. Through the apex the seminiferous tubules are the continuation of the tubuli recti, i.e., the initial part of the rete testis.

The tunica albuginea is formed early, immediately after the appearance of the primitive testis cords [1]. One fibrous basement membrane immediately under the coelomic epithelium as a result of cell differentiation of coelomic epithelium and testicular interstitium and possible migration of extragonadal cells is formed [2, 3]. In the newborn the structure closely resembles that of an adult. The early formation of the tunica albuginea seems to be under the control of the anti-Müllerian hormone produced by Sertoli cells [4].

Histology

In the adult, the tunica albuginea has three layers: the outer layer (tunica vaginalis) is thin and consists of a mesothelial lining resting on a basement membrane. The middle or thicker layer is dense connective tissue, and the inner layer (tunica vasculosa) is loose connective tissue. In the middle layer, the cells, fibroblasts, myofibroblasts, and smooth muscle cells and the fibers, mostly collagenous fibers, are arranged in planes parallel to the surface [5] (Fig. 1.1). From the outer to the inner layers, the amount of collagen fibers decreases, whereas the number of cells increases. This phenomenon is parallel to changes in the phenotype of contractile cells. A secretory phenotype predominates in the most superficial zone and a contractile phenotype in the deepest one [6]. The density of the smooth muscle cells varies in different parts of the tunica albuginea, being higher in the lower pole and the posterior edge of the testicle. Among muscle cells and in their immediate apposition, axon varicosities containing vesicles are distributed suggesting functional innervations of the smooth muscle. The tunica at the lower pole of the testis is crossed by arteries, and nerves that pierce the tunica vasculosa and advance along it reach the parenchyma through the interlobular septa, and in the opposite direction is crossed by veins and lymphatics.

The tunica albuginea, like all testicular structures, is subject to changes throughout life. These changes affect the thickness as well as cell differentiation and the degree of collagenization. During the first 6 years, the thickness hardly changes although a progressive collagenization of the outer part of the middle layer occurs. From

M. Nistal et al., *Clues in the Diagnosis of Non-tumoral Testicular Pathology*,
DOI 10.1007/978-3-319-49364-0_1

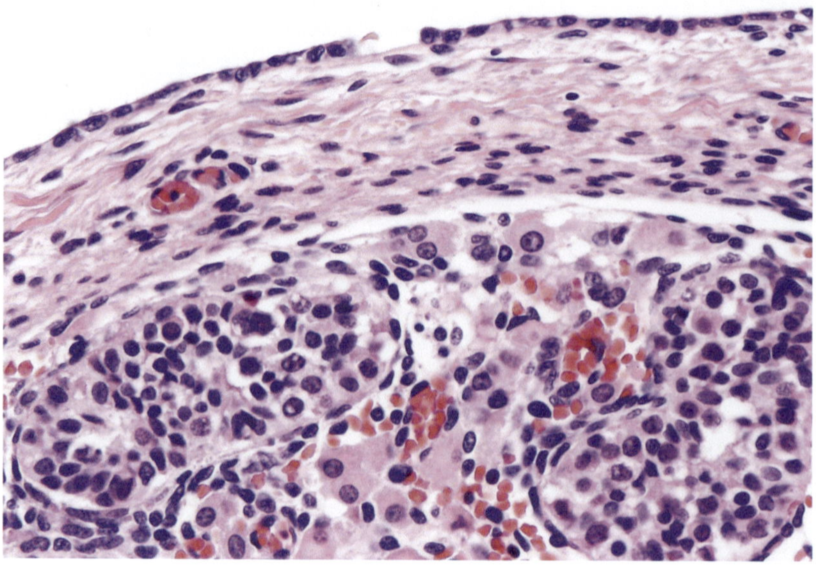

Fig. 1.1 Testis of a newborn baby. The tunica albuginea shows mesothelial lining. Beneath there are two layers, the external one is poorly cellular with abundant collagenous fibers while the internal layer is more cellular. Two sections of seminiferous tubules and abundant Leydig cells are recognized in a deeper location

these 6 years onward, the thickening process continues and accelerates in puberty and goes from 400 microns in young men to over 900 microns in some older men.

Physiology
The functions of the tunica albuginea are multiple. To classic functions such as protection of testis against traumas or acting as a semipermeable membrane that produces the fluid of the vaginalis cavity, a contractile function is added. It is spontaneously able to contract and relax due to the presence of abundant contractile cells showing high concentrations of guanosine monophosphate (GMP), and thus the testicular size and the propelling of sperm from the seminiferous tubules into the head of the epididymis are regulated [7]. This process is dominated by the adrenergic system in association with a smaller purinergic component [8].

1.2 Persistence of Testicular Blastema

Testicular blastema represents the next step in male differentiation of gonadal blastema. It is identified by the presence of poorly defined immature sexual cords with germ cells and little mesenchyma without differentiated Leydig cells [9, 10]. It is the result of the expression of *SRY* gene by Sertoli cells that trigger the expression of other Sertoli cell-specific genes that cause Sertoli-primordial germ cell aggregation and proliferation of Sertoli cells in the underlying mesenchyme [11].

The presence of testicular blastema has been observed in both testes of three newborn babies from a total of 3228 consecutive autopsies at the La Paz University Hospital [12]. These patients had the following conditions: one was the result of a spontaneous abortion due to chorioamnionitis; one was an elective abortion due to a neural tube defect, omphalocele, and asymmetrical arthrogryposis; and the third case had trisomy 18 and the classic features of the Edwards' syndrome.

Histology The persistence of testicular blastema (PBT) takes the form of a crescent, is located in the upper pole of the testis in the vicinity of the epididymis, and occupies an area of several millimeters. There is no tunica albuginea at this level, although the rest of the tunica and the testicular parenchyma and epididymis are normal for the age.

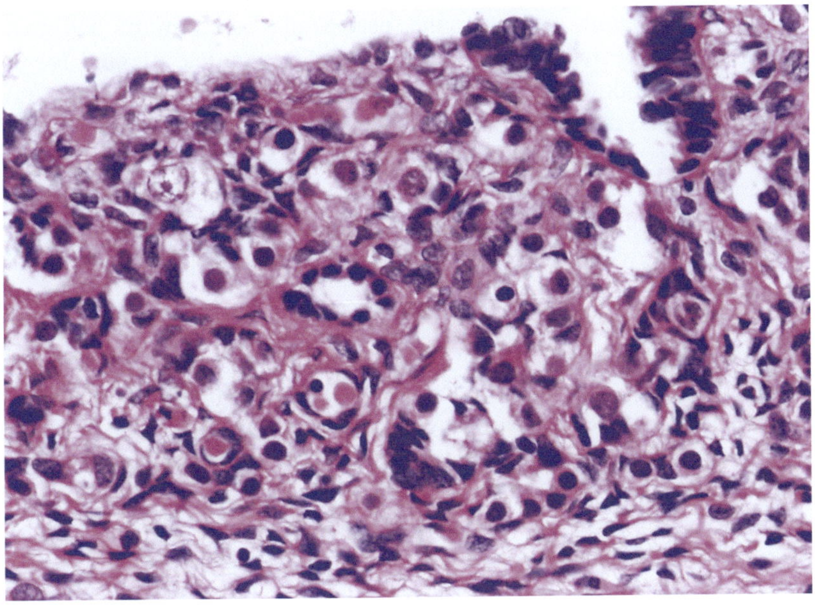

Fig. 1.2 Testicular blastema. Under the coelomic lining formed by cylindrical cells, there is a cellular proliferation in which two cell types are identified; one, the less abundant, has a large and clear cytoplasm; the other is smaller and tends to be arranged around the former cells

The appearance of PBT in low power field is a densely cellular tissue without internal architecture in which at least two cell types are distinguished; one, the most abundant, in continuity with the lining epithelium is polygonal to oval-shaped cells with scant cytoplasm and prominent nucleoli; the other is larger with clear cytoplasm, vesicular nucleus, and central nucleolus in small numbers randomly distributed among the above (Fig. 1.2).

Immunohistochemistry Immunohistochemistry techniques show that the first cell type is derived from the lining epithelial and is being incorporated into the lesion. These cells are strongly positive for cytokeratin AE1/AE3 and calretinin as the epithelial lining. This positivity decreases as the cells take deeper positions until eventually disappearing. The second cell type is represented by primordial germ cells or gonocytes for their positive expression of PLAP and OCT3/4. When the lesion is studied with immunostaining for laminin and collagen IV, a startup organization is revealed inside, unsuspected with H&E, of short, rough, and thick cords surrounded by laminin and collagen IV that are in continuity with the coelomic epithelium. Peritubular myoid cells stained for smooth muscle actin or Leydig cells expressing calretinin are not observed.

The immunohistochemical study supports an early testicular differentiation. Cellular cords probably correspond to pre-Sertoli cells that begin to synthesize components of the basal lamina as laminin and collagen IV, but these cells are still unable to differentiate into myoid cells to form tunica propria, and neither are they able to induce Leydig cell differentiation, both functions related to early differentiation of Sertoli cells [13, 14].

Differential Diagnosis The most important differential diagnosis of this lesion arises with the persistence of "undifferentiated gonadal tissue" (UGT) and secondly with ovotestes. The UGT is a characteristic lesion of patients with disorders of sexual differentiation (DSD) with streak gonads with epithelial cords, dysgenetic testis, streak testis, and ovotestis. UGT represents a gonad in which the arrest of further differentiation is even earlier as ovarian or testicular differentiation is not recognized and does not take a surface distribution like a band in the gonad. These testes, in opposition to those who are UGT carriers, do not have a higher incidence of transformation into gonadoblastoma.

PBT shares with ovotestes the peripheral arrangement on a crescent in a testis but the difference is the following: in the ovarian component of ovotestes there is no tubular organization; the size of germ cells, oocytes, is much higher than that of gonocytes; among female germ cells, there is an abundant stroma similar to that in the ovarian cortex, which is absent in PBT; PBT is not clinically associated with DSD.

Biological Behavior It is very likely that the evolution of PBT, although very delayed in time, would be toward testicular parenchyma both with seminiferous tubules and Leydig cells. The last lesion commented has been observed in infants, children, and adults in this same area of the testis as ectopia of the seminiferous tubules with normal tunica albuginea.

1.3 Persistence of Seminiferous Tubules in Normal Tunica Albuginea

These are seminiferous tubules in formation, directly in connection with the mesothelium externally lining the albuginea. There are short and twisty epithelial cords with scarce interstitium. The extent of the surface of the tunica affected is very variable, and it is not exceptional that almost all of it is involved. It is noteworthy that in all cases under this lesion, the normal structure of the deepest part of the tunica and the delimitation with testicular parenchyma remain clear (Figs. 1.3, 1.4, and 1.5).

Histology Forming seminiferous tubules are constituted by both Sertoli cells, the most numerous, and by gonocytes, numbering two or three per tube. They are surrounded by a thin basement membrane with linear positivity for collagen IV and laminin and externally by a layer of myoid cells. Some Leydig cells develop between the tubular formations.

Immunohistochemistry Immunohistochemistry allows following all the steps of this newly formed tubules. The onset of formation of the seminiferous tubules begins at the surface with changes in morphology and immunophenotype of the mesothelium. The usually cuboidal or squamous epithelium becomes cylindrical and loses the expression of characteristic mesothelial cytokeratins except for cytokeratin 18. Seminiferous tubules, in the form of epithelial

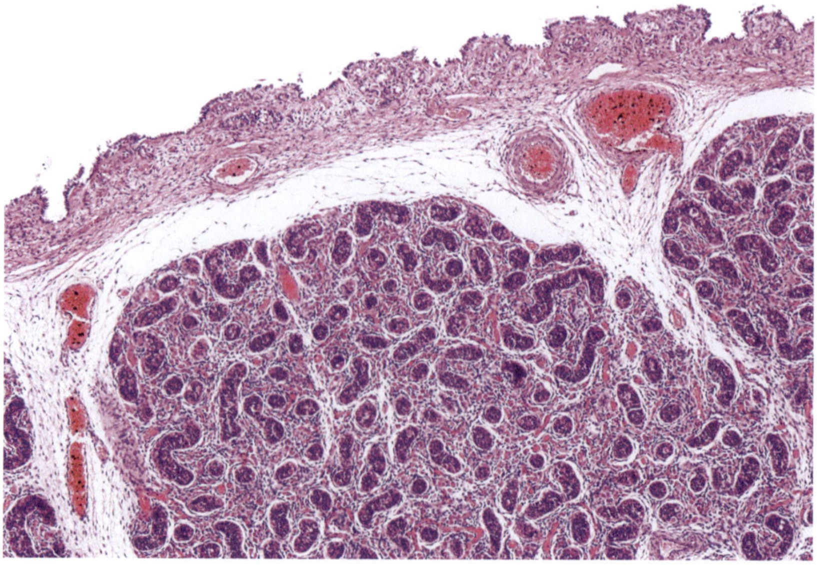

Fig. 1.3 Persistence of seminiferous tubules in formation in the surface of tunica albuginea. The outer contour of the testis has a wavy surface caused by protrusions of different groups of seminiferous tubules in development

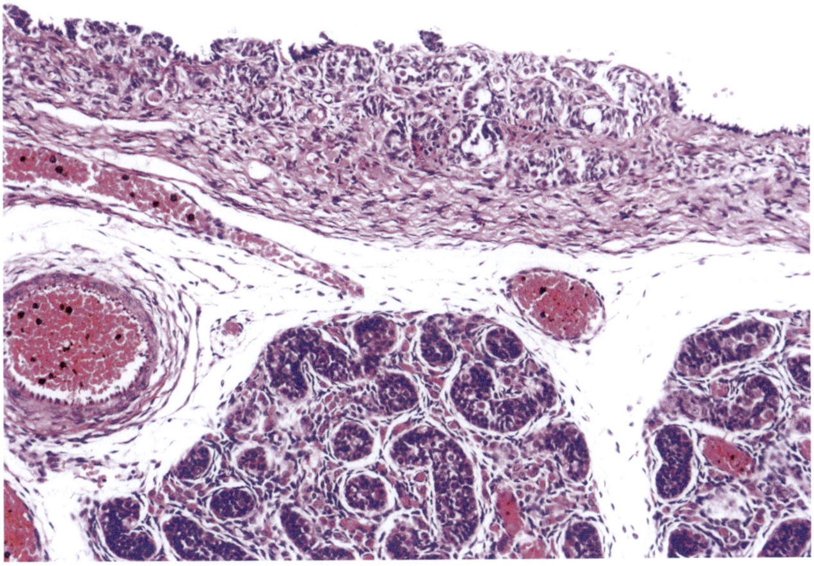

Fig. 1.4 Seminiferous tubules continue their development in the most superficial zone of the tunica respecting the deeper more cellular area and the vasculosa tunic

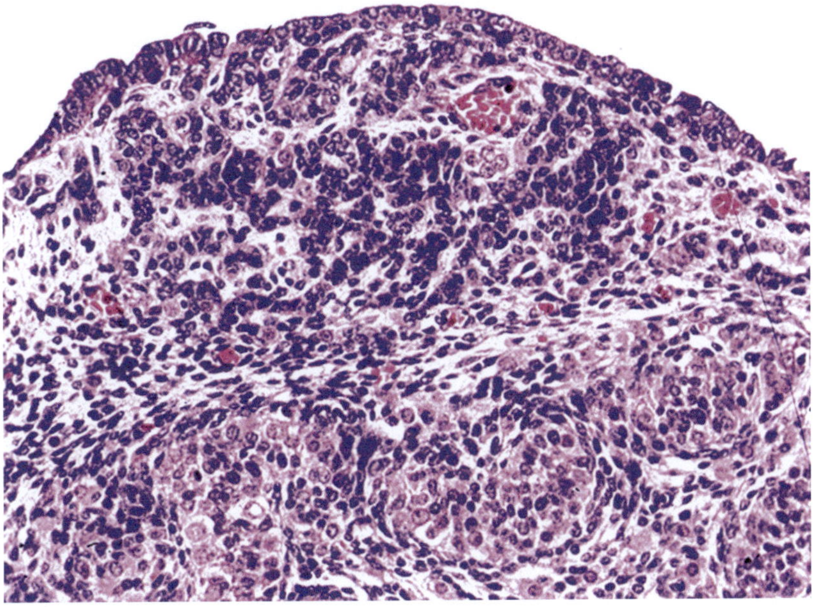

Fig. 1.5 Tunica albuginea is replaced by cell cords that appear connected with the epithelial lining. In depth there is a good delimitation with the seminiferous tubules

cords, still retain calretinin positive expression that the mesothelium used to have and show an important coexpression of inhibin in Sertoli cells. Germ cells are identified as gonocytes (positive for PLAP and OCT3/4).

Differential Diagnosis The differential diagnosis of persistent seminiferous tubules in formation in the normal tunica as well as in the persistence of testicular blastema arises with the UGT and has already been discussed in previous paragraphs. This lesion is interpreted as a late tubular neoformation, uncoupled in time, which starts after the collagenization of the tunica occurred by the action of AMH. And therefore there is a perfect demarcation between the tunica and normal testicular parenchyma. In the newborn child, it coincides with a delay in the maturation of germ cells with persistently high number of gonocytes in the lumen of the seminiferous tubules of the remaining testis. Both findings are characteristic of trisomy 18.

1.4 Ectopia of Testicular Parenchyma in the Normal Tunica Albuginea

It is a focal lesion, generally single, in which the testicular parenchyma extends through the entire thickness of a histologically normal tunica. The presence of testicular parenchyma in the thickness of the tunica is rarely observed; in 0.8 % of pediatric and 0.3 % of adult autopsies, it is probably related to the number of slices studied [15]. It is more common in undescended testes than in normal testes and can be bilateral. It is not associated with DSD.

Histopathology Grossly, this lesion has been reported in the child as rounded macules on the surface of the testicle [16]. In the adult, it is described as a bunch of grapes emerging through a thin tunica albuginea of several millimeters in diameter [17]. But in most cases, it is an incidental histological finding.

The seminiferous tubules have a degree of development similar to the rest of the testicular parenchyma, and among the seminiferous tubules, there are Leydig cells in cases of newborn and in adult testes (Fig. 1.6). Ectopic tubules in adult testes can show spermatogenesis, hyalinization, or cystic transformation (Fig. 1.7). The ectopic seminiferous tubules may or may not be connected to the seminiferous tubules of the testicular parenchyma [4].

The origin of ectopic testicular parenchyma is speculative. It is a process that probably happens between gestation days 44–48, when the sexual cords are formed, and days 48–60, when the tunica albuginea is formed [18]. A delay in growth and maturation of the sex cords would cause them to get trapped inside the tunica albuginea in formation.

Differential Diagnosis The most important differential diagnosis has to be done with the gonad known as dysgenetic testis, the typical gonad of patients with male undermasculinization and Müllerian remnants. The three most important

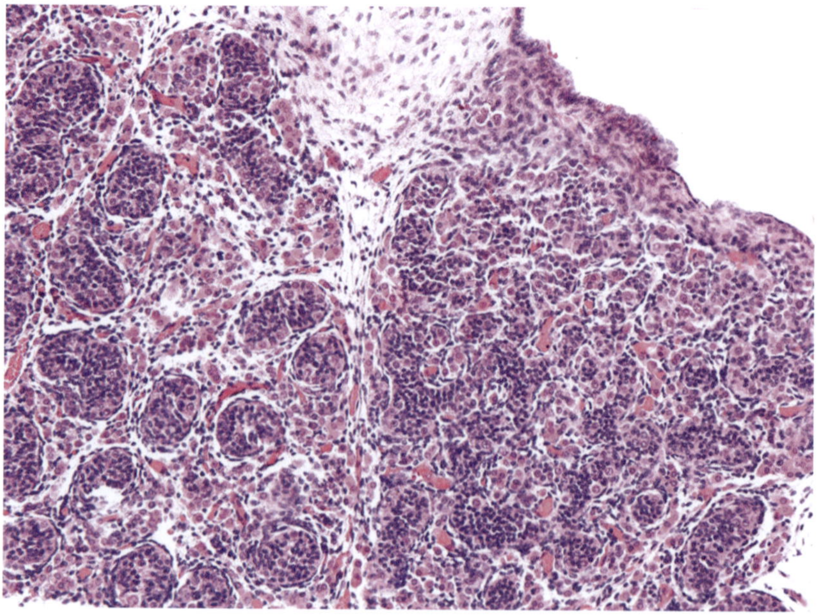

Fig. 1.6 Ectopia testicular parenchyma in the tunica albuginea of a newborn baby. The tunica albuginea is very thickened and contains testicular parenchyma formed by cell cords, seminiferous tubules, and abundant Leydig cells in the interstitium

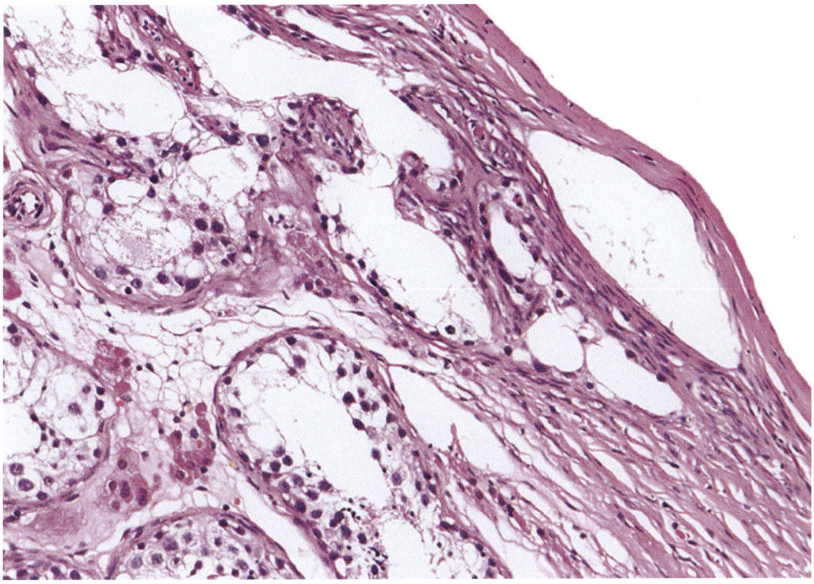

Fig. 1.7 Ectopia of seminiferous tubules present in the thickness of normal tunica albuginea in adult testis. Ectopic tubules show cystic transformation and partially preserved spermatogenesis

criteria are a tunica that is normal in thickness and collagenization, absence of a similar ovarian stroma, and clear delineation between the normal tunica albuginea and testicular parenchyma. In the adult testicles when the seminiferous tubules have undergone a cystic transformation, albuginea cysts must be discarded. These cysts sometimes are mesothelial, and other mesonephric remnants are easily identifiable by immunohistochemical techniques, positive for D2–40 and calretinin in the first case and CD10 in the second one.

1.5 Ectopia of Seminiferous Tubules in an Ovarian-Like Stroma

Testes with this lesion show two distinct areas consisting of a well-developed central testicular parenchyma and another peripheral one in which the tubular density is lower, and the stroma is similar to the ovarian stroma. Both areas may be separated by a loose connective tissue. These gonads are known as dysgenetic testis.

The albuginea is generally thick and lacks the structure and organization characteristic of the tunica of a normal testis. Cells and fibers are not parallel to the surface layers but are arranged in a swirling pattern. The tunica is not well defined from the testicular parenchyma.

The seminiferous tubules of the testicular peripheral area often show anastomosis and penetrate deep into the tunica albuginea, even reaching its surface (Fig. 1.8). Germ cells are rare, and some intratubular eosinophilic bodies and microliths can be observed [4].

Testes with these lesions are associated with the presence of Müllerian structures. The defect in the development of this albuginea is interpreted as the result of a defect in the synthesis or action of AMH, and it is the most common finding in one or both testicles that enables the pathologist to suggest that the patient has one of the following clinical syndromes: dysgenetic male pseudohermaphroditism, mixed gonadal dysgenesis (Sohval syndrome or asymmetric gonadal differentiation), and persistent Müllerian duct syndrome (male with uterus) [19] (see Chap. 4).

Patients with this type of ectopia of the seminiferous tubules require monitoring due to the high proportion of germ cell tumors that develop in the adult [20].

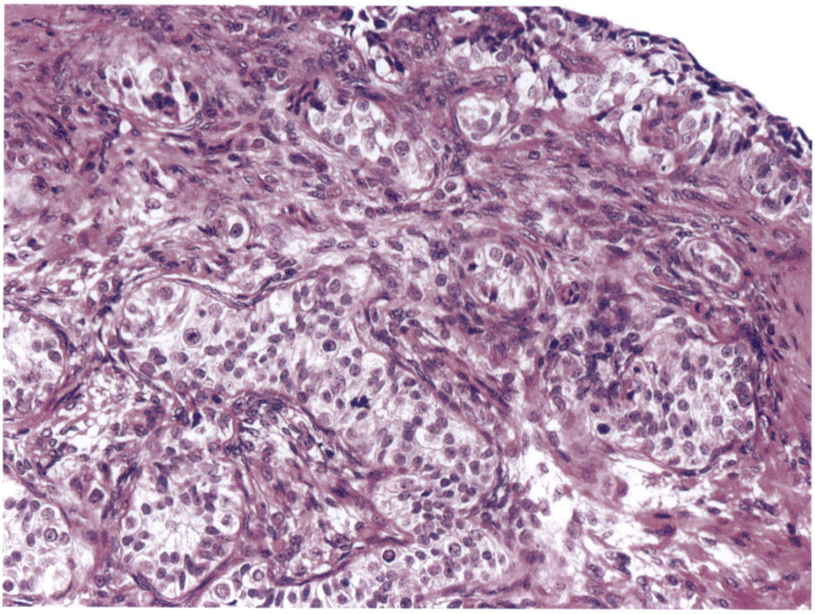

Fig. 1.8 Ectopia of seminiferous tubules present in the thickness of the tunica albuginea with ovarian-like stroma in the testis of a patient with defective AMH

References

1. Waters BL, Trainer TD. Development of the human fetal testis. Pediatr Pathol Lab Med. 1996;16:9–23.
2. Karl J, Capel B. Sertoli cells of the mouse testis originate from the coelomic epithelium. Dev Biol. 1998;203:323–33.
3. Carmona FD, Lupianez DG, Martin JE, Burgos M, Jimenez R, Zurita F. The spatio-temporal pattern of testis organogenesis in mammals—insights from the mole. Int J Dev Biol. 2009;53:1035–44.
4. Jirásek JE. Testicular dysgenesis syndromes. Birth Defects Orig Artic Ser. 1971;7:159–65.
5. Langford GA, Heller CG. Fine structure of muscle cells of the human testicular capsule: basis of testicular contractions. Science. 1973;179:573–5.
6. Middendorff R, Müller D, Mewe M, Mukhopadhyay AK, Holstein AF, Davidoff MS. The tunica albuginea of the human testis is characterized by complex contraction and relaxation activities regulated by cyclic GMP. J Clin Endocrinol Metab. 2002;87:3486–99.
7. Hargrove JL, MacIndoe JH, Ellis LC. Testicular contractile cells and sperm transport. Fertil Steril. 1977;28:1146–57.
8. Banks FC, Knight GE, Calvert RC, Turmaine M, Thompson CS, Mikhailidis DP, Morgan RJ, Burnstock G. Smooth muscle and purinergic contraction of the human, rabbit, rat, and mouse testicular capsule. Biol Reprod. 2006;74:473–80.
9. Jost A, Magre S, Agelopoulou R. Early stages of testicular differentiation in the rat. Hum Genet. 1981;58:59–63.
10. Magre S, Jost A. The initial phases of testicular organogenesis in the rat. An electron microscopy study. Arch Anat Microsc Morphol Exp. 1980;69:297–318.
11. Albrecht KH, Eicher EM. Evidence that Sry is expressed in pre-Sertoli cells and Sertoli and granulosa cells have a common precursor. Dev Biol. 2001;240:92–107.
12. Cajaiba MM, García-Fernández E, Reyes-Múgica M, Nistal M. The spectrum of persistence of testicular blastema and ectopic testicular parenchyma: a possible result of focal delay in gonadal development. Virchows Arch. 2007;451:89–94.
13. Merchant-Larios H, Taketo T. Testicular differentiation in mammals under normal and experimental conditions. J Electron Microsc Tech. 1991;19:158–71.
14. Tilmann C, Capel B. Mesonephric cell migration induces testis cord formation and Sertoli cell differentiation in the mammalian gonad. Development. 1999;126:2883–90.
15. Nistal M, Paniagua R, León L, Regadera J. Ectopic seminiferous tubules in the tunica albuginea of normal and dysgenetic testes. Appl Pathol. 1985;3:123–8.
16. Sanjuán Rodríguez S, Catalina Fernández I, Reyes Mondragón AL, Moreno Hurtado C, Torres de Aguirre A. Ectopic testicular parenchyma in albuginealtunic. Cir Pediatr. 2012;25:211–2.
17. Schmidt SS, Minckler TM. Pseudocysts of the tunica albuginea: benign invasion by testicular tubules. J Urol. 1987;138:151.
18. Wartenberg H. Human testicular development and the role of the mesonephros in the origin of a dual Sertoli cell system. Andrologia. 1978;10:1–21.
19. Chemes H, Muzulin PM, Venara MC, Mulhmann Mdel C, Martínez M, Gamboni M. Early manifestations of testicular dysgenesis in children: pathological phenotypes, karyotype correlations and precursor stages of tumour development. APMIS. 2003;111:12–23.
20. Jørgensen A, Johansen ML, Juul A, Skakkebaek NE, Main KM, Meyts ER. Pathogenesis of germ cell neoplasia in testicular dysgenesis and disorders of sex development. Semin Cell Dev Biol. 2015;45:124–37.

2 Disorders of Sexual Development from the Pathologist's Perspective

Manuel Nistal, Pilar González-Peramato, and Álvaro Serrano

2.1 Introduction

Disorders of sexual development (DSD) [1] are defined as those congenital conditions in which the development of chromosomal, gonadal, and anatomical sex is atypical [2]. Their frequency is estimated at 1 in 4.500–5.500 of the global population [3], but if we include all congenital genital anomalies, including cryptorchidism and hypospadias, it rises to 1:200–1:300 [4]. To solve such important issues as gender assignment, genital surgery, functional outcome, lifelong care, and psychosexual adjustments, DSD requires to be approached from different points of view such as genetic, endocrinological, histological, and surgical [5, 6]. Until just over 10 years ago, diagnoses such as hermaphroditism, pseudohermaphroditism, or intersex still persisted in literature. The consensus classification issued by the Chicago Meeting in 2005 [2] had the good sense to consider these terms obsolete and reunite all of them under the term "disorders of sexual development." It also introduced a classification based on the karyotype, as it was not possible to make a classification based on the underlying genetic error (Fig. 2.1). And certainly, it was most important to create a way of working that allows to standardize the information in order to determine the therapeutic behavior that such a varied pathology produces [7]. In itself, the classification based on the karyotype does not represent a real advance in the knowledge of the DSD for two reasons: (a) the same karyotype may result in different phenotypes with different biological behaviors and the possibility of different tumor development, and (b) very often patients are not 46,XX DSD or 46,XY DSD but have more than one cell line or a complex chromosomal constitution. Other patients as ovotesticular DSD are considered within any of the groups as the karyotype, among others, can be 46,XX, 46,XY, or 46,XY/46,XY (Fig. 2.1).

Not least important is the problem that arises when we have to explain the DSD as pathologists. There is no logical reason to use the karyotype as a starting point as the gonads grouped under the same karyotype have little histological similarities. Therefore, it is imperative to present a more didactic classification. A classification based on histology has many advantages as it allows to know the gonad leading to different genotypes, to assess its functional capacity, and to evaluate the risk of developing a germ cell tumor.

M. Nistal et al., *Clues in the Diagnosis of Non-tumoral Testicular Pathology*,
DOI 10.1007/978-3-319-49364-0_2

Sex chromosome DSD	46,XY DSD		46,XX DSD		
	Disorders of testicular development	Disorders of androgen synthesis / action	Disorders of ovarian development	Fetal androgen excess: CAH	Fetal androgen excess: Non CAH
- 45,X Turner and variants - 47,XXY Klinefelter and variants - 45,X/46,XY MGD - Chromosomal ovotesticular DSD	- Complete gonadal dysgenesis - Partial gonadal dysgenesis - Gonadal regression - Ovotesticular DSD	- Androgen synthesis defect - LH-receptor defect - Androgen insensitivity - 5α–reductase deficiency - Disorders AMH - Timing defect - Endocrine disrupters - Cloacal extrophy	- Ovotesticular DSD - Testicular DSD - Gonadal dysgenesis	- 21-OH-deficiency - 11-OH deficiency	- Aromatase deficiency - POR gene defect - Maternal luteoma - Iatrogenic

DSD: Disorders of sex development, MGD: Mixed Gonadal Dysgenesis, AMH: anti-Müllerian hormone, CAH: Congenital adrenal hyperplasia

Fig. 2.1 Classification based on the karyotype of DSD

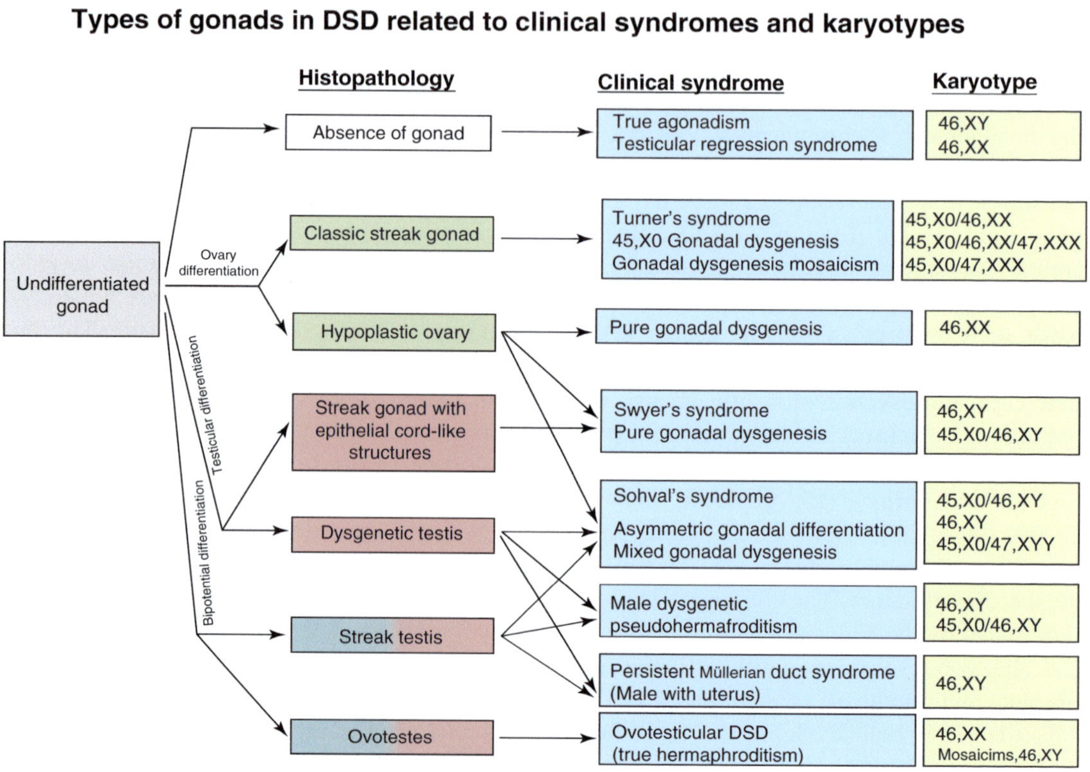

Fig. 2.2 The different types of gonads observed in DSD, the most frequent clinical patterns, and the characteristic karyotypes are shown in the figure. The structurally normal testis present in some DSD such as fetal androgen excess insensitivity syndromes, a 5-alpha-reductase defect is not included in this scheme

2.2 Histological Classification

The DSD show gonads whose structure is in different stages of development or suffer the consequence of a failure of the hormones they should have produced. When the gonad starts to differentiate into ovaries, it may develop as a streak gonad with or without ovarian follicles or become a hypoplastic ovary. If it differentiates into testes, it can be detained forming a structure similar to the streak gonad but with cords of epithelial-looking cells inside (streak testis with epithelial cords), or it may come to acquire a differentiation that grossly simulates a testicle but still presents major defects in its differentiation (dysgenetic testes). If the gonad has a double differentiation into testis and ovary, an ovotestis is formed, but if it partially stops its differentiation, a streak testis results. If the undifferentiated gonad undergoes involution a real agonadism occurs [8–10]. Figure 2.2 shows the different types of gonads observed in DSD, the most frequent clinical patterns, and the characteristic karyotypes.

2.3 Types of Gonads

Undifferentiated Gonadal Tissue (UGT) It is characterized by the presence of germ cells which are similar to gonocytes mixed with smaller cells with hyperchromatic nucleus. There is no cordonal, tubular, or follicular formation. The immunophenotype of the germ cell is similar to that described in the gonads known as streak gonad with epithelial cords. Companion cells have Sertoli/granulosa cell characteristics. UGT is observed not only in this type of streak gonad but also in dysgenetic testis, streak testis, or ovotestis. Gonads with UGT are at high risk of gonadoblastoma and other germ cell tumor development [11].

Classical Streak Gonad A streak gonad is elongated and whitish. It consists of connective tissue that is arranged in bundles reminiscent of ovarian stroma. It is the characteristic gonad of 45,XO gonadal dysgenesia or Turner's syndrome (Fig. 2.3). The streak gonads of some of these patients contain primordial follicles, primary follicles, atretic follicles, small cysts, and clusters of hilar cells in adults (Fig. 2.4). These gonads are characteristic of Turner's syndrome with chromosomal mosaicism and of 46,XX pure gonadal dysgenesis patients (Figs. 2.5 and 2.6).

Hypoplastic Ovary The gonads are ovoid shaped, whitish, and have a smooth surface. Histologically, they show isolated primordial follicles, some primary follicles, and sometimes developing follicles. It is the characteristic gonad of 46,XX pure gonadal dysgenesis and also can be observed in some patients with ovotesticular DSD.

Streak Gonad with Epithelial Cord-Like Structures Macroscopically these gonads resemble the classical streak gonads, but their histological structure is completely different. Instead of isolated follicles, cellular cords are observed in an ovarian-like stroma. These cords do not have a specific spatial orientation, but they are anastomosing and branching. Their thickness is very variable. Histologically, they are formed by two cell types, pre-Sertoli cells and germ cells. The pre-Sertoli cells are the most numerous and notable for their small and hyperchromatic nucleus. They are supported by a basal membrane of varying thickness.

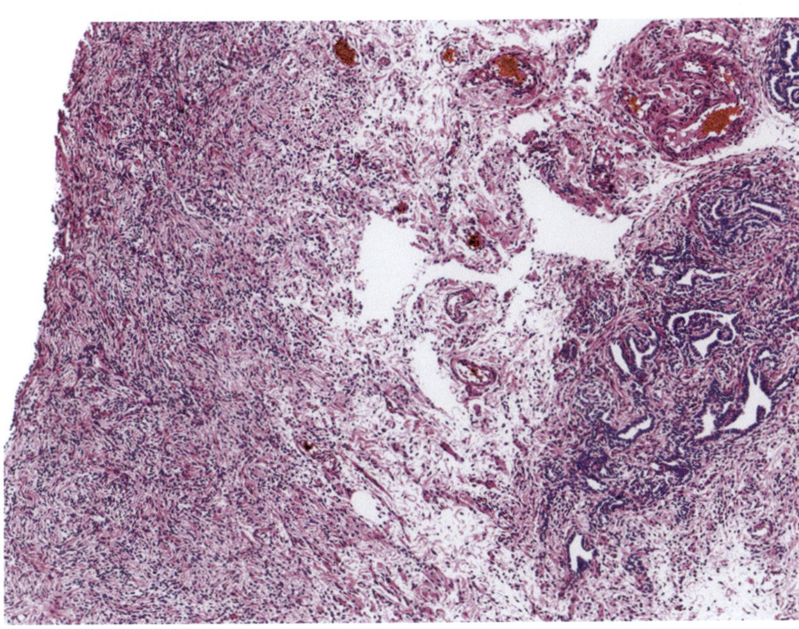

Fig. 2.3 Classical streak gonad in a patient with Turner's syndrome and karyotype 45,X0. The outer area shows a connective tissue reminiscent of ovarian stroma. Deeply, the glandular-like formations correspond to the rete ovarii

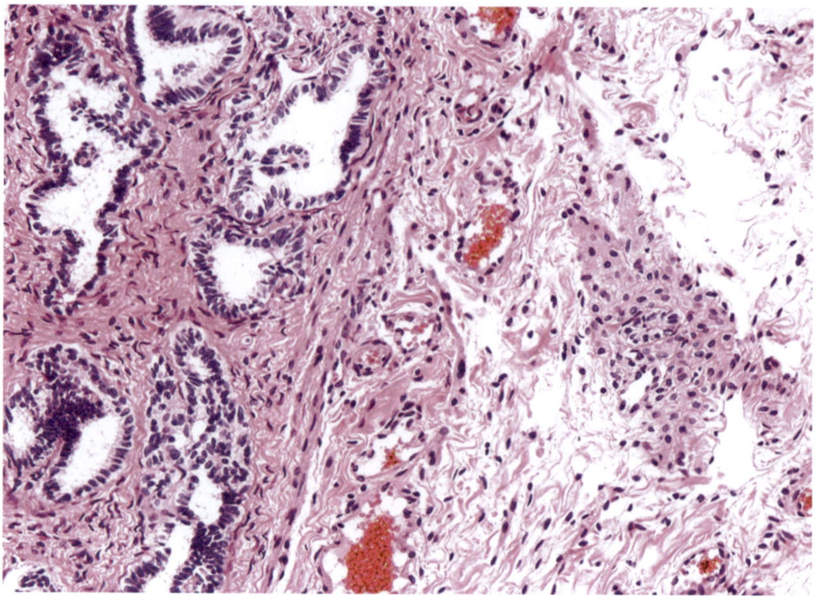

Fig. 2.4 Classical streak gonad. Beside the rete ovarii cavities, there is a cluster of hilar cells surrounding a vessel

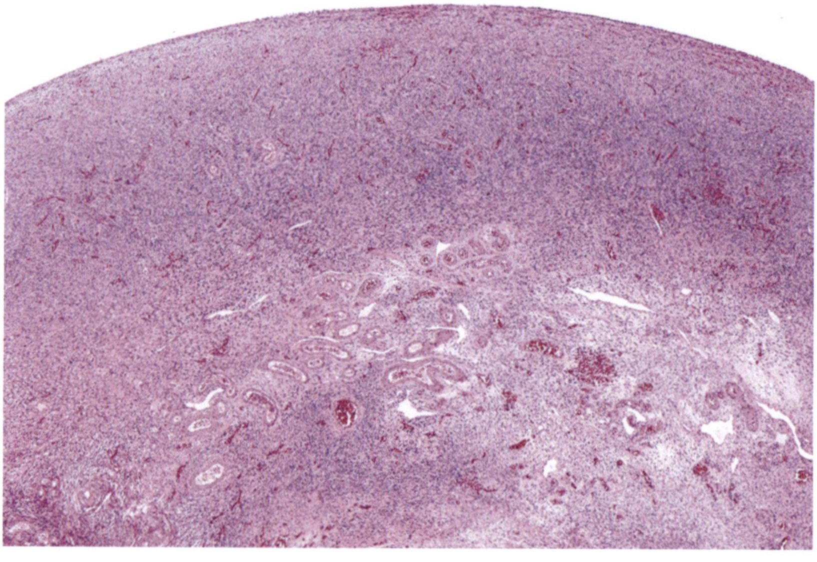

Fig. 2.5 Classical streak gonad in a 46,XX pure gonadal dysgenesis patient

Germ cells resemble gonocytes. They are located inside the epithelial cords or isolated in the stroma and have a large, vesicular nucleus, a central nucleolus, and a pale cytoplasm. Epithelial cells are strongly positive for cytokeratins AE1/AE3, moderately positive for inhibin and D2–40, and weak to AMH. The immunophenotype of germ cells is as follows: OCT3/4 +, c-Kit +, PLAP +, TSPY + (testis-specific protein Y-encoded), and VASA +. It is the characteristic gonad of 46,XY pure gonadal dysgenesis or Swyer syndrome.

Dysgenetic Testis They are small testes formed by a solid tubular grouping in the center of the gonad and a peripheral area in which the tubules are scarce and separated by an abundant stroma. The tunica albuginea is poorly collagenized, and the border with the testicular parenchyma is not well delimited. Its structure recalls the ovarian cortex. The seminiferous tubules of the peripheral zone are often anastomosed and extend through the tunica albuginea until contacting the surface. Sertoli cells of the peripheral tubules express calretinin plus inhibin and AMH. The

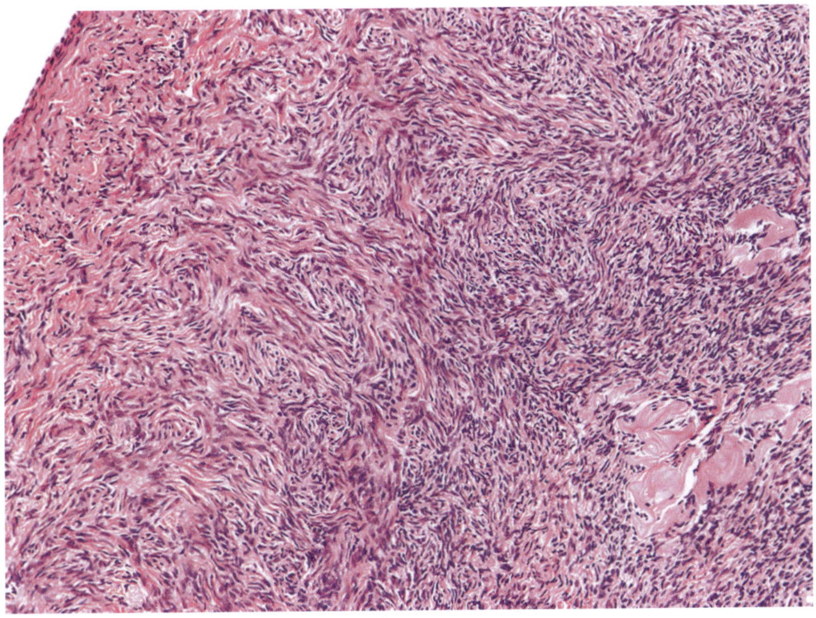

Fig. 2.6 Classical streak gonad in 46,XX pure gonadal dysgenesis patient. Areas of eosinophilic very collagenized fibrosis immersed in a swirling stroma are shown

germ cell phenotype is VASA +, TSPY +, and D2–40 +, and a subpopulation is OCT3/4 +, c-Kit +, and PLAP +. In dysgenetic testis of postpubertal patient's incomplete maturation of Sertoli cells, the absence of spermatogenesis and the hyperplasia of the Leydig cells are observed. The testicles retain the stroma similar to ovarian stroma in peripheral areas. In many cases in situ germ cell neoplasia is observed. This gonad is observed in three syndromes: mixed gonadal dysgenesis (Sohval's syndrome), male dysgenetic pseudohermaphroditism, and Müllerian duct persistence syndrome (male with uterus).

Streak Testis This gonad comprises two areas, the bulkier one corresponds to a dysgenetic testis, and the other one is an elongated structure continuous with the testicular tunica albuginea. It can contain epithelial cords with germ cells in some cases, ovarian follicles in others, or no germ cells at all. It can be seen in the same group of patients with dysgenetic testis.

Ovotestis This is a gonad containing testicular and ovarian tissue. It may take the form of a bilobed structure with separation of the testicular and the ovarian parenchyma, or else it may constitute a single structure standing ovarian parenchyma as a half moon over the testicle. It is a gonad characteristic of the ovotesticular DSD.

Structurally Normal Testes They are architecturally well-formed testicles but with abnormalities at the level of the seminiferous tubules (defects in Sertoli cells and germ) or in the Leydig cells. Their evaluation in childhood requires quantitative studies and immunohistochemical markers. Morphological details allow to individualize different entities. The absence of Leydig cells suggests defect receptivity to LH; persistence of clusters of microvacuolated fetal Leydig cells suggests lipoid congenital adrenal hyperplasia due to STAR mutations, androgen insensitivity, and a 5-alpha-reductase defect. For deeper knowledge of this pathology and postpubertal changes of these testicles, see Chap. 13 (Testicular Dysgenesia Syndrome) and Chap. 18 (Chromosomal Abnormalities and Infertility).

2.4 True Agonadism

True agonadism is defined by the absence of gonads in phenotypically female patients. It was first described in two sisters by Overzier and Linden [12]. The most common karyotype is 46,XY, rarely 46,XX. It can occur sporadically or as a family trait. Inheritance is autosomal recessive [13]. The complaint is short height, lack of breast development, or amenorrhea. The internal genitalia, depending on the time when the gonad disappeared, can be female or persist as Müllerian or Wolffian remnants. In some cases the cause is heterozygous WT1 mutation [14] or a Y-chromosome structural rearrangement [15], but in most cases it remains unknown. Agonadism can be associated with various syndromes: PAGOD (acronym for hypoplasia of the lung and pulmonary artery, agonadism, omphalocele/diaphragmatic defect, dextrocardia) [16], Kennerknecht's [13], Seckel's [17], and Charge's syndromes [18]. Patients with testicular regression syndrome usually show male internal genitalia and a variable grade of external genitalia development related to the moment of testicular involution.

2.5 Gonadal Dysgenesis with Classical Streak Gonad

2.5.1 Turner's Syndrome

Patients with Turner's syndrome are phenotypically short women with sexual childishness, streak gonads, and numerous dysmorphic signs such as a low hairline, a triangular face, a high-arched palate, a small mandible, a webbed neck, a broad chest with widely spaced nipples, cubitus valgus, short four metacarpals, multiple pigmented nevi, congenital lymphedema of hands and feet, and cardiac and renal anomalies [19]. The incidence is 1:2500 live born females. The etiology of Turner's syndrome in 50–60 % of cases is the chromosome monosomy 45,X0, whereas the remaining patients display other chromosome anomalies with or without mosaicism [20].

Patients *with X monosomy* have female development. The gonads are the classic streak gonads that consist of ovarian-like stroma. Clusters of hilar cells and rete ovarii cysts can be observed in adults. Gonads develop normally until the third month of fetal life. From that moment gonocytes begin to disappear due to widespread meiotic pairing errors. Apoptosis of germ cells is maximal between 15 and 20 weeks of pregnancy. The majority of the oocytes have disappeared at birth. Only 3 % of patients in adulthood have ovarian follicles that are responsible for the presence of menses for a short period of time. Keep in mind that a 45,X0 karyotype in peripheral blood leukocytes does not preclude the coexistence of a mosaic 45,X0/46,XY in the gonad. In these cases the gonadal function remains better preserved. The prevalence of Y-chromosome sequences in patients who present with a nonmosaic 45,X0 karyotype is 6–11 % [21].

The most frequent *chromosomal mosaicism* in Turner's syndrome is 45,X0/46,XX. Karyotypes 45,X0/47,XXX; 45,X0/46,XX/47,XXX, and 45,X0/46,XY are rare [22]. Patients with mosaic 45,X0/46,XX present important differences as compared with 45,X0 patients. They are taller, they have spontaneous puberty (menarche 12 %), and their fertility is more frequent than in the monosomy 45,X0. Eighteen percent have breast development compared to 5 % of 45,X0 patients. Pregnancies either spontaneous or after oocyte donation have been reported although with high rates of miscarriages and fetal anomalies (intrauterine growth restriction, low birth weight, prematurity) and important maternal complications [23].

Patients with Turner's syndrome and Y-chromosomal material have a high risk of developing a germ cell tumor in their gonads (10–30 %) which makes it imperative to carry out molecular studies and FISH, in addition to the classic cytogenetic studies. Gonadoblastoma is the most common tumor. In these patients gonadectomy with or without prophylactic salpingectomy is recommended [24]. Prolonged estrogen treatments are also a risk for endometrial carcinoma [25].

2.5.2 46,XX Pure Gonadal Dysgenesis

Patients with this syndrome have a female phenotype with absence of spontaneous pubertal development, primary amenorrhea, normal height, absence of turner stigma and hypergonadotropic hypogonadism as a result of primary gonadal failure. The presentation can be sporadic or genetic [26]. 46,XX pure gonadal dysgenesis is caused by autosomal mutations in the genes encoding the follicle-stimulating hormone (FSH) receptor, *WNT4*, *R-Spondin*, *PSMC3IP*, *MCM9*, *MCM8*, *STAG3*, *SYCE1*,and *NUP107* or by X-linked recessive mutations in *BMP15* [27]. The internal genitalia consist of uterus and streak gonads or severe ovarian hypoplasia.

The risk of developing tumors, not being carriers of Y-chromosome sequences, is low, and only isolated cases of gonadoblastoma and dysgerminoma have been observed. So the need for bilateral gonadectomy is questioned [28].

46,XX pure gonadal dysgenesis is associated with the following anomalies: neurosensory hearing loss (Perrault's syndrome) [29], achondroplasia [30], and fatal lung fibrosis with immunodeficiency [31].

References

1. Dreger AD, Chase C, Sousa A, Gruppuso PA, Frader J. Changing the nomenclature/taxonomy for intersex: a scientific and clinical rationale. J Pediatr Endocrinol Metab. 2005;18:729–33.
2. Lee PA, Houk CP, Ahmed SF, Hughes IA. Consensus statement on management of intersex disorders. International Consensus Conference on Intersex. Pediatrics. 2006;118:e488–500.
3. Sax L. How common is intersex? A response to Anne Fausto-Sterling. J Sex Res. 2002;39:174–8.
4. Nordenvall AS, Frisén L, Nordenström A, Lichtenstein P, Nordenskjöld A. Population based nationwide study of hypospadias in Sweden, 1973 to 2009: incidence and risk factors. J Urol. 2014;191:783–9.
5. Ostrer H. Disorders of sex development (DSDs): an update. J Clin Endocrinol Metab. 2014;99:1503–9.
6. Mieszczak J, Houk CP, Lee PA. Assignment of the sex of rearing in the neonate with a disorder of sex development. Curr Opin Pediatr. 2009;21:541–7.
7. Lee PA, Nordenström A, Houk CP, Ahmed SF, Auchus R, Baratz A, Baratz Dalke K, Liao LM, Lin-Su K, Looijenga 3rd LH, Mazur T, Meyer-Bahlburg HF, Mouriquand P, Quigley CA, Sandberg DE, Vilain E, Witchel S, Global DSD Update Consortium. Global disorders of sex development update since 2006: perceptions, approach and care. Horm Res Paediatr. 2016;85:158–80.
8. Nistal M, Gonzalez-Peramato P. Las disgenesias gonadales. Aproximación a través de la anatomía patológica al diagnóstico. Rev Horm Crecim. 2010;XIII:77–88.
9. Nistal M, Gonzalez-Peramato P. Disorders of sex development. In: Davor J, editor. Atlas on the human testis. Normal morphology and pathology. London: Springer; 2012. p. 265–80. ISBN:978-1-4471-2762-8.
10. Nistal M, Paniagua R, Gonzalez-Peramato P. Nonneoplastic diseases of the testis. In: Bostwick DG, Cheng L, editors. Urologic surgical pathology. 3rd ed. Philadelphia: Elsevier Saunders; 2014. p. 560–735. ISBN: 978-1-4557-4327-8.
11. Cools M, Stoop H, Kersemaekers AM, Drop SL, Wolffenbuttel KP, Bourguignon JP, Slowikowska-Hilczer J, Kula K, Faradz SM, Oosterhuis JW, Looijenga LH. Gonadoblastoma arising in undifferentiated gonadal tissue within dysgenetic gonads. J Clin Endocrinol Metab. 2006;91:2404–13.
12. Linden H, Overzier C. True agonadism (anorchism) in siblings. Gynaecologia. 1956;142:215–33.
13. Kennerknecht I, Sorgo W, Oberhoffer R, Teller WM, Mattfeldt T, Negri G, Vogel W. Familial occurrence of agonadism and multiple internal malformations in phenotypically normal girls with 46,XY and 46,XX karyotypes, respectively: a new autosomal recessive syndrome. Am J Med Genet. 1993;47:1166–70.
14. Devriendt K, Deloof E, Moerman P, Legius E, Vanhole C, De Zegher F, Proesmans W, Devlieger H. Diaphragmatic hernia in Denys-Drash syndrome. Am J Med Genet. 1995;57:97–101.
15. Cui YX, Shi YC, Liu Q, Xia XY, Lu HY, Shao HF, Jia L, Yao B, Ge YF, Li XJ, Huang YF. A case of agonadism associated with y-chromosome rearrangement: cytogenetic and molecular studies. J Androl. 2009;30:650–4.
16. Takahashi K, Miyake A, Nakayashiro M. Hypoplastic left heart syndrome in PAGOD syndrome. Pediatr Int. 2014;56:422–4.
17. Silengo M, Del Monaco A, Linari A, Lala R. Low birth-weight, microcephalic malformation syndrome in a 46,XX girl and her 46,XY sister with agonadism: third report of the Kennerknecht syndrome or autosomal recessive Seckel-like syndrome with previously undescribed genital anomalies. Am J Med Genet. 2001;101:275–8.
18. Kushnick T, Wiley JE, Palmer SM. Agonadism in a 46,XY patient with CHARGE association. Am J Med Genet. 1992;42:96–9.
19. Sybert VP, McCauley E. Turner's syndrome. N Engl J Med. 2004;351:1227–38.
20. Bispo AV, Dos Santos LO, Burégio-Frota P, Galdino MB, Duarte AR, Leal GF, Araújo J, Gomes B, Soares-Ventura EM, Muniz MT, Santos N. Effect of chromosome constitution variations on the expression of Turner phenotype. Genet Mol Res. 2013;12: 4243–50.
21. Zelaya G, López Marti JM, Marino R, Garcia de Dávila MT, Gallego MS. Gonadoblastoma in patients with Ullrich-Turner síndrome. Pediatr Dev Pathol. 2015;18:117–21.
22. Tauchmanovà L, Rossi R, Pulcrano M, Tarantino L, Baldi C, Lombardi G. Turner's syndrome mosaicism 45X/47XXX: an interesting natural history. J Endocrinol Invest. 2001;24:811–5.
23. Chevalier N, Letur H, Lelannou D, Ohl J, Cornet D, Chalas-Boissonnas C, Frydman R, Catteau-Jonard S, Greck-Chassain T, Papaxanthos-Roche A,

Dulucq MC, Couet ML, Cédrin-Durnerin I, Pouly JL, Fénichel P. French Study Group for Oocyte Donation. Materno-fetal cardiovascular complications in Turner syndrome after oocyte donation: insufficient prepregnancy screening and pregnancy follow-up are associated with poor outcome. J Clin Endocrinol Metab. 2011;96:E260–7.
24. Kanakatti Shankar R, Inge TH, Gutmark-Little I, Backeljauw PF. Oophorectomy versus salpingo-oophorectomy in Turner syndrome patients with Y-chromosome material: clinical experience and current practice patterns assessment. J Pediatr Surg. 2014;49:1585–8.
25. McCarty Jr KS, Barton TK, Peete Jr CH, Creasman WT. Gonadal dysgenesis with adenocarcinoma of the endometrium: an electron microscopic and steroid receptor analyses with a review of the literature. Cancer. 1978;42:512–20.
26. Kohmanaee S, Dalili S, Rad AH. Pure gonadal dysgenesis (46 XX type) with a familial pattern. Adv Biomed Res. 2015;4:162.
27. Weinberg-Shukron A, Renbaum P, Kalifa R, Zeligson S, Ben-Neriah Z, Dreifuss A, Abu-Rayyan A, Maatuk N, Fardian N, Rekler D, Kanaan M, Samson AO, Levy-Lahad E, Gerlitz O, Zangen D. A mutation in the nucleoporin-107 gene causes XX gonadal dysgenesis. J Clin Invest. 2015;125:4295–304.
28. Kanagal DV, Prasad K, Rajesh A, Kumar RG, Cherian S, Shetty H, Shetty PK. Ovarian gonadoblastoma with dysgerminoma in a young girl with 46, XX karyotype: a case report. J Clin Diagn Res. 2013;7:2021–2.
29. Sampathkumar G, Veerasigamani N. Perrault syndrome – a rare case report. J Clin Diagn Res. 2015;9:OD01–2.
30. Gokce C, Atabek ME, Kaynar L, Torun E, Kurtoglu S, Bayram F. Achondroplasia associated with gonadal dysgenesis. J Int Med Res. 2008;36:605–8.
31. Somech R, Somers GR, Chitayat D, Grunebaum E, Atkinson A, Kolomietz E, Roifman CM. Fatal lung fibrosis associated with immunodeficiency and gonadal dysgenesis in 46XX sisters–a new syndrome. Am J Med Genet A. 2008;146A:8–14.

3 Clinical Syndromes Associated with Streak Gonads with Epithelial Cords

Manuel Nistal, Pilar González-Peramato, and Álvaro Serrano

3.1 46,XY Gonadal Dysgenesis

This disorder is also known as Swyer syndrome [1]. It is a disorder of sexual development (DSD) in which patients with 46,XY chromosomal constitution have a female phenotype and absence of Turner stigmata. Most patients with 46,XY gonadal dysgenesis are sporadic. In some family cases, the inheritance may be X chromosome-linked recessive, autosomal dominant limited to the male in other cases, or even autosomal recessive in other patients [2]. Two variants of 46,XY gonadal dysgenesis, complete and incomplete, are distinguished.

Complete 46,XY Gonadal Dysgenesis The external genitalia are female with or without labia fusion and clitoral hypertrophy, and the internal genitalia include the vagina, uterus, Fallopian tubes, and fibrous tracts. Its estimated incidence is 1:80,000 births [3]. The diagnosis is usually made after adolescence. Patients consult for primary amenorrhea and delayed puberty. They develop hypergonadotropic hypogonadism with low estrogen levels, high stature, and poor development of axillary and pubic hair. Pregnancies have been achieved after treatment with estrogen and egg donation.

The etiology of this disorder is known in only 10–15 % of cases. Mutations and deletions in the *SRY* gene have been identified [4] and in a small number of cases also *DHH* gene mutation, duplication of *DAX1* (also known as *NROB1*) and *WNT4* genes, as well as haploinsufficiency of the *SOX9*, *SF1*, *WT1*, and *WMRT1-WMRT2* genes [5].

Incomplete (Partial) 46,XY Gonadal Dysgenesis It is characterized by ambiguity of the external genitalia ranging from a female phenotype with clitoromegaly to a male phenotype in patients with 46,XY karyotype. In most cases (80 %), no mutations in major genes required for gonadal development, *SRY* and *WT1*, are observed [6]. Some cases associated with *NR5A1* mutation have been reported [7].

Patients may or may not have uterus and Fallopian tubes. Most of them grow up as males, have a spontaneous puberty, develop hypergonadotropic hypogonadism, and are infertile [8].

Pathology of 46,XY Gonadal Dysgenesis The histology of the gonads is quite varied. Patients with female phenotype and clitoromegaly often have incipient ovarian differentiation with classic streak gonads and hilar cells [9] or hypoplastic

M. Nistal et al., *Clues in the Diagnosis of Non-tumoral Testicular Pathology*,
DOI 10.1007/978-3-319-49364-0_3

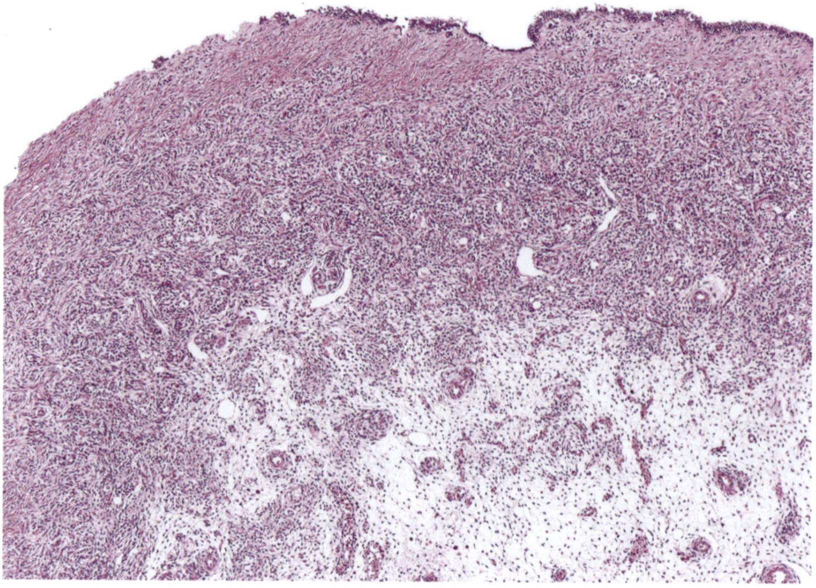

Fig. 3.1 Streak gonad with epithelial cords in a patient with incomplete (partial) 46,XY gonadal dysgenesis. The epithelial cords may go unnoticed when observed at low magnification

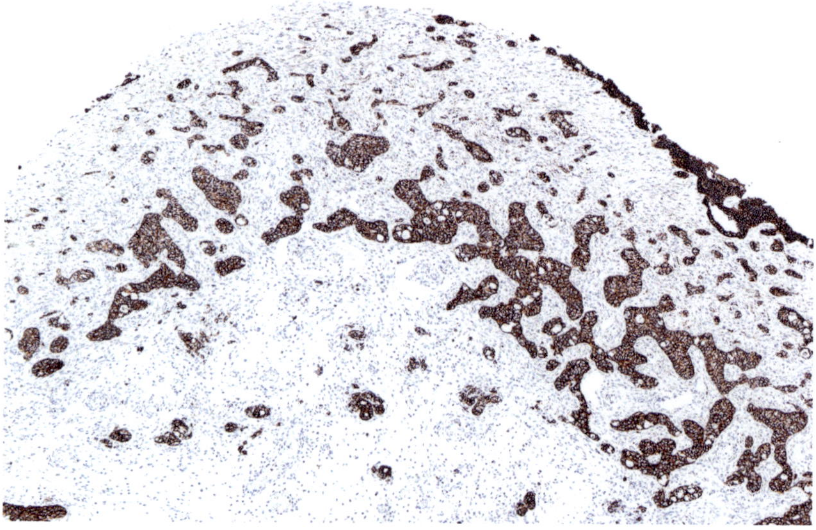

Fig. 3.2 Streak gonad with epithelial cords is immunostained for AE1/AE3 cytokeratin. The epithelial cords extend throughout the thickness of the gonad. They are thicker and anastomosing in the deeper zone

ovaries. Gonads showing differentiation toward testis as streak gonads with epithelial cords predominate in patients with ambiguous genitalia. Epithelial cells are strongly positive for cytokeratins AE1/AE3, moderately positive for inhibin and D2-40, and weak to AMH (Figs. 3.1, 3.2, 3.3, and 3.4). There are cases of partial 46,XY gonadal dysgenesis with ambiguous external genitalia, well-developed Müllerian structures coexisting with testicles similar to dysgenetic testes. This situation has been interpreted as a decoupling in time between the time of AMH and testosterone production and maximum responsiveness of target structures [10]. Patients with complete 46,XY gonadal dysgenesis and absence of internal genitalia, whose gonads were testicles with Sertoli cell only, have also been reported. In some of these patients, *NR5A1* gene mutation has been shown [11].

The tumor risk is very variable – it is estimated at 5 % during the first decade of life and between 25–30 % throughout life [12]. In principle, gonadectomy as soon as the diagnosis is made seems desirable. The most common tumors

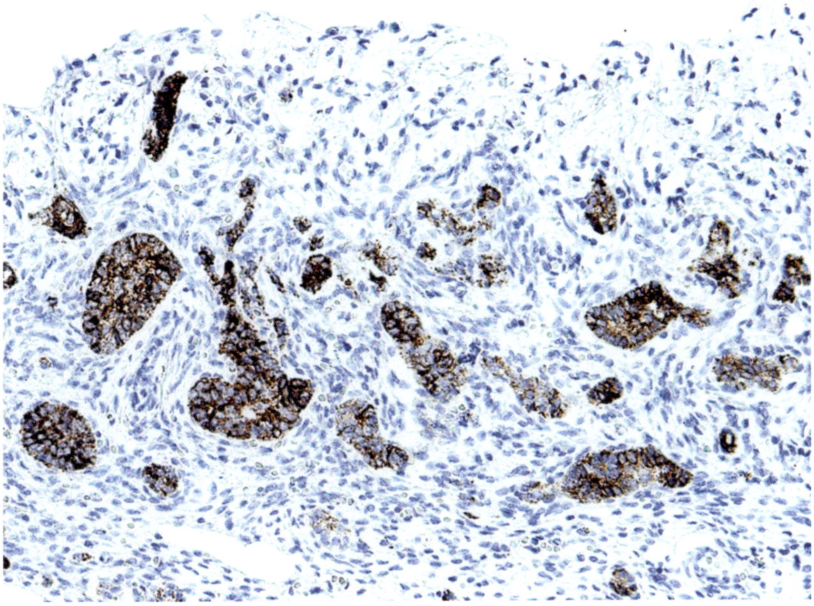

Fig. 3.3 Streak gonad with epithelial cords. Many cells in epithelial cords show immunoexpression for inhibin

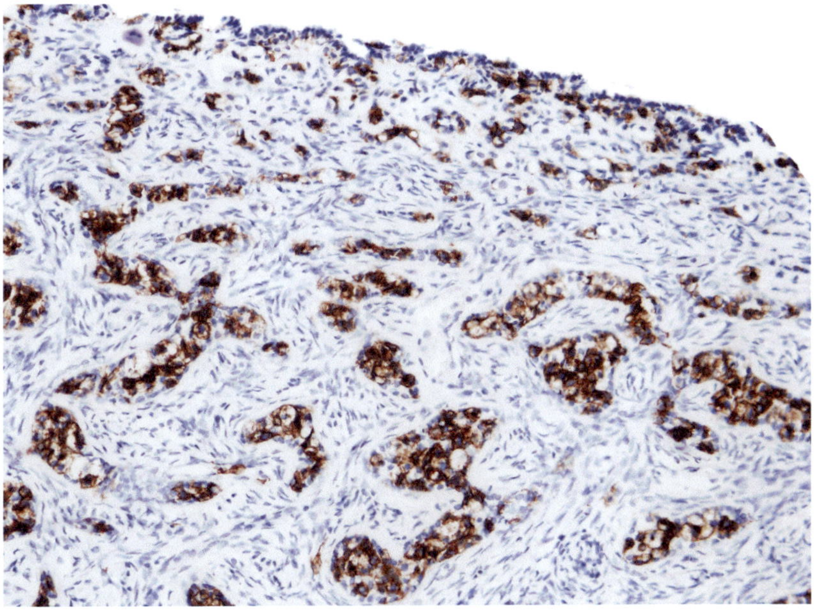

Fig. 3.4 Streak gonad with epithelial cords. The cells in cords that are negative for inhibin are germ cells (the majority gonocytes). Germ cells show immunoexpression for PLAP

are gonadoblastomas (Fig.3.5), dysgerminomas (Fig.3.6), teratoma, and choriocarcinoma [13, 14]. In case the gonads are testes and are lodged in labioscrotal folds, provided the follow-up is assured, they can be maintained until puberty. The presence of germinal tumors has been associated in some cases with the development of a peripheral precocious puberty [15].

Extragonadal Anomalies in 46,XY Gonadal Dysgenesis The most common forms are campomelic dysplasia and renal disorder; myotonic dystrophy plus renal disease; progressive renal insufficiency (Frasier syndrome); associated renal insufficiency and Wilms tumor (Denys-Drash syndrome); mental retardation with or without facial anomalies and with or without

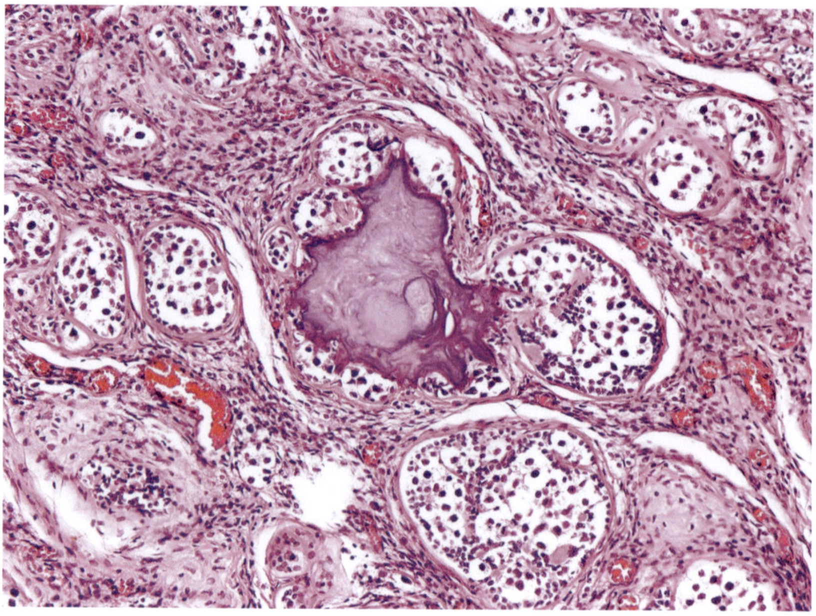

Fig. 3.5 Streak gonad of a Swyer syndrome patient. The streak gonad shows numerous oval formations of different sizes characteristic of gonadoblastoma. One nodular formation with extensive calcification of geographical boundaries can be identified in the central part of the figure

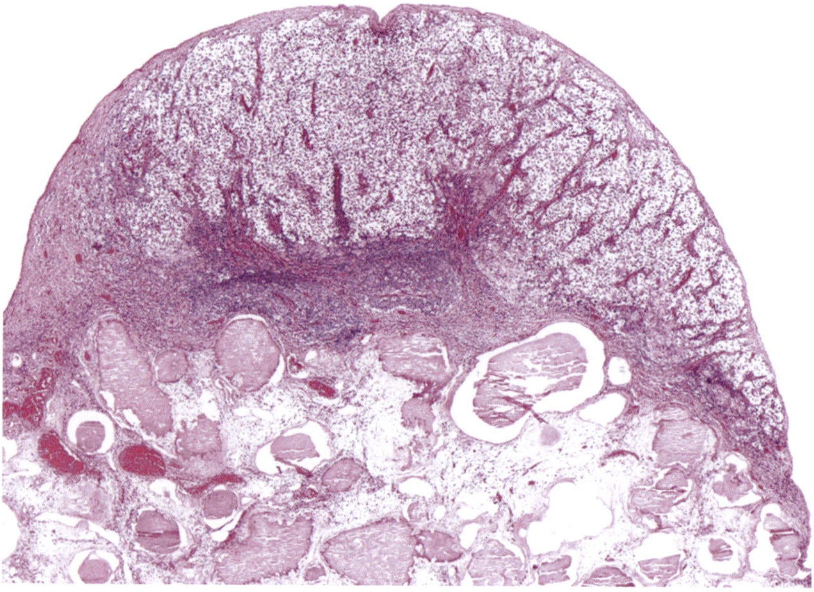

Fig. 3.6 Streak gonad of a Swyer syndrome patient. The streak gonad is markedly thickened. The outer half moon corresponds to a dysgerminoma. At the bottom standout numerous calcifications in which remains of a gonadoblastoma are still recognized

short height; cleft palate, micrognathia, kyphoscoliosis and clubfoot (Gardner-Silengo-Wachtel syndrome or genito-palato-cardiac syndrome); pterygium multiple syndrome; Graves' disease; congenital universal alopecia, microcephalia, cutis marmorata, and short height; and peripheral neuropathy among others [16].

3.2 Syndromes Associated with 46,XY Gonadal Dysgenesis

3.2.1 Denys-Drash Syndrome

Denys-Drash syndrome was described as the association of pseudohermaphroditism, nephroblastoma, and glomerular disease in patients with 46,XY karyotype [17]. Patients may have from external female genitalia to male genitalia with perineal hypospadias and undescended testes. The most common nephropathy is diffuse mesangial sclerosis, which causes rapid renal failure [18].

In most cases, this syndrome is produced by point mutations in exons 6–9 and 6–9 introns of the Wilms tumor suppressor gene (*WT*1) [19, 20]. *WT1* gene is expressed in the gonadal ridge in the sixth week of embryonal development. Gene mutations lead to the abnormal development of kidneys and gonads leading to a diffuse mesangial sclerosis, gonadal dysgenesis, and increased risk of Wilms tumor.

It may present with different clinical manifestations, 46,XY gonadal dysgenesis [21], mixed gonadal dysgenesis [22], and dysgenetic male pseudohermaphroditism, and there are even cases of ovotesticular DSD.

Mutations of *WT1* can give rise to streak gonads with epithelial cords in most cases [23] followed in a few cases by testes [24] and, if a delay in testicular determination occurs, normal testes.

3.2.2 Frasier Syndrome

The Frasier syndrome is a rare inherited disease characterized by a steroid-resistant nephrotic syndrome (focal and segmental glomerulosclerosis), gonadal tumor, and male pseudohermaphroditism. These patients do not have a predisposition toward Wilms tumor.

Eighty percent of patients are characterized by external female genitalia with 46,XY karyotype, 10 % with male external genitalia with 46,XY, and 10 % with female external genitalia with 46,XX. In the first two groups (patients with 46,XY), gonads are formed by structures with testicular differentiation such as streak gonads with epithelial cords or even testes. In the third group (patients 46,XX), classic streak gonads or hypoplastic ovaries are observed. Patients with 46,XY and female external genitalia have a high risk of germ cell tumor (67 %), which is not the case in patients with 46,XX whose risk is very low [25].

Similarly to the Denys-Drash syndrome, the Frasier syndrome is caused by mutations in the *WT1* gene, which differs in renal injury. In this case, it is a focal segmental glomerulosclerosis, with no predisposition to Wilms tumor, and increased risk for germ cell tumor in the gonads. Since some symptoms overlap with the Denys-Drash syndrome, some authors consider both syndromes part of the same spectrum and not two different entities.

Although most males with Frasier syndrome have the typical male chromosome pattern (46,XY), they have gonadal dysgenesis, in which external genitalia do not look either clearly male or clearly female (ambiguous genitalia), or else the genitalia appear to be completely feminine. The gonads are typically undeveloped and referred to as streak gonads [26].

3.2.3 WARG Syndrome

The acronym WARG for this syndrome means Wilms tumor (W), aniridia (A), genitourinary anomalies (G), and mental retardation (R). The prevalence of the WARG syndrome is 1:500,000 to 1:1,000,000, and the prevalence of Wilms tumors is 7:1000. Most cases are identified in childhood due to sporadic aniridia. Patients with aniridia have a 45–60 % chance to develop Wilms tumor. Patients with female phenotype often have bicournuate uterus and streak gonads. Affected males have undescended testes [27].

The cause of the symptoms of this syndrome is the loss of multiple genes located on the short arm of chromosome 11 [28, 29]. WAGR syndrome is described as a contiguous gene deletion syndrome because it results from the loss of several genes neighboring – and including – *WT1* and *PAX6* [30].

3.2.4 Campomelic Dysplasia

This is a serious genetic disorder that affects the development of the skeleton and the genitalia. It is characterized by the following symptoms: bowed long bones, particularly the femur and the tibia, winged scapulae, fewer ribs, narrow iliac wings, clubbed feet, the Robin's sequence, and ambiguous genitals. The incidence is estimated at 0.5–1 for every 100,000 live newborns. Two-thirds of patients with 46,XY constitution have ambiguous or female external genitalia [31]. The gonadal histology includes streak gonads [32], testis [33], ovarian hypoplasia [34], and even ovotestes [35].

In 90 % of cases, the disease is the result of mutations in gene *SOX9*, and in 5 % there are partial or complete deletions of 17q24.3-25.1. This gene encodes a transcription factor which is a gene with pleiotropic effects on ossified cartilage and testes [36]. Death usually occurs by respiratory insufficiency during the neonatal period. Only 5–10 % of the patients survive. The disorder is inherited in an autosomal dominant manner, but in most cases, the mutation is de novo in the family. The risk of gonadoblastoma is low [37].

References

1. Swyer GIM, Phil D. Male pseudohermaphroditism: a hitherto undescribed form. Br Med J. 1955;2:709–12.
2. Simpson JL, Blagowidow N, Martin AO. XY gonadal dysgenesis: Genetic heterogeneity based upon clinical observations, H-Y antigen status and segregations analysis. Hum Genet. 1981;58:91–7.
3. Lee DG, Han DH, Park KH, Baek M. A novel WT1 gene mutation in a patient with Wilms' tumor and 46, XY gonadal dysgenesis. Eur J Pediatr. 2011;170:1079–82.
4. Andonova S, Robeva R, Sirakov M, Mainhard K, Tomova A, Ledig S, Kumanov P, Savov A. A novel SRY gene mutation p.F109 L in a 46,XY female with complete gonadal dysgenesis. Sex Dev. 2015;9:333–7.
5. King TF, Conway GS. Swyer syndrome. Curr Opin Endocrinol Diabetes Obes. 2014;21:504–10.
6. Tagliarini EB, Assumpcao JG, Scolfaro MR, Mello MP, Marciel-Guerra AT, Guerra Junior G, Hackel C. Mutations in SRY and WT1 genes required for gonadal development are not responsible for XY partial gonadal dysgenesis. Braz J Med Res. 2005;38:17–25.
7. Pedace L, Laino L, Preziosi N, Valentini MS, Scommegna S, Rapone AM, Guarino N, Boscherini B, De Bernardo C, Marrocco G, Majore S, Grammatico P. Longitudinal hormonal evaluation in a patient with disorder of sexual development, 46,XY karyotype and one NR5A1 mutation. Am J Med Genet A. 2014;164A:2938–46.
8. Gabriel Ribeiro de Andrade J, Marques-de-Faria AP, Fabbri HC, de Mello MP, Guerra-Júnior G, Maciel-Guerra AT. Long-term follow-up of patients with 46,XY partial gonadal dysgenesis reared as males. Int J Endocrinol. 2014;2014:480724.
9. Zarate A, Karchmer S, Esteves R, Teter J. Gonadal dysgenesis with isolated clitoromegalia, XY karyotype, and bilateral gonocytoma with massive Leydig cell hyperplasia. Am J Obstet Gynecol. 1971;110:875–8.
10. Fuqua JS, Sher ES, Perlman EJ, Urban MD, Ghahremani M, Pelletier J, Migeon CJ, Brown TR, Berkovitz GD. Abnormal gonadal differentiation in two subjects with ambiguous genitalia, Müllerian structures, and normally developed testes: evidence for a defect in gonadal ridge development. Hum Genet. 1996;97:506–11.
11. Werner R, Mönig I, August J, Freiberg C, Lünstedt R, Reiz B, Wünsch L, Holterhus PM, Kulle A, Döhnert U, Wudy SA, Richter-Unruh A, Thorns C, Hiort O. Novel insights into 46,XY disorders of sex development due to NR5A1 gene mutation. Sex Dev. 2015;9:260–8.
12. Ramani P, Yeung CK, Habeebu SSM. Testicular intratubular germ cell neoplasia in children and adolescents with intersex. Am J Surg Pathol. 1993;17:1124–33.
13. Michala L, Goswami D, Creighton SM, Conway GS. Swyer syndrome: presentation and outcomes. BJOG. 2008;115:737–41.
14. Du X, Zhang X, Li Y, Han Y. 46,XY female sex reversal syndrome with bilateral gonadoblastoma and dysgerminoma. Exp Ther Med. 2014;8:1102–4.
15. Santalha M, Amaral B, Pereira J, Ribeiro L, João Oliveira M, Figueiredo S, Cardoso H, Peixoto C, Borges T, Cidade-Rodrigues JA. Peripheral precocious puberty: 46, XY complete gonadal dysgenesis. An Pediatr (Barc). 2014;81:246–50.
16. Nistal M, Paniagua R, González-Peramato P, Reyes-Múgica M. Perspectives in pediatric pathology, Chapter 5. Gonadal dysgenesis. Pediatr Dev Pathol. 2015;18:259–78.

17. Drash A, Sherman F, Hartmann WH, Blizzard RM. A syndrome of pseudohermaphroditism, Wilms' tumor, hypertension, and degenerative renal disease. J Pediatr. 1970;76:585–93.
18. Nso Roca AP, Peña Carrión A, Benito Gutiérrez M, García Meseguer C, García Pose A, Navarro M. Evolutive study of children with diffuse mesangial sclerosis. Pediatr Nephrol. 2009;24:1013–9.
19. Niaudet P, Gubler MC. WT1 and glomerular diseases. Pediatr Nephrol. 2006;21:1653–60.
20. Furtado LV, Pysher T, Opitz J, Lamb R, Comstock J, Batish S, Mauch T, Nelson R, Zhou H. Denys-Drash syndrome with neonatal renal failure in monozygotic twins due to c.1097G>A mutation in the WT1 gene. Fetal Pediatr Pathol. 2011;30:266–72.
21. McTaggart SJ, Algar E, Chow CW, Powell HR, Jones CL. Clinical spectrum of Denys-Drash and Frasier syndrome. Pediatr Nephrol. 2001;16:335–9.
22. Shapiro O, Welch TR, Sheridan M, Stred S, Upadhyay J. Mixed gonadal dysgenesis and Denys-Drash syndrome: urologists should screen for nephrotic syndrome. Can J Urol. 2007;14:3767–9.
23. Coppes MJ, Huff V, Pelletier J. Denys-Drash syndrome: relating a clinical disorder to genetic alterations in the tumor suppressor gene WT1. J Pediatr. 1993;123:673–8.
24. Clarkson PA, Davies HR, Williams DM, Chaudhary R, Hughes IA, Patterson MN. Mutational screening of the Wilms's tumor gene, WT1 in males with genital abnormalities. J Med Genet. 1993;30:767–72.
25. Ezaki J, Hashimoto K, Asano T, Kanda S, Akioka Y, Hattori M, Yamamoto T, Shibata N. Gonadal tumor in Frasier syndrome: a review and classification. Cancer Prev Res (Phila). 2015;8:271–6.
26. Gwin K, Cajaiba MM, Caminoa-Lizarralde A, Picazo ML, Nistal M, Reyes-Múgica M. Expanding the clinical spectrum of Frasier syndrome. Pediatr Dev Pathol. 2008;11:122–7.
27. Fischbach BV, Trout KL, Lewis J, Luis CA, Sika M. WAGR syndrome: a clinical review of 54 cases. Pediatrics. 2005;116:984–8.
28. Riccardi VM, Sujansky E, Smith AC, Francke U. Chromosomal imbalance in the Aniridia-Wilms' tumor association: 11p interstitial deletion. Pediatrics. 1978;61:604–10.
29. Andrade JG, Guaragna MS, Soardi FC, Guerra-Júnior G, Mello MP, Maciel-Guerra AT. Clinical and genetic findings of five patients with WT1-related disorders. Arq Bras Endocrinol Metabol. 2008;52:1236–43.
30. Sinha A, Sharma S, Gulati A, Sharma A, Agarwala S, Hari P, Bagga A. Frasier syndrome: early gonadoblastoma and cyclosporine responsiveness. Pediatr Nephrol. 2010;25:2171–3274.
31. Dahdaleh NS, Albert GW, Hasan DM. Campomelic dysplasia: a rare cause of congenital spinal deformity. J Clin Neurosci. 2010;17:664–6.
32. Lecointre C, Pichon O, Hamel A, Heloury Y, Michel-Calemard L, Morel Y, David A, Le Caignec C. Familial acampomelic form of campomelic dysplasia caused by a 960 kb deletion upstream of SOX9. Am J Med Genet A. 2009;149A:1183–9.
33. Chen SY, Lin SJ, Tsai LP, Chou YY. Sex-reversed acampomelic campomelic dysplasia with a homozygous deletion mutation in SOX9 gene. Urology. 2012;79:908–11.
34. Foster JW, Dominguez-Steglich MA, Guioli S, Kwok C, Weller PA, Stevanović M, Weissenbach J, Mansour S, Young ID, Goodfellow PN, et al. Campomelic dysplasia and autosomal sex reversal caused by mutations in an SRY-related gene. Nature. 1994;372:525–30.
35. Beaulieu Bergeron M, Lemyre E, Rypens F, Scherer G, Lemieux N, Fournet JC. Diagnosis of true hermaphroditism in a fetus with acampomelic campomelic dysplasia. Prenat Diagn. 2009;29:528–30.
36. Kobayashi A, Chang H, Chaboissier MC, Schedl A, Behringer RR. Sox9 in testis determination. Ann N Y Acad Sci. 2005;1061:9–17.
37. Hong JR, Barber M, Scott CI, Guttemberg M, Wolfson PJ. Three-year-old phenotypic female with campomelic dysplasia and bilateral gonadoblastoma. J Pediatr Surg. 1995;30:1735–7.

Clinical Syndromes Associated with Dysgenetic Testis

4

Manuel Nistal, Pilar González-Peramato, and Álvaro Serrano

4.1 Introduction

Until the sixth week of gestation, the gonads of both sexes are indistinguishable. When the chromosome constitution is 46,XY, the testes develop due to the effect of the *SRY* gene. At sixth to seventh week of development (8–9 weeks of gestation), Sertoli cells starting to produce AMH are recognized. AMH is a large glycoprotein that acts locally by diffusion causing regression of the Müllerian ducts between 56 and 62 days after fertilization. The whole process must be finished by day 77, after which the Müllerian ducts become insensitive to AMH [1]. A proper functioning prevents the development of the uterus, Fallopian tubes, and proximal vagina. Another important function of AMH is the correct formation of the tunica albuginea with a stroma with bundles of cells and fibers parallel to the surface with a sharp boundary between it and the testicular parenchyma planes. Sertoli cells stimulate differentiation of Leydig cells. The Leydig cells produce androgens that induce differentiation of Wolff ducts in epididymis, vas deferens, ejaculatory ducts, and seminal vesicles. Differentiation of the external genitalia begins around the ninth week of gestation and is under the influence of androgens, mainly dihydrotestosterone.

4.2 Mixed Gonadal Dysgenesis

The asymmetrical gonadal differentiation was first observed in 1962 by Bergada [2]. A year later, Sohval [3] proposed the term mixed gonadal dysgenesis to what is now known as DSD characterized by the presence in the same patient of a streak gonad on one side and dysgenetic testis on the opposite. The incidence is estimated at 15 % of DSD in 0.23/1000 amniocentesis or 1.7 per 10,000 newborn babies [4, 5].

Etiology The most frequent karyotype is 45,X/45,XY (55.6 % of patients) [6]. Other observed karyotypes are 46,XY (13.6 %), and 45,X/47,XYY [7], 45,X/46,XX/46,XY, 45,X/46, XYq-, 45,X/46,XYp-, 45,X/46,X add (Y) (p11.3), and 45,X/46,X dic (Yp). More than 80 % of patients bear Y chromosome [8]. Mutations in *SRY* gene have not been reported. The complexity of karyotypes is even higher in peripheral blood and gonadal tissue. 45,X/46,XY is produced by chromosome loss and due to nondisjunction subsequent to the normal disomic fertilization. In patients with 45,X/46,XY, there are two cell lines, one with monosomy X (45,X) and one with a normal male constitution (46,XY). The distribution of each line in the various tissues determines the variety of phenotypes.

M. Nistal et al., *Clues in the Diagnosis of Non-tumoral Testicular Pathology*, DOI 10.1007/978-3-319-49364-0_4

Clinically The phenotype is very heterogeneous. There are three situations. Patients with male phenotype can first consult for infertility, patients with ambiguous genitalia and female phenotype, and patients with or without short height and Turner's syndrome. Patients with 45,X/46,XY and normal male external genitalia, probably due to dominance of the line 46,XY, have bilateral testes [9]. They consult for infertility and azoospermia. Some patients have structural Y chromosome abnormalities, including deletions of the AZF region. Spermatogenesis has been observed in other patients [10]. Cryptorchidism and hypospadias are frequent. Patients with 45,X/46,XY and ambiguous external genitalia are subject to study in the postnatal stage. The gonads are usually dysgenetic testis or streak gonad in one side and dysgenetic testis in the contralateral side [11]. Patients with 45,X/46,XY and female phenotype may be indistinguishable from patients 45,X, which have been linked to the predominance of the line 45,X. In these patients, both gonads are streak gonads. Other common diseases are heart and kidney abnormalities [12].

Histology Gonads can be of three types: dysgenetic testis, streak testis, and streak gonads. In the streak testis, the degree of development of streak gonad is highly variable from a classic streak gonad with or without isolated ovarian follicles to a streak gonad with epithelial cords (Fig. 4.1). When the streak gonad contains ovarian follicles, it should be considered ovotestis instead of streak testis, but given the clinically limited functionality of ovarian differentiation, there is a tendency not to include these patients in ovotesticular DSD.

The internal genitalia are usually aligned with the nature of the ipsilateral gonad. Coincident with the streak gonad, in 95 % of cases, there is a Fallopian tube. And if the opposite side shows a dysgenetic testis besides epididymis and vas deferens, a Fallopian tube can be observed in 74 % of cases. The degree of development of the testicular parenchyma is related to the degree of Müllerian duct regression [13]. Gonads in mixed gonadal dysgenesis are lacking the ability to inhibit the growth of the Müllerian duct, acquire a complete differentiation of the Wolffian ducts, properly virilize the external genitalia, promote testicular descent, and develop spermatogenesis.

Tumors The incidence of tumors in 45,X/46,XY patients is estimated to be between 15 % and 20 % [11]. The most common tumor is gonadoblastoma, although all germ cell tumors

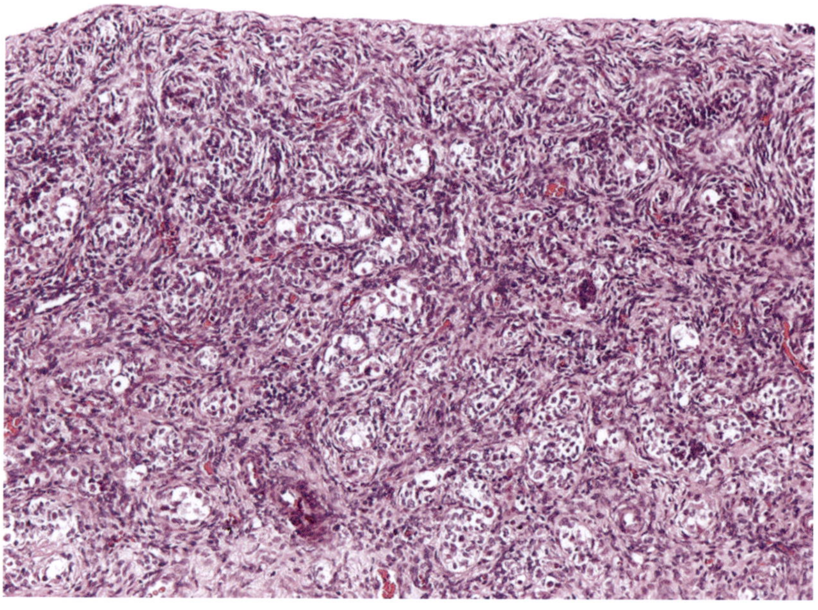

Fig. 4.1 Mixed gonadal dysgenesis. Streak gonad with epithelial cords. Germ cells stand out by their pale cytoplasm in a stroma reminiscent of ovarian stroma

except spermatocytic tumor have been observed, including specialized gonadal stromal tumors such as juvenile granulosa cell tumor. The majority of tumors occur during the second decade of life.

There are no guidelines for management *of these patients*. Conservative attitudes are recommended in patients with male phenotype. Also, histological verification of the nature of the gonads and, in the case of being testes perform orchidopexy, teaching testicular self-examination and performing ultrasound annually are suggested. In the case of ambiguous external genitalia and in patients with female phenotype, gonadectomy should be considered [14].

4.3 Dysgenetic Male Pseudohermaphroditism

This is a DSD characterized by the presence in a patient of two dysgenetic testis or streak testis, Müllerian derivatives, cryptorchidism, incomplete virilization, and in some cases Turner stigmata. This disorder was described by Federman in 1967 [15], and it is considered a variant of the mixed gonadal dysgenesis. The most common karyotypes are 46,XY and 45,X/46,XY [16]. In childhood, and additionally to the characteristic anomalies of the tunica albuginea, the dysgenetic testes have a decreased tubular diameter, an increased number of Sertoli cells, and a diminution of the germ cells. In adulthood, only some patients develop spermatogenesis, and this is very low. The interstitium shows Leydig cell hyperplasia. The tumor risk is very high (46 %) [17].

4.4 Persistent Müllerian Duct Syndrome (PMDS)

PMDS is a syndrome characterized by the presence of Müllerian structures in patients with normal male genotype and phenotype. It was described by Nilson in 1939 [18] and called hernia uteri inguinalis. Since then, 262 cases have been reported [19]. The syndrome may be sporadic or inherited in an autosomal recessive manner in some cases [20] and X linked in others [21].

Etiology The molecular basis is heterogeneous. The following hypothesis has been proposed: In 45 % of cases, it could be due to a mutation in the *AMH* gene located on the short arm of chromosome 19 [22]. In 39 % of cases, it is a resistance to AMH in the target organs due to a deficit of the type II receptor of this hormone located on chromosome 12 [23]. In these cases, the AMH hormone is high. In the remaining cases (16.5 %), the cause could be a mismatch between the time of onset of secretion and maximum responsiveness.

Clinical Findings Patients with PMDS are often asymptomatic. The most frequent reasons for consultation are inguinal hernia, cryptorchidism, infertility, and tumor. Cryptorchidism in 25 % of cases is unilateral and 75 % bilateral. The situation of the testes and the associated pathology are varied, but most cases can be included in the following three groups [24]:

1. Patients with bilateral abdominal cryptorchidism (60–70 % of cases). The testes are located in a similar position as that of the ovaries; each has epididymis, vas deferens, and a Fallopian tube and is accompanied by a centrally located hypoplastic uterus [25].
2. Patients with unilateral cryptorchidism (20–30 %). The contralateral testis is placed in a hernia sac or scrotum, and there is a Fallopian tube and a uterus adhered to it [26].
3. Patients with transverse testicular ectopy (10 %). Both testes share the same scrotal bag inside a hernia sac. The bag also contains a Fallopian tube and a uterus [27] (Fig. 4.2).

Histology The most characteristic feature observed in both childhood and adulthood is the abnormal development of the tunica albuginea. It consists of a whirled stroma reminiscent of an ovarian stroma with a thickness supporting seminiferous tubes; the boundary between tunica albuginea and testicular parenchyma is not clear

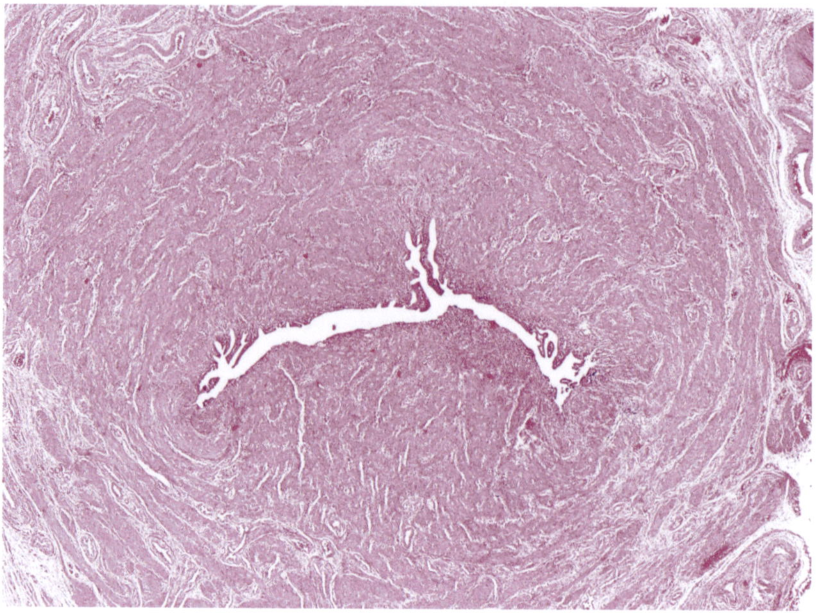

Fig. 4.2 Persistent Müllerian duct syndrome. Hypoplastic uterus in a hernia sac

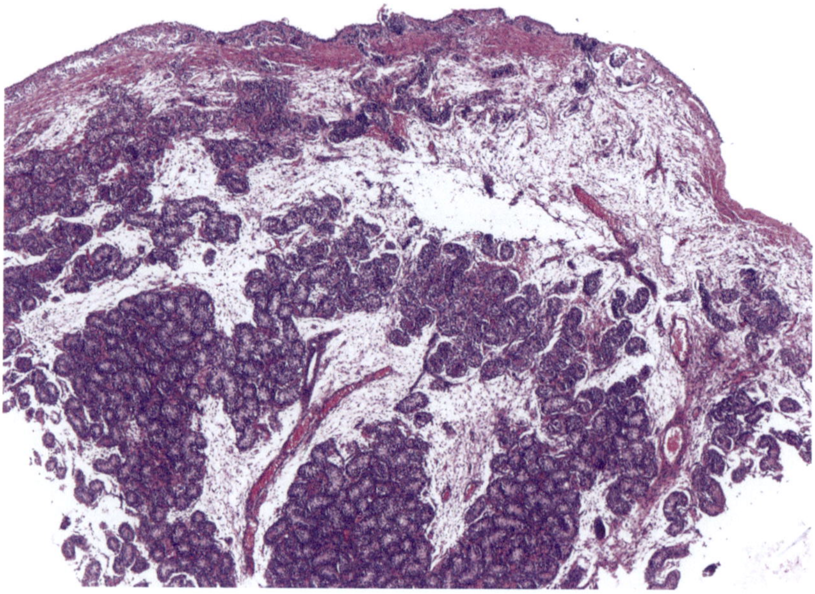

Fig. 4.3 Dysgenetic testis. The central zone is formed by several lobules with compactly arranged seminiferous tubules in each lobule. In the peripheral zone, the tubules are arranged in the thickness of the tunica albuginea adopting varied shapes and sizes

(Figs. 4.3, 4.4, and 4.5). In infancy, both the tubular diameter and the tubular fertility rate are low. In adulthood, no spermatogenesis develops in most cases, or else it is only focal and associated with Sertoli cell-only tubules (mixed atrophy) or tubules with different degrees of hyalinization. Most patients have oligozoospermia or azoospermia. Paternity is achieved in 11 % of the cases [28].

Tumors The risk of malignancy is high – estimated at 18 %. The most common tumor is seminoma. Germ cell neoplasia in situ (GCNIS) (Fig. 4.6), embryonal cell carcinoma, yolk sac tumor, and teratomas have also been reported [29]. Most tumors develop in the undescended testicle and in some cases in the scrotal one [30]. In some patients, tumors have been observed in malignant Müllerian derivatives [31].

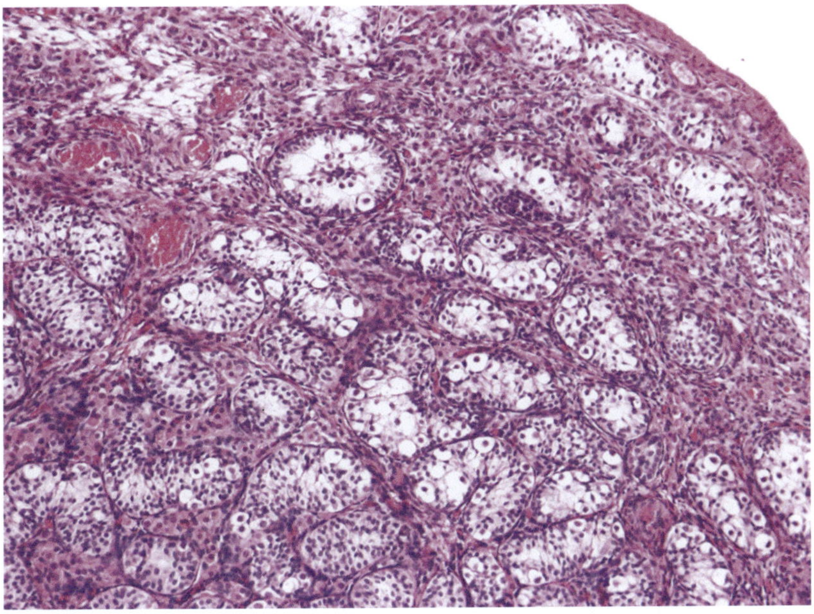

Fig. 4.4 Dysgenetic testis. Some seminiferous tubules are placed in the thickness of a tunica albuginea with ovarian-like stroma. The boundary between the testicular parenchyma and tunica albuginea is not clear

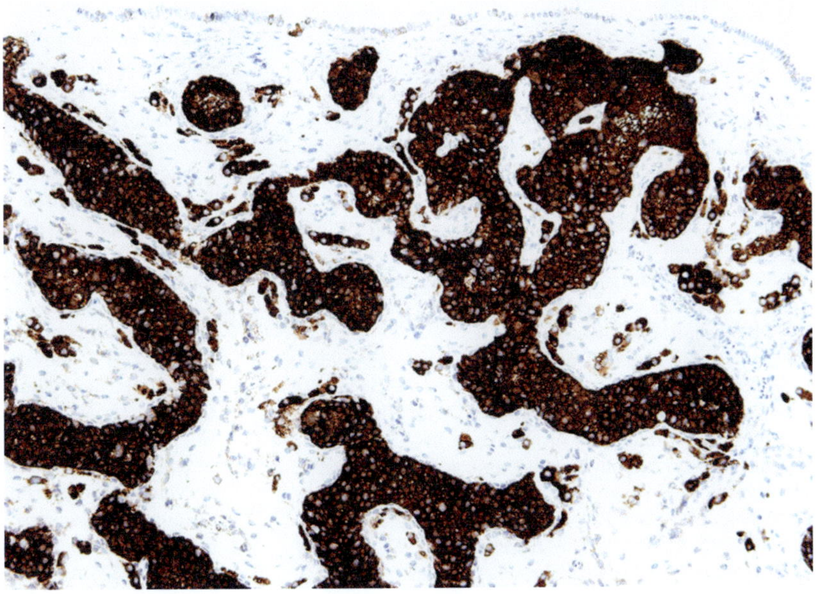

Fig. 4.5 Dysgenetic testis. Inhibin immunostaining stand out the form and arrangement of the seminiferous tubules in the surface of the testis. Among the seminiferous tubules, positive expression is observed also in Leydig cells

The *management of these patients* is complicated and aimed at the descent of the testes, removal of Müllerian structures, and patient monitoring. The descent of the testes must be achieved as early as possible, and a testicular biopsy should be performed at this moment. Preserving the testes keeps the endogenous source of hormone and a fertility potential. Orchiectomy is relegated only to the testes that have not been able to descend. The Müllerian structures must be removed to prevent their malignant transformation, but the risk of damaging structures of the genitourinary tract should be considered. The surveillance is aimed mainly to control the testes by means of testicular self-examination and annual ultrasound, which can detect tumor development [19].

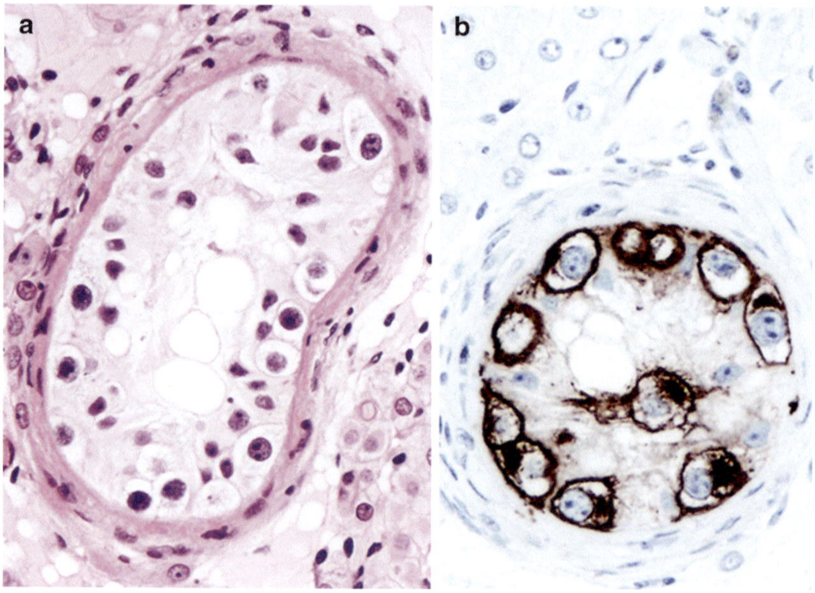

Fig. 4.6 Persistent Müllerian duct syndrome in a postpubertal patient. Germ cell neoplasia in situ (GCNIS). (**a**) Atypical germ cells are large and are arranged over the basement membrane, while Sertoli cells are moved toward the lumen. (**b**) Immunostaining for PLAP in the peripheral cytoplasm and perinuclear dot in GCNIS cells

References

1. Rajpert-De Meyts E, Jørgensen N, Graem N, Müller J, Cate RL, Skakkebaek NE. Expression of anti-Müllerian hormone during normal and pathological gonadal development: association with differentiation of Sertoli and granulosa cells. J Clin Endocrinol Metab. 1999;84:3836–44.
2. Bergada C, Cleveland WW, Jones HW, Wilkins L. Gonadal histology in patients with male pseudohermaphroditism and atypical gonadal dysgenesis: relation to theories of sex differentiation. Acta Endocrinol. 1962;40:493–520.
3. Sohval AR. "Mixed" gonadal dysgenesis: a variety of hermaphroditism. Am J Hum Genet. 1963;15:155–8.
4. Huang B, Thangavelu M, Bhatt S, J Sandlin C, Wang S. Prenatal diagnosis of 45,X and 45,X mosaicism: the need for thorough cytogenetic and clinical evaluations. Prenat Diagn. 2002;22:105–10.
5. Chang HJ, Clark RD, Bachman H. The phenotype of 45,X/46,XY mosaicism: an analysis of 92 prenatally diagnosed cases. Am J Hum Genet. 1990;46:156–67.
6. Andrade JG, Guerra-Júnior G, Maciel-Guerra AT. 46,XY and 45,X/46,XY testicular dysgenesis: similar gonadal and genital phenotype, different prognosis. Arq Bras Endocrinol Metabol. 2010;54:331–4.
7. Ragg S, Härle M, Scherthan H. Analysis of sex chromosome distribution in the gonadal tissue of a 45,X/47,XYY mosaic by fluorescence in situ hybridization. Mod Pathol. 1995;8:295–8.
8. Shinawi M, Cain MP, Vanderbrink BA, Grignon DJ, Mensing D, Cooper ML, Bader P, Cheung SW. Mixed gonadal dysgenesis in a child with isodicentric Y chromosome: does the relative proportion of the 45,X line really matter? Am J Med Genet A. 2010;152A:1832–7.
9. Tosson H, Rose SR, Gartner LA. Description of children with 45,X/46,XY karyotype. Eur J Pediatr. 2012;171:521–9.
10. Flannigan RK, Chow V, Ma S, Yuzpe A. 45,X/46,XY mixed gonadal dysgenesis: a case of successful sperm extraction. Can Urol Assoc J. 2014;8:E108–10.
11. Verp MS, Simpson JL. Abnormal sexual differentiation and neoplasia. Cancer Genet Cytogenet. 1987;25:191–218.
12. Farrugia MK, Sebire NJ, Achermann JC, Eisawi A, Duffy PG, Mushtaq I. Clinical and gonadal features and early surgical management of 45,X/46,XY and 45,X/47,XYY chromosomal mosaicism presenting with genital anomalies. J Pediatr Urol. 2013;9:139–44.
13. Chemes H, Muzulin PM, Venara MC, Mulhmann MC, Martinez M, Gamboni M. Early manifestations of testicular dysgenesis in children: pathological phenotypes, karyotype correlations and precursor stages of tumor development. APMIS. 2003;111:12–23.
14. Cools M, Pleskacova J, Stoop H, Hoebeke P, Van Laecke E, Drop SL, Lebl J, Oosterhuis JW, Looijenga LH, Wolffenbuttel KP, Mosaicism Collaborative Group. Gonadal pathology and tumor risk in relation to clinical characteristics in patients with 45,X/46,XY mosaicism. J Clin Endocrinol Metab. 2011;96:E1171–80.
15. Federman DD. Abnormal sexual development. Philadelphia: W.B. Saunders Co.; 1967.
16. Proença E, Freitas S, Fonseca M, Figueiredo S, Rodrigues C. Dysgenetic male pseudohermaphroditism. Acta Med Port. 2001;14:511–4.
17. Mandell J, Stevens PS, Fried FA. Childhood gonadoblastoma and seminoma in a dysgenetic cryptorchid gonad. J Urol. 1977;117:674–5.

18. Nilson O. Hernia uteri inguinalisbeim Manne. Acta Chir Scand. 1939;83:231–49.
19. Shalaby MM, Kurkar A, Zarzour MA, Faddan AA, Khalil M, Abdelhafez MF. The management of the persistent Müllerian duct syndrome. Arab J Urol. 2014;12:239–44.
20. Imbeaud S, Belville C, Messika-Zeitoun L, Rey R, di Clemente N, Josso N, Picard JY. A 27 base-pair deletion of the anti-müllerian type II receptor gene is the most common cause of the persistent Müllerian duct syndrome. Hum Mol Genet. 1996;5:1269–77.
21. Carré-Eusèbe D, Imbeaud S, Harbison M, New MI, Josso N, Picard JY. Variants of the anti-Müllerian hormone gene in a compound heterozygote with the persistent Müllerian duct syndrome and his family. Hum Genet. 1992;90:389–94.
22. Belville C, Josso N, Picard J-Y. Persistence of Müllerian derivatives in males. Am J Med Genet. 1999;89:218–23.
23. Belville C, Maréchal JD, Pennetier S, Carmillo P, Masgrau L, Messika-Zeitoun L, Galey J, Machado G, Treton D, Gonzalès J, Picard JY, Josso N, Cate RL, di Clemente N. Natural mutations of the anti-Mullerian hormone type II receptor found in persistent Mullerian duct syndrome affect ligand binding, signal transduction and cellular transport. Hum Mol Genet. 2009;18:3002–13.
24. Clarnette TD, Sugita Y, Hutson JM. Genital anomalies in human and animal models reveal the mechanisms and hormones governing testicular descent. Br J Urol. 1997;79:99–112.
25. Nayak VJ, Kamath AS, Krishnappa MH, Bylappa SK. Persistent mullerian duct syndrome: a case report and review of the literature. Int J Appl Basic Med Res. 2014;4:125–7.
26. Imbeaud S, Faure E, Lamarre L, Mattei MG, Di Clemente N, Tizard R, Carré-Eusèbe D, Belville C, Tragethon L, Tonkin C, Nelson J, McAuliffe M, Bidart JM, Lababidi A, Josso N, Cate RL, Picard JY. Insensitivity to anti-Müllerian hormone due to a spontaneous mutation in the human anti-Múllerian hormone receptor. Nat Genet. 1995;11:382–8.
27. Kamble RS, Gupta RK, Gupta AR, Kothari PR, Dikshit KV, Kesan KK. Laparoscopic management of transverse testicular ectopia with persistent Mullerian duct syndrome. J Minim Access Surg. 2015;11: 213–5.
28. Farag TI. Familial persistent müllerian duct syndrome in Kuwait and neighboring populations. Am J Med Genet. 1993;47:432–4.
29. Yamada K, Takahata A, Ichijo Y, Akazawa K, Goto M, Terayama K, Yamada K. A case of testicular seminoma in persistent Mullerian duct syndrome with transverse testicular ectopia. Abdom Imaging. 2015;40:475–9.
30. Nistal M, Paniagua R, Isorna S, Mancebo J. Diffuse intratubular undifferentiated germ cell tumor in both testes of a male subject with a uterus and ipsilateral testicular dysgenesis. J Urol. 1980;124:286–9.
31. Thiel DD, Erhard MJ. Uterine adenosarcoma in a boy with persistent Müllerian duct syndrome: first reported case. J Pediatr Surg. 2005;40:e29–31.

5 True Hermaphroditism (Ovotesticular DSD)

Manuel Nistal, Pilar González-Peramato, and Álvaro Serrano

5.1 Introduction

Ovotesticular DSD is defined on basis of the histology of the gonads after verifying that the patient has both ovarian and testicular differentiation. It represents approximately 10 % of the DSD [1], with an incidence of 1/100,000 live births [2]. Around 500 cases have been reported. True hermaphrodites are more common in Africa. Even though hermaphroditism should be suspected in any patient with ambiguous genitalia, the diagnosis is often delayed for many years. Only 25 % of patients are diagnosed before the age of 20, and in many cases, they have already undergone major corrective surgeries both for undescended testes and for the external genitalia [3, 4].

5.2 Karyotype

The most frequent karyotype of true hermaphrodites is 46,XX (60 %), followed by several chromosomal mosaicisms in decreasing order of frequency (46,XX/46,XY, 46,XY/47,XXY, 45,X0/46,XY, 46XX/45,X0, 46,XX/47,XXY [33 %], and 46,XY karyotype [7 %]). Isolated karyotype cases with 47,XYY/46,XY/45,X0 [5, 6], and 46,XderY/45,X0 with rearranged Y chromosome [7], have been reported.

The incidence of different karyotypes is related to different ethnic groups and geographic areas. Most of the true hermaphrodites in Africa (96.6 %) have karyotype 46,XX. The 46,XY karyotype frequency is similar in Europe, Asia, and North America [8]. In Europe, a chromosomal mosaicism is found in 40.5 % of cases, and in North America, such mosaicism appeared in only 21 % of cases. Most of true hermaphroditism cases are sporadic.

5.3 Pathogenetic Theories

There are different pathogenetic theories that explain the presence of testis in the absence of the Y chromosome and therefore the TDF (testicular determining factor produced by the *SRY* gene): (a) a hidden mosaicism including a line with the Y chromosome [9], (b) translocation of paternal Y chromosomal material that includes the *SRY* gene to the X chromosome, (c) an autosomal mutation with variable penetrance, and (d) by X chromosome-linked mutations that either is coupled with a rare X chromosome inactivation [10]

M. Nistal et al., *Clues in the Diagnosis of Non-tumoral Testicular Pathology*,
DOI 10.1007/978-3-319-49364-0_5

or permits testicular differentiation in the absence of *SRY* [11] or mutations in genes such as *SOX9* and *FGF9* that regulate the action of *SRY* [12]. Other causes are partial deletion of *DMRT1* [13] and mutations in *RSPO1* [14].

5.4 Phenotype

The phenotype of true hermaphrodites varies from male to female. Most of the patients consult at puberty by the first time. Seventy-five percent of patients grow up as males, and in 80 % of them, chordee, hypospadias, cryptorchidism, and gynecomastia can be seen [15, 16]. Infertility is the complaint of some patients [17]. Normal male phenotype does not exceed 10 % [18]. Twenty-five percent of them grow up as women; they consult due to menstrual disorders or clitoromegaly and more rarely because of a cyclic pain in the descended or undescended gonad [19]. Almost all patients have a urogenital sinus remnant and most also have a uterus. Some isolated cases consult because of an irreducible hernia, which contained a uterus (hernia uteri inguinalis), and phenotype similar to type 1 persistent Müllerian duct syndrome but obviously with a different type of gonad [20].

Correlation Between Genotype and Phenotype

The phenotype is related to the presence of the *SRY* gene. In patients with 46,XY chromosome constitution, the presence of testis and male development is well understood. Several theories have been proposed to explain masculinization of XX patients. The phenotype could depend on two features, the length of Y translocated material (the higher the length of the Yp fragment, the more complete is the masculinization), or the X chromosome where the *SRY* gene is the translocated one. If the translocation is in the active X chromosome, the phenotype will be XX male (with masculinized external genitalia), while if the translocation is made to the inactive X chromosome, the phenotype will be ambiguous genitalia. The presence of a prostate has been reported in 46,XX male patients without *SRY* and complete male phenotype with absence of female internal genitalia [21].

5.5 Gonadal Types

The gonadal types observed in true hermaphrodites can be the ovotestis (44 %), ovary (33 %), and testis (22 %).

The gonad nature can be suspected during physical examination. Hormonal determinations are inconclusive. There are few data of Leydig cell function in children. More than 60 % show a normal testosterone response to stimulation with hCG. This response does not correlate with the presence of the Y chromosome [22].

In adults, high serum testosterone levels suggest the presence of Leydig cells and therefore the occurrence of a testis. High levels of E2 after human menopausal gonadotropin (hMG) stimulation suggest the presence of an ovary [23].

Ovotestis

The ovotestis is the most frequent gonad (44.4 %), and its preferential localization is the right side. Fifty percent of the ovotestis are found in an abdominal position and 25 % in the inguinal region, and 25 % are labioscrotal. Complete gonad descent occurs in 5 % of patients with bilateral ovotestis [17]. Macroscopically, the ovotestis can consist of two pieces joined by a pedicle or forming a single structure. In the first case, the ovary has the shape of a cap on top of the testis. In the second case, it occupies the outer part and is crescent shaped [24]. The proportion ovarian/testicular tissue varies widely from one to another patient.

In childhood, the ovarian part shows abundant primordial follicles and some primary follicles (Fig. 5.1). Secondary follicles of Graff, the presence of a corpus luteum, and numerous albicans bodies are frequent in adulthood (Figs. 5.2, 5.3, and 5.4). In childhood, the testis part consists of seminiferous tubules with a few germ cells in a dense stroma. Anastomosing tubules are frequent.

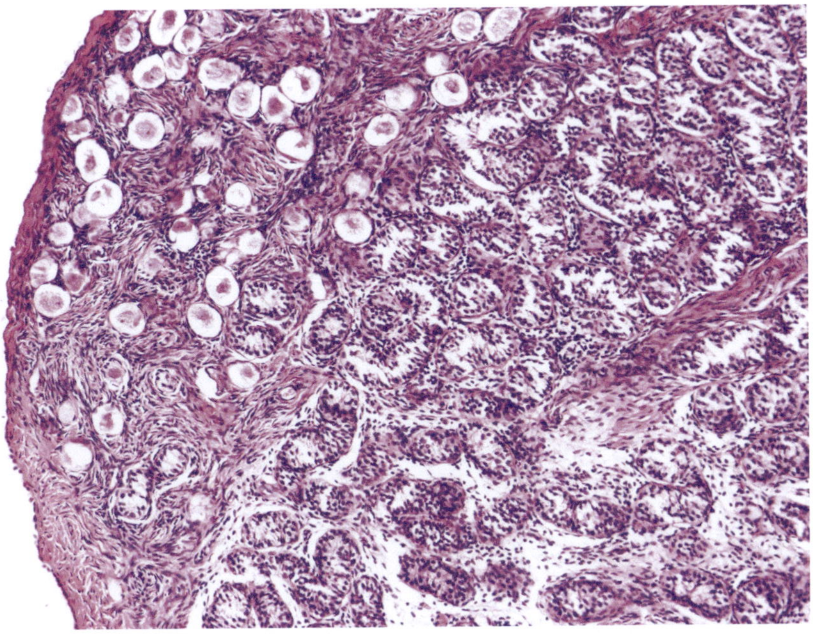

Fig. 5.1 Ovotestis in a 6-month-old patient. The ovarian parenchyma is peripherally located. It consists of numerous primordial follicles in a dense stroma. The seminiferous tubules are of normal size

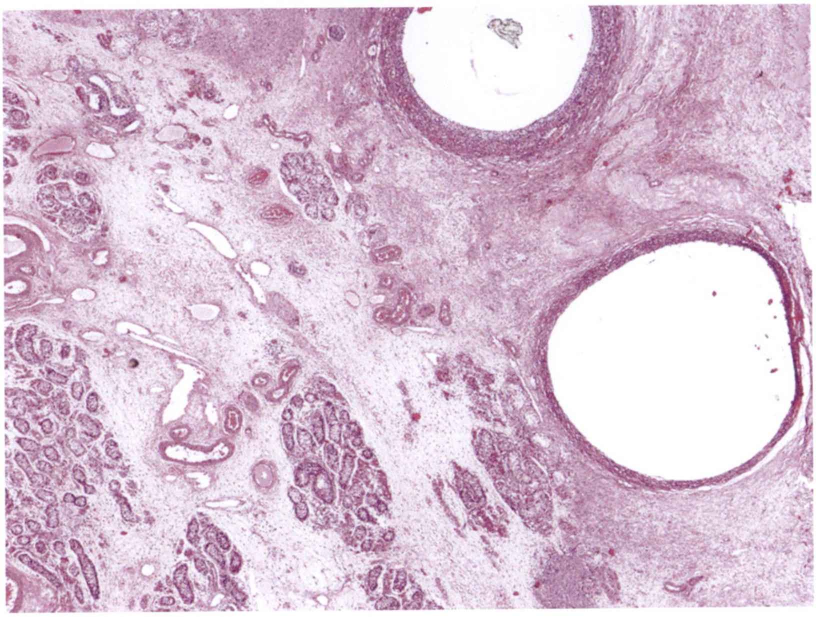

Fig. 5.2 Ovotestis of an 18-year-old patient. Cystic formations correspond to tertiary follicles. The groups of seminiferous tubules are separated by abundant stroma

In the adult, tubules with spermatogenesis are rare, and usually small dysgenetic tubules predominate. The Sertoli cells show immature characteristics with hyperchromatic nuclei, focal immunostaining for calretinin and D2-40, and focal absence of androgen receptors. These tubules have no lumen. The presence of fully hyalinized seminiferous tubules is common. Leydig cells are present, sometimes forming large clumps (Fig. 5.5).

The complexity of the structure of ovotestis may be greater as it has been observed in a large series of South African patients [25].

In the transition between testicular parenchyma and ovotestis, at the level of the tunica albuginea, some seminiferous tubules can be

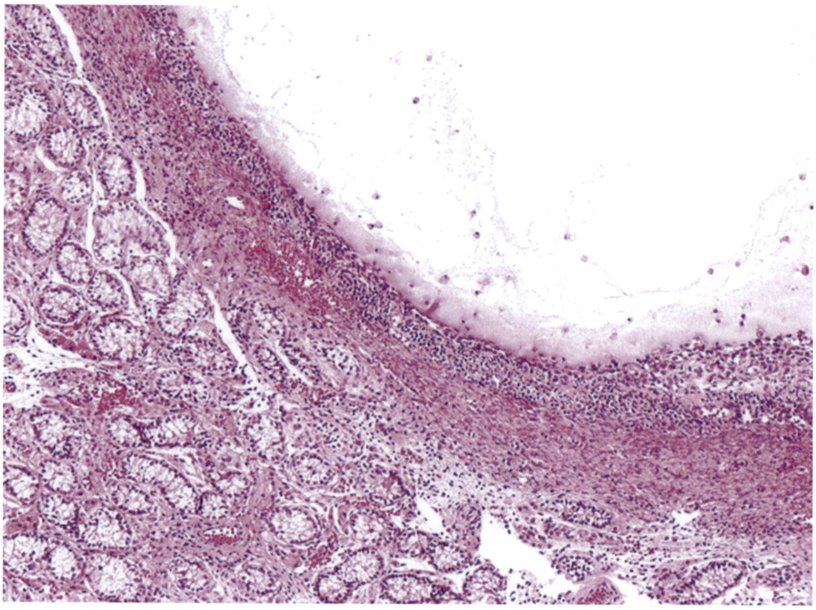

Fig. 5.3 Ovotestis of the same patient. The seminiferous tubules are in intimate relationship with an ovarian follicle

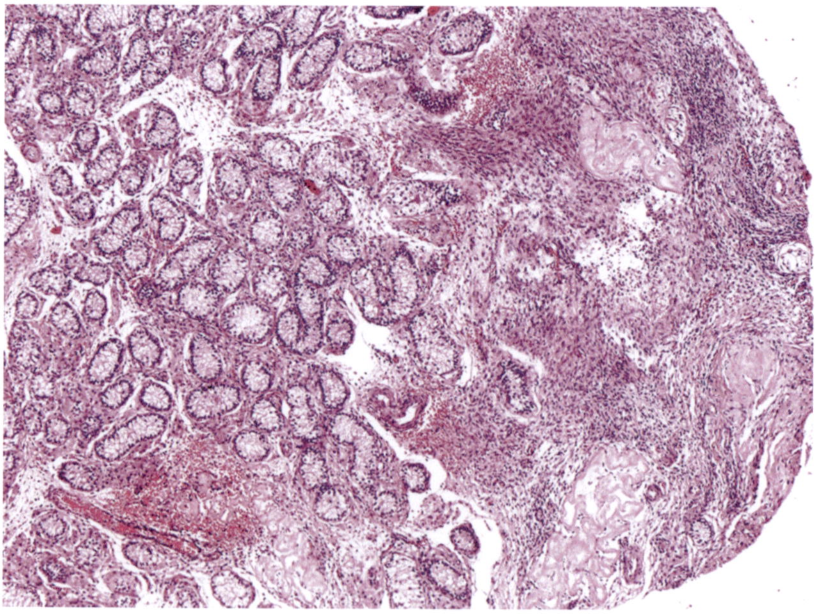

Fig. 5.4 Ovotestis of an adult patient. In the peripheral zone, eosinophilic areas of irregular contours that probably correspond with atretic follicles stand out

seen located in its thickness and surrounded by an ovarian-like stroma reminiscent of the testes of DSD with Müllerian remnants.

The ovotestis is associated with Fallopian tubes in 65 % of cases and with ductus deferens in the rest of cases (Fig. 5.6). The uterus is completely developed if the patient has ovotestis/ovary. When ovotestis is bilateral, uterine agenesis is frequent (13 % of cases) [26]. Many times microcystic transformation of ductuli efferentes is observed in the epididymis that accompanies the ductus deferens.

Testis

The testis is preferentially located in the right side (60 %), at any level between the abdomen and the scrotal pouch or labia. Fifty percent of the testes

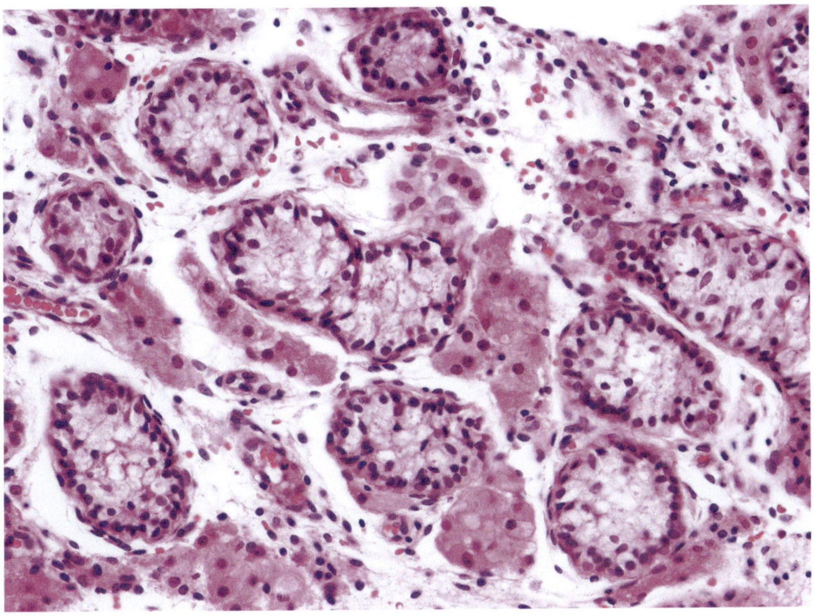

Fig. 5.5 Ovotestis of the same adult patient of the previous figure. The seminiferous tubules have an infantile maturational pattern which contrasts with the abundant clusters of Leydig cells

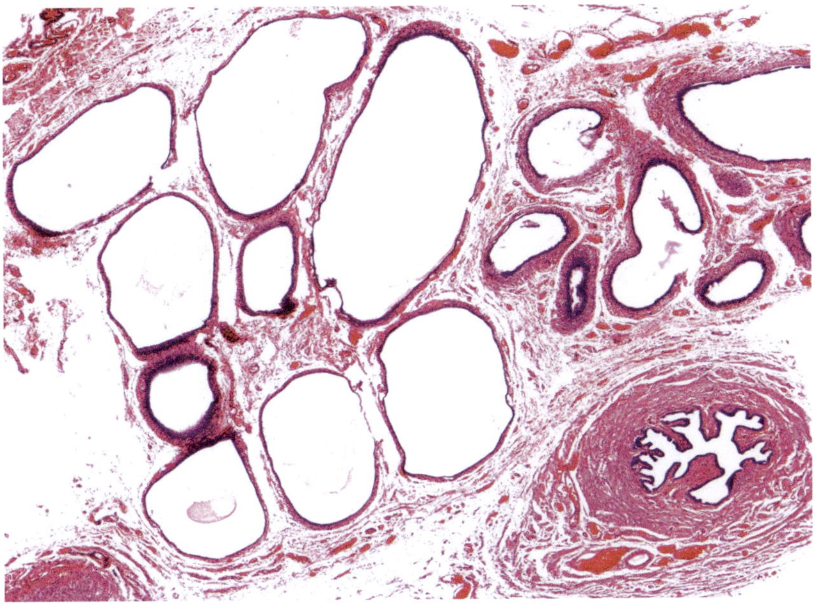

Fig. 5.6 Epididymis with cystic transformation besides a hypoplastic Fallopian tube

are labioscrotal. Since infancy, the testis shows a low tubular fertility index. At puberty, the seminiferous tubules do not develop to the normal diameter, and often they consist of dysgenetic Sertoli cells only, similar to what is observed in many cryptorchidic testes. Incomplete spermatogenesis can be observed in some cases, and complete spermatogenesis is exceptional. Although some testicular lesions may be primary, others could be caused by the increased level of estrogens that the testicular parenchyma undergoes.

Ovary

The ovary is most frequent in the left side (63 %) and is usually abdominal (85 %). Most times the ovary is hypoplastic and shows scant primordial follicles, although, in a reduced number of patients, the ovary is histologically and functionally normal.

5.6 Types of True Hermaphroditism

Patients with ovotesticular DSD are classified into three types depending on the location and histology of the gonads: unilateral, bilateral, and lateral. Most of ovotesticular DSD are of the unilateral type with ovotestis in one side and a normal gonad in the other side. Forty percent of them show a combination of the ovotestis and ovary, and 15 % combine the ovotestis and testicle. In bilateral type, both gonads are ovotestes (34 %). Eleven percent of patients are ovotesticular DSD lateral type: one gonad is a testis and the other gonad is an ovary [25–27]. Other rare presentations are patients with an ovotestis and a contralateral streak gonad [28] and patients with crossed ectopy, consisting of a left side ovotestis that is displaced to the right scrotum [29]. Patients with Y chromosome have a testis more frequently than those who do not have such chromosome (55.8 % vs. 22.7 %). The degree of gonadal descent is parallel to the amount of functional testicular tissue present.

5.7 Biological Behaviour of the Gonads

More than two dozens of pregnancies in true hermaphrodites have been reported [30]. This contrasts with the exceptional cases of paternity even with assisted reproductive techniques [31, 32]. The origin of the ovules might be an ovotestis [33] or an ovary [34]. Most patients develop hypergonadotropic hypogonadism.

The incidence of tumors has been estimated between 4 % for those with 46,XX karyotype and 10 % when the karyotype is 46,XY or mosaicism 46,XX/XY [8, 35]. The most frequent tumors are gonadoblastoma, dysgerminoma/seminoma [36, 37], choriocarcinoma [38], and yolk sac tumor. Other reported tumors are mature teratoma and carcinoid and granulose cell tumor.

5.8 Patient Management

There are two main problems with ovotesticular DSD patients: sex assignment and actions to take with this type of gonads. The decision on sex reassignment must take into account the genetic sex, gonadal sex, social sex, and psychological sex, as well as the desires of the patients and their families [39].

The treatment of ovotesticular DSD is complex because it involves several specialists. In principle, the genetic sex determined by karyotype and/or Y chromosome sequence detection is not considered a useful criterium [40]. These are considered important factors: age of the patient at diagnosis, nature and location of the gonads, and development of the external genitalia [41]. The risk of germ cell tumors and the potential for future fertility should also be considered. Bilateral castration might be justified by the risk of gonadal neoplasia. However, the maintenance of gonads presents some advantages, principally if the hermaphrodite is growing as a girl, who may have a spontaneous puberty, and even be fertile. The risk of tumor can be minimized if several precautions are taken: removal of a testis that cannot be descended to the scrotal pouch and periodical survey of the residual gonad by ultrasonography.

References

1. Krstic ZD, Smoljanic Z, Vukanic D, Varinac D, Janjic G. True hermaphroditism: 10 years' experience. Pediatr Surg Int. 2000;16:580–3.
2. Blackless M, Charuvastra A, Derryck A, Fausto-Sterling A, Lauzanne K, Lee E. How sexually dimorphic are we? Review and synthesis. Am J Hum Biol. 2000;12:151–66.
3. Matsumoto F, Yamauchi K, Matsui F, Shimada K, Ida S. Acquired cryptorchidism in a boy with disorder of sex development. Clin Pediatr Endocrinol. 2012;21:1–3.
4. Wettasinghe KT, Sirisena ND, Andraweera PH, Jayasekara RW, Dissanayake VH. A case series of five srilankan patients with ovotesticular disorder of sex development. Clin Pediatr Endocrinol. 2012;21:69–73.
5. Dutta D, Shivaprasad KS, Das RN, Ghosh S, Chatterjee U, Chowdhury S, Dasgupta R. Ovotesticular disorder of sexual development due to 47,XYY/46,XY/45,X mixed gonadal dysgenesis in a phenotypic male

presenting as cyclical haematuria: clinical presentation and assessment of long-term outcomes. Andrologia. 2014;46:191–3.

6. Becker RE, Akhavan A. Prophylactic bilateral gonadectomy for ovotesticular disorder of sex development in a patient with mosaic 45,X/46,X,idic (Y)q11.222 karyotype. Urol Case Rep. 2016;5:13–6.
7. Zannoni GF, Vellone VG, Cordisco EL, Sangiorgi E, Grimaldi ME, Neri C, Nanni L, Neri G. Morphology and immunophenotyping of a monolateral ovotestis in a 46,Xder Y/45,X mosaic individual with ambiguous genitalia. Int J Gynecol Pathol. 2010;29:33–8.
8. Krob G, Braun A, Kuhnle U. True hermaphroditism: geographical distribution, clinical findings, chromosomes and gonadal histology. Eur J Pediatr. 1994;153:2–10.
9. Kojima Y, Hayashi Y, Asai N, Maruyama T, Sasaki S, Kohri K. Detection of the sex-determining region of the Y chromosome in 46,XX true hermaphroditism. Urol Int. 1998;60:235–8.
10. Kolon TF, Ferrer FA, Mckenna PH. Clinical and molecular analysis of XX sex reversed patients. J Urol. 1998;160:1169–72.
11. Berkovitz GD, Fechner PY, Marcantonio SM, Bland G, Stetten G, Goodfellow PN, Smith KD, Migeon CJ. The role of the sex-determining region of the Y chromosome (SRY) in the etiology of 46,XX true hermaphroditism. Hum Genet. 1992;88:411–6.
12. Kojima Y, Hayashi Y, Mizuno K, Sasaki S, Fukui Y, Koopman P, Morohashi K, Kohri K. Up-regulation of SOX9 in human sex-determining region on the Y chromosome (SRY)-negative XX males. Clin Endocrinol (Oxf). 2008;68:791–9.
13. Ledig S, Hiort O, Wünsch L, Wieacker P. Partial deletion of DMRT1 causes 46,XY ovotesticular disorder of sexual development. Eur J Endocrinol. 2012;167:119–24.
14. Tomaselli S, Megiorni F, De Bernardo C, Felici A, Marrocco G, Maggiulli G, Grammatico B, Remotti D, Saccucci P, Valentini F, Mazzilli MC, Majore S, Grammatico P. Syndromic true hermaphroditism due to an R-spondin1 (RSPO1) homozygous mutation. Hum Mutat. 2008;29:220–6.
15. Morel Y, Rey R, Teinturier C, Nicolino M, Michel-Calemard L, Mowszowicz I, Jaubert F, Fellous M, Chaussain JL, Chatelain P, David M, Nihoul-Fekete C, Forest MG, Josso N. A etiological diagnosis of male sex ambiguity: a collaborative study. Eur J Pediatr. 2002;161:49–59.
16. Ouhilal S, Turco J, Nangia A, Stotland M, Manganiello PD. True hermaphroditism presenting as bilateral gynecomastia in an adolescent phenotypic male. Fertil Steril. 2005;83:1041.
17. Kropp BP, Keating MA, Moshang T, Duckett JW. True hermaphroditism and normal male genitalia: an unusual presentation. Urology. 1995;46:736–9.
18. Yordam N, Alikasifoglu A, Kandemir N, Caglar M, Balci S. True hermaphroditism: clinical features, genetic variants and gonadal histology. J Pediatr Endocrinol Metab. 2001;14:421–7.
19. Olsson CA, Tessier PA, Brown ML, Austen Jr G. True hermaphroditism. J Urol. 1971;105:586–90.
20. Venkataram A, Shivaswamy S, Babu R, Santhosh S. Hernia uteri inguinalis in a case of ovotesticular disorder of sexual differentiation. J Pediatr Adolesc Gynecol. 2013;26:e17–9.
21. Irkilata HC, Basal S, Taslipinar A, Gur A, Piskin MM, Kurt B, Tahmaz L, Bolu E, Dayanc M. Ovotesticular disorder of sex development with a prostatic gland and review of literature. Andrologia. 2009;41:387–91.
22. Matsui F, Shimada K, Matsumoto F, Itesako T, Nara K, Ida S, Nakayama M. Long-term outcome of ovotesticular disorder of sex development: a single center experience. Int J Urol. 2011;18:231–6.
23. Mendez JP, Schiavon R, Diaz-Cueto L, Ruiz AI, Canto P, Diaz-Sanchez V, Ulloa-Aguirre A. A reliable endocrine test with human menopausal gonadotropins for diagnosis of true hermaphroditism in early infancy. J Clin Endocrinol Metab. 1998;83: 3523–6.
24. Iqbal MZ, Jam MR, Saleem M, Ahmad M. True hermaphrodite: a case report. APSP J Case Rep. 2011;2:16.
25. Wiersma R, Ramdial PK. The gonads of 111 South African patients with ovotesticular disorder of sex differentiation. J Pediatr Surg. 2009;44:556–60.
26. Van Niekert WA, Retief AE. The gonads of human true hermaphrodites. Hum Genet. 1981;58:117–22.
27. Aaronson IA. True hermaphroditism. A review of 41 cases with observations on testicular histology and function. Br J Urol. 1985;57:775–9.
28. Tran CN, Semins MJ, Epstein JI, Gearhart JP. Ovotesticular disorder of sex development with mosaic 45,X/46,X,idic (Y) (q11.23) karyotype and streak gonad. Urology. 2011;78:1178–81.
29. Lim DJ, Mullins DL, Stevens PS. Crossed ectopia of ovotestis in a case of true hermaphroditism. J Pediatr Surg. 1996;31:1440–2.
30. Schultz BA, Roberts S, Rodgers A, Ataya K. Pregnancy in true hermaphrodites and all male offspring to date. Obstet Gynecol. 2009;113:534–6.
31. Younis JS, Radin O, Kerner H, Ben-Ami M. Successful monozygotic twin pregnancy fathered by a male 46,XY true hermaphrodite. Reprod Biomed Online. 2011;22:80–2.
32. Sugawara N, Kimura Y, Araki Y. Successful second delivery outcome using refrozen thawed testicular sperm from an infertile male true hermaphrodite with a 46, XX/46, XY karyotype: case report. Hum Cell. 2012;25:96–9.
33. Tiltman AJ, Sweerts M. Multiparity in a covert true hermaphrodite. Obstet Gynecol NY. 1982; 60:752–4.
34. Minowada S, Fukutani K, Hara M, Shinohara M, Kamioka J, Isurugi K, Nijima T. Childbirth in true hermaphrodite. Eur Urol. 1984;10:414–5.
35. Verp MS, Simpson JL. Abnormal sexual differentiation and neoplasia. Cancer Genet Cytogenet. 1987;25:191–218.

36. Malik V, Gupta D, Gill M, Salvi AL. Seminoma in a male phenotype 46XX true hermaphrodite. Asian J Surg. 2007;30:85–7.
37. Kini U, Bantwal G, Ayyar V, Idiculla J. Bilateral gonadoblastomas with a left sided dysgerminoma in a true hermaphrodite (disorder of sexual differentiation) with 46 XY karyotype. J Assoc Physicians India. 2008;56:549–51.
38. Wang D, Hu Y, He Y, Xie C, Yin R. Pure ovarian choriocarinoma mimicking ectopic pregnancy in true hermaphroditism. Acta Obstet Gynecol Scand. 2009;88:850–2.
39. Jingde Z, Xin X, Entan G, Junhui L, Chunyu X, Xiaoyun W. Surgical treatment of hermaphroditism: experience with 25 cases. Ann Plast Surg. 2009;63:543–51.
40. Parada-Bustamante A, Ríos R, Ebensperger M, Lardone MC, Piottante A, Castro A. 46,XX/SRY-negative true hermaphrodite. Fertil Steril. 2010;94:2330.
41. Nihoul-Fekete C, Lortat-Jacob S, Cachin O, Josso N. Preservation of gonadal function in true hermaphroditism. J Pediatr Surg. 1984;19:50–5.

6 Usefulness of Histological Studies in Patients with the Androgen Insensitivity Syndrome

Manuel Nistal, Pilar González-Peramato, and Álvaro Serrano

6.1 Introduction

Androgen insensitivity syndrome (AIS) is a 46,XY DSD. The incidence is estimated at 15–20 % of all DSD (one in every 20,000–64,000 newborn males). It is caused by inactivation or deletion of the X-linked androgen receptor gene, resulting in the decrease or the abolishment of the androgenic effects on target tissues. Over 1000 mutations of the androgen receptor gene are known [1]. Depending on the degree of response of the external genitalia to androgens, three clinical forms are distinguished: complete androgen insensitivity (CAIS), partial androgen insensitivity (PAIS), and mild androgen insensitivity (MAIS). Patients with CAIS have a normal female phenotype and generally consult in childhood for inguinal hernia or swollen labia that contain a testicle; during adolescence they consult for primary amenorrhea. They have a regular pubertal growth spurt, breast development, scarce or absent development of axillary and pubic hair, a short vagina, and absence of Müllerian derivatives (uterus, cervix, and proximal vagina) [2, 3]. The testes can be abdominal, inguinal, or labial. Patients with PAIS may have variable phenotypes: from women with clitoromegaly and/or posterior labial fusion to males with gynecomastia, cryptorchidism, and infertility, including intermediate situations such as micropenis, severe hypospadias, and bifid scrotum which may contain the testes [4]. MAIS patients have a normal male phenotype, and most of them consult for infertility. Additionally to infertility, some patients with PAIS also have bulbar and spinal muscular atrophy (Kennedy's disease). Ninety-five percent of patients with CAIS versus 25 % of patients with PAIS have mutations of the *AR* [1]. Most of the histological data collected in the literature refer to patients with CAIS, and this chapter is focused on them.

6.2 CAIS in Fetal Age

The study of the gonads of fetuses with AIS is very limited. Only one case of well-documented CAIS is known [5]. The study was done in a 20-week fetus coming from an abortion. The study has not only served to know the morphology of the gonads at this time of development but to highlight the limited role of androgens in the development of the testis up to the second quarter of pregnancy. The size of both testes was increased and reached the major axis diameter of 12 mm, as compared to 6 mm in the control. The development of the seminiferous tubules was similar. Sertoli cells had an intense expression of AMH. Peritubular cells showed a lower expression of AMHR2 than the controls. In the interstitium, hypertrophy and hyperplasia of the Leydig cells were outstanding. The patient had uterus, vagina, and Fallopian tube remnants.

M. Nistal et al., *Clues in the Diagnosis of Non-tumoral Testicular Pathology*,
DOI 10.1007/978-3-319-49364-0_6

6.3 CAIS in Prepubertal Patients

6.3.1 Histological Findings

The location of the testes does not seem to influence their morphology [6]. In the first 4 years, the histological findings are only suggestive, as they are common to other diseases. Only when paratesticular structures are studied in some cases the diagnosis is definitive. From 4 years of age onwards, when under normal conditions most Sertoli cells express androgen receptor, the diagnosis is facilitated [7].

Seminiferous Tubules There is a decrease in the tubular diameter. The number of Sertoli cells also appears decreased [8]. Ring-shaped tubules with eosinophilic bodies and microliths can be observed. The number of germ cells declines rapidly after the first year of life [9]. Multinucleated

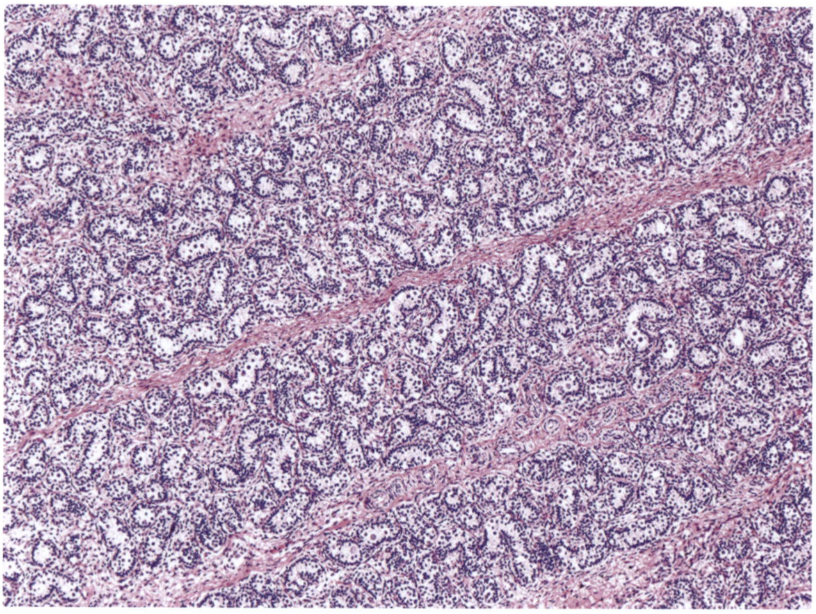

Fig. 6.1 CAIS. Patient of 1 year of age. Testicular lobules are separated by thick cellular septa

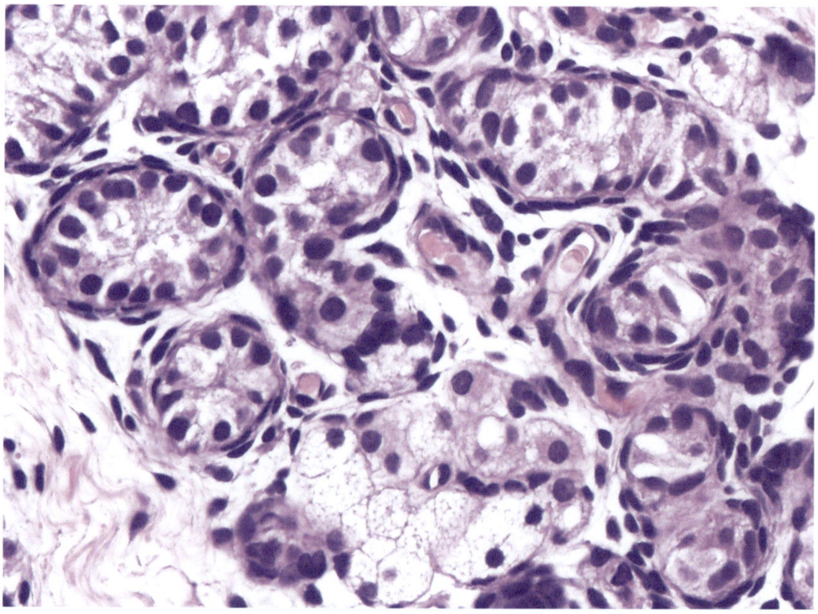

Fig. 6.2 CAIS. Testis of a child with small seminiferous tubules with marked reduction in Sertoli cell and germ cell number. Presence of Leydig cell groups with multivacuolated cytoplasm

spermatogonia can be present. The tubular wall shows no alterations.

Interstitium is loose and abundant in younger patients, while in older ones, it tends to be fibrous (Fig. 6.1). Fetal Leydig cells do not disappear and form small clusters between the seminiferous tubules or on the periphery of the testicular lobules. They are large and their cytoplasm is vacuolated (Fig. 6.2). Calretinin makes it very clear that there are not only isolated Leydig cells as it would correspond to the age but groups of four to eight cells. The lymphatic vessels of the tunica vasculosa and interlobular septa are distended in most cases.

6.3.2 Differential Diagnosis

Throughout childhood, the differential diagnosis is made with the following entities: cryptorchidism, persistent Müllerian duct syndrome, defect in 5-alpha-reductase type II, and *NR5A1* gene mutations. Before 4 years of age, the diagnosis is difficult, but subsequently, demonstration of the absence of androgen receptors in Sertoli cells facilitates the diagnosis. Which histological data can be useful before 4 years of age? The first one is the appearance of the interstitium. A broad and cellular interstitium and thickened interlobular septa are more characteristic of AIS. A tunica albuginea similar to ovarian stroma with tubular formations inside is characteristic of the defects seen in AMH [10]. The absence or severe reduction of Leydig cells (assessment with calretinin is required) is characteristic of cryptorchidism. However, the presence of Leydig cell groups considered characteristic of *NR5A1* mutations [11] can be observed in other pathologies as well. Markedly hypoplastic or absent epididymis suggest AIS. The presence of smooth muscle forming a mass in the lower pole of the testis is characteristic of AIS [12].

6.3.3 Associated Pathology

It is very important to know that the following facts can be observed in these testes in childhood: delayed maturation of germ cells, germ cell neoplasia in situ, and presence of a variable development of the Wolffian and Müllerian structures.

Delayed Maturation of Germ Cells AIS patients often show a delay in the maturation of germ cells. This is characterized by persistent gonocytes in the center of the seminiferous tube until 1 year of age (Fig. 6.3). They are morphologically identifiable as large cells with spherical nucleus and prominent nucleoli. They retain

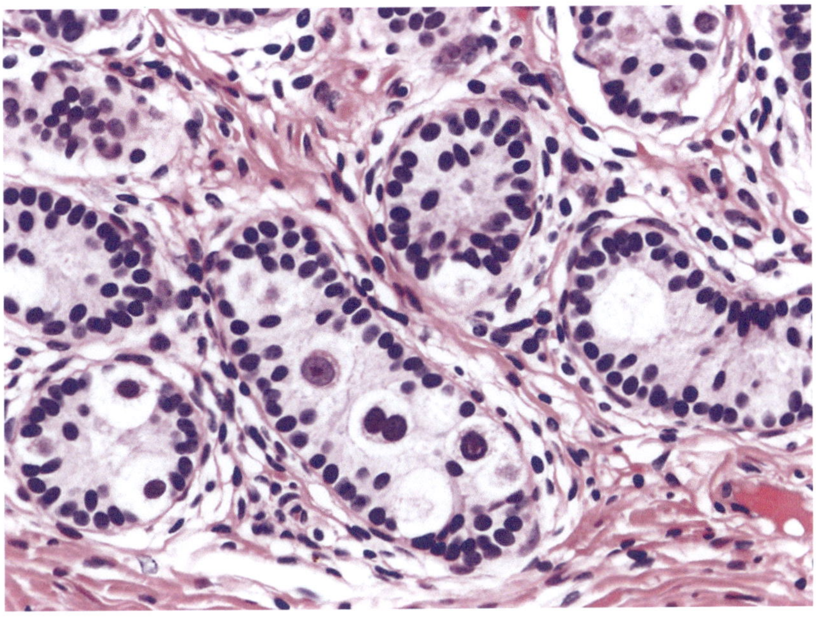

Fig. 6.3 CAIS patient of one and a half year of age. Delayed maturation of germ cells is shown with persistence of gonocytes in the central part of a seminiferous tubule

immunohistochemical positivity for OCT3/4, PLAP, or c-KIT. The tubules with gonocytes are regularly distributed throughout the testis [13].

Germ Cell Neoplasia in Situ Some patients have GCNIS. GCNIS diagnosis in childhood requires evaluating several facts such as patient age, germ cell morphology, distribution of germ cells, and immunohistochemical pattern.

From 1 year old, when there is a delay in the maturation of germ cells, in most cases, the cells that do not reach the basement membrane undergo a process of apoptosis. In some patients, this regression does not occur and then GCNIS should be suspected.

Morphologically, it is necessary to note that during childhood, the seminiferous tubules of patients with AIS can have a variety of germ cells besides gonocytes and spermatogonia type A; there are hypertrophic spermatogonia and tumor cells. Hypertrophic spermatogonia may be confused with GCNIS cells. They are large cells with large nuclei of circular contours and compact chromatin that does not allow to distinguish a nucleolus. They are usually located on the basement membrane. They are polyploid cells that are unable to complete their division and probably degenerate. GCNIS cells are large cells, similar to gonocytes; they are placed inside the tube but are also found on the basal membrane. The most important differences are a nucleus of irregular contours, coarse granular heterochromatin, and the presence of one or two bulky nucleoli. The same seminiferous tubule may have spermatogonia and tumor cells.

Distribution of gonocyte-like cells: when these cells do not have a regular arrangement in the testicular parenchyma but are found only in a group of seminiferous tubules, or only in a testicular lobule, the suspicion of GCNIS is very high.

Immunohistochemically, spermatogonia are *TSPY1* positive. GCNIS cells show nuclear expression of OCT3/4 or TSPY expression in cytoplasm and membrane and can also show expression of c-kit and PLAP.

Presence of Wolffian Structures Epididymis/vas deferens is present in 36 % of cases and shows various degrees of maturation at puberty [14]. It is interpreted that these patients harbor mutant receptors showing a residual response to high concentrations of androgens. Most cases are hypoplastic Wolffian derivatives.

Müllerian Remnants The presence, even grossly, of smooth muscle tissue is observed in 80 % of the testes out of the tunica at the lower pole of the

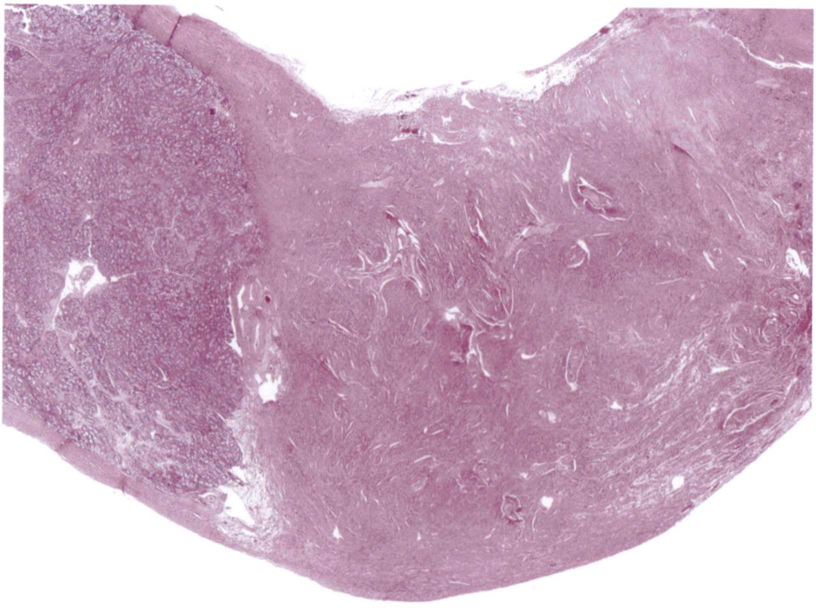

Fig. 6.4 Smooth muscle hamartoma. A mass of smooth muscle cells rests directly on the tunica albuginea

testis. Most often it is bilateral [15]. In some cases there are formations constituted by thick bundles of smooth muscle cells described sometimes as muscle hamartomas and also as leiomyomas [16] (Fig. 6.4). On other occasions, the muscle tissue is more organized. It may form cordonal structures that fuse in the midline simulating a bicornis uterus. Other patients have hypoplastic uterine tubes.

6.4 CAIS in Pubertal and Adult Patients

6.4.1 Histological Findings

There are differences depending on the expected residual AR activity. When there is no androgen activity, the diameter of the seminiferous tubules is very small and lacks germ cells. The seminiferous tubes are reminiscent of a child's testicle, but there are even smaller groups of tubules comprising only three or four Sertoli cells per cross tubular section (Fig. 6.5). These data correlate well with the conservation of immunoexpression calretinin and D2-40. When AR residual activity is retained, the tubular diameter is greater, but it lacks tubular lumen, or this is only present in isolated tubules. A considerable number of seminiferous tubules have germinal cells [9]. Even in the best cases, Sertoli cells retain immature signs as spherical nuclei, absence of Charcot-Bötther crystals, annulated lamellae, or well-developed Sertoli-Sertoli joints. They express strong cytoplasmic immunostaining for AMH, nuclear for SOX-9, and weak cytoplasmic expression for PGDS and absence of AR immunostaining [17]. In 14 % of the testicles, there are granular changes in Sertoli cells. Among the seminiferous tubules, large clusters of Leydig cells lacking Reinke crystals are observed. The interstitium contains thick bundles of spindle cells simulating ovarian stroma. Most of these cells express SMA [18]. Lymphangiectasis in tunica vasculosa and interlobular septa can be observed (Fig. 6.6).

6.4.2 Associated Pathology

Sertoli-Leydig Hamartomas They are lesions ranging in size from 1 to 5 mm, usually multiple, well defined, unencapsulated (Fig. 6.7). They are present in 63 % of cases [19]. They consist of seminiferous tubules and Leydig cells similar to the rest of the parenchyma but with a disrupted

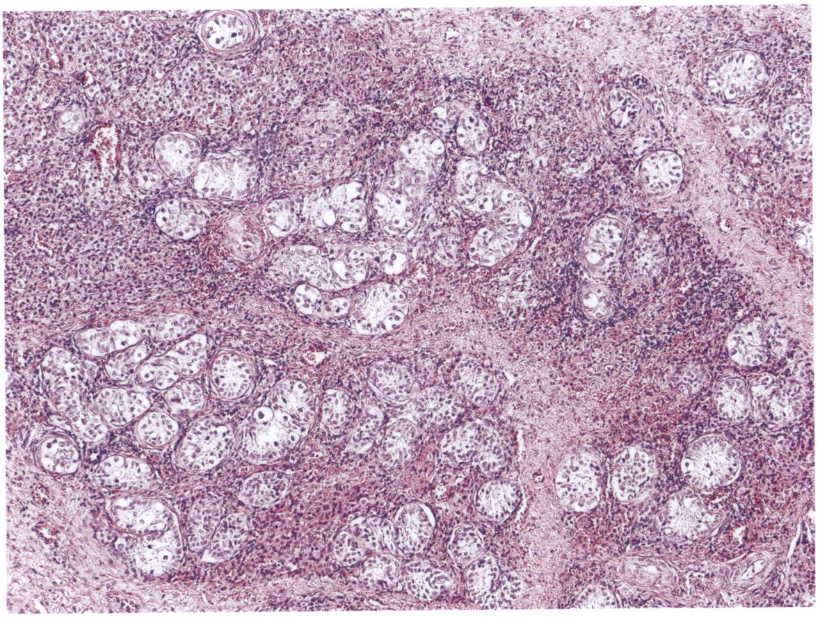

Fig. 6.5 CAIS in a postpubertal patient. Seminiferous tubules showing an infantile development contrasting with Leydig cell hyperplasia

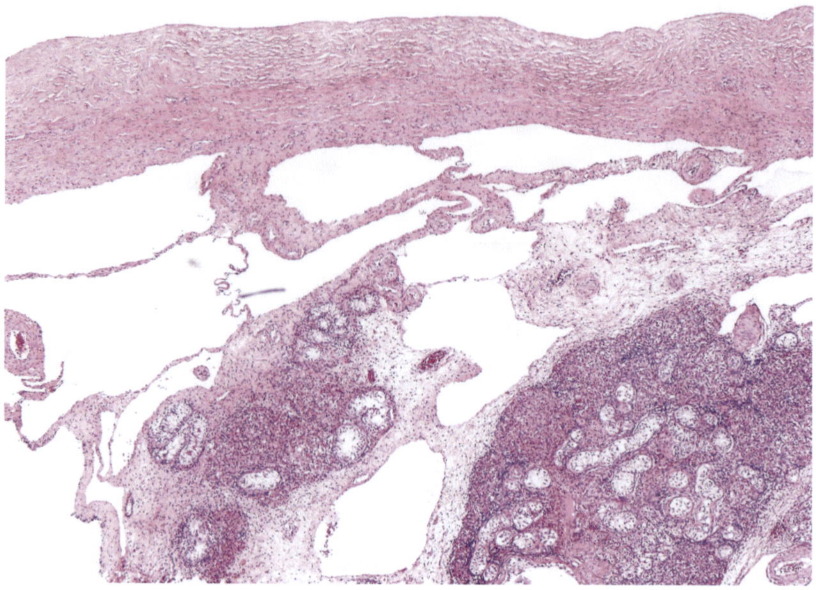

Fig. 6.6 CAIS in a postpubertal patient. Lymphangiectasis in tunica vasculosa and interlobular septa

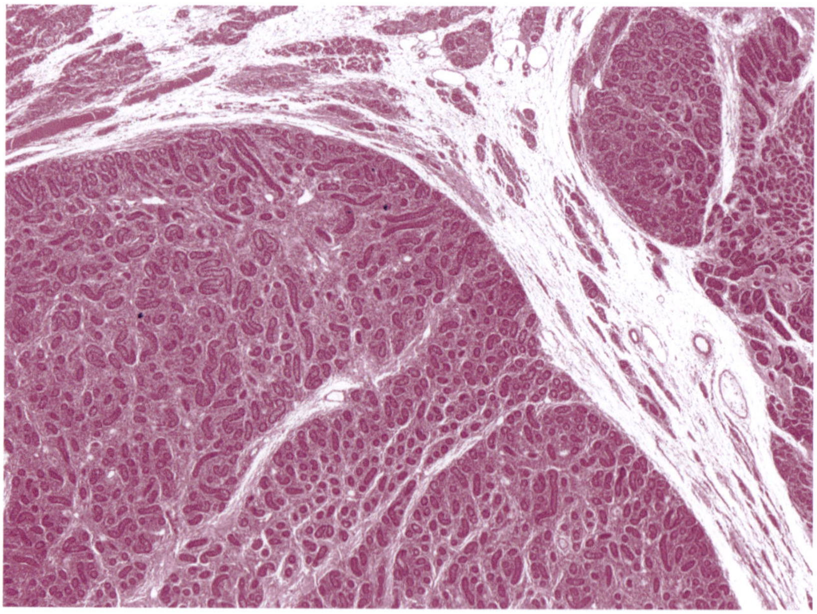

Fig. 6.7 CAIS. Adult patients with Sertoli/Leydig hamartomas. Nodular formations are well defined but unencapsulated

architecture. Seminiferous tubules have a fetal or child development. Sertoli cells have signs of both morphological and immunohistochemical immaturity. Their nucleus is spherical, and inhibin bodies and positivity for calretinin are observed in the cytoplasm. The tubular wall can be thin, but in some tubules, it may show concentric hyalinization. The intertubular space is occupied by Leydig cells showing a marked hyperplasia [20]. Leydig cells lack Reinke crystals. These hamartomas cannot be considered well-differentiated Sertoli-Leydig tumors, as occasionally it erroneously appears in some publications.

Sertoli Cells Adenomas They are observed in 23 % of the adult testes. They are unencapsulated formations whose diameter can exceed

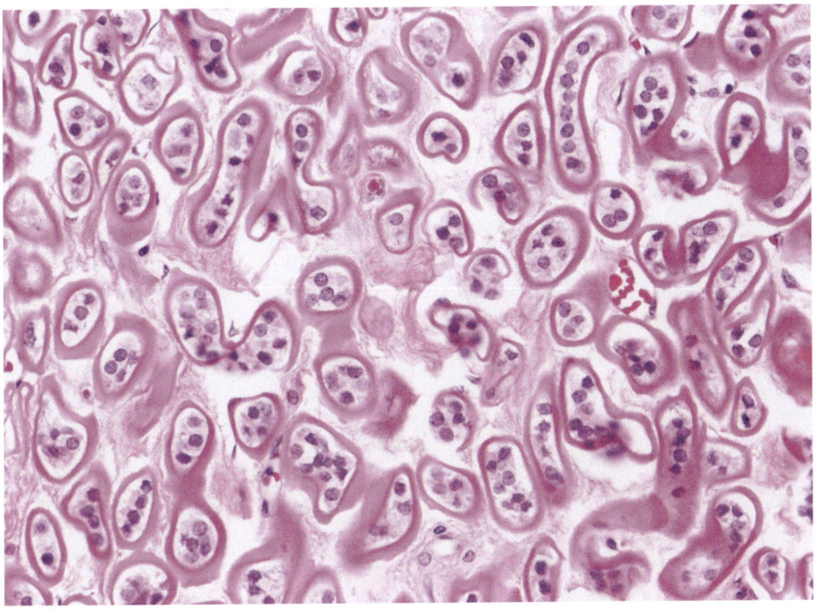

Fig. 6.8 CAIS. Sertoli cell adenoma in an adult patient. The tubular formations show a much thickened wall and contain scant Sertoli cells. Among the tubular formations, no Leydig are observed

10 cm. They consist of tubular formations devoid of lumen whose diameter does not exceed that of a seminiferous tube in childhood. The cells that constitute them are cubic and have a spherical nucleus, small nucleoli, and finely granular cytoplasm. The number of cells per tubular section, although variable, is less than half that of a child seminiferous tubule. The cells rest on a basement membrane whose thickness is highly variable even in the various sectors of the tubule. Thickening does become rings leaving within two or three Sertoli cells. The tubular wall lacks myoid cells. The interstitium is scarce and does not show Leydig cells (Fig. 6.8). The cells of the tubular formations are positive for inhibin alpha and WT1, focally for calretinin, and the proliferation rate is very low. They are negative for estrogen, progesterone, and Melan A [21].

6.5 PAIS

Most studies of PAIS on testicular histology refer to patients with a male phenotype as the Reifenstein's syndrome (micropenis, hypospadias, cryptorchidism, testicular atrophy, poor virilization, gynecomastia, azoospermia or oligozoospermia, and infertility) [22, 23] and the Rosewater's syndrome (males with gynecomastia and infertility). The fact that patients with slight undervirilization had azoospermia, and patients with hypospadias and gynecomastia were fertile, suggests that androgens can influence spermatogenesis and genital differentiation through different routes [24, 25]. Histological findings vary from tubules with marked wall hyalinization and absence of spermatogenesis to seminiferous tubules that focally retain germline. Leydig cells are increased in all cases.

6.6 MAIS

It is the least common form of AIS. Most fertile patients with mild impaired AR activities have slight signs of undervirilization such as gynecomastia and/or a small penis, simple coronal hypospadias, or prominent raphe of the scrotum [4]. Investigations of AR anomalies in infertile men have revealed that a significant percentage of them carry abnormalities in the AR gene [26–28]. Histologically, the most important finding is diffuse Leydig cell hyperplasia that is associated with some seminiferous tubules with poor spermatogenesis.

6.7 Tumors in AIS

Among the benign tumors, tumors of large Sertoli cells with calcifications, sex cord with annular tubules, Leydig cell tumors, leiomyomas (or smooth muscle hamartoma), and fibromas have been reported [19]. The classical malignancy has been estimated at 3.6 % at 25 years and 33 % at 50 years of age, with the greatest incidence of intra-abdominal testes. The incidence in CAIS is low when compared with PAIS, and the gonads must be maintained until puberty is complete [29–31]. GCNIS, various types of germ cell tumors both unilateral and bilateral, and malignant sex cord tumors have also been reported.

References

1. Gottlieb B, Beitel LK, Nadarajah A, Paliouras M, Trifiro M. The androgen receptor gene mutations database: 2012 update. Hum Mutat. 2012;33:887–94.
2. Botella Llusia J, Nogales F. Pseudohermafroditismo masculino con feminización total. Acta Ginecol. 1952;3:379–30.
3. Morris JM. The syndrome of testicular feminization in male pseudohermaphrodites. Am J Obstet Gynecol. 1953;65:1192–211.
4. Quigley CA, Tan JA, He B, Zhou ZX, Mebarki F, Morel Y, Forest MG, Chatelain P, Ritzén EM, French FS, Wilson EM. Partial androgen insensitivity with phenotypic variation caused by androgen receptor mutations that disrupt activation function 2 and the NH(2)- and carboxyl-terminal interaction. Mech Ageing Dev. 2004;125:683–95.
5. Corbetta S, Muzza M, Avagliano L, Bulfamante G, Gaetti L, Eller-Vainicher C, Beck-Peccoz P, Spada A. Gonadal structures in a fetus with complete androgen insensitivity syndrome and persistent Müllerian derivatives: comparison with normal fetal development. Fertil Steril. 2011;95:1119.e9–14.
6. Kaprova-Pleskacova J, Stoop H, Brüggenwirth H, Cools M, Wolffenbuttel KP, Drop SL, Snajderova M, Lebl J, Oosterhuis JW, Looijenga LH. Complete androgen insensitivity syndrome: factors influencing gonadal histology including germ cell pathology. Mod Pathol. 2014;27:721–30.
7. Chemes HE, Rey RA, Nistal M, Regadera J, Musse M, González-Peramato P, Serrano A. Physiological androgen insensitivity of the fetal, neonatal, and early infantile testis is explained by the ontogeny of the androgen receptor expression in Sertoli cells. J Clin Endocrinol Metab. 2008;93:4408–12.
8. Müller J. Morphometry and histology of gonads from twelve children and adolescents with the androgen insensitivity (testicular feminization) syndrome. J Clin Endocrinol Metab. 1984;59:785–9.
9. Hannema SE, Scott IS, Rajpert-De Meyts E, Skakkebaek NE, Coleman N, Hughes IA. Testicular development in the complete androgen insensitivity syndrome. J Pathol. 2006;208:518–27.
10. Nistal M, Paniagua R, González-Peramato P, Reyes-Múgica M. Perspectives in Pediatric Pathology, Chapter 5 Gonadal Dysgenesis. Pediatr Dev Pathol. 2015;18:259–78.
11. Camats N, Pandey AV, Fernández-Cancio M, Andaluz P, Janner M, Torán N, Moreno F, Bereket A, Akcay T, García-García E, Muñoz MT, Gracia R, Nistal M, Castaño L, Mullis PE, Carrascosa A, Audí L, Flück CE. Ten novel mutations in the NR5A1 gene cause disordered sex development in 46,XY and ovarian insufficiency in 46,XX individuals. J Clin Endocrinol Metab. 2012;97(7):E1294–306.
12. Nistal M, Paniagua R, Gonzalez-Peramato P, Reyes-Múgica M. Perspectives in pediatric pathology, Chapter 6. Male undermasculinization. Pediatr Dev Pathol. 2015;18:279–96.
13. Cools M, van Aerde K, Kersemaekers AM, Boter M, Drop SL, Wolffenbuttel KP, Steyerberg EW, Oosterhuis JW, Looijenga LH. Morphological and immunohistochemical differences between gonadal maturation delay and early germ cell neoplasia in patients with undervirilization syndromes. J Clin Endocrinol Metab. 2005;90:5295–303.
14. Hannema SE, Scott IS, Hodapp J, Martin H, Coleman N, Schwabe JW, Hughes IA. Residual activity of mutant androgen receptors explains wolffian duct development in the complete androgen insensitivity syndrome. J Clin Endocrinol Metab. 2004;89:5815–22.
15. Güven A, Dursun F, Özkanlı S, Güçlüer B, Kuru Lİ. Complete androgen insensitivity syndrome and discordant Müllerian remnants: two cases with novel mutation in the androgen receptor. J Pediatr Endocrinol Metab. 2013;26:909–14.
16. Krichen Makni S, Mnif Hachicha L, Ellouze S, Mnif M, Khabir A, Ketata H, Abid M, Sellami Boudawara T. Feminizing testicular syndrome with multiple hamartomas and bilateral paratesticular leiomyomas. Rev Med Interne. 2005;26:980–3.
17. Papanastasopoulos P, Panagidis A, Verras D, Repanti M, Georgiou G. A case of complete androgen insensitivity syndrome presenting with incarcerated inguinal hernia: an immunohistochemical study. Fertil Steril. 2009;92:1169.e11–4.
18. Regadera J, Martínez-García F, Paniagua R, Nistal M. Androgen insensitivity syndrome: an immunohistochemical, ultrastructural, and morphometric study. Arch Pathol Lab Med. 1999;123:225–34.
19. Rutgers JL. Advances in the pathology of intersex conditions. Hum Pathol. 1991;22:884–91.
20. Nistal M, De La Roza C, Cano J. Síndrome de feminización testicular completa. Patología. 1979;12:119–25.
21. Fernandez-Vega I, Santos-Juanes J, García-Pravia C. Bilateral Sertoli cell adenoma in gonads, associated with serous cystadenoma. Pol J Pathol. 2014;65:154–6.

22. Tordjman KM, Yaron M, Berkovitz A, Botchan A, Sultan C, Lumbroso S. Fertility after high-dose testosterone and intracytoplasmic sperm injection in a patient with androgen insensitivity syndrome with a previously unreported androgen receptor mutation. Andrologia. 2014;46:703–6.
23. Lee SW, Kwak DS, Jung IS, Kwak JH, Park JH, Hong SM, Lee CB, Park YS, Kim DS, Choi WH, Ahn YH. Partial androgen insensitivity syndrome presenting with gynecomastia. Endocrinol Metab (Seoul). 2015;30:226–30.
24. Chu J, Zhang R, Zhao Z, Zou W, Han Y, Qi Q, Zhang H, Wang JC, Tao S, Liu X, Luo Z. Male fertility is compatible with an Arg(840) Cys substitution in the AR in a large Chinese family affected with divergent phenotypes of AR insensitivity syndrome. J Clin Endocrinol Metab. 2002;87:347–51.
25. O'Hara L, Smith LB. Androgen receptor roles in spermatogenesis and infertility. Best Pract Res Clin Endocrinol Metab. 2015;29:595–605.
26. Hiort O, Holterhus PM, Horter T, Schulze W, Kremke B, Bals-Pratsch M, Sinnecker GH, Kruse K. Significance of mutations in the androgen receptor gene in males with idiopathic infertility. J Clin Endocrinol Metab. 2000;85:2810–5.
27. Lombardo F, Sgro P, Salacone P, Gilio B, Gandini L, Dondero F, Jannini EA, Lenzi A. Androgens and fertility. J Endocrinol Invest. 2005;28:51–5.
28. Massin N, Bry H, Vija L, Maione L, Constancis E, Haddad B, Morel Y, Claessens F, Young J. Healthy birth after testicular extraction of sperm and ICSI from an azoospermic man with mild androgen insensitivity syndrome caused by an androgen receptor partial loss-of-function mutation. Clin Endocrinol (Oxf). 2012;77:593–8.
29. Hersmus R, de Leeuw BH, Wolffenbuttel KP, Drop SL, Oosterhuis JW, Cools M, Looijenga LH. New insights into type II germ cell tumor pathogenesis based on studies of patients with various forms of disorders of sex development (DSD). Mol Cell Endocrinol. 2008;291:1–10.
30. Wünsch L, Holterhus PM, Wessel L, Hiort O. Patients with disorders of sex development (DSD) at risk of gonadal tumour development: management based on laparoscopic biopsy and molecular diagnosis. BJU Int. 2012;110:E958–65.
31. Patel V, Casey RK, Gomez-Lobo V. Timing of gonadectomy in patients with complete androgen insensitivity syndrome-current recommendations and future directions. J Pediatr Adolesc Gynecol. 2016;29:320–5.

7 Differential Diagnosis of Tumors in the Adrenogenital Syndrome

Manuel Nistal, Pilar González-Peramato, and Álvaro Serrano

7.1 Introduction

Congenital adrenal hyperplasia (CAH) is an autosomal recessive disorder of the adrenal steroid synthesis caused by defects in the enzymes involved in the production of cortisol, aldosterone, and sex hormones. There are two forms of CAH, the classical form with salt-wasting and simple virilizing subtypes and the nonclassical form that is more frequent. The classic form is severe while the nonclassical form is mild and of late onset. Ninety percent of the cases are associated with loss-of-function mutations or translocations involving the *CYP21* gene that encodes the 21-alpha-hydroxylase enzyme, and 5–8 % are associated with loss-of-function mutations in the *CYP11B1* gene encoding the 11-beta-hydroxylase enzyme. Less frequent are the defects in enzyme 17α-hydroxylase (mutations in the gene *CYP17A1*) and 3β-hydroxysteroid dehydrogenase (mutations in the gene *HSD3β2*). Loss of function of these enzymes determines impaired production of cortisol and other steroid hormones. As a result, an increased secretion of hypothalamic corticotropin-releasing hormone (CRH) and an increase in pituitary ACTH production occur which leads to bilateral adrenal gland hyperplasia [1].

One of the most important complications in patients with congenital adrenal hyperplasia is the development of testicular tumors. Testicular tumors in adrenogenital syndrome are clinically observed in 27 % to 47 % of patients with congenital adrenal hyperplasia [2]. Testicular tumors of the adrenogenital syndrome resemble histologically Leydig cell tumors, which poses a difficulty to differential diagnosis [3].

7.2 Development of Tumors of the Adrenogenital Syndrome

When patients with CAH are diagnosed late or not treated properly, they develop testicular lesions. High plasma levels of ACTH stimulate possible adrenal rests as well as pluripotential cells, "steroid" cells normally present in the testicular hilum [4, 5]. Hyperplasia of these cells leads to the formation of tumor nodules between the rete testis cavities or between the rete testis and the testicular parenchyma (Fig. 7.1). This highly selective localization justifies the infertility (by obstructive azoospermia) which some patients consult for as the first symptom of the disease [6]. The infertility is caused by the hypogonadotropic hypogonadism secondary to the increased production of adrenal androgens [7]. These nodules are known by different names: "bilateral nodular hyperplasia of testicular adrenal rests," "testicular adrenal rest tumors (TART)" [8], "testicular tumors in congenital adrenal hyperplasia," "testicular adrenogenital tumors" [9], "adrenogenital syndrome-associated

M. Nistal et al., *Clues in the Diagnosis of Non-tumoral Testicular Pathology*,
DOI 10.1007/978-3-319-49364-0_7

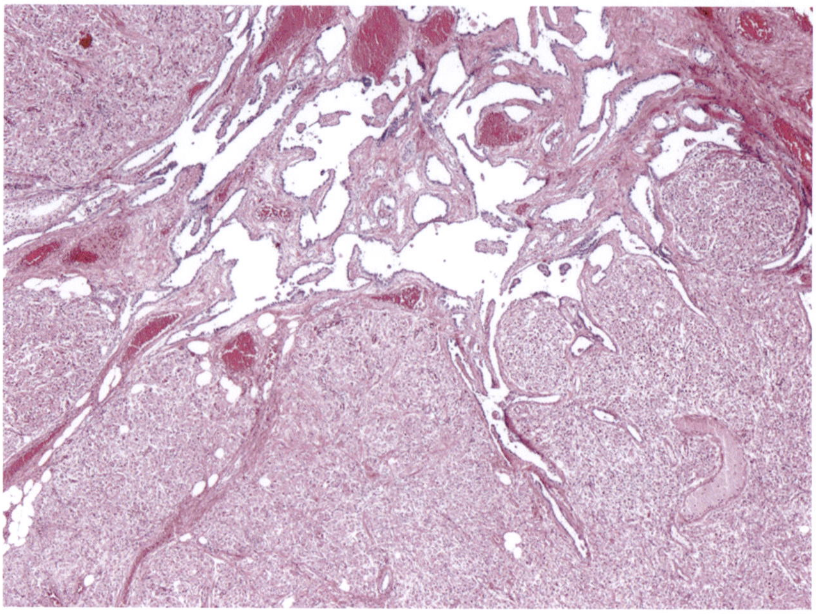

Fig. 7.1 Tumor of the adrenogenital syndrome. Nodular formations located in the vicinity of testicular mediastinum. Among the different nodules, tubuli recti and marked dilation of the rete testis cavities are observed

tumors" [10], and "testicular tumors of the adrenogenital syndrome (TTAGS)" [11, 12].

The first case of TTAGS was published by Wilkins in 1940 [13] and concerned the autopsy of a 3-year-old child whose major symptoms were a marked salt craving, an enlarged penis and scrotum, and bilateral testicular tumors similar to those observed in the adrenal cortex.

TTAGS are present in 94 % of patients with CAH [14]. Classically, the development of TTAGS is synchronous in both testicles [15]; however since ultrasound has been used routinely in the study of testicular tumors, unilateral lesions are found more often which if untreated could lead to bilateral tumors [14]. The size of these tumors varies from microscopic to several cms, being able to affect the entire testicular parenchyma. Given their initial location in the mediastinum, only those tumors larger than 2 cm are palpable.

Five stages have been described in the development of TTAGS. Stage 1: adrenal rest cells are present within the rete testis. Stage 2 is characterized by hyperplasia and hypertrophy of the rest cells. Stage 3: the rest cells compress the rete testis. Stage 4: the cell nests induce fibrosis and lymphoid infiltrates in the neighboring testicular parenchyma. Stage 5: there is irreversible damage to the testicular parenchyma. The testicular parenchyma lesions are considered secondary to the obstruction of the seminiferous tubules where they flow into the rete testis [16].

7.3 Clinical and Laboratory Diagnostic Clues

The differential diagnosis between TTAGS and LCT is particularly important as the treatments are quite different (cortisol and/or mineralocorticoid replacement therapy for CAH versus enucleation or orchiectomy for LCT). Difficulties are added when TTAGS have a unilateral or metachronous presentation in adults with milder forms of CAH; moreover correctly treated TTAGS do not regress, but become autonomous. The most important key for differential diagnosis between TTAGS and LCT must be sought in the clinical and laboratory data to support hyperandrogenism and testicular mass. The most important clues are the following:

- Most common age of TTAGS in children is under 4 years (ranging from 2 to 32 years) [17]. Most Leydig cell tumors in children are seen between 5 and 10 years [18].

- The bilateral lesions are observed in 80 % of TTAGS [2]. The scrotal skin hyperpigmentation associated with hyperandrogenism and bilateral testicular masses suggests an increase in the levels of ACTH secondary to congenital adrenal hyperplasia.
- TTAGS rarely have any estrogenic activity (gynecomastia) [19], while it is present in 30 % of patients with Leydig cell tumors.
- The presence of extratesticular nodules in a patient with bilateral macroorchidism favors TTAGS.
- Serum testosterone levels are not as high in TTAGS as in Leydig cell tumors [20].
- The elevation of 11-deoxycortisol associated with the increase in androgens suggests a defect in 11-beta-hydroxylase, the second most common cause of congenital adrenal hyperplasia [21].
- Preoperative determination of serum ACTH allows a differential diagnosis between TTAGS and testicular tumors.
- The TTAGS represent a reactive hyperplasia that develops after a supraphysiological stimulation of ACTH. The Leydig cell tumors are not ACTH responsive and are not associated with an elevation of ACTH.
- Hydrocortisone treatment suppresses the secretion of ACTH and produces a decrease in TTAGS.

7.4 Diagnostic Imaging

Imaging tests are useful for diagnosis, management, and follow-up of the patients [22]. The most common sonographic finding is bilateral intratesticular hypoechoic masses of spikelike appearance, with no sound attenuation surrounding the testicular mediastinum [23]. The prevalence is 94 % of CAH adults. In some cases nodules are heterogeneous or hyperechoic. The echogenicity is related to the size of the lesions, all lesions under 2 cm being hypoechoic, while lesions larger than 2 cm are heterogeneous and hyperechoic. The hyperechoic areas may represent fibrosis or calcification. The small nodules may be unilateral and the larger ones are usually bilateral. Bilateral lesions may extend from the mediastinum to the testicular parenchyma. LCT are intraparenchymal [14].

The prevalence of TTAGS is similar in MRI and ultrasound [14]. Just as the adrenal cortex, the TTAGS are isointense with muscle on T1- and T2-weighted images. Regarding the testicular parenchyma, it is described as iso- or hyperintense on T1-weighted images and hypointense on T2-weighted images with well-defined margins without capsule or pseudocapsule. Homogenous enhancement occurs after the injection of gadolinium [24]. CT of the adrenal glands shows increased size in patients with TTAGS.

7.5 Histological and Immunohistochemical Clues

Histological Data Differential diagnosis between TTAGS and LCT is not possible by means of a single datum [25].

- Location in the testicular hilum favors TTAGS and only rarely they are intraparenquimal [26].
- TTAGS are macroscopically firm and multinodular with a dark brown color against the presence of a single yellow nodule in the LCT on cut sections.
- TTAGS are well defined but not encapsulated. LCT shows an infiltrating border.
- TTAGS resemble adrenocortical tissue although typical zonation of adrenal cortex is absent.
- TTAGS show sheets of large polygonal cells with abundant eosinophilic cytoplasm intersected by broad fibrous bands (Figs. 7.2 and 7.3). LCT may have fiber tracts but they are thin.
- The absence of cellular atypia except for, in some cases, cells with large pleomorphic nuclei, with one or two prominent nucleoli.
- The absence of mitotic activity in TTAGS [26]. In LCT multinucleated cells are frequent, and most have focal large pleomorphic nuclei. Isolated mitoses are observed.
- Abundant lipofuscins pigment in TTAGS (Fig. 7.3), compared to the small amount in LCT.
- No Reinke crystals in TTAGS, but bear in mind that they are only observed in 40 % of LCT.

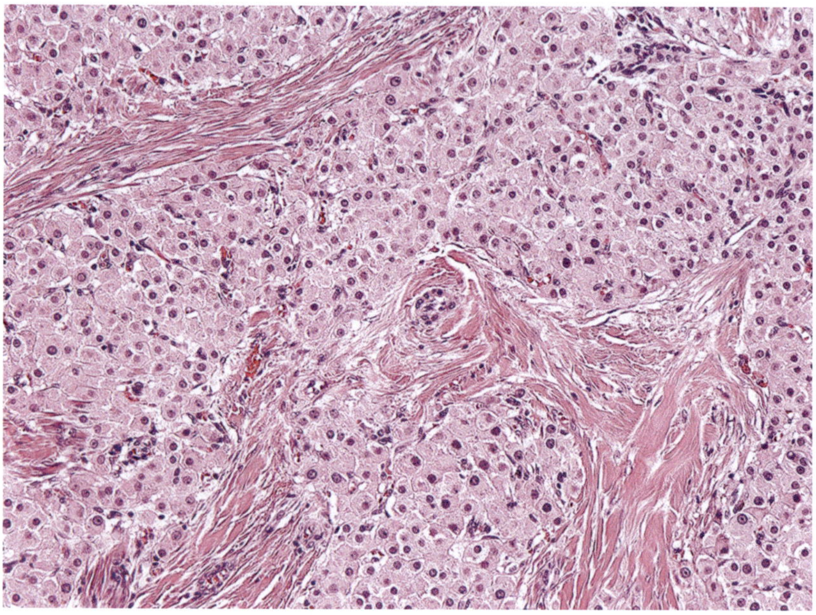

Fig. 7.2 Tumor of the adrenogenital syndrome. Cellular proliferation arranged in sheets intersected by broad fibrous bands of very collagenized connective tissue

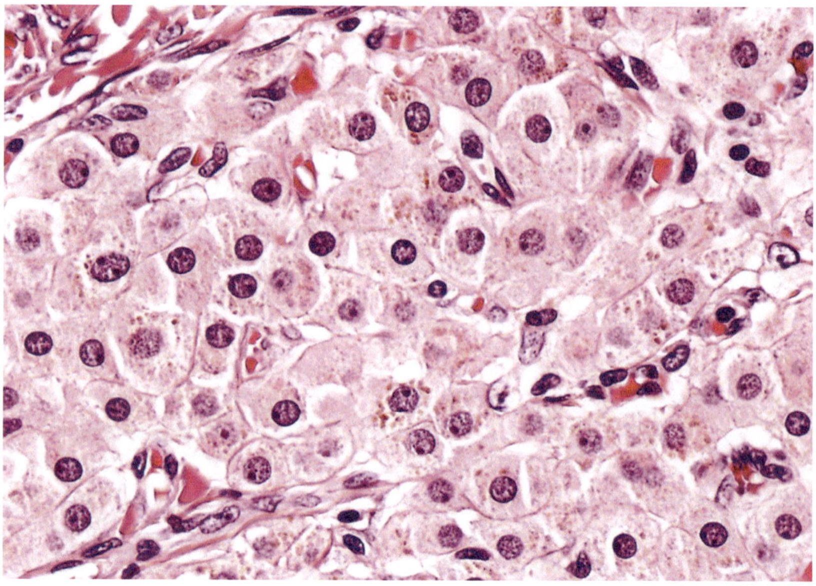

Fig. 7.3 Tumor of the adrenogenital syndrome. Cells are polyhedral with a central nuclei and abundant granular cytoplasm with lipofuscins

- Focal lymphocytic infiltration in TTAGS (Fig. 7.4).
- Adipose metaplasia in 56 % of TTAGS (Fig. 7.4) compared to the rarity with which it appears in LCT [27, 28].
- Atrophy of the seminiferous tubules versus the advanced maturation – even with spermatogenesis – in LCT (Figs. 7.5 and 7.6).

Among other differential diagnostics from the histological point of view, it would also include nodular hyperplasia of Leydig cells. This is a multifocal lesion that has no features of expansive growth; seminiferous tubules are included inside the lesion; and it is often associated with familial male-limited precocious puberty [29].

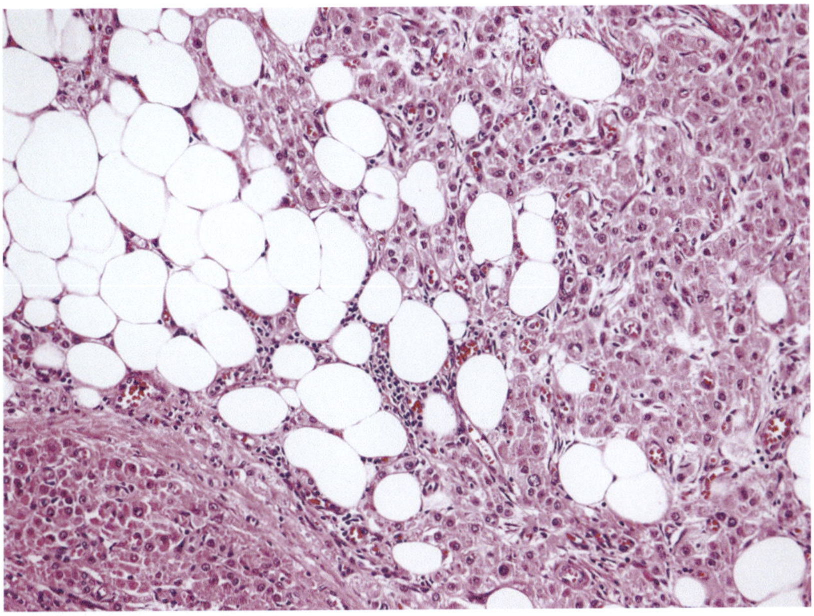

Fig. 7.4 Tumor of the adrenogenital syndrome. On the periphery of nodules, adipose metaplasia and lymphocyte infiltration are observed

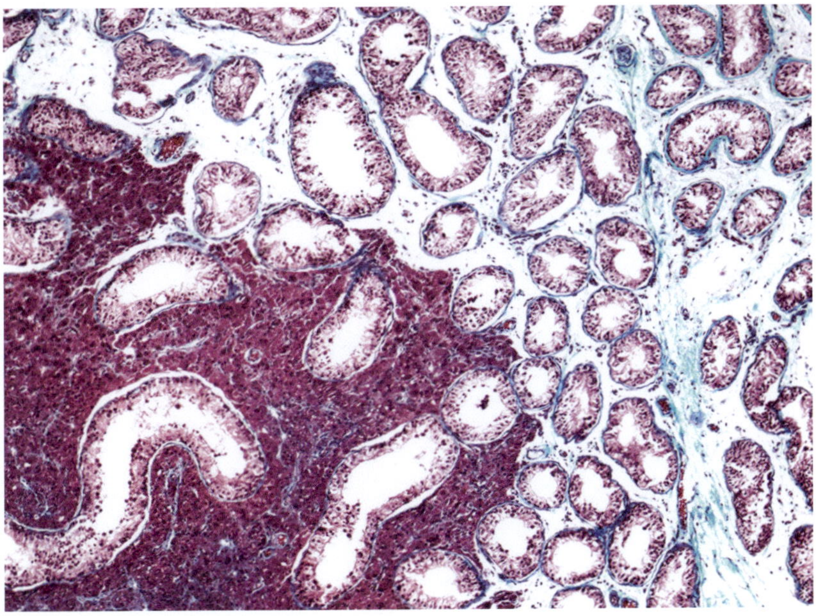

Fig. 7.5 Functionating Leydig cell tumor in a 7-year-old boy. Several seminiferous tubules have been trapped by tumor cells in the periphery of the tumor. These seminiferous tubules show larger diameter and the presence of lumen in contrast to the development of the farthest seminiferous tubules

Immunohistochemical Data

- Synaptophysin expression in 88 % of TTAGS against 8 % LCT [26].
- CD56 is strongly and diffusely positive in TTAGS and only weak or moderate in LCT [30].
- Androgen receptor immunoexpression is negative in TTAGS (Fig. 7.7) and positive in 85 % of LCT.
- TTAGS have angiotensin II and ACTH receptors.
- Positivity for inhibin, Melan A, vimentin, and calretinin is considered nonspecific as they are also expressed in LCT [31].
- The most useful marker in this differential is the absence of expression in TTAGS of a Leydig cell marker such as insulin-like 3 (INSL3) [32].

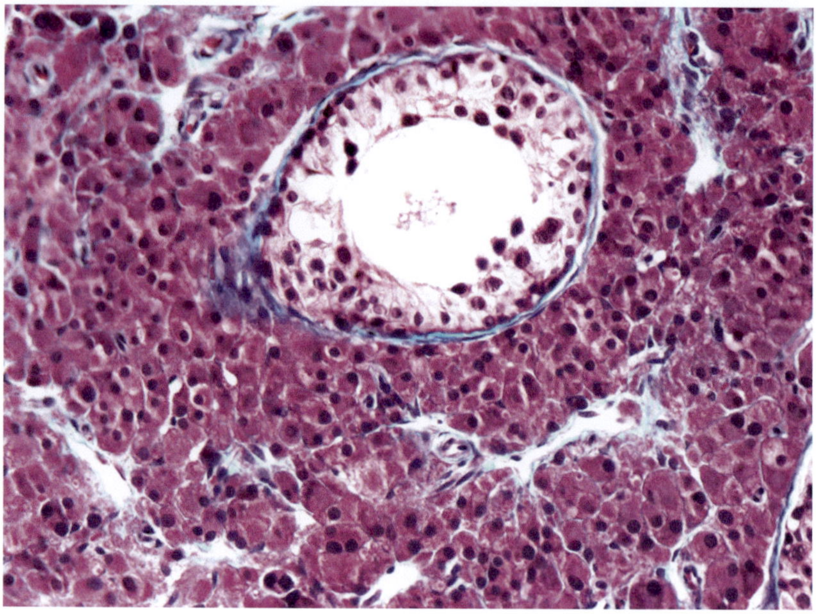

Fig. 7.6 Seminiferous tubule with marked dilatation of its lumen and the presence of spermatogenesis. It is surrounded by Leydig tumor cells of the same case of the previous figure

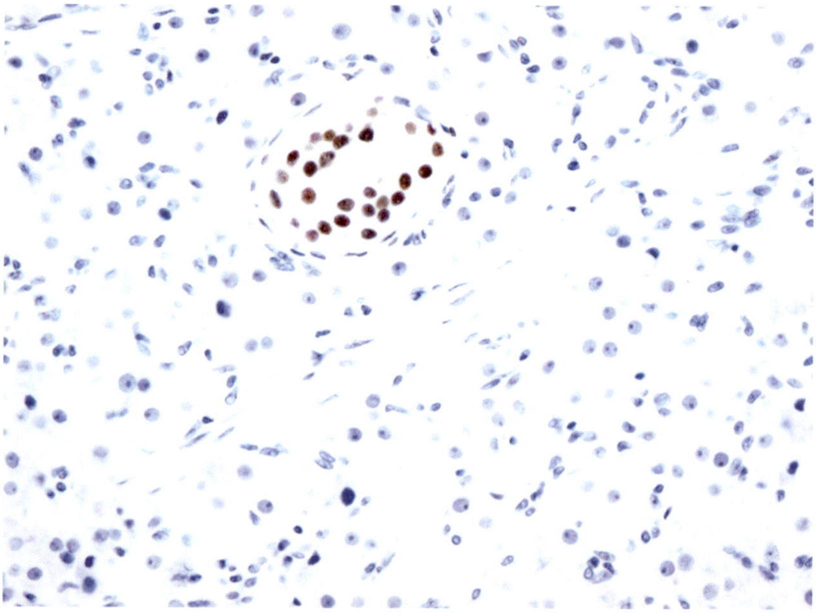

Fig. 7.7 Tumor of the adrenogenital syndrome. Cellular proliferation has engulfed a seminiferous tubule. Note positivity for androgen receptor in the nucleus of the Sertoli cells which contrasts with its negativity in tumor cells

Summarizing, diagnosis of TTAGS may require the sum of clinical, laboratory, imaging, and histological and immunohistochemical studies, particularly in their less severe forms of presentation in adults and in patients claiming infertility. The establishment of an adequate treatment not only corrects the hormonal failure but in some cases can restore fertility. In other cases the selective localization of tumor nodules leads to irreversible testicular atrophy through the obstructive mechanism.

References

1. Forest MG. Recent advances in the diagnosis and management of congenital adrenal hyperplasia due to 21-hydroxylase deficiency. Hum Reprod Update. 2004;10:469–85.
2. Bercovici JP, Fiet J, Gibault L, Volant A, Abalain JH, Floch HH, Sonnet E, Fournier G. Testicular adrenal rest tumours in salt wasting congenital adrenal hyperplasia (in vivo and in vitro studies). J Steroid Biochem Mol Biol. 2005;93:67–72.

3. Ulbright TM, Young RH. Tumors of the testis and adjacent structures, AFIP atlas of tumor pathology series 4, fascicle, 18th ed. Silver Spring, Maryland: American Registry of Pathology; 2013.
4. Val P, Jeays-Ward K, Swain A. Identification of a novel population of adrenal-like cells in the mammalian testis. Dev Biol. 2006;299:250–6.
5. Paner GP, Kristiansen G, McKenney JK, Amin MB. Rete testis-associated nodular steroid cell nests: description of putative pluripotential testicular hilus steroid cells. Am J Surg Pathol. 2011;35:505–11.
6. Murphy H, George C, De Kretser D, Judd S. Successful treatment with ICSI of infertility caused by azoospermia associated with adrenal rest in the testes: case report. Hum Reprod. 2001;16:263–7.
7. Stikkelbroeck NM, Otten BJ, Pasic A, Jager GJ, Sweep CG, Noordam K, Hermus AR. High prevalence of testicular adrenal rest tumors, impaired spermatogenesis, and Leydig cell failure in adolescent and adult males with congenital adrenal hyperplasia. J Clin Endocrinol Metab. 2001;86:5721–8.
8. Hicks MJ, Cipriani N, Pytel P, Shimada H. The pineal, pituitary, parathyroid, thyroid and adrenal glands. In: Husain AN, Stocker JT, Dehmer LP, editors. 4rd ed. Stocker and Dehner's pediatric pathology. Wolters Kluger: Philadelphia; 2016.
9. Lack E, Paal E. Neoplasm of the testis. In: Bostwick DG, Cheng L, editors. Urologic surgical pathology. 3rd ed. Philadelphia: Elsevier Health Sciences; 2014.
10. Sabine N, Malone M, Ashworth M, et al. Diagnostic pediatric surgical pathology. Edinburgh: Elsevier; 2010.
11. Al-Ahmadie H. "Testicular tumors," in pediatric pathology. Alphen aan den Rijn: Wolters Kluwer; 2011.
12. Ulbright TM, Young RH. Testicular and paratesticular tumors and tumor-like lesions in the first 2 decades. Semin Diagn Pathol. 2014;31:323–81.
13. Wilkins L, Fleischmann W, Howard JE. Macrogenitosomiaprecox associated with hyperplasia of the androgenic tissue of the adrenal and death from cortico adrenal insufficiency. Case report. Endocrinology. 1940;26:385–3.
14. Stikkelbroeck NM, Suliman HM, Otten BJ, Hermus AR, Blickman JG, Jager GJ. Testicular adrenal rest tumours in postpubertal males with congenital adrenal hyperplasia: sonographic and MR features. Eur Radiol. 2003;13:1597–603.
15. Rutgers JL, Young RH, Scully RE. The testicular "tumor" of the adrenogenital syndrome. A report of six cases and review of the literature on testicular masses in patients with adrenocortical disorders. Am J Surg Pathol. 1988;12:503–13.
16. Claahsen-van der Grinten HL, Otten BJ, Hermus AR, Sweep FC, Hulsbergen-van de Kaa CA. Testicular adrenal rest tumors in patients with congenital adrenal hyperplasia can cause severe testicular damage. Fertil Steril. 2008;89:597–601.
17. Claahsen-van der Grinten HL, Sweep FC, Blickman JG, Hermus AR, Otten BJ. Prevalence of testicular adrenal rest tumours in male children with congenital adrenal hyperplasia due to 21-hydroxylase deficiency. Eur J Endocrinol. 2007;157:339–44.
18. Al-Agha OM, Axiotis CA. An in-depth look at Leydig cell tumor of the testis. Arch Pathol Lab Med. 2007; 131:311–7.
19. Souverijns G, Peene P, Keuleers H, Vanbockrijck M. Ectopic localization of adrenal cortex. Eur Radiol. 2000;10:1165–8.
20. Charfi N, Kamoun M, Feki Mnif M, Mseddi N, Mnif F, Kallel N, Ben Naceur B, Rekik N, Fourati H, Daoud E, Mnif Z, Hadj Sliman M, Sellami-Boudawara T, Abid M. Leydig cell tumor associated with testicular adrenal rest tumors in a patient with congenital adrenal hyperplasia due to 11β-hydroxylase deficiency. Case Rep Urol. 2012;2012:648643.
21. Rich MA, Keating MA. Leydig cell tumors and tumors associated with congenital adrenal hyperplasia. Urol Clin North Am. 2000;27:519–28.
22. Teixeira SR, Elias PC, Andrade MT, Melo AF, Elias Junior J. The role of imaging in congenital adrenal hyperplasia. Arq Bras Endocrinol Metabol. 2014;58:701–8.
23. Avila NA, Premkumar A, Shawker TH, Jones JV, Laue L, Cutler Jr GB. Testicular adrenal rest tissue in congenital adrenal hyperplasia: findings at Gray-scale and color Doppler US. Radiology. 1996;198:99–104.
24. Fitoz S, Atasoy C, Adiyaman P, Berberoglu M, Erden I, Ocal G. Testicular adrenal rests in a patient with congenital adrenal hyperplasia: US and MRI features. Comput Med Imaging Graph. 2006;30:465–8.
25. Young RH. Testicular tumors–some new and a few perennial problems. Arch Pathol Lab Med. 2008;132:548–64.
26. Ashley RA, McGee SM, Isotaolo PA, Kramer SA, Cheville JC. Clinical and pathological features associated with the testicular tumor of the adrenogenital syndrome. J Urol. 2007;177:546–9.
27. Santonja C, Varona C, Burgos FJ, Nistal M. Leydig cell tumor of testis with adipose metaplasia. Appl Pathol. 1989;7:201–4.
28. Ulbright TM, Srigley JR, Hatzianastassiou DK, Young RH. Leydig cell tumors of the testis with unusual features: adipose differentiation, calcification with ossification, and spindle-shaped tumor cells. Am J Surg Pathol. 2002;26:1424–33.
29. Leschek EW, Chan WY, Diamond DA, Kaefer M, Jones J, Barnes KM, Cutler Jr GB. Nodular Leydig cell hyperplasia in a boy with familial male-limited precocious puberty. J Pediatr. 2001;138:949–51.
30. Wang Z, Yang S, Shi H, Du H, Xue L, Wang L, Dong Y, Han A. Histopathological and immunophenotypic features of testicular tumour of the adrenogenital syndrome. Histopathology. 2011;58:1013–8.
31. Vukina J, Chism DD, Sharpless JL, Raynor MC, Milowsky MI, Funkhouser WK. Metachronous bilateral testicular leydig-like tumors leading to the diagnosis of congenital adrenal hyperplasia (adrenogenital syndrome). Case Rep Pathol. 2015;2015:459318.
32. Lottrup G, Nielsen JE, Skakkebæk NE, Juul A, Rajpert-De Meyts E. Abundance of DLK1, differential expression of CYP11B1, CYP21A2 and MC2R, and lack of INSL3 distinguish testicular adrenal rest tumours from Leydig cell tumours. Eur J Endocrinol. 2015;172:491–9.

8 Fetal Gonadoblastoid Testicular Dysplasia: An Early Defect in Testicular Tubulogenesis

Manuel Nistal, Pilar González-Peramato, and Álvaro Serrano

8.1 Introduction

Fetal gonadoblastoid testicular dysplasia was described by Martin in 1986 and also by Spear [1] in a 28-week old newborn baby of that weighed 950 g and died 1 h after delivery due to multiple malformations. FGTD appears early and is related to the Walker-Warburg's syndrome (WWS), as in the case reported by Weinberg in 1989 [2] and in the same year in the three cases provided by Hung et al. [3]. In two cases published by Nistal et al. in 2007 [4], it was not associated with WWS, although one patient had muscle lesions suggesting a mitochondrial myopathy, and in two more cases published by Reischer et al. in 2016 [5], it was associated with a lethal type of Noonan's syndrome.

8.2 Histology

Except for their small size, the testes do not show macroscopic abnormalities, neither are these observed in the epididymis. All testicles show a well-collagenized tunica albuginea, lobular organization, and seminiferous tubules that, although few in number, have a development consistent with age. The number of Leydig cells is the expected one for the age. The data characterizing the FGTD is the presence of solid, spherical, or ovoid formations up to 300 microns in diameter (Fig. 8.1). When these formations are abundant, they are arranged throughout the testicle, but when they are scarcer, they are located preferably in the periphery of the testicle.

Each nodular formation is externally well delimited by a basal membrane and separated from the testicular parenchyma by several layers of fusiform cells (Fig. 8.2). It contains three types of cells. The first cell type corresponds to cells with vesicular nucleus and pale cytoplasm, the second type includes cells with elongated, hyperchromatic nucleus, and scant cytoplasm, and the third one includes germ cell-like cells (Fig. 8.3). Among the cells there are one or more PAS-positive eosinophilic bodies reminiscent of Call-Exner bodies of the ovary. In the periphery, small arterioles which are situated between the spindle cells and the basement membrane are observed. Sometimes these arterioles penetrate into the nodules, and the serial sections show that they are inside only until they are recognized as a mass of nuclei, three to five, inside or in the vicinity of eosinophilic bodies. Some nodular formations are in continuity with seminiferous tubules.

Immunohistochemistry shows positivity for vimentin, cytokeratin (AE1/AE3), and inhibin (Fig. 8.4) that are focal in the first two cell types that form the nodular formations and PLAP positivity in isolated germ cells. No germ-like cell was positive for OCT3/4. Positivity for specific muscle actin in perinodular fusiform cells was observed. Collagen IV stained linearly in the basement membrane and on the wall forming

M. Nistal et al., *Clues in the Diagnosis of Non-tumoral Testicular Pathology*,
DOI 10.1007/978-3-319-49364-0_8

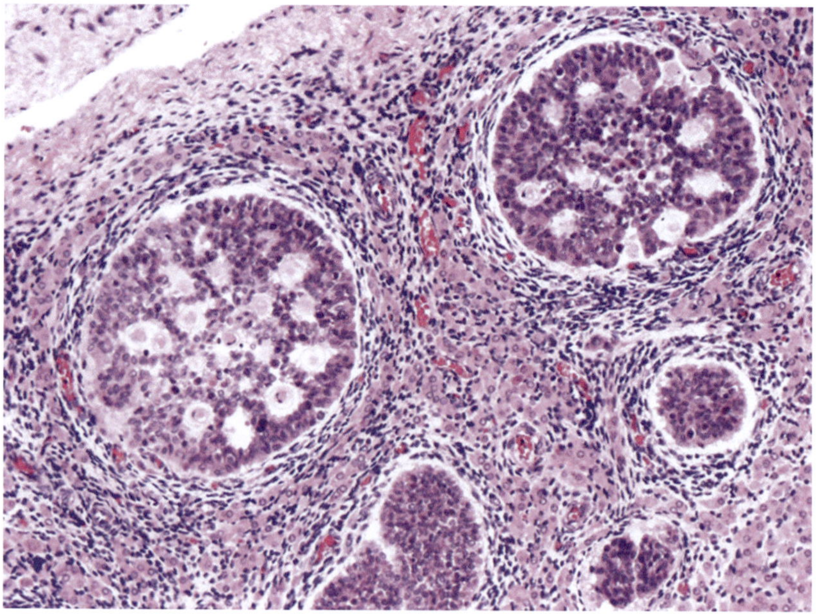

Fig. 8.1 Fetal gonadoblastoid testicular dysplasia. Two spherical formations surrounded and separated from normal seminiferous tubules by abundant cellular stroma

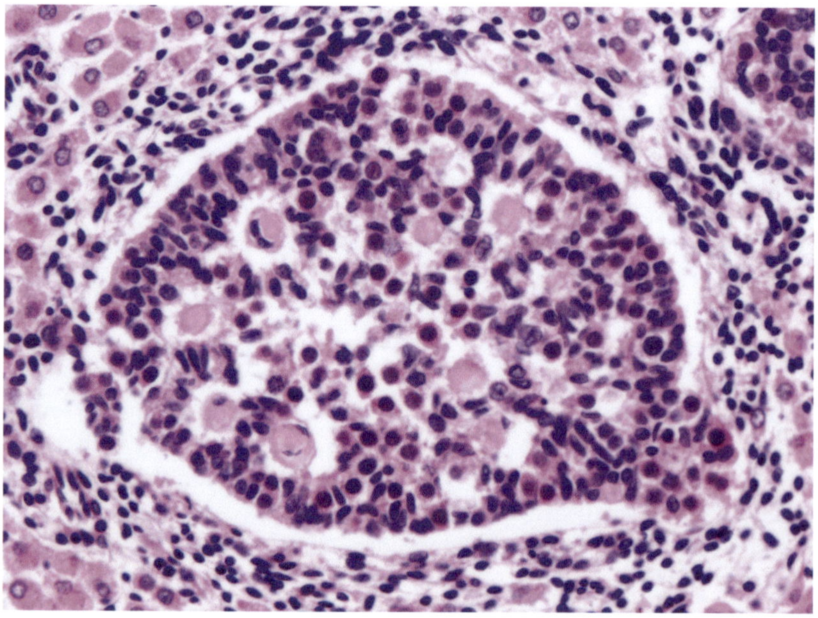

Fig. 8.2 Fetal gonadoblastoid testicular dysplasia. Nodular formation surrounded by fusiform cells and more externally by Leydig cells. Inside the nodular formation, there are abundant eosinophilic bodies

subendothelial accumulations of arterioles penetrating the nodules and constituting the eosinophilic Call-Exner-like bodies (Figs. 8.5 and 8.6). Laminin is observed in the basal lamina of seminiferous tubules and nodules (Fig. 8.7). In the rest of the testicular parenchyma, inhibin expression in Sertoli cells and Leydig was normal.

8.3 Differential Diagnosis

There are two processes that may constitute a differential diagnosis with this lesion, and both only occur in patients with testicular development disorders such as testicular dysgenesis and gonadoblastoma.

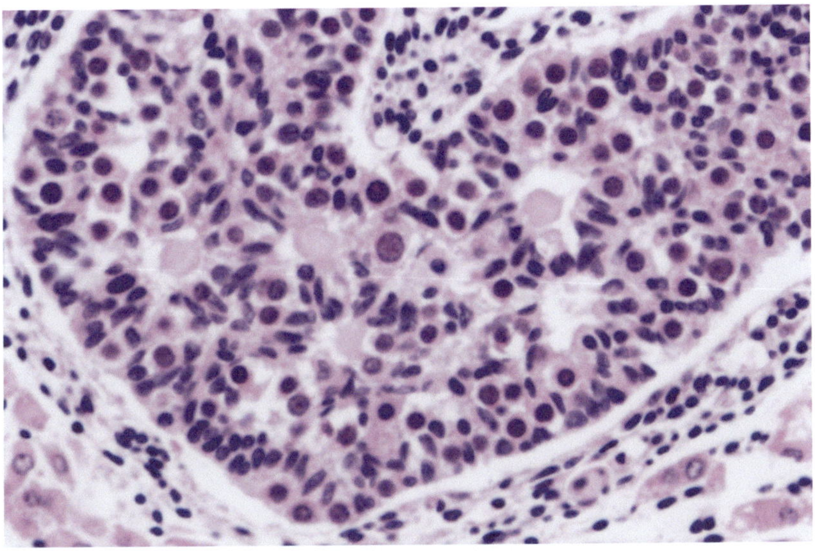

Fig. 8.3 Nodular formation composed of different cell types. Small cells (the most numerous) have elongated and hyperchromatic nuclei, while large cells have spherical nuclei and pale cytoplasm

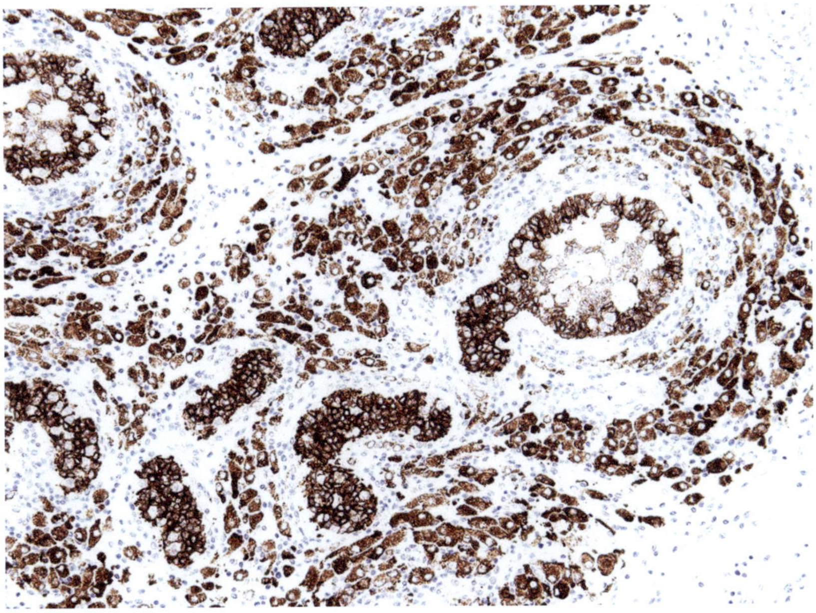

Fig. 8.4 Most cells in nodular formations show immunostaining for inhibin. Intense positive expression is also observed in Sertoli cells of neighboring tubules and in abundant Leydig cells

In *testicular dysgenesis* a testis with a central part consisting of seminiferous tubules arranged compactly and a peripheral zone of seminiferous tubules irregular in shape and size with frequent anastomoses is observed. In the more peripheral areas, these tubules are attached to an ovarian-like stroma and reach the surface of the gonad. Coinciding with these areas, the tunica albuginea does not show the structure and constitution of a normal testicle. The appearance and the swirling arrangement of the cells simulate an ovarian stroma. Despite the differences in the size of the tubules, they never form solid nodules. Testicular dysgenesis is the characteristic gonad of DSD by default AMH. No cases of FGTD associated with DSD have been reported.

At first sight FGTD has a strong resemblance to *gonadoblastoma*. This likeness is even higher if it originates on a dysgenetic testis since malformed seminiferous tubules can be seen beside gonado-blastoma nodules. Two facts are important for differential diagnosis. Germ cells in gonadoblastoma

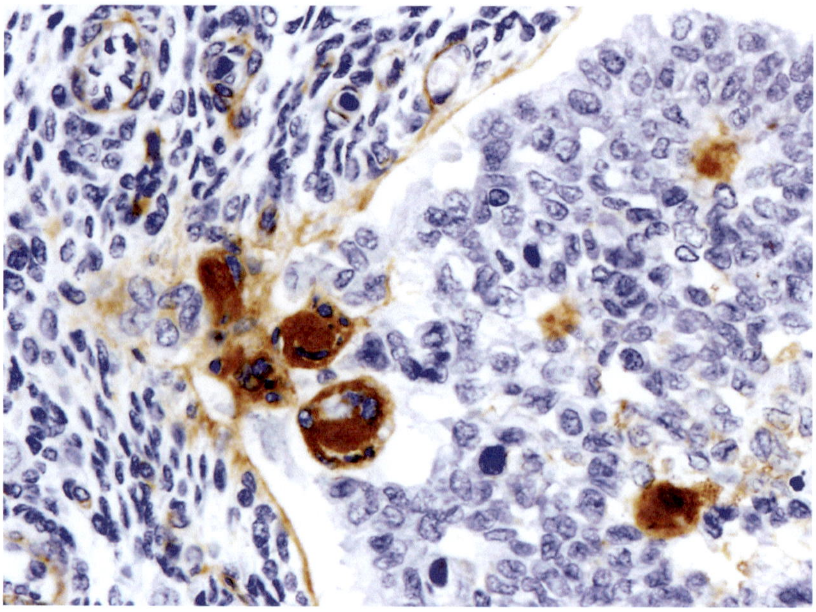

Fig. 8.5 Fetal gonadoblastoid testicular displasia. Collagen IV deposit in an arteriole which has penetrated the nodular formation

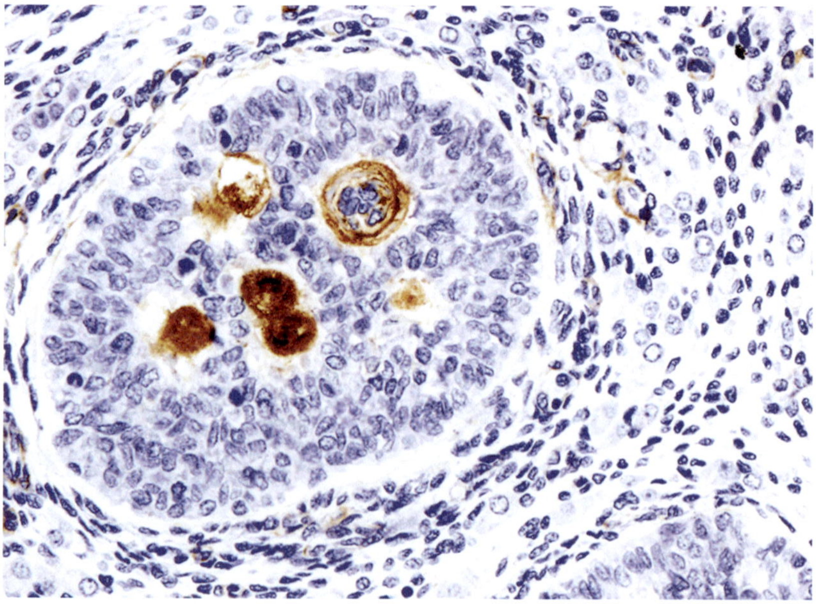

Fig. 8.6 Fetal gonadoblastoid testicular displasia. Collagen IV deposit inside a nodule. Positive expression is observed around a group of nuclei and eosinophilc bodies

are OCT3/4 positive, and internodal stroma characteristics are similar to those of the ovarian stroma. All patients with gonadoblastoma have a DSD.

8.4 Etiopathogenesis

Even though its intimate mechanisms are not known, several non-exclusive hypotheses are suggested by the symptoms and by histology – vascular hypothesis, an alteration in the basal lamina of testicular cords, and *PTPN11* gene mutations.

Vascular Hypothesis The first morphological indicator of testicular differentiation is the formation of the seminiferous cords. Precursors of Sertoli cells derive from the coelomic epithelium. The coelomic epithelium thickens as it differentiates. Primordial germ cells have already reached the cords before Sertoli cells differentiate,

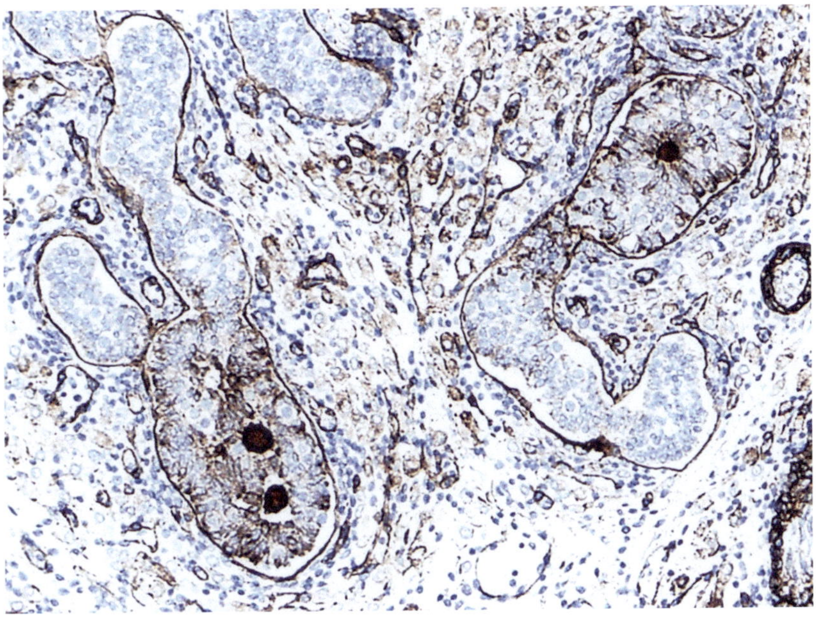

Fig. 8.7 Fetal gonadoblastoid testicular dysplasia. Deposit of laminin in eosinophilic bodies. Note the continuity between the basal lamina of the seminiferous tubules and that of nodules

although germ cells are not needed to form the testicular cords. The first step is the formation of clusters of pre-Sertoli and germ cells, after transformation of the clusters into primitive testis cord network (proto-cords), and finally transformation into definitive testis cord occurs.

The interaction between Sertoli cells and peritubular myoid cells leads to the polarization of the pre-Sertoli cells and the production of several extracellular matrix proteins and cells in which the two cell types are involved [6, 7]. The primitive testis cords have a toroid (cylindric ring) configuration that resembles a stack of donuts [8]. The looped cords are aligned in parallel along the major axis, perpendicular to the gonad. When the formation of the primitive cord starts, they vary in shape and size, and there are pictures of transition between the clusters and the final cords [9]. The testicular cords of the central area of the testicle, although irregular in shape and size, are more advanced in their development than the polar cords. Fusions and blind-ended branch cords can be seen at all levels [10]. Most cordonal structures originate and terminate in the mesonephric edge. In the dorsomedial area of the gonad, the cords converge and connect with each other forming a plexus that will be the future rete testis that will connect with the mesonephric tubules. This plexus has perforations through which vessels penetrate the mesonephros. Among the different factors involved in tubulogenesis, there is one that is essential: vascularization of the gonad [11].

The primitive gonad has a vascular system consisting of microvessels from the mesonephric vessels extending radially inside. In XY gonads the mesonephric plexus dissolves, and the migration of individual endothelial cells from the antimesonephric region or to the coelomic domain begins. In the course of this migration, it secretes over a dozen areas and induces the arrangement of the Sertoli cells in the primitive cords. This migration is likely induced by factors secreted by the Sertoli cells [12, 13], and it is *SRY* dependent [14].

In the XY gonad, when the endothelial cells reach the coelomic domain, the coelomic vessel originates beneath the coelomic epithelium. The primordial blood vessel system of the testis is formed from the coelomic vessel. Coelomic vessel branches penetrate between the testicular cords and participate in tubulogenesis. Tubulogenesis occurs through a process of partitioning and remodeling cord branches to transform into independent loops [15].

Alteration in the migration of endothelial cells from the mesonephros disrupts cord formation

[16]. The arterial blood supply is not only important to supply blood to the gonad, but it also intervenes in the testicular morphogenesis, especially in testis cord partitioning. Several mutant mouse models relate vascular anomalies and defects in the formation of the cords [17–19]. The presence of vessels penetrating into the nodules forming FGTD could be the image of the failure of endothelial cells to induce tubulogenesis and development in number and length of the seminiferous tubules.

Alteration in the Basal Lamina of the Testicular Cords Half of FGTD cases have been observed in patients with WWS. WWS is a rare autosomal recessive form of congenital muscular dystrophy associated with brain and eye malformations [20]. It is the most severe form of the dystroglycanopathies [21]. In patients with WWS, there is an abnormal glycosylation of dystroglycan. Dystroglycan (DS) is a key protein for maintaining the muscle cell architecture by bridging the basal lamina with the cytoskeleton. DG is the central component of the dystrophin-glycoprotein complex; it contributes to the structure of the basement membrane and stabilizes it through its function as a receptor for proteins of the extracellular matrix such as laminin, agrin, and perlecan in a variety of tissues. It is well known that Sertoli cells interact with peritubular myoid cells to produce a polarized secretion of various extracellular matrix proteins such as laminin, type IV collagen and IXa3 collagen, and heparan sulfate. These molecules are required for the formation of the basal lamina surrounding the seminiferous tubules and to maintain their structural integrity [22]. A failure in the formation of the basement membrane would make the transformation of pre-Sertoli and germ cells clusters into the primitive testicular cords impossible. Proliferation of pre-Sertoli and germ cells clusters would lead to FGTD nodules.

Mutations in the *PTPN11* Gene The fact that two of the patients with FGTD had mutations in this gene and were carriers of the Noonan's syndrome adds an interesting fact. It is well known that the testes of patients with the Noonan's syndrome are carriers of primary lesions that often cause infertility. The high prevalence of cryptorchidism in these patients, up to 80 %, could be the explanation, but infertility is observed also in patients with descended testicles [23]. Hormonal and histological data suggest a defect in the number and function of Sertoli and Leydig cells [24]. Most *PTPN11* functions on the testicle have been studied in adults, highlighting its role on cell adhesion, which is necessary for the formation of the blood-testis barrier and regulation of the population of germ cells [25]. It is more than likely that mutations in this gene are also responsible for cases of FGTD.

References

1. Spear GS, Martin CG. Fetal gonadoblastoid testicular dysplasia. Hum Pathol. 1986;17:531–3.
2. Weinberg AG. Walker-Warburg syndrome. Pediatr Pathol. 1989;9:749–55.
3. Hung NA, Silver MM, Chitayat D, Provias J, Toi A, Jay V, Becker LE. Gonadoblastoid testicular dysplasia in Walker-Warburg syndrome. Pediatr Dev Pathol. 1998;1:393–404.
4. Nistal M, Rodríguez JI, García-Fernández E, Cajaiba MM, Reyes-Múgica M. Fetal gonadoblastoid testicular dysplasia: a focal failure of testicular development. Pediatr Dev Pathol. 2007;10:274–81.
5. Reischer T, Schmid M, Vodopiutz J, Krampl-Bettelheim E, Popitsch N, Streubel B. A case of Noonan syndrome with gonadoblastoid testicular dysplasia. 14th World Congress in Fetal Medicine. 2015 21-25th June. Crete. Greece.
6. Pelliniemi LJ, Paranko J, Grund SK, Fröjdman K, Foidart JM, Lakkala-Paranko T. Extracellular matrix in testicular differentiation. Ann N Y Acad Sci. 1984;438:405–16.
7. Fröjdman K, Paranko J, Virtanen I, Pelliniemi LJ. Intermediate filaments and epithelial differentiation of male rat embryonic gonad. Differentiation. 1992;50:113–23.
8. Svingen T, Koopman P. Building the mammalian testis: origins, differentiation, and assembly of the component cell populations. Genes Dev. 2013;27:2409–26.
9. Harikae K, Miura K, Kanai Y. Early gonadogenesis in mammals: significance of long and narrow gonadal structure. Dev Dyn. 2013;242:330–8.
10. Nel-Themaat L, Gonzalez G, Akiyama H, Behringer RR. Illuminating testis morphogenesis in the mouse. J Androl. 2010;31:5–10.

11. Sargent KM, McFee RM, Spuri Gomes R, Cupp AS. Vascular endothelial growth factor A: just one of multiple mechanisms for sex-specific vascular development within the testis? J Endocrinol. 2015;227:R31–50.
12. Merchant-Larios H, Moreno-Mendoza N, Buehr M. The role of the mesonephros in cell differentiation and morphogenesis of the mouse fetal testis. Int J Dev Biol. 1993;37:407–15.
13. Tilmann C, Capel B. Mesonephric cell migration induces testis cord formation and Sertoli cell differentiation in the mammalian gonad. Development. 1999;126:2883–90.
14. Brennan J, Karl J, Capel B. Divergent vascular mechanisms downstream of Sry establish the arterial system in the XY gonad. Dev Biol. 2002;244:418–28.
15. Combes AN, Lesieur E, Harley VR, Sinclair AH, Little MH, Wilhelm D, Koopman P. Three-dimensional visualization of testis cord morphogenesis, a novel tubulogenic mechanism in development. Dev Dyn. 2009;238:1033–41.
16. Coveney D, Cool J, Oliver T, Capel B. Four-dimensional analysis of vascularization during primary development of an organ, the gonad. Proc Natl Acad Sci U S A. 2008;105:7212–7.
17. Brennan J, Tilmann C, Capel B. Pdgfr-a mediates testis cord organization and fetal Leydig cell development in the XY gonad. Genes Dev. 2003;17:800–10.
18. Bott RC, McFee RM, Clopton DT, Toombs C, Cupp AS. Vascular endothelial growth factor and kinase domain region receptor are involved in both seminiferous cord formation and vascular development during testis morphogenesis in the rat. Biol Reprod. 2006;75:56–67.
19. Yao HH, Aardema J, Holthusen K. Sexually dimorphic regulation of inhibin beta B in establishing gonadal vasculature in mice. Biol Reprod. 2006;74:978–83.
20. Whitley CB, Thompson TR, Mastri AR, Gorlin RJ. Warburg syndrome: lethal neurodysplasia with autosomal recessive inheritance. J Pediatr. 1983;102:547–51.
21. Trkova M, Krutilkova V, Smetanova D, Becvarova V, Hlavova E, Jencikova N, Hodacova J, Hnykova L, Hroncova H, Horacek J, Stejskal D. ISPD gene homozygous deletion identified by SNP array confirms prenatal manifestation of Walker-Warburg syndrome. Eur J Med Genet. 2015;58:372–5.
22. Jeanes A, Wilhelm D, Wilson MJ, Bowles J, McClive PJ, Sinclair AH, Koopman P. Evaluation of candidate markers for the peritubular myoid cell lineage in the developing mouse testis. Reproduction. 2005;130:509–16.
23. Nistal M, Paniagua R, Pallardo LF. Testicular biopsy and hormonal study in a male with Noonan's syndrome. Andrologia. 1983;15:415–25.
24. Ankarberg-Lindgren C, Westphal O, Dahlgren J. Testicular size development and reproductive hormones in boys and adult males with Noonan syndrome: a longitudinal study. Eur J Endocrinol. 2011;165:137–44.
25. Puri P, Walker WH. The regulation of male fertility by the PTPN11 tyrosine phosphatase. Semin Cell Dev Biol. 2016;59:27–34.

9 Differential Diagnosis of Sertoli Cell Nodules

Manuel Nistal, Pilar González-Peramato, and
Álvaro Serrano

9.1 Introduction

Sertoli cell nodules consist of a conglomerate of seminiferous tubules with fetal or infantile development, well delimited from the rest of the parenchyma [1]. They are usually multiple lesions, ranging in size from microscopic to 3 mm [2]. They are observed in more than 50 % of undescended testes in adults, in the peripheral parenchyma of germ cell tumors, and in infertile patients. They are rare in normal testes although isolated tubules with similar characteristics can be observed (hypoplastic tubules or dysgenetic tubules). A Sertoli cell nodule in the epididymis has been reported [3]. Sertoli cell nodules are considered one of the most common histological findings in the testicular dysgenesis syndrome (see Chap. 13).

9.2 Histology

The most common image is that of a group of tubules without lumen, small size (usually microscopic), irregularly shaped, and arranged back to back with one another [4]. The tubules are surrounded by a basement membrane showing variable thicknesses from one tube to another [5]. The basement membrane gives out fingerlike projections. Sertoli cells have small, spherical, hyperchromatic nuclei of antipodal distribution, on the periphery of the tubules and surrounding projections of the basement membrane. The arrangement of Sertoli cells around the central mass, derived from the basal membrane, gives the tubules a ringed aspect. The cells may show mitosis. The tubular wall has no elastic fibers. The intertubular stroma is scarce and often lacks Leydig cells (Fig. 9.1).

Immunohistochemical studies noted immature Sertoli cells, which express in addition to diffuse inhibin, inhibin bodies, D2-40, AMH, cytokeratin 18, connexin 43, and partial or total absence of androgen receptors. Some are PCNA + and Ki-67 + [6]. The material of the basement membrane and nodular formations are strongly PAS-positive laminin and collagen IV [7].

9.3 Variability of Sertoli Cell Nodules

There are a number of variations that affect the size, the boundaries, the Sertoli cell differentiation, the presence of germ cells, the presence of Leydig cells between the tubular formations, the degree of tubular hyalinization, and the presence of calcification.

The size of the nodules, usually microscopic, can reach 10 mm. At least 10 cases have been reported of these "macroscopic" Sertoli cell nodules. They are nodules that may be palpable and are sonographically revealed as a testicular tumor [8, 9] (Fig. 9.2).

M. Nistal et al., *Clues in the Diagnosis of Non-tumoral Testicular Pathology*,
DOI 10.1007/978-3-319-49364-0_9

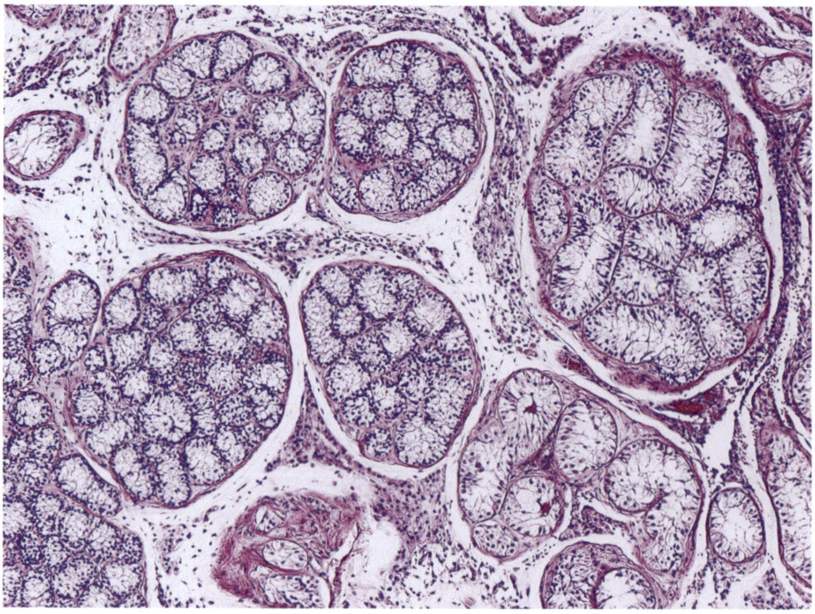

Fig. 9.1 Multiple spherical formations with cribriform pattern by the presence of tubular formations resembling fetal seminiferous tubules. Among the tubular formations, a loose stroma with Leydig cells can be observed

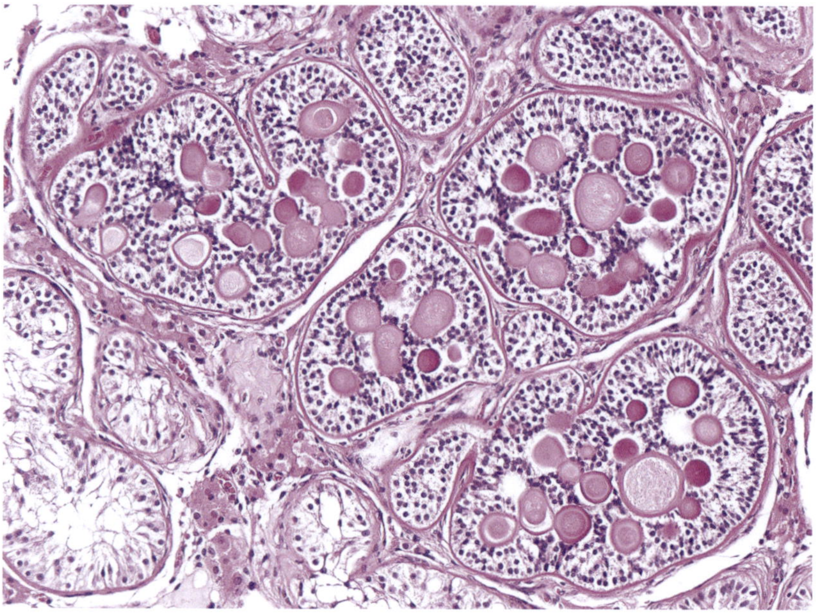

Fig. 9.2 Giant Sertoli cell nodule. Tubular formations of different shapes and sizes with multiple irregularly anastomosing PAS-positive bodies. The nodule is well delimited from the surrounding testicular parenchyma

The delimitation of the nodules with the parenchyma is generally good (Fig. 9.2), and even some Sertoli cell nodules are partially or fully encapsulated. In other cases peripheral hypoplastic tubes are less cohesive and mixed with seminiferous tubules of the neighboring testicular parenchyma.

In some nodules Sertoli cells do not always show a fetal or infantile appearance, but they have some differentiation. These cells are larger, with elongated and vesicular nuclei and a central nucleolus. The cytoplasm can display one or more large vacuoles that displace the nuclei (Fig. 9.3). The tubules in these cases are larger with smaller deposits of basement membrane. Sertoli cells resemble the dysgenetic variety and are seen in adult undescended testes and in some infertile patients with dysgenetic Sertoli cell-only

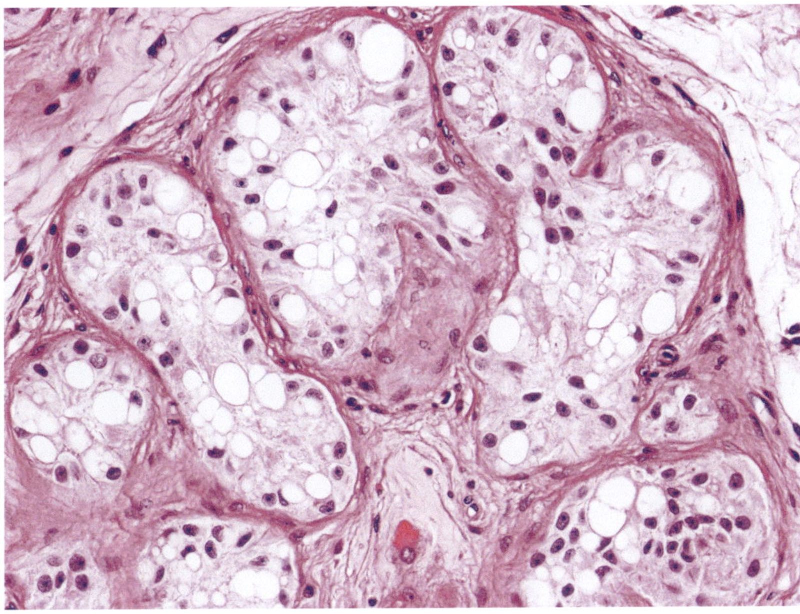

Fig. 9.3 Sertoli cell nodule composed of cells that show some degree of pubertal maturation. The nuclei show a central nucleolus, and the cytoplasms are large and vacuolated

syndrome. Even in these tubules, the Sertoli cells do not reach full maturation.

The degree of thickening of the basement membrane not only varies within the same lesion but between the different lesions that could be present in the same testicle. The hyalinization tends to increase with age and may become so important that the tubular formations are reduced to thick, coarse rings or anastomosing cords made only of basement membrane material.

The tubular formations of Sertoli cell nodules usually lack germ cells, but in some cases, the presence of spermatogonia and even some first-order spermatocytes can be observed. When the testicle carries a germ cell tumor, the nodules may contain a germ cell neoplasia in situ.

Sertoli cell nodules are the result of the inability of differentiation of the cells that constitute them. Sertoli cells and myoid peritubular cells do not respond, or do so improperly, to hormonal stimuli to which they are subject, in contrast with the development of the rest of the parenchyma. The low expression of inhibin, the absence of androgen receptors, and the presence of inhibin bodies are immunohistochemical markers that support the immaturity of Sertoli cells. The absence of elastic fibers in adult testes suggests immaturity of the peritubular myoid cells [10]. Based on these facts, Sertoli cell nodules can be considered a primary testicular anomaly, and as such, this lesion is included among the lesions observed in the testicular dysgenesis syndrome [11].

An unresolved issue is the correct identification of Sertoli cell nodules in childhood. The importance of correct identification is great because if we consider that these lesions are dysgenetic, they must somehow be present in the prepubertal testicles. And their observation would provide more information when assessing the fertility potential in a biopsy in childhood. In retrospective, a study trying to identify the presence of hypoplastic areas has observed a lesion that could be the precursor. It is a focal lesion that consists of seminiferous tubules with numerous anastomoses that can show granular changes in Sertoli cells and lack of androgen receptors in the testes of patients older than 5 years.

9.4 Differential Diagnosis

The variety of histological patterns of the Sertoli cell nodules may pose a differential diagnosis with the following entities: intratubular large cell hyalinizing Sertoli cell neoplasia, gonadoblastoma, sex cord tumor with annular tubules, and Sertoli cell tumor "not otherwise specified"

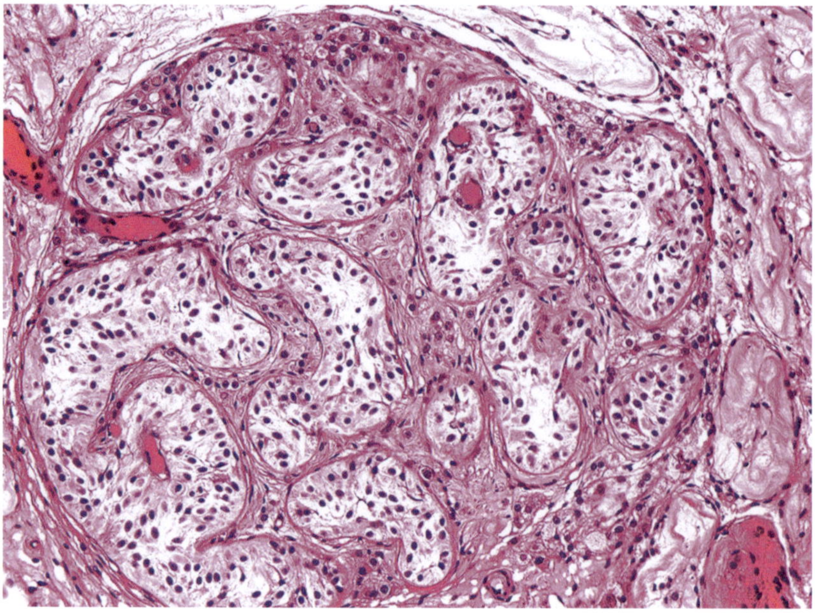

Fig. 9.4 Sertoli cell nodule surrounded by atrophic seminiferous tubules. Among the tubular sections, there are numerous Leydig cells simulating a well-differentiated Sertoli/Leydig cell tumor

(Fig. 9.4). The differential diagnosis can also arise with fetal gonadoblastoid testicular dysplasia (see Chap. 8), Sertoli-Leydig hamartoma, and Sertoli cell adenoma in patients with androgen insensitivity (see Chap. 6).

9.4.1 Sertoli Cell Nodules Versus Intratubular Large Cell Hyalinizing Sertoli Cell Neoplasia

Sertoli cell nodules share with this neoplasm the multifocality; the small size, none of them usually causing testicular enlargement; the maintenance of a tubular structure; the thickening of the basement membrane; the intratubular protrusions; and the presence of calcifications (Fig. 9.5). The most important differences are in intratubular large cell hyalinizing Sertoli cell neoplasia, the tubules are more individualized, they rarely anastomose, and they may be in continuity with normal tubes. The diameter is larger. Sertoli cells are larger. The nuclei are spherical, they are not polarized, they are euchromatic, and they have a central nucleolus [12, 13]. They do not contain germ cells (Fig. 9.6).

In childhood, seminiferous tubules of the peritumoral testicular parenchyma in this neoplasia have a more advanced maturation not only with the presence of a greater number of spermatogonia but even spermatids [14]. Immunohistochemically cells of the intratubular hyalinizing large Sertoli cells neoplasia express the following markers: calretinin, cytokeratin AE1/AE3, Melan A, and synaptophysin. Many of these neoplasias are diagnosed in childhood, at an age in which Sertoli cell nodules are not well developed, in undescended testes and in patients with Peutz-Jeghers syndrome or Carney complex [14, 15].

9.4.2 Sertoli Cell Nodules with GCNIS Versus Gonadoblastoma

When Sertoli cell nodules contain germ cells, they adopt a strong resemblance to nodular formations of gonadoblastoma (Figs. 9.7 and 9.8). The differential diagnosis is important among other data because 40 % of gonadoblastomas are bilateral cases that can progress to an infiltrating tumor. Macroscopically, cell nests of gonadoblastomas are larger without an inner tubular architecture.

Hyalinization of the tubular wall, inward basement membrane protrusions, and double

Fig. 9.5 Sertoli cell nodule. Numerous fingerlike projections of the basement membrane material into the seminiferous tubules stained with PAS

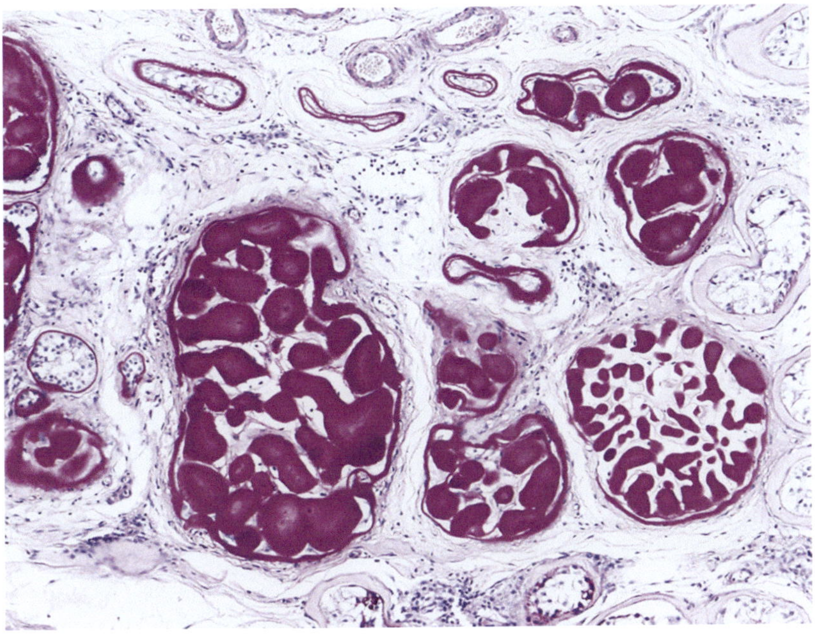

Fig. 9.6 Intratubular large cell hyalinizing Sertoli cell neoplasia. The tubules have both focal and diffuse thickening of the basement membrane and projections inside of the same material; some tumor Sertoli cells are preserved (PAS stain)

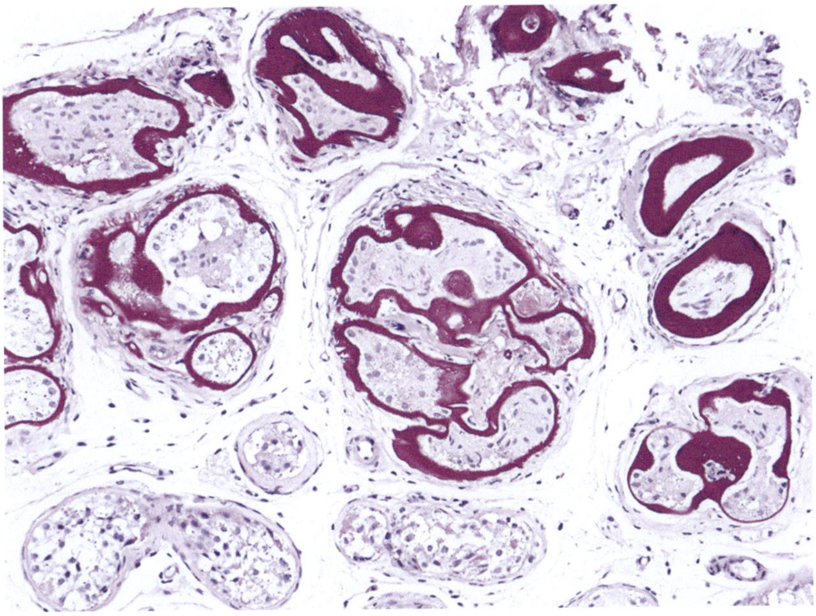

cell type, one of hyperchromatic nucleus and germ cells, may be observed in both disorders. The first one has a more angulated nucleus and little cytoplasm and shares with Sertoli cell inhibin expression in the Sertoli cell nodules, WT1 and SOX9, but differ from them by the nuclear expression FOXL2, which permits us to say that these sex cord cells are more undifferentiated, which justifies its interpretation sometimes as Sertoli cell and in other occasions as granulosa cells [16].

In Sertoli cell nodules, the germ cells can be spermatogonia or gonocyte-like cells. The presence of the second type of cells makes diagnosis more difficult. In both cases there are tumor germ cells (cells positive for PLAP and OCT3/4).

Distribution of germ cells, the findings in the neighboring parenchyma, and the pathology being suffered by the patient are considered important differential criteria. In Sertoli cell nodules with tumor cells, these are not as abundant, they adopt a patchwork distribution, and they are located peripherally or centrally. No preferred distribution exists in a gonadoblastoma. The neighboring parenchyma shows a germ cell tumor or germ cell neoplasia in situ, and the interstitium is scarce and loose in the Sertoli cell nodules. Patients with Sertoli cell nodules are phenotypically normal males which often have cryptorchidism, while carriers of a gonadoblastoma have a disorder of sexual development. In these cases, the gonadoblastoma can settle on a streak gonad, on dysgenetic testes, or on streak testes or ovotestes.

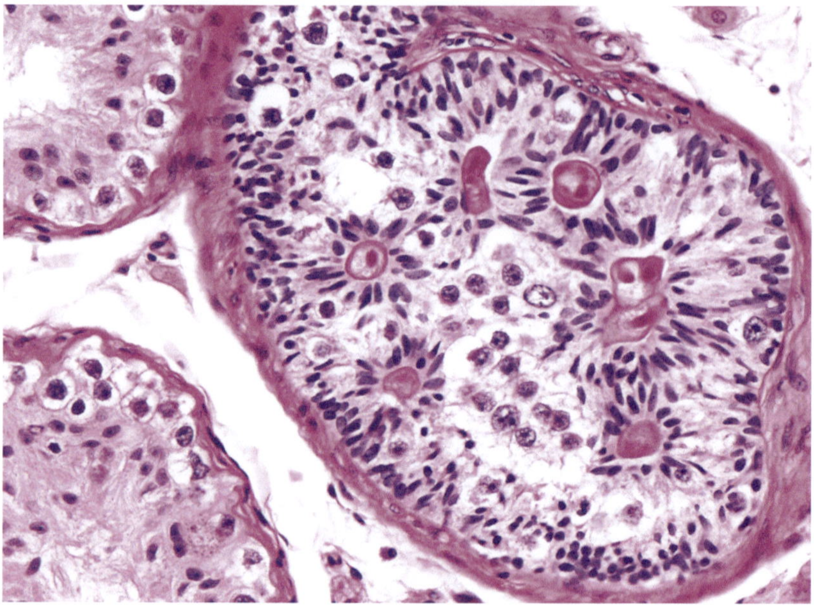

Fig. 9.7 Sertoli cell nodule located infiltrated by GCNIS cells on the periphery of a germ cell tumor. In the central part of the tube, atypical germ cells are outstanding. Adjacent tubules also show GCNIS

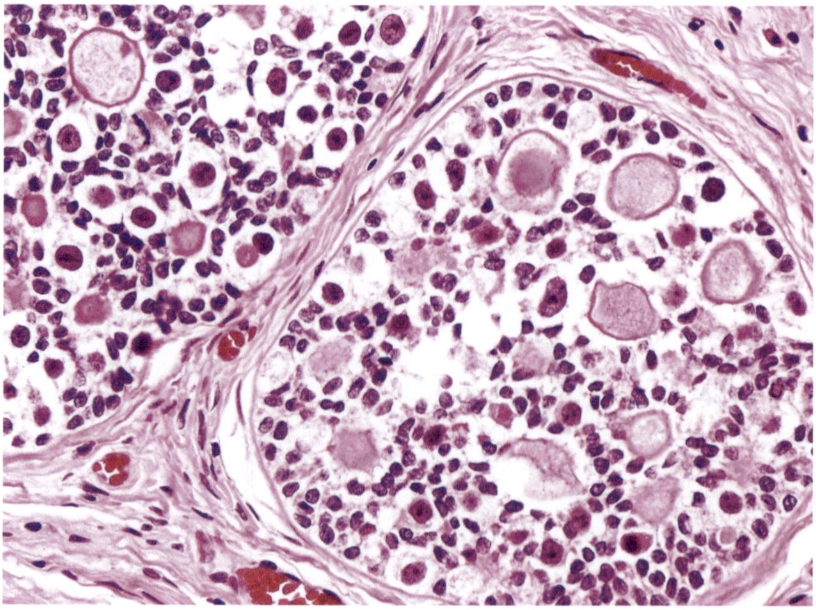

Fig. 9.8 Gonadoblastoma. The figure shows two nodular formations that have a significant resemblance to those of the previous figure. The more regular distribution of germ cells between the Sertoli/granulosa cells and separation of the nodules by dense connective tissue are important clues for differential diagnosis

9.4.3 Sertoli Cell Nodules Versus Sex Cord Tumor with Annular Tubules (SCTAT)

Ring-shaped tubules can be seen in the Sertoli cell nodules, in large cell intratubular hyalinizing Sertoli cell neoplasia, in the periphery of the calcifying large cell Sertoli cell tumor, and in sex cord tumor with annular tubules. While diagnosis of the first one is relatively easy, the morphological differential diagnosis of sex cord tumor with annular tubules is more difficult because the images can be superimposed. A useful criterion, in addition to the size, is the absence in Sertoli cell nodules in the large islet of cells surrounding multiple bodies derived from the basement membrane that is one of the main components of tumors with annular tubules [17] (Figs. 9.9 and 9.10).

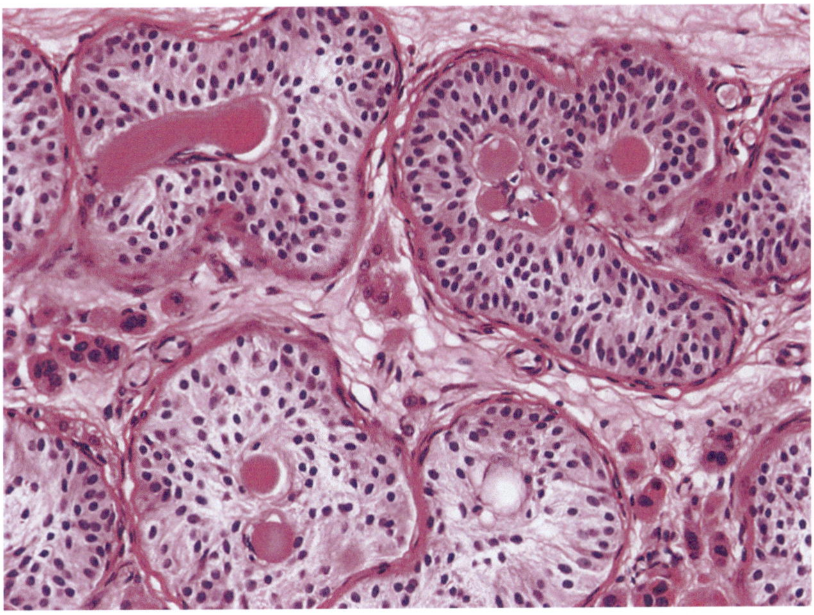

Fig. 9.9 Sertoli cell nodule in which the distribution of cells over the basement membrane and over the eosinophilic material of the bodies simulates sex cord tumor with annular tubules

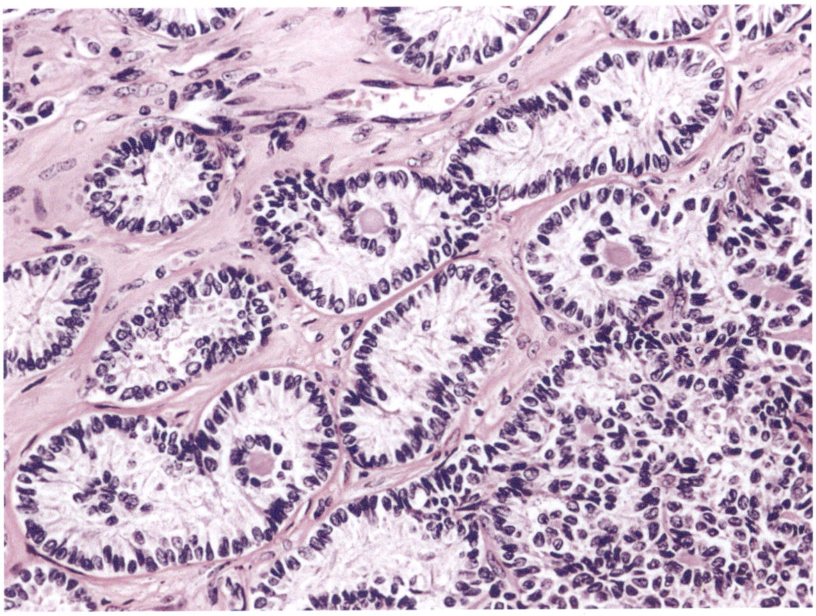

Fig. 9.10 Sex cord tumor with annular tubules. The complexity of tubular formations with numerous annular formations inside is an important data for differential diagnosis

9.4.4 Macroscopic Sertoli Cell Nodules Versus Sertoli Cell Tumors "Not Otherwise Specified"

Cases have been reported in which the size of Sertoli cell nodules reaches 10 mm. On the other hand, the size of Sertoli cell tumors ranges from 0.3 to 15 cm [18, 19]. Consequently, the size is not an absolute criterion. This Sertoli cell tumor has a strong tubular structure. Basement membranes are neither thickened nor have inward PAS-positive protrusions. The cells have ovoid, vesicular nuclei and an important cytoplasmic vacuolization. The intertubular stroma is generally fibrous, often hyalinized. The most important immunohistochemical data for distinguishing them are positivity in tumor cells for calretinin, cytokeratins, beta-catenin, S100, chromogranin, and EMA.

References

1. Mostofi F, Price EJ. Atlas of tumor pathology: tumors of the male genital system. Second series, fascicle 8. Washington, DC: Armed Forces Institute of Pathology; 1973.
2. Govender D, Sing Y, Chetty R. Sertoli cell nodules in the undescended testis: a histochemical, immunohistochemical, and ultrastructural study of hyaline deposits. J Clin Pathol. 2004;57:802–6.
3. Harbaum L, Langner C. Epididymal Sertoli cell nodule–a diagnostic pitfall. Histopathology. 2009;55:475–7.
4. Hedinger CE, Huber R, Weber E. Frequency of so-called hypoplastic or dysgenetic zones in scrotal and otherwise normal human tests. Virchows Arch Pathol Anat Physiol Klin Med. 1967;342:165–8.
5. Schulze C, Schütte B. Concretions in the human testis are derived from the basal lamina of seminiferous cords. Cell Tissue Res. 1990;260:1–12.
6. Hayrabedyan S, Todorova K, Pashova S, Mollova M, Fernández N. Sertoli cell quiescence–new insights. Am J Reprod Immunol. 2012;68:451–5.
7. Nistal M, Pastrián LG, González-Peramato P, De Miguel MP. Inhibin bodies: a new marker for immature Sertoli cells. Histopathology. 2011;58:1019–27.
8. Barghorn A, Alioth HR, Hailemariam S, Bannwart F, Ulbright TM. Giant Sertoli cell nodule of the testis: distinction from other Sertoli cell lesions. J Clin Pathol. 2006;59:1223–5.
9. Vallangeon BD, Eble JN, Ulbright TM. Macroscopic sertoli cell nodule: a study of 6 cases that presented as testicular masses. Am J Surg Pathol. 2010;34:1874–80.
10. Regadera J, Martínez-García F, González-Peramato P, Serrano A, Nistal M, Suárez-Quian C. Androgen receptor expression in Sertoli cells as a function of seminiferous tubule maturation in the human cryptorchid testis. J Clin Endocrinol Metab. 2001;86:413–21.
11. Wohlfahrt-Veje C, Main KM, Skakkebaek NE. Testicular dysgenesis syndrome: foetal origin of adult reproductive problems. Clin Endocrinol (Oxf). 2009;71:459–65.
12. Venara M, Rey R, Bergadá I, Mendilaharzu H, Campo S, Chemes H. Sertoli cell proliferations of the infantile testis: an intratubular form of Sertoli cell tumor? Am J Surg Pathol. 2001;25:1237–44.
13. Armijo B, Bocklage T, Heideman R. Intratubular large cell hyalinizing sertoli cell tumor of the testes in a 4-year-old male with Peutz-Jeghers syndrome. J Pediatr Hematol Oncol. 2015;37:e184–7.
14. Ros P, Nistal M, Alonso M, Calvo de Mora J, Yturriaga R, Barrio R. Sertoli cell tumour in a boy with Peutz-Jeghers syndrome. Histopathology. 1999;34:84–6.
15. Ulbright TM, Amin MB, Young RH. Intratubular large cell hyalinizing sertoli cell neoplasia of the testis: a report of 8 cases of a distinctive lesion of the Peutz-Jeghers syndrome. Am J Surg Pathol. 2007;31:827–35.
16. Kao CS, Ulbright TM, Idrees MT. Gonadoblastoma: an immunohistochemical study and comparison to Sertoli cell nodule with intratubular germ cell neoplasia, with pathogenetic implications. Histopathology. 2014;65:861–7.
17. Ramaswamy G, Jagadha V, Tchertkoff V. A testicular tumor resembling the sex cord with annular tubules in a case of the androgen insensitivity syndrome. Cancer. 1985;55:1607–11.
18. Young RH, Koelliker DD, Scully RE. Sertoli cell tumors of the testis, not otherwise specified: a clinicopathologic analysis of 60 cases. Am J Surg Pathol. 1998;22:709–21.
19. Nagata M, Kurimoto S, Takeuchi T, Ohta N, Minowada S, Kitamura T. Tiny nodule in the testicle: case report of a sertoli cell tumor. Int J Urol. 2004;11:61–2.

10 Meaning of the Finding of Testicular and Paratesticular Calcifications

Manuel Nistal, Pilar González-Peramato, and Álvaro Serrano

10.1 Testicular Calcifications

10.1.1 Testicular Microlithiasis

Incidence The presence of microliths is a common finding in patients with cryptorchidism; infertility; testicular tumors; genetic syndromes such as Down, Klinefelter's, and McCune-Albright; and congenital adrenal hyperplasia and even in testicles considered normal. The most interesting problem is to separate the cases where it has no clinical relevance from those others that can actually be a manifestation of an underlying pathology as it occurs in the testicular dysgenesis syndrome.

Historical data of the impact of microlithiasis were based on histological and radiographic studies. In histological studies, testicular microlithiasis is found in about 0.16 % of pediatric testicular biopsies [1], 1 % of biopsies of infertile men [2], and 4 % of adult male autopsies [3]. The incidence found in two radiological series varied from 0.6 % [4] to 74 % [5].

Studies based on ultrasound show an incidence that is related to the following variables: age, symptomatic or asymptomatic populations, and testicular disease studied. The incidence in asymptomatic boys is 2.4 % for classical microlithiasis and 1.8 % for limited microlithiasis [6]. In pediatric patients with any of the following conditions: cryptorchidism, hydrocele, scrotal swelling, chromosomal anomalies, orchalgia, and testicular torsion, the incidence of microlithiasis varies from 2.8 % [6] to 8.7 % [7]. In undescended testes it is related to the location of the testes (1 % in inguinal testes, 5 % intra-abdominal testes) and bilateralism (25 % in bilateral cryptorchid testes). Microlithiasis incidence tends to increase with age.

Sonographic incidence of classical microlithiasis in asymptomatic adults varies from 2.4 % [8] to 5.6 %, and 66 % of them were bilateral [9]. There are significant ethnic differences (white 4 %, black 14.1 %, and Hispanic 8.5 %) and geographic differences (Asian or Pacific Island men 5.6 %). In adults the incidence varies greatly depending on the disease studied: 9.52 % of patients with excryptorchidic testes [10], from 1.5 to 18 % in infertile patients [11, 12], and 30–50 % of adult testes with germ cell tumors [13]. It can be seen both in tumoral and contralateral testis whether or not this one has a tumor [14]. Both the number of microliths and their distribution pattern are very variable (Fig. 10.1). Characteristic patterns as a diffuse symmetrical distribution, unilateral foci, and peripheral clumping have all been described [15].

The most common clinical symptom for which ultrasound is prescribed is pain (48 %), and cryptorchidism is the most frequently associated clinical pathology (11 %). The pain has been associated with seminiferous tubule dilatation secondary to the obstruction caused by microliths [16].

M. Nistal et al., *Clues in the Diagnosis of Non-tumoral Testicular Pathology*,
DOI 10.1007/978-3-319-49364-0_10

Histology In prepubertal testis, microliths stand out both by their concentric laminar structure and by being surrounded by a double crown of Sertoli cells (Fig. 10.2). The difference in size of the tubules with microliths and those in the rest of the parenchyma is very large. This fact is further highlighted by the already decreased tubular diameter caused by the underlying testicular pathology [1].

In adults, microliths can be seen in the lumen of the seminiferous tubules, but also within the seminiferous epithelium of the seminiferous tubules or outside them (Figs. 10.2 and 10.3). Also other common locations are the Sertoli cell nodules, frequent in undescended testes, and inside the seminiferous tubules with germ cell neoplasia in situ (Figs. 10.4 and 10.5). X-ray diffraction [17] and Raman spectroscopy [18] studies suggest that the mineralized material corresponds to hydroxyapatite crystals.

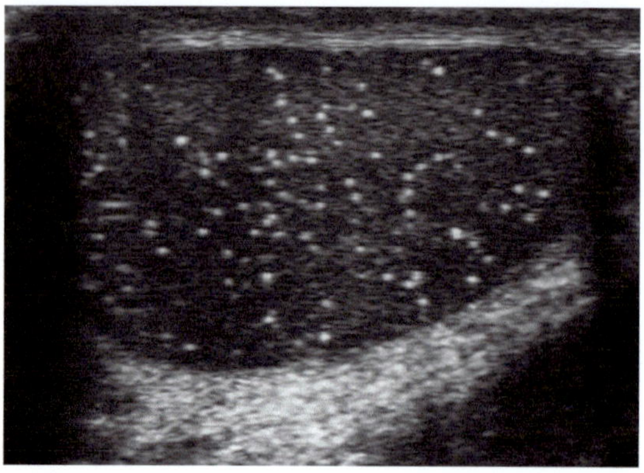

Fig. 10.1 Classic microlithiasis in a 5-year-old child. Ultrasound image showing numerous regularly distributed microliths in the testicular parenchyma

Origin of the Microliths There are two schools of thought. The first one believes that microliths originate intratubularly. The second one thinks they are formed in the tubule wall and removed through the tubular epithelium into the lumen. Inside the tubule they would originate in sloughed germ cell debris on which concentric rings of glycoproteins are deposited [19]. The second hypothesis, an extratubular origin, is supported by morphological and immunohistochemical facts [20]. Both in childhood and adulthood, spherical eosinophil bodies in the wall of the seminiferous tubules can be seen in the testis with microlithiasis. This material is surrounded by abundant laminin and collagen IV, two constitutive basal lamina materials produced by Sertoli cells. In childhood, serialization of the tubules with microliths known as "ring-shaped tubules" shows

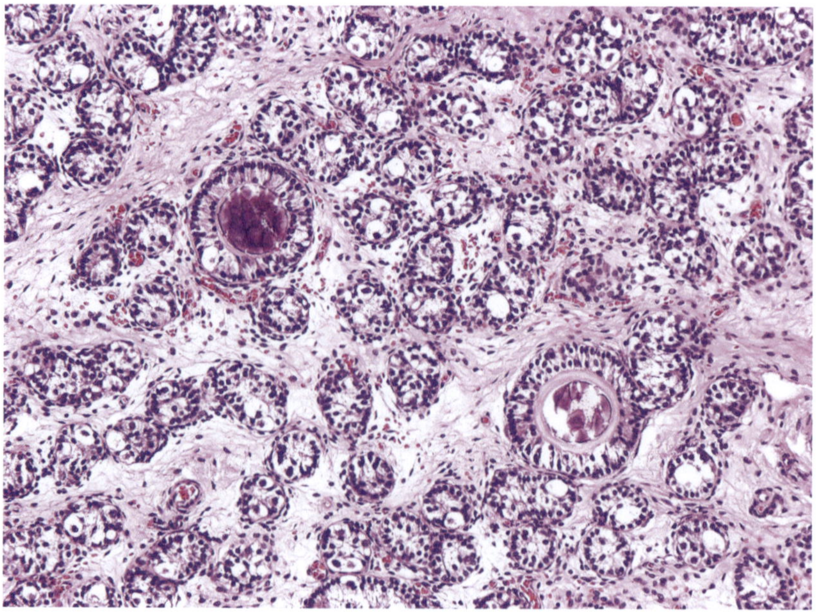

Fig. 10.2 Two microliths surrounded by a double crown of Sertoli cells in a child with cryptorchidism

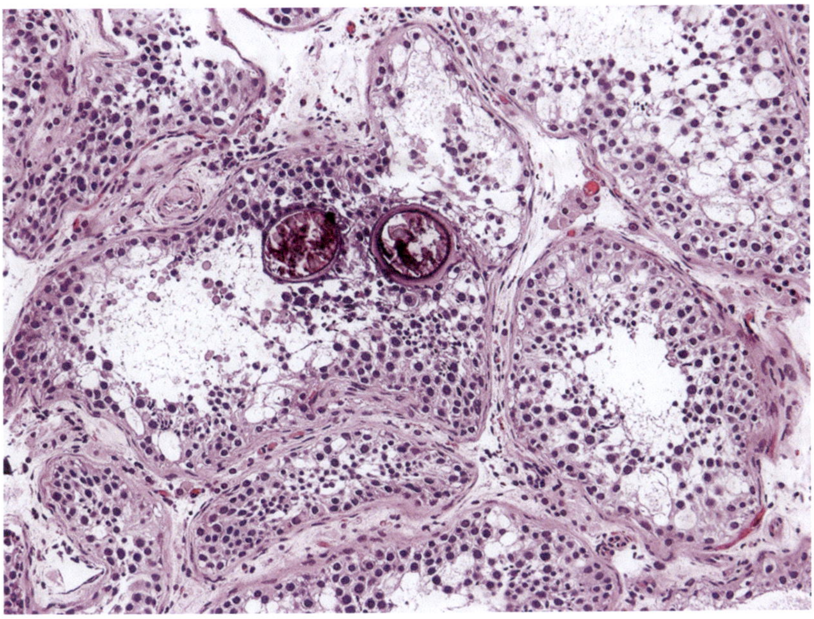

Fig. 10.3 Microliths in one seminiferous tubule with spermatogenesis in an infertile patient. One microlith appears in the lumen of the tubule, while the other is still connected to the tubular wall

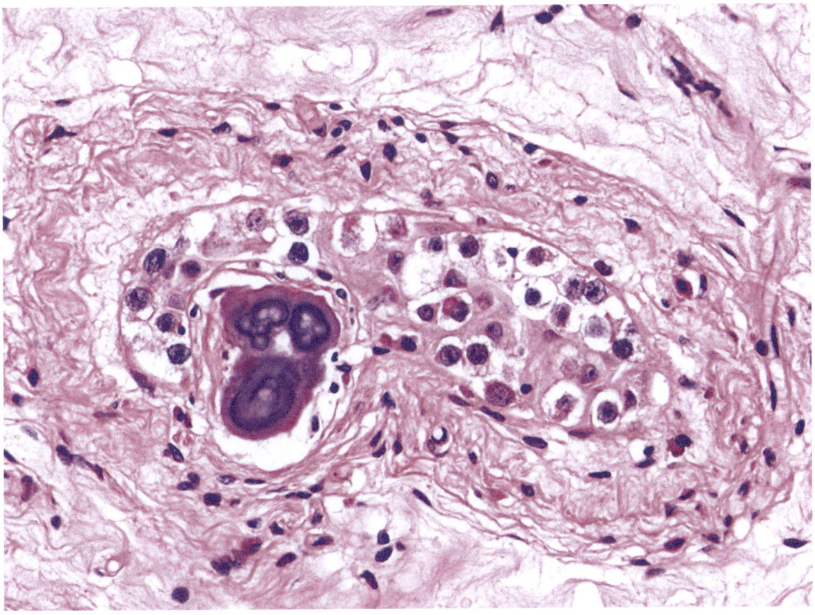

Fig. 10.4 Microlithiasis and GCNIS. Seminiferous tubule with marked thickening of the wall and forming microliths located between the wall and the tumor cells. The microliths are still surrounded by some flattened cells of the wall that they have probably been dragged inward

that they are bell shaped, and it is in the central part, extratubularly, where the microlith is located. Some are even surrounded by a layer of flattened cells of the tubular wall. In the adult, a whole sequence of images showing migration from the tubular wall to the lumen can be seen; first they protrude inwardly, then they lift the seminiferous epithelium, and finally they get located in the lumen. The seminiferous tubules suffer cystic transformation probably secondary to obstruction by microliths. The participation of Sertoli cells and structures of the tubular wall in the formation of microliths links different histological lesions observed in the testicular dysgenesis syndrome.

Microlithiasis and Testicular Cancer The association of microlithiasis and testicular can-

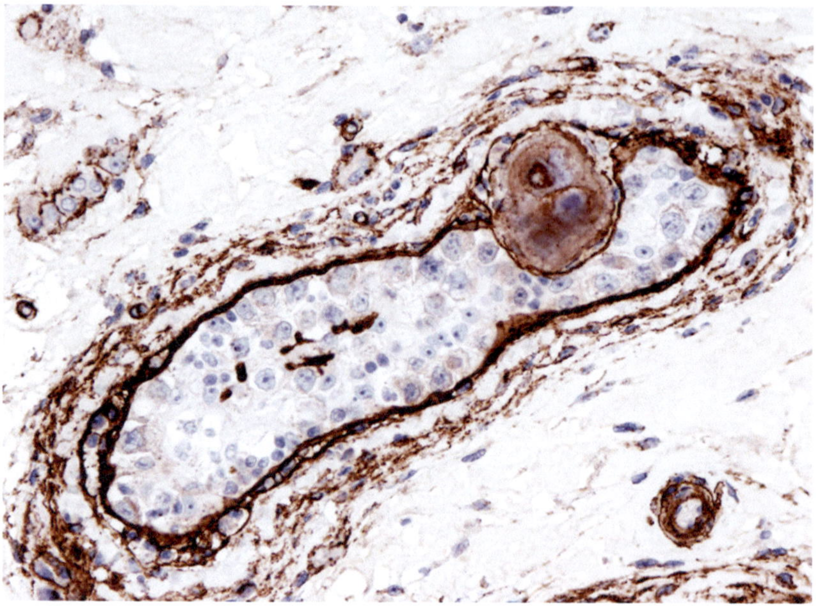

Fig. 10.5 Microlith in formation present in one seminiferous tubule with GCNIS. The microlith with laminated structure is placed in a splitting of the tubular wall. Immunostaining for laminin

cer is still an unresolved problem [21]. While in childhood there is no concern about the microlithiasis, unless there is another associated pathology, in adults the evidence of this association grows over the basis on the following facts: half of the patients with germ cell tumors have microlithiasis, some patients diagnosed with microlithiasis develop testicular tumor, and there are patients with retroperitoneal or mediastinal germ cell tumors showing testicular microlithiasis. There is an increased incidence of testicular microlithiasis in men with familial testicular germ cell tumors and their relatives. Not all germ cell tumors are associated with microlithiasis with the same frequency; seminomas are having the highest association and embryonal carcinomas the lowest one [22].

Monitoring of patients with testicular microlithiasis but no other illness would be enough with an annual ultrasound [23] or could even do without it [24]. Annual ultrasonography and testicular biopsy would be indicated in patients with any of the following associated pathologies: cryptorchidism, infertility, testicular atrophy, and microlithiasis in the testis contralateral to the one with germ cell tumor [25]. Do not forget that all these conditions are included in the testicular dysgenesis syndrome (see Chap. 13).

10.1.2 Macrolithiasis Separated from Any Intratesticular Mass

Macroliths have been defined as calcifications with a size between 2 and 10 mm in diameter. They are more frequent in adults than in children. Most calcifications correspond to old processes such as testicular infarcts, hematomas, and granulomatous orchitis. In other cases they are associated with vascular pathologies such as phleboliths in the varicoceles or calcification of the vascular wall with age.

A very interesting calcification is described in adults as calcified “clumps” or calcified “scars.” This intraparenchymatous macrocalcification is observed in patients presenting with a mediastinal or retroperitoneal germ cell tumor. Upon exploring the testicle, a retracted area stands out with a scarred aspect that can show multiple calcifications. This type of calcification is related to the sequel of a “burnt-out” testicular germ cell tumor that has previously originated metastases. In the histological study of a testicular tumor, often some tumor rests are still recognized such as germ cell neoplasia in situ or small cysts [26].

10.1.3 Tumor-Associated Calcifications

Intratesticular calcifications are observed in tumoral and pseudotumoral lesions. Calcifications are typical of gonadoblastoma, the most frequent tumor of the gonads in DSD patients. Calcification can become so massive that it prevents the histological recognition of tumor rests. Germ cell tumors that most often show calcifications are teratomas (Fig. 10.6) followed by embryonal carcinomas and choriocarcinomas, in the latter two in relation to areas of necrosis. Gonadal stromal tumors may also show calcifications which are common in some variants of Sertoli cell tumors such as large cell calcifying Sertoli cell tumors [27] (Fig. 10.7) and intratubular large cell hyalinizing Sertoli cell neoplasia [28]. Leydig

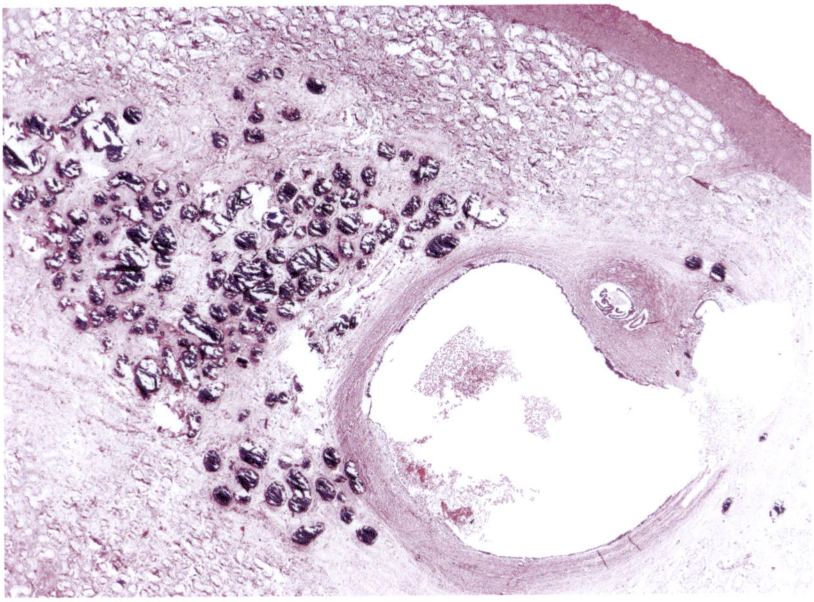

Fig. 10.6 Conglomerate of multiple calcifications in the testicular parenchyma is next to a residual cystic formation in a patient with a burned-out germ cell tumor

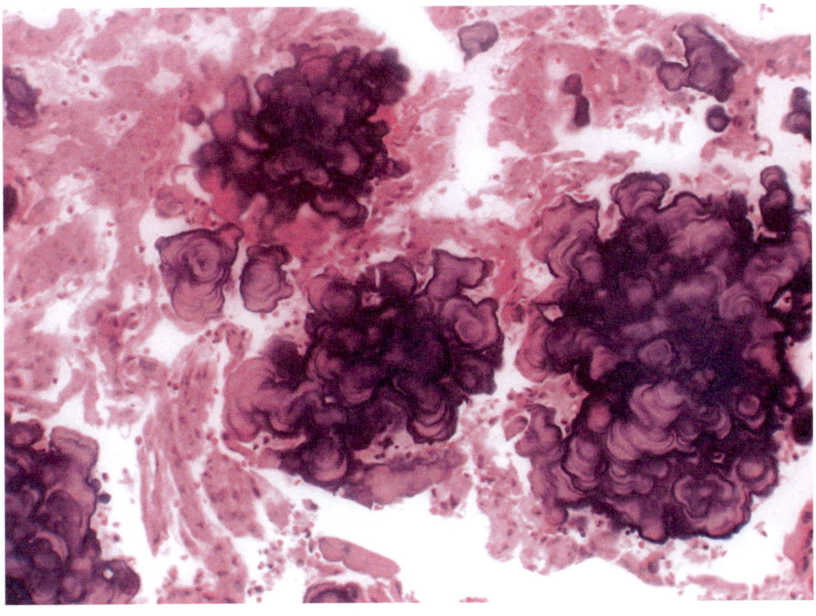

Fig. 10.7 Laminated calcifications of varied shapes and sizes surrounding cell cords in large cell calcifying Sertoli cell tumor

cell tumors rarely show calcifications [29]. Calcifications in the wall of different types of intraparenchymal cysts such as epidermoid cysts, or simple testicular cysts, have also been reported.

10.2 Paratesticular Calcifications

Paratesticular calcifications are more common than testicular ones and are generally associated with benign processes [30]. They can be located in the epididymis, epididymal or testicular appendix, tunica vaginalis, or intravaginal cavity (see Chaps. 31, 35, and 37).

10.2.1 Calcifications of the Epididymis

Etiology The etiology of calcifications of the epididymis is varied: post-inflammatory (chronic bacterial epididymitis, tuberculosis, genital filariasis), post-traumatic (riding, extreme mountain bikers), vascular (arteriosclerosis, hematoma, and varicocele), and post-obstructive (sperm granuloma). Ultrasound images of some calcifications are characteristic. In granulomatous and tuberculous epididymitis and secondary to repeated microtrauma (mountain bikers), calcifications are unique and large (up to 1 cm diameter) and cast an acoustic shadow. Calcification hematomas have a curvilinear appearance.

An extremely common condition is epididymal calcifications secondary to hemodialysis. These calcifications are mostly bilateral and have the sonographic features of microliths. They are described as multiple comet-shaped foci of microcalcifications throughout the epididymis [31]. They are present in 70 % of patients undergoing dialysis [32] and in 77 % in the population of young adult kidney transplant recipients [33]. The calcification is due to cell-mediated mechanisms secondary to an imbalance in calcium and phosphorus metabolism [33].

Histology Histologically calcifications can adopt two patterns, amorphous and laminated concentric (microlithiasis). Amorphous calcifications are characteristic of post-inflammatory, post-traumatic, vascular, and post-obstructive injuries. Most calcium deposits are related to interstitial and sperm extravasation or chronic inflammation. Idiopathic epididymal microlithiasis is a rare, asymptomatic disease not related to testicular microlithiasis or testicular cancer [34, 35]. In 0.8 % of histological autopsy studies of normal subjects, idiopathic calcifications are

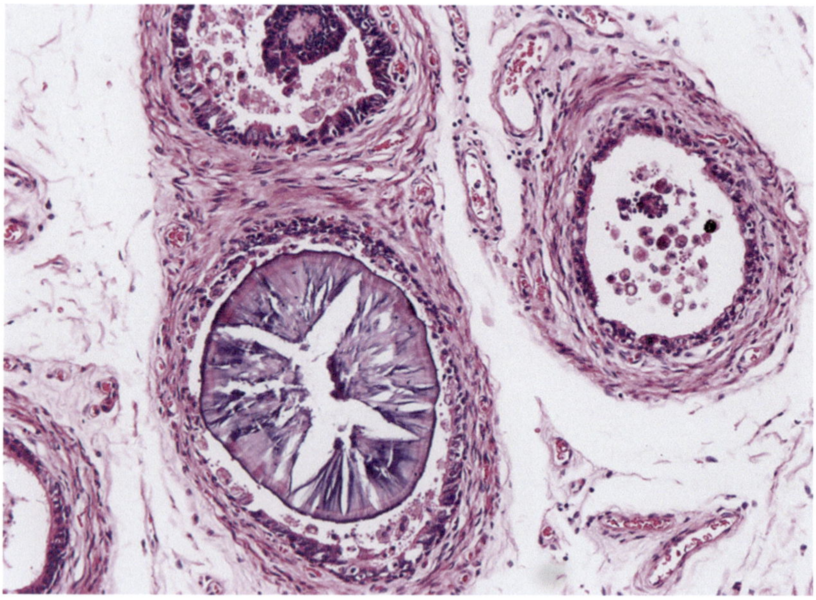

Fig. 10.8 Idiopathic microlithiasis of the epididymis. The tubular lumen is completely occupied by a fully calcified microlith

observed, a figure that rises up to 3 % of the epididymis removed due to scrotal diseases [34].

Microliths are found in three different locations: intraluminal, subepithelial, and interstitial. Intraluminal microliths have three origins: microliths originated in the testicle or in the rete testis that are expelled through the spermatic ducts; microliths originated under the epithelium and secondarily eliminated into the lumen, as it occurs in testicular microlithiasis; and calcification of intraluminal eosinophil bodies described as Liesegang rings [36] (Fig. 10.8).

Interstitial microliths are located in the body and the tail of the epididymis and associated with rich infiltrated macrophages simulating malacoplakia. Some originate directly in the interstitium coinciding with ischemic lesions; others, especially those of the cauda epididymis, reach the interstitium through breaks in the wall of diverticula that are frequent at this level [37].

10.2.2 Epididymal Stones

They constitute an incidental finding in the study of surgical specimens removed due to different pathologies or in routine autopsy studies of elderly testes. They are preferably located in the tail, a dilated epididymal duct, or inside a diverticulum. Its size can reach several mm. The shape is ovoid or lobed. Histologically they lack the radial and laminar structure of microliths. Epididymal lithiasis is associated with testicular parenchyma lesions of obstructive pattern (see Chap. 17).

References

1. Nistal M, Paniagua R, Diez-Pardo JA. Testicular microlithiasis in 2 children with bilateral cryptorchidism. J Urol. 1979;121:535–7.
2. Sasagawa I, Nakada T, Kazama T, Satomi S, Katayama T, Matuda S. Testicular microlithiasis in male infertility. Urol Int. 1988;43:368–9.
3. Renshaw AA. Testicular calcifications: incidence, histology and proposed pathological criteria for testicular microlithiasis. J Urol. 1998;160:1625–8.
4. Höbarth K, Susani M, Szabo N, Kratzik C. Incidence of testicular microlithiasis. Urology. 1992;40:464–7.
5. Ikinger U, Wuster K, Terwey B, Mohring K. Microcalcifications in testicular malignancy: diagnostic tool in occult tumor? Urology. 1982;19:525–8.
6. Goede J, Hack WW, van der Voort-Doedens LM, Sijstermans K, Pierik FH. Prevalence of testicular microlithiasis in asymptomatic males 0 to 19 years old. J Urol. 2009;182:1516–20.
7. Deganello A, Svasti-Salee D, Allen P, Clarke JL, Sellars ME, Sidhu PS. Scrotal calcification in a symptomatic paediatric population: prevalence, location, and appearance in a cohort of 516 patients. Clin Radiol. 2012;67:862–7.
8. Serter S, Orguc S, Gumus B, Ayyildiz V, Pabuscu Y. Doppler sonographic findings in testicular microlithiasis. Int Braz J Urol. 2008;34:477–82. discussion 482–4.
9. Peterson AC, Bauman JM, Light DE, Mcmann LP, Costabile RA. The prevalence of testicular microlithiasis in an asymptomatic population of men 18 to 35 years old. J Urol. 2001;166:2061–4.
10. Nicolas F, Dubois R, Laboure S, Dodat H, Canterino L, Rouviere O. Testicular nicrolithiasis and cryptorchidism: ultrasound analysis after orchidopexy. Prog Urol. 2001;11:357–61.
11. Kessaris DN, Mellinger BC. Incidence and implication of testicular microlithiasis detected by scrotal duplex sonography in selected group of infertile men. J Urol. 1994;152:1560–1.
12. Aizenstein RI, Didomenico D, Wilbur AC, O'Neil HK. Testicular microlithiasis: association with male infertility. J Clin Ultrasound. 1998;26:195–8.
13. Rashid HH, Cos LR, Weinberg E, Messing EM. Testicular microlithiasis: a review and its association with testicular cancer. Urol Oncol. 2004;22:285–9.
14. Holm M, Hoei-Hansen CE, Rajpert-De Meyts E, Skakkebaek NE. Increased risk of carcinoma in situ in patients with testicular germ cell cancer with ultrasonic microlithiasis in the contralateral testicle. J Urol. 2003;170:1163–7.
15. Backus ML, Mack LA, Middleton WD, King BF, Winter 3rd TC, True LD. Testicular microlithiasis: imaging appearances and pathologic correlation. Radiology. 1994;192:781–5.
16. Moran JM, Moreno F, Climent V, Nistal M. Idiopathic testicular microlithiasis ultrastructural study. Br J Urol. 1993;72:252–3.
17. Smith GD, Steele L, Barnes RB, Levine LA. Identification of seminiferous tubule aberrations and a low incidence of testicular microliths associated with the development of azoospermia. Fertil Steril. 1999;72:467–71.
18. De Jong BW, De Gouveia Brazao CA, Stoop H, Wolffenbuttel KP, Oosterhuis JW, Puppels GJ, Weber RF, Looijenga LH, Kok DJ. Raman spectroscopic analysis identifies testicular microlithiasis as intratubular hydroxyapatite. J Urol. 2004;171:92–6.
19. Vegni-Talluri M, Bigliardi E, Vanni MG, Tota G. Testicular microliths: their origin and structure. J Urol. 1980;124:105–7.

20. Nistal M, Martinez-Garcia C, Paniagua R. The origin of testicular microliths. Int J Androl. 1995;18:221–9.
21. Tan IB, Ang KK, Ching BC, Mohan C, Toh CK, Tan MH. Testicular microlithiasis predicts concurrent testicular germ cell tumors and intratubular germ cell neoplasia of unclassified type in adults: a meta-analysis and systematic review. Cancer. 2010;116: 4520–32.
22. Sharmeen F, Rosenthal MH, Wood MJ, Tirumani SH, Sweeney C, Howard SA. Relationship between the pathologic subtype/initial stage and microliths in testicular germ cell tumors. J Ultrasound Med. 2015;4:1977–82.
23. Dagash H, Mackinnon EA. Testicular microlithiasis: what does it mean clinically? BJU Int. 2007;99: 157–60.
24. Ravichandran S, Smith R, Cornford PA, Fordham MV. Surveillance of testicular microlithiasis? Results of an UK based national questionnaire survey. BMC Urol. 2006;6:8.
25. Meissner A, Mamoulakis C, de la Rosette JJ, Pes MP. Clinical update on testicular microlithiasis. Curr Opin Urol. 2009;19:615–8.
26. Harris RD. Extragonadal tumor and testicular microlithiasis. J Ultrasound Med. 2011;30:868.
27. Plata C, Algaba F, Andújar M, Nistal M, Stocks P, Martínez JL, Nogales FF. Large cell calcifying Sertoli cell tumour of the testis. Histopathology. 1995;26: 255–9.
28. Ulbright TM, Amin MB, Young RH. Intratubular large cell hyalinizing sertoli cell neoplasia of the testis: a report of 8 cases of a distinctive lesion of the Peutz-Jeghers syndrome. Am J Surg Pathol. 2007;31: 827–35.
29. Woodward PJ, Sohaey R, O'Donoghue MJ, Green DE. From the archives of the AFIP: tumors and tumorlike lesions of the testis: radiologic-pathologic correlation. Radiographics. 2002;2:189–216.
30. Martin B, Tubiana JM. Significance of scrotal calcifications detected by sonography. J Clin Ultrasound. 1988;6:545–52.
31. Vandervelde C, Varghese A, Mason A, Howlett D. Sonographic appearance of epididymal microlithiasis. J Clin Ultrasound. 2007;35:413–5.
32. Guvel S, Pourbagher MA, Torun D, Egilmez T, Pourbagher A, Ozkardes H. Calcification of the epididymis and the tunica albuginea of the corpora cavernosa in patients on maintenance hemodialysis. J Androl. 2004;25:752–6.
33. Bozzini G, Lunelli L, Berlingheri M, Groppali E, Carmignani L. Epididymis microlithiasis and semen abnormalities in young adult kidney transplant recipients. Andrologia. 2013;45:357–60.
34. Nistal M, García-Cabezas MA, Regadera J, Castillo MC. Microlithiasis of the epididymis and the rete testis. Am J Surg Pathol. 2004;28:514–22.
35. Mathew M, Thomas J. Microlithiasis of the epididymis: a case report and review of literature. Indian J Pathol Microbiol. 2008;51:534–5.
36. Liesegang RE. Uber einige eigerschaften von Gallerton. Nat Wochenschr. 1896;11:353–62.
37. Nistal M, Iñiguez L, Paniagua R, Regadera J. Diverticula of the ductus epididymis in men. J Urol. 1986;136:1224–7.

Helpful Data for Evaluating an Undescended Testis in Childhood

11

Manuel Nistal, Pilar González-Peramato, and Álvaro Serrano

11.1 Hypothalamic-Pituitary-Testicular Axis

The hypothalamic-pituitary-testicular axis (HPT) undergoes three activations throughout life: in fetal life, in the first months of postnatal life (mini-puberty) and at puberty.

The HPT Axis in Fetal Life At 15 weeks of gestation, GnRH neurons from the nasal placode have already reached the hypothalamus. Stimulation of gonadotropic cells of the anterior lobe of the hypophysis leads to secretion of FSH and LH, which can be detected between 12 and 14 weeks. Circulating levels reach a peak between 20 and 25 weeks of gestation. Early in fetal life, the placenta secretes hCG that reaches a peak in the fetal circulation between 12 and 17 weeks. This gonadotropin is structurally and biologically similar to LH. The three gonadotropins decrease throughout pregnancy to be probably suppressed by high estrogen production by the placenta [1].

From week 8 fetal testes produce two hormones: the antimüllerian hormone (AMH) and testosterone. AMH secreted by Sertoli cells forces the regression of the Müllerian ducts. Testosterone comes from conversion of androstenedione secreted by Leydig cells by the Sertoli cells [2] and induces the development of the male internal genitalia. The conversion of testosterone in dihydrotestosterone by the 5-alpha-reductase enzyme leads to the development of the prostate, the penis, and the scrotum. Higher testosterone levels are reached between 10 and 20 weeks and then decline throughout gestation. Testosterone secretion depends on the hCG in the first and second quarters of pregnancy.

The testicular descent begins early. The first phase of testicular descent is known as transabdominal and completed in the 15th week of gestation. It depends on insulin-like peptide 3 (INSL-3) produced by the Leydig cells, which reaches peak levels during the first half of gestation [3]. The second phase of descent, also known as inguinoscrotal, is completed in the 35th week of gestation and is androgen dependent. Androgens act indirectly via the genitofemoral nerve that produces calcitonin gene-related peptide that controls the elongation of the gubernaculum until reaching the scrotum [4].

The HPT Axis in Postnatal Life Very low levels of FSH and LH are found during the first days of life. HCG disappears after the first few days. From this moment, a new activation of HPT axis known as mini-puberty starts [5]. After the first week, a rapid rise of LH and FSH in smaller proportion occurs to reach a peak within 3 months. Hormonal rates are similar to those of puberty or even to adulthood. The consequence of elevated LH is an activation of the Leydig cells with increased testosterone and INSL-3 production. The elevation of FSH produces increased number

M. Nistal et al., *Clues in the Diagnosis of Non-tumoral Testicular Pathology*,
DOI 10.1007/978-3-319-49364-0_11

of Sertoli cells and their markers, inhibin B and AMH, as well as renewal and differentiation of germ cells with an increase in their number. As a result of this hormonal activation, the testicular volume increases temporarily. FSH and LH levels begin to decrease between the 6 and the 9 months of life, which correlates with a diminution of testicular size that occurs by the second year of life.

11.2 Basic Data to Evaluate an Undescended Testis

11.2.1 Clinical Data

Among the clinical data, the following are particularly significant: age, location of the testicle, bilateralism, testicular volume, hormonal rates, associated malformations, associated syndromes, and chromosomal abnormalities.

Age Testicular alterations in undescended testes are considered early so that delaying treatment beyond the first year supposes a risk of lesion worsening [6].

Location of the Testis Abdominal testes develop more serious lesions than those in the inguinal canal. The most consistent alteration is the loss of germ cells [7].

Bilateralism Bilateralism is a sign of poor prognosis. The incidence of azoospermia in patients with unilateral cryptorchidism is 13 %, while in patients with bilateral undescended testes, it is 89 % [6]. Patients with bilateral undescended testis in adulthood generally have lower sperm concentration, lower sperm motility, smaller testicular volume, and lower inhibin B levels.

Testicular Volume The seminiferous tubules are responsible for 90 % of the testicular volume in childhood. Of all the methods for measuring testicular volume, including orchidometry [8, 9], rulers, calipers, and ultrasonography, this is the most accurate system for measuring testicular size in children [10]. The testicular volume in cubic cm is calculated with the following formula: length × width × height × 0.71 [11]. In the first 5 months of life, testicular volume increases 0.27 cm^3 (±0, 002) to 0.44 cm^3 (±0.03). The volume decreases to 0.31 cm^3 (±0.02) at 9 months. The greater testicular size in this period occurs in the mini-puberty [12]. During the following years, the volume remains constant until the age of 6 years. In undescended testicles the tubular diameter remains below normal values.

Another method used is the *testicular atrophy index*, introduced by Niedzielski in 2003 [13]. It is defined as less affected testis volume/contralateral testis volume × 100, expressed as a percent that is useful for unilateral cryptorchidic testes, and the variant introduced by Spinelli in 2014 [14] for bilateral ones. With these methods it is possible to identify patients amenable to medical treatment in addition to surgery.

Hormonal Rates There is ample evidence to suggest that many cryptorchidic boys have a deficit at the hypothalamic or pituitary level. Cryptorchidic patients show low inhibin B and low LH levels and testosterone and free androgen deficiency early after birth. The response to stimulation with hCG of Leydig cells is decreased. Treatment prior to orchiopexy with GnRH improves tubular fertility index in both bilateral and unilateral cryptorchidism [15], elongates the spermatic cord structures, and enlarges the inguinal canal [16].

Associated Malformations Sixty-two to Ninety percent of cryptorchidic patients have an ipsilateral patent vaginal process, and 65–75 % of cryptorchidic males have a hernial sac. Urological malformations are present in 10 % of patients and include hypospadias, complete duplication of the urinary tract, nonobstructive urethral dilation, kidney malrotation, and posterior urethral valves. Anomalies in the relationship between testis and epididymis are frequent in the undescended testes. Some of them consist of fusion anomalies and others of suspension anomalies [17].

Associated Syndromes Although cryptorchidism usually appears as an isolated anomaly, this disorder is often associated with congenital, endocrine, or chromosomal disorders and also with disorders in sexual differentiation. Cryptorchidism is a common finding in patients with GnRH deficit, Kallman's syndrome, Prader-Willi's syndrome, testicular feminization syndromes caused by androgen receptor anomalies, 5-α-reductase deficiency, several types of undermasculinization caused by AMH absence, Klinefelter's syndrome, and Noonan's syndrome.

11.2.2 Histological Data

The procedure that has contributed most to the knowledge of lesions in the undescended testis has been the testicular biopsy. Today it continues to be indicated in all undescended testes that do not respond to LHRH therapy. Many histological data evaluated as a whole allow us to suggest the nature of the lesions and venture a fertility prognosis in patients with cryptorchidism. The tubular diameter, the number and type of germ cells, the distribution of germ cells in the seminiferous tubules, the number of Sertoli cells by transverse tubular section, and the state of the Leydig cells are considered particularly important.

The *tubular diameter* in childhood depends primarily on the number of Sertoli cell and their trophic status, data that correlate with FSH levels, and rates of responsiveness to them. The contribution of germ cells to the tubular diameter at this stage of development is scarce. The tubular diameter varies throughout childhood, reaches 80 microns at the 6th month of life and reaches its lowest at the end of the third year, and then it increases slowly until 9 years and then abruptly at puberty with the appearance of tubular lumen and spermatogenesis; it finally goes up to 180 microns in adults.

The decrease of the tubular diameter or tubular hypoplasia is very common in undescended testicles. It can be graduated as mild tubular hypoplasia (tubular diameter loss of no more than 10 % of the average value for age), moderate tubular hypoplasia (tubular diameter loss is >10 % but <30 % of the normal diameter for age) (Fig. 11.1), and severe tubular hypoplasia (tubular diameter loss is >30 % of the normal value for age).

Germ Cells The number of germ cells can be estimated by two methods: (1) the tubular fertility index and (2) the germ cell number per cross-sectioned tubules.

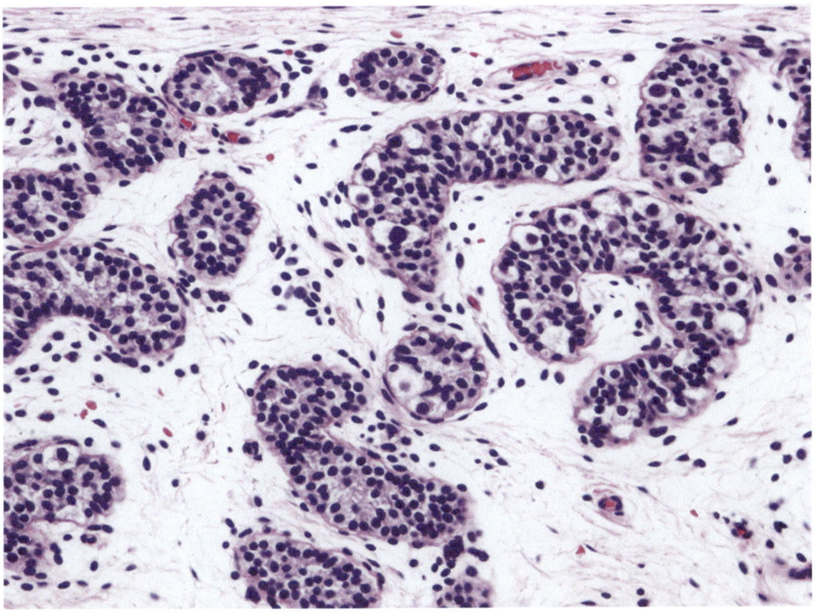

Fig. 11.1 Cryptorchidism type II. Moderate decrease of the diameter tubular and the presence of spermatogonia in approximately 50 % of the tubular sections are shown

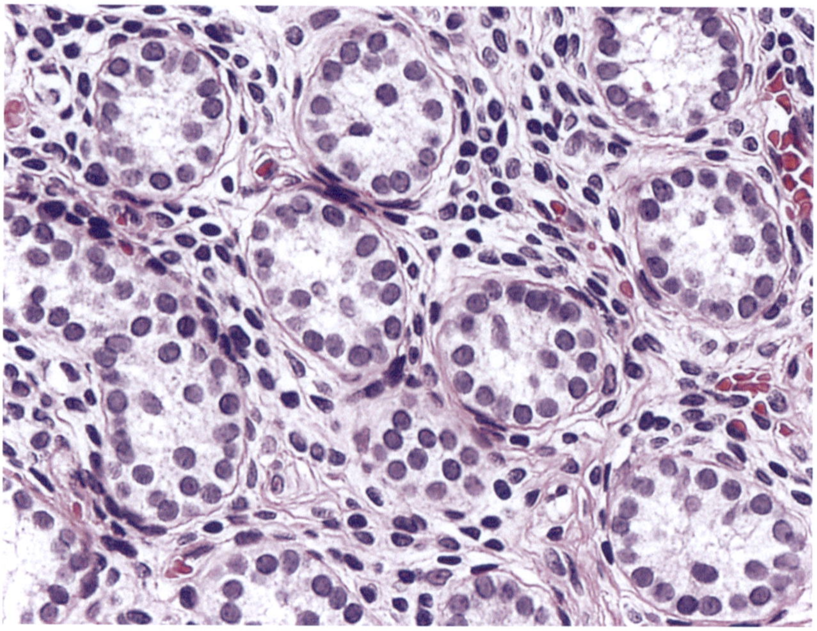

Fig. 11.2 Cryptorchidism type III. The absence of germ cells in a 3-year-old child. The seminiferous tubules have reduced diameter and a low number of Sertoli cells

The *tubular fertility index (TFI)* [18] is the percentage of tubular sections shown by at least one germ cell. In normal testicles this number decreases from birth (68 %) until the end of 3 years of age (50 %) and, slowly, increases again to reach 100 % at puberty [19]. TFI decreases can be slight (TFI higher than 50 %), marked (TFI between 50 and 30 %), and intense (TFI lower than 30 %). Marked and intense decreases are very frequent in undescended testes, often associated with low tubular diameters [20] (Fig. 11.2).

Germ Cell Number per Cross-Sectioned Tubule In normal testes, the number of spermatogonia decreases from birth to the end of 3 years of life, increases slowly up to 8 years of age, decreases again between 9 and 10 years, and markedly increases once more from 12 years of age to the end of puberty [21, 22]. In most undescended testes, this parameter is decreased.

Distribution of Spermatogonia in the Testicular Parenchyma Undescended testes frequently show an irregular distribution of germ cells. There are tubules devoid of them that have the peculiarity, as found in serial sections, to belong to the same lobule. These tubules will probably never develop spermatogenesis.

Germ Cell Types Changes in the number of spermatogonia and gonocytes can be observed in cryptorchidic testes, as well as the appearance of hypertrophic and multinucleated spermatogonia. The differential count of spermatogonia and gonocytes enables to differentiate two groups of undescended testes. One of these groups shows the following changes: complete migration of gonocytes and fetal spermatogonia from the center of the seminiferous tubules to the periphery, transformation of gonocytes into A dark spermatogonia, and the absence of gonocytes after the first year of life. In the second group of undescended testes, these events have not occurred. The transformation of gonocytes in Ad spermatogonia that occurs in late pregnancy and the first months of life is an androgen-dependent phenomenon, and it is not present in many undescended testicles [23].

The first group has a similar-to-testis normal behavior and therefore has undergone mini-puberty. In the second group, mini-puberty does not occur and patients are carrier of hypogonadotropic hypogonadism [24, 25]. A mini-puberty defect may be present in up to 50 % of cryptorchidic boys [26]. The presence of Ad spermatogonia in childhood in both testes is positively correlated with fertility [27].

Appearance of First-Order Spermatocytes Throughout the fourth year of life, some spermatocytes that are located in the central part of the tubule appear in many seminiferous tubules of the control testes [28]. This initial spermatogenesis does not progress and is a transient event. It is not related to any increase in FSH, LH, or testosterone but most likely depends on the appearance of androgen receptors in the Sertoli cells that would optimize the small amounts of androgens produced by the Leydig cells. First-order spermatocytes are absent in many undescended testicles [29].

Hypertrophic and Multinucleated Spermatogonia Hypertrophic spermatogonia are observed in most undescended testes. They are interpreted as cells unable to complete mitosis once they were able to duplicate the DNA [30]. Multinucleated spermatogonia appear in 8 % of undescended testicles. The nuclei may be all Ad or Ap spermatogonia or a combination of the two types. They are considered the product of amitotic divisions and a feature of cellular degeneration [31] (Figs. 11.3 and 11.4).

Sertoli Cells In childhood the Sertoli cells are mainly responsible for the testicular volume and represent 93–95 % of cells in the tubule [32]. The increase in testicular volume is linked to growth in length of the seminiferous tubules, facilitated by the displacement of the Sertoli cells along same, rather than to an increase of the tubular diameter. The number of Sertoli cells per tubular cross section suffers only moderate changes throughout childhood.

However, in half of the cases of undescended testes, the number of Sertoli cells is lower than normal (<26 ±3 per cross tubular section at the time of birth) [33]. This number decreases to 16±2 at the end of the third year. Sertoli cells often do not acquire androgen receptors at 4 years of age, or do so irregularly, and they are present in some children but not in others (Fig. 11.5); this situation is usually prolonged beyond puberty. Two-point-six percent of undescended testes show focal granular changes in the Sertoli cells. These granular changes represent an accumulation of large lysosomes in their cytoplasm [34]. Sertoli cell-only tubules frequently express D2-40 (Fig. 11.6).

Leydig Cells Based on the number of Leydig cells and their differentiation throughout childhood, there are two types of undescended testi-

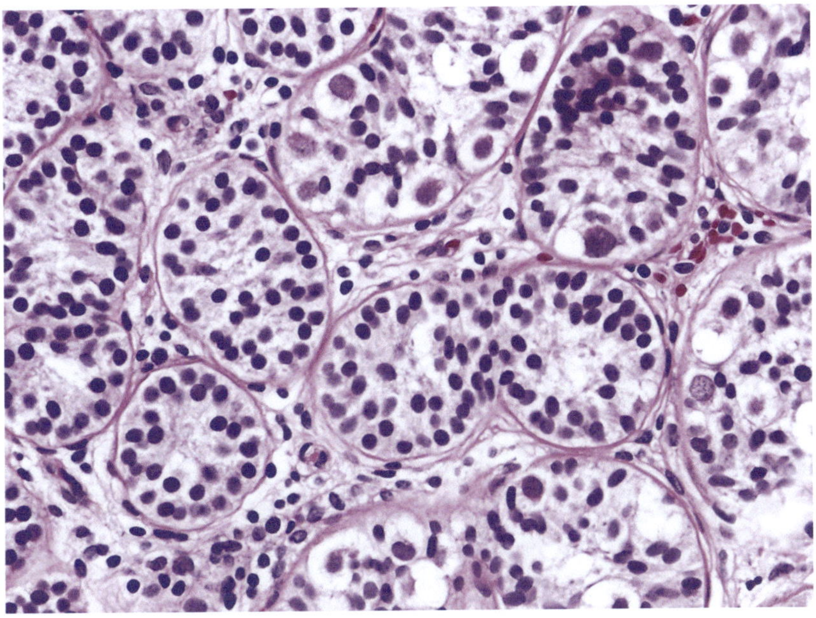

Fig. 11.3 Hypertrophic spermatogonia in an undescended testicle of a 3-year-old child

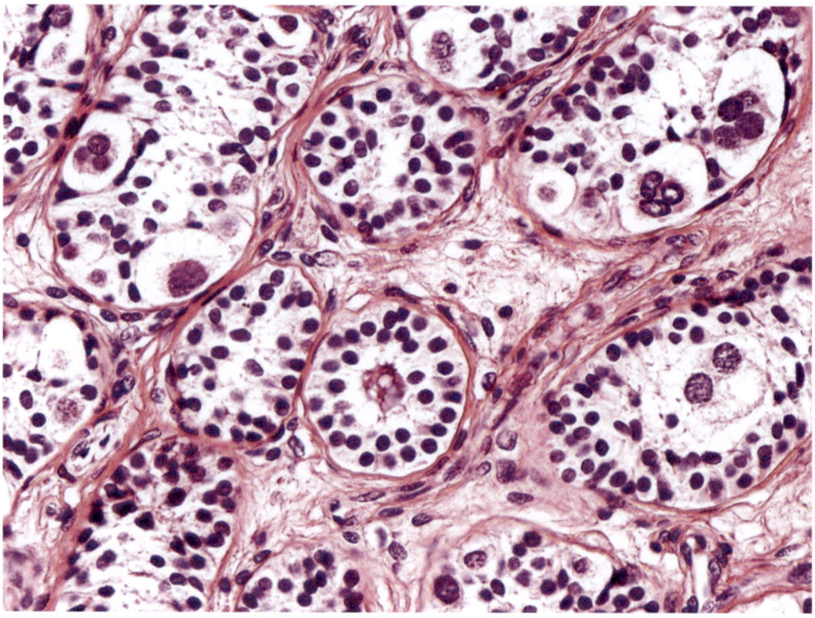

Fig. 11.4 Undescended testicle of a 3-year-old child showing multinucleated spermatogonia located both over the basement membrane and within the seminiferous tubules

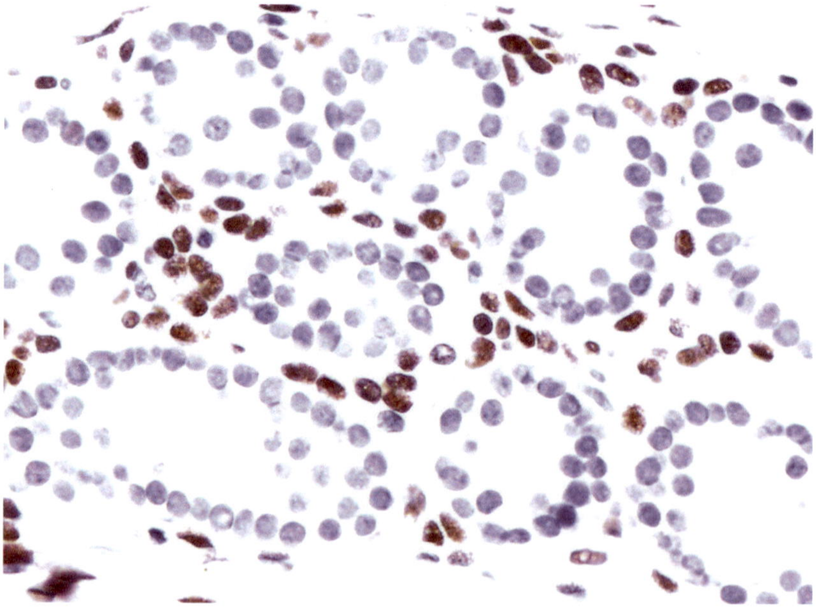

Fig. 11.5 Undescended testicle of a 9-year-old boy. The absence of androgen receptor expression in the nuclei of Sertoli cells in contrast to the presence of androgen receptor staining in myoid cells of the tubular walls can be seen

cles. In one of these types, the Leydig cells show marked atrophy [35, 36]. These testes are associated with the absence of Ad spermatogonia and suboptimal testosterone secretion. Other testes show normal secretion of testosterone and the presence of Ad spermatogonia. The first group supports the idea of an endocrine disease as an etiological factor in cryptorchidism [6].

Contralateral Testis In many cases the contralateral testis shows lesions similar to the undescended testis, reinforcing the idea that cryptorchidism is a bilateral disease [37, 38].

Development of Epididymis Histological studies have revealed a delay in the development of the epididymis in all prepubertal undescended testicles. The height of the epithelium, the development of the muscular layer, and the amplitude of light are affected [39].

11.3 Classification of Undescended Testis

The frequency with which the previously described histological lesions are grouped allows to classify most testicular biopsies from cryptorchidic testis of children younger than 4 years of age in three types: type I, testes with slight alterations (31 % of undescended testes); type II, testes with marked germinal hypoplasia (29 %); and type III, testes with severe germinal hypoplasia (40 %) [40] (Table 11.1).

Ninety-five percent of the testicles with type I lesions have spermatogonia type Ad, suggesting that they have undergone mini-puberty. About 8 % show many multinucleated spermatogonia. Type I lesions are comparable to the lesions seen in experimental cryptorchidism and also in normal testes with lesions induced by increased temperature [38].

The testicles with type II lesions show a slight thickening of the lamina propria. Twenty percent also show Ad spermatogonia, but their number is very limited by the presence of abundant tubules devoid of germ cells. Most testes with type III lesions lack Ad spermatogonia and have marked thickening of the tunica propria and in 30 % of cases microliths (Fig. 11.7).

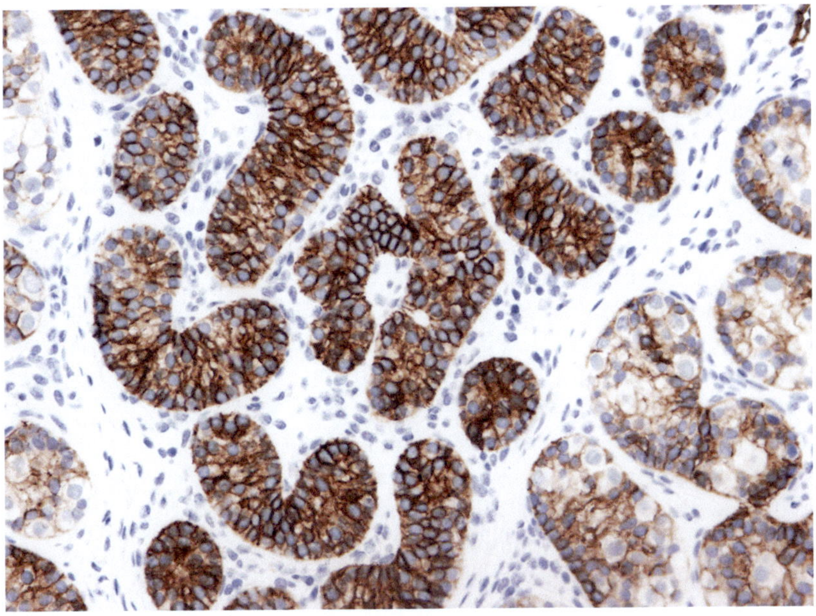

Fig. 11.6 Testicular lobule of an undescended testis with Sertoli cell-only tubules positive for D2-40 is side by side with other seminiferous tubule with germ cells

Table 11.1 Classification of histological lesions in prepubertal cryptorchidic testis according to morphometric parameters

Type of lesion (incidence)	MTD	TFI (%)	SCN	Spermatogonia distribution	Spermatogonia Ad
Type I (31 %)	Slightly decreased (90 % normal values)	>50	Normal	Regular	95 %
Type II (29 %)	Markedly decreased (90–60 % normal values)	30–50	Decreased	Irregular	29 %
Type III (40 %)	Severely decreased (<60 % normal values)	0–30	Very low	Irregular	Isolated

MTD mean tubular diameter, *TFI* tubular fertility index (percentage of germ cell-containing tubules), *SCN* Sertoli cell number (average Sertoli cell number per cross-sectioned tubule)

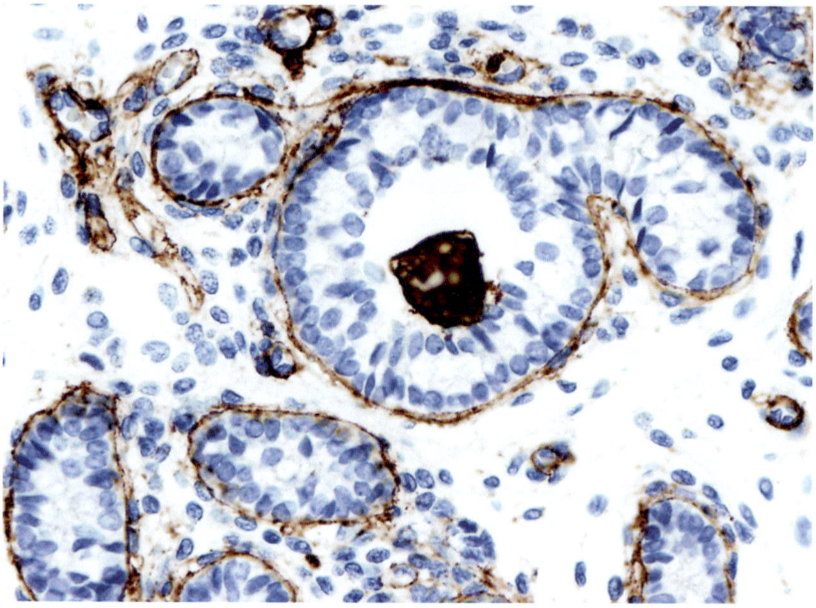

Fig. 11.7 A microlith is inside a large seminiferous tubule in a child with cryptorchidism type III. Immunostaining with type IV collagen

The contralateral testis in unilateral cryptorchidism often presents lesions. Generally these lesions are of lower degree than those of the undescended testis, but they may be similar and in some cases even more severe. In unilateral cryptorchidism 71 % of scrotal testes have a small number of germ cells and 75 % have impaired transformation of gonocytes in Ad spermatogonia [27]. The most frequent lesions in patients with bilateral cryptorchidism are types II and III.

Fifty percent of acquired undescended testes develop lesions similar to those of congenital cryptorchidism, and the same occurs with retractile testicles [41, 42]. This has led to consider that congenital cryptorchidism, retractile testicles, and acquired undescended testes are part of the spectrum of the same process in which hormonal factors play a very important role [43, 44].

References

1. Scott HM, Mason JI, Sharpe RM. Steroidogenesis in the fetal testis and its susceptibility to disruption by exogenous compounds. Endocr Rev. 2009;30: 883–925.
2. Shima Y, Miyabayashi K, Haraguchi S, Arakawa T, Otake H, Baba T, Matsuzaki S, Shishido Y, Akiyama H, Tachibana T, Tsutsui K, Morohashi K. Contribution of Leydig and Sertoli cells to testosterone production in mouse fetal testes. Mol Endocrinol. 2013;27:63–73.
3. Anand-Ivell R, Ivell R, Driscoll D, Manson J. Insulin-like factor 3 levels in amniotic fluid of human male fetuses. Hum Reprod. 2008;23:1180–6.
4. Hutson JM, Li R, Southwell BR, Newgreen D, Cousinery M. Regulation of testicular descent. Pediatr Surg Int. 2015;31:317–25.
5. Kuiri-Hänninen T, Sankilampi U, Dunkel L. Activation of the hypothalamic-pituitary-gonadal axis in infancy: minipuberty. Horm Res Paediatr. 2014;82:73–80.
6. Hadziselimovic F. Cryptorchidism, its impact on male fertility. Eur Urol. 2002;41:121–3.
7. Wilkerson ML, Bartone FF, Fox L, Hadziselimovic F. Fertility potential: a comparison of intra-abdominal and intracanalicular testes by age groups in children. Horm Res. 2001;55:18–20.
8. Prader A. Testicular size: assessment and clinical importance. Triangle. 1966;7:240–3.
9. Takihara H, Sakatoku J, Fujii M, Nasu T, Cosentino MJ, Cockett AT. Significance of testicular size measurement in andrology. I. A new orchiometer and its clinical application. Fertil Steril. 1983;39:836–40.
10. Taskinen S, Taavitsainen M, Wikström S. Measurement of testicular volume: comparison of 3 different methods. J Urol. 1996;155:930–3.
11. Lambert B. The frequency of mumps and of mumps orchitis and the consequences for sexuality and fertility. Acta Genet Stat Med. 1951;2:1–166.
12. Kuijper EA, van Kooten J, Verbeke JI, van Rooijen M, Lambalk CB. Ultrasonographically measured testicular volumes in 0- to 6-year-old boys. Hum Reprod. 2008;3:792–6.
13. Niedzielski J, Pisarska K, Przewratil P. The usefulness of testicular atrophy index in the assessment of unde-

scended testicle–preliminary report. Rocz Akad Med Bialymst. 2003;48:112–4.
14. Spinelli C, Strambi S, Busetto M, Pucci V, Bianco F. Effects on normalized testicular atrophy index (TAIn) in cryptorchid infants treated with GnRHa pre and post-operative vs surgery alone: a prospective randomized trial and long-term follow-up on 62 cases. Pediatr Surg Int. 2014;30:1061–7.
15. Jallouli M, Rebai T, Abid N, Bendhaou M, Kassis M, Mhiri R. Neoadjuvant gonadotropin-releasing hormone therapy before surgery and effect on fertility index in unilateral undescended testes: a prospective randomized trial. Urology. 2009;73:1251–4.
16. Schwentner C, Oswald J, Kreczy A, Lunacek A, Bartsch G, Deibl M, Radmayr C. Neoadjuvant gonadotropin-releasing hormone therapy before surgery may improve the fertility index in undescended testes: a prospective randomized trial. J Urol. 2005;173:974–7.
17. Caterino S, Lorenzon L, Cavallini M, Cavaniglia D, Ferro F. Epididymal-testicular fusion anomalies in cryptorchidism are associated with proximal location of the undescended testis and with a widely patent processus vaginalis. J Anat. 2014;225:473–8.
18. Mack WS, Scott LS, Ferguson-Smith MA, Lennox B. Ectopic testis and true undescended testis: a histological comparison. J Pathol Bacteriol. 1961;82: 439–43.
19. Müller J, Skakkebaek NE. Quantification of germ cells and seminiferous tubules by stereological examination of testicles from 50 boys who suffered from sudden death. Int J Androl. 1983;6:143–56.
20. Queizán de la Fuente A, Nistal M. Contribution to the study and treatment of cryptorchism. Cir Pediatr. 1989;2:157–67.
21. Paniagua R, Nistal M. Morphological and histometric study of human spermatogonia from birth to the onset of puberty. J Anat. 1984;139:535–52.
22. Cortes D, Thorup JM, Beck BL. Quantitative histology of germ cells in the undescended testes of human fetuses, neonates and infants. J Urol. 1995;154: 1188–92.
23. Zivkovic D, Bica DT, Hadziselimovic F. Relationship between adult dark spermatogonia and secretory capacity of Leydig cells in cryptorchidism. BJU Int. 2007;100:1147–9.
24. Hadziselimovic F, Zivkovic D. Is the prohibition of hormonal treatment for cryptorchidism, as suggested by the Nordic consensus group, justifiable? Acta Paediatr. 2007;96:1368–9.
25. Docampo MJ, Hadziselimovic F. Molecular pathology of cryptorchidism-induced infertility. Sex Dev. 2015;9:269–78.
26. Bilius V, Verkauskas G, Dasevicius D, Kazlauskas V, Malcius D, Hadziselimovic F. Incidence of high infertility risk among unilateral cryptorchid boys. Urol Int. 2015;95:142–5.
27. Hadziselimovic F, Hoecht B. Testicular histology related to fertility outcome and postpubertal hormone status in cryptorchidism. Klin Padiatr. 2008;220:302–7.
28. Nistal M, Paniagua R. Occurrence of primary spermatocytes in the infant and child testis. Andrologia. 1984;16:532–6.
29. Huff DS, Hadziselimovic F, Snyder 3rd HM, Duckett JW, Keating MA. Postnatal testicular maldevelopment in unilateral cryptorchidism. J Urol. 1989;142: 546–8.
30. Codesal J, Nistal M, Queizan A, Carretero JL, de Vega RM, Perez A, Paniagua R. Number and DNA content of hypertrophic spermatogonia in normal and cryptorchid human testes. Arch Androl. 1992;29: 157–62.
31. Cortes D, Thorup J, Visfeldt J. Multinucleated spermatogonia in cryptorchid boys: a possible association with an increased risk of testicular malignancy later in life? APMIS. 2003;111:25–30.
32. Chemes HE. Infancy is not a quiescent period of testicular development. Int J Androl. 2001;24:2–7.
33. Nistal M, Abaurrea MA, Paniagua R. Morphological and histometric study on the human Sertoli cell from birth to the onset of puberty. J Anat. 1982;134: 351–63.
34. Nistal M, Regadera J, Winitzky P, Tejerina E, Chemes H. Granular changes in Sertoli cells in children and pubertal patients. Fertil Steril. 2005;83:1489–99.
35. Hadziselimovic F, Herzog B, Seguchi H. Surgical correction of cryptorchism at 2 years: electron microscopic and morphometric investigations. J Pediatr Surg. 1975;10:19–26.
36. Nistal M, Paniagua R, Regadera J, Santamarìa L, Amat P. A quantitative morphological study of human Leydig cells from birth to adulthood. Cell Tissue Res. 1986;246:229–36.
37. Salle B, Hedinger C, Nicole R. Significance of testicular biopsies in cryptorchidism in children. Acta Endocrinol. 1968;58:67–76.
38. Huff DS, Fenig DM, Canning DA, Carr MG, Zderic SA, Snyder 3rd HM. Abnormal germ cell development in cryptorchidism. Horm Res. 2001;55:11–7.
39. De Miguel MP, Mariño JM, Gonzalez-Peramato P, Nistal M, Regadera J. Epididymal growth and differentiation are altered in human cryptorchidism. J Androl. 2001;22:212–25.
40. Nistal M, Paniagua R, Díez-Pardo JA. Histologic classification of undescended testes. Hum Pathol. 1980;11:666–74.
41. Herruzo A, Sánchez Corral F, Nistal M, Ruíz Balda JA, Cuadrado C. Seminal pathology in patients with retractile testes. Acta Obstet Ginecol Hisp Lusit. 1979;27:181–93.
42. Nistal M, Paniagua R. Infertility in adult males with retractile testes. Fertil Steril. 1984;41:395–403.
43. Tanyel FC. The descent of testis and reason for failed descent. Turk J Pediatr. 2004;46(Suppl):7–17.
44. van Brakel J, Kranse R, de Muinck Keizer-Schrama SM, Hendriks AE, de Jong FH, Hack WW, van der Voort-Doedens LM, Bangma CH, Hazebroek FW, Dohle GR. Fertility potential in a cohort of 65 men with previously acquired undescended testes. J Pediatr Surg. 2014;49:599–605.

The Most Frequent Histological Findings in the Adult Testis When Testicular Descent Was Performed in Childhood

12

Manuel Nistal, Pilar González-Peramato, and Álvaro Serrano

12.1 Most Frequent Testicular Lesions Observed in Adulthood

The extensive use of in vitro fertilization techniques has indirectly contributed to a resurgence of testicular biopsy. The material obtained from patients with azoospermia or oligozoospermia is useful not for extracting sperm but also for immunohistochemical or genetic histological studies. The results from three series of patients studied in our Department of Pathology of Hospital La Paz are discussed in this chapter: (Group A) undescended testicles biopsied or removed in the adult; (Group B) patients who consulted for infertility and had two biopsies, one at the time of surgical descent in childhood and another one in adulthood during the study of infertility; and (group C) patients with undescended testes who had been treated surgically in childhood and now consulted for infertility.

Group A: Undescended Testes Biopsied or Removed in the Adult This group consisted of 19 testes of patients aged 16–54 years. Cryptorchidism was unilateral in 18 and bilateral in one. All were located in the inguinal canal except for three that were abdominal. All testes were smaller than normal, 12 were removed, and the rest had been descended. All had histological lesions affecting the seminiferous tubules and interstitium. The seminiferous epithelium lesions were mixed atrophy in six cases with less than 50 % of tubes with spermatogenesis (spermatogenesis was very poor in most of them) (Fig. 12.1), two cases with maturation arrest in spermatogonia (the number of spermatogonia per seminiferous tube was very small) (Fig. 12.2), five cases with Sertoli cell- only (Fig. 12.3), and six cases with variable degrees of tubular hyalinization until the total disappearance of the seminiferous epithelium (Fig. 12.4). The lesions were similar to those of other series [1]. An obstructive pattern was recognized in four cases (Table 12.1).

Sertoli cells in the tubules with Sertoli cell-only often show cytological signs of immaturity [2]. This immaturity manifests immunohistochemically in different ways, in the basal cytoplasm for positivity for cytokeratins and vimentin [3, 4] and in the apical cytoplasm by the presence of inhibin bodies [5] and decreased or absent expression of the androgen receptor [6]. In the tubular wall, immaturity is recognized by a decrease in elastic fibers [7], increased collagenization and irregular deposits of laminin and collagen IV [8, 9], and a partial loss of contractile marker proteins in the peritubular cells [10].

Sertoli cell nodules were observed in 7 out of the 12 removed testes and granular changes in Sertoli cells in three of them. Leydig cells were scarce in eight, they formed large clusters in the vicinity of the rete testis and subalbuginea areas in five, and the remaining cases showed cytoplasmic microvacuolization [11]. The rete testis of 7 out of

M. Nistal et al., *Clues in the Diagnosis of Non-tumoral Testicular Pathology*,
DOI 10.1007/978-3-319-49364-0_12

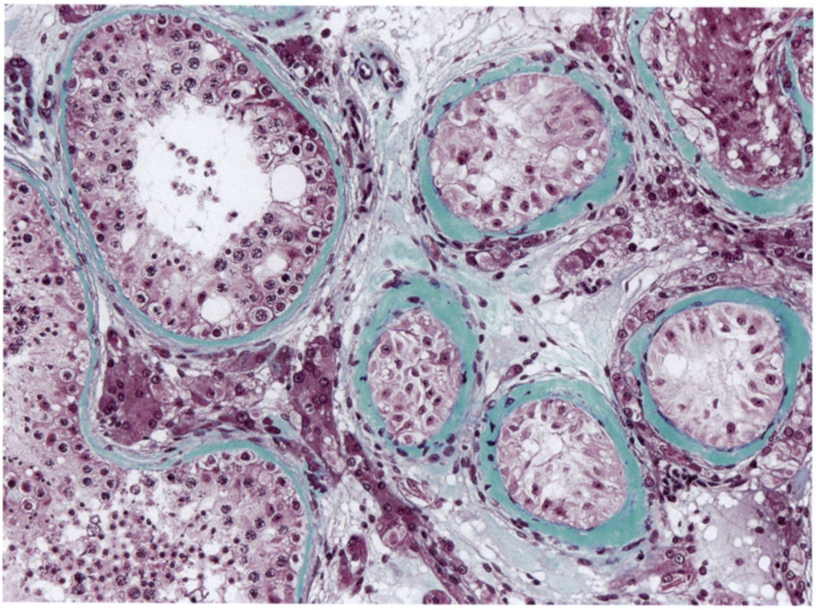

Fig. 12.1 Mixed atrophy. Tubules with complete spermatogenesis are adjacent to other smaller Sertoli cell-only tubules devoid of the lumen with marked wall thickening

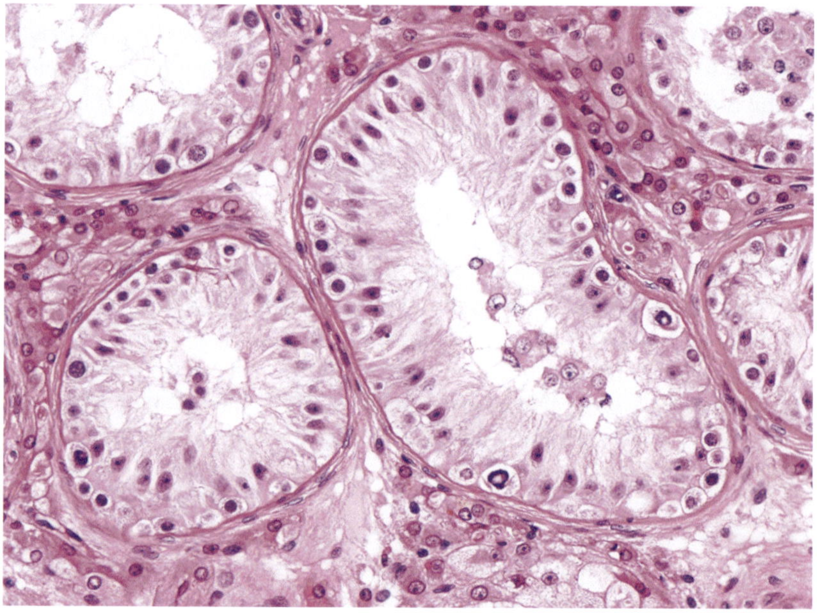

Fig. 12.2 Seminiferous tubules showing maturation arrest in spermatogonia. The seminiferous tubules only have spermatogonia, most of them type A dark, and Sertoli cells. The interstitium shows mild Leydig cell hyperplasia

the 12 specimens of orchiectomy was hyperplasic (rete testis dysgenesis) [12].

Group B: Patients with Pre- and Postpubertal Bilateral Biopsies This group consisted of 25 patients. The size of the undescended testes was normal in 5 and decreased in 20. The results of biopsies of ex-cryptorchidic adult testis were as follows: 21 showed mixed atrophy (tubules with spermatogenesis were less than 50 % in 20 cases). Two had late spermatocyte sloughing (Fig. 12.5), one had early first-order spermatocyte sloughing (Fig. 12.6), and one had Sertoli cell-only. Eleven testes (six patients with corrected bilateral cryptorchidism) had Leydig cell hyperplasia.

Of the 16 contralateral testes studied, 13 were of normal size, two were smaller than normal, and one was larger than normal due to a germ cell tumor. Histologically, seven cases had mixed atrophy with complete spermatogenesis in over 50 % of the seminiferous tubule biopsy, four cases had

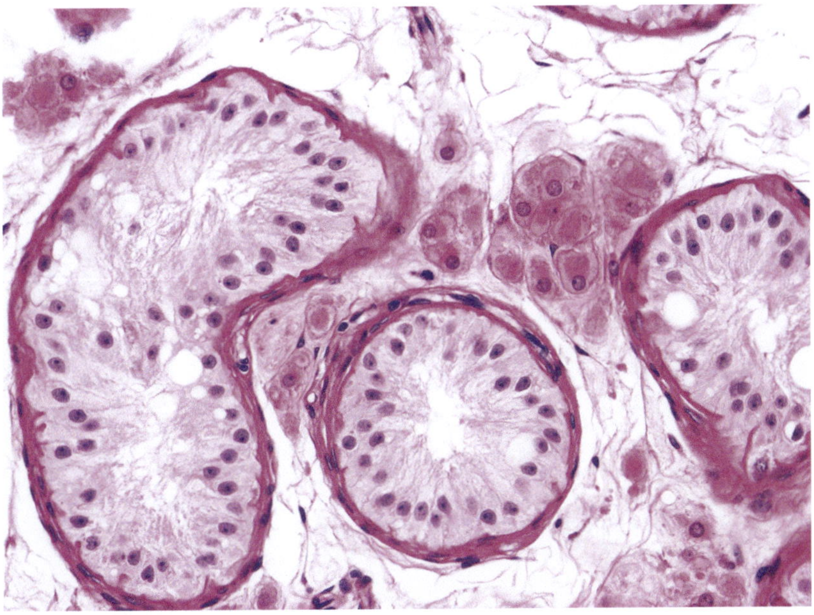

Fig. 12.3 Seminiferous tubules with Sertoli cell-only. Seminiferous tubules lack lumen, have thickening of the tubular wall, and are lined by Sertoli cells preferably with oval nuclei and central nucleolus

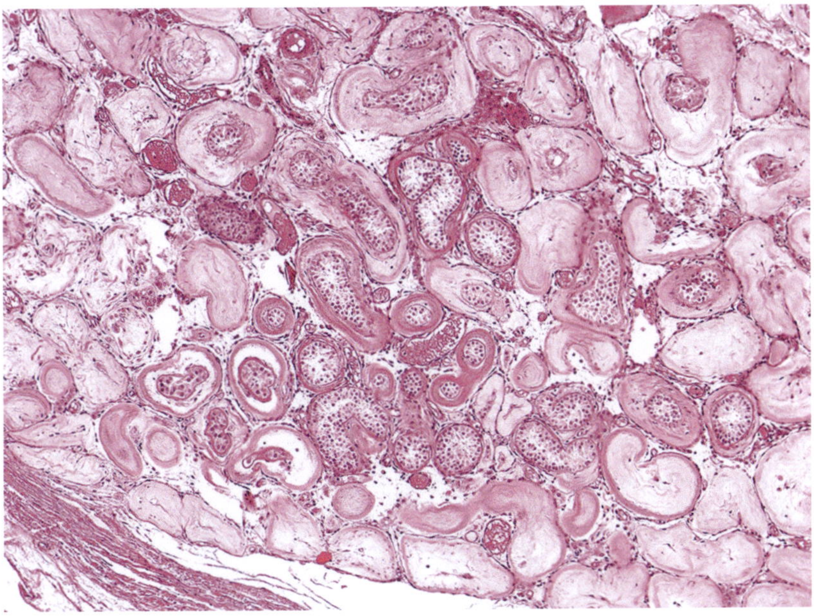

Fig. 12.4 Diffuse tubular hyalinization. Most seminiferous tubules have concentric hyalinization. Some Sertoli cells still persist inside seminiferous tubules

late spermatocyte sloughing, one had early first-order spermatocyte sloughing, three cases had hypospermatogenesis associated with first-order spermatocyte sloughing (Fig. 12.7), and one case had Sertoli cell-only. Leydig cell hyperplasia was observed in two biopsies (the data are taken from previously published work: [13]).

Group C: Patients with Undescended Testes Who Had Been Treated Surgically in Childhood and Now Consulted for Infertility Eighteen biopsies were studied. In all cases only the primitively scrotal testes were biopsied due to their larger size. Three patients had consulted for azoospermia and 15 for severe oligozoospermia. In five cases the serum levels of FSH and LH were elevated. Serum testosterone levels were within normal limits. The size of the testicle that was descended was decreased in 13 cases, and in five cases, the decreased size also affected the contralateral testis, even though to a lesser

Table 12.1 Seminiferous tubule lesions in patients with undescended testes

	Group A 19 testes	Group B 41 testes		Group C 18 testes
		Patients with pre- and postpubertal bilateral biopsies		
Seminiferous tubule lesions	Undescended testes biopsied or removed in the adult	Ex-cryptorchidic testis 25 testes	Contralateral testes 16 testes	Contralateral to the testis descended in childhood
Mixed atrophy	6 All have <50 % tubules with spermatogenesis	21 20 have <50 % tubules with spermatogenesis	7 All have complete spermatogenesis in >50 % tubules	9 All have complete spermatogenesis in >50 % tubules
Late sloughing of spermatocyte I		2	4	7
Early sloughing of spermatocyte I		1	1	1
Hypospermatogenesis + spermatocyte I sloughing			3	
Maturation arrest in spermatogonia	2			
Sertoli only-cell	5	1	1	1
Diffuse tubular hyalinization	6			
Obstructive pattern	4	9	6	5

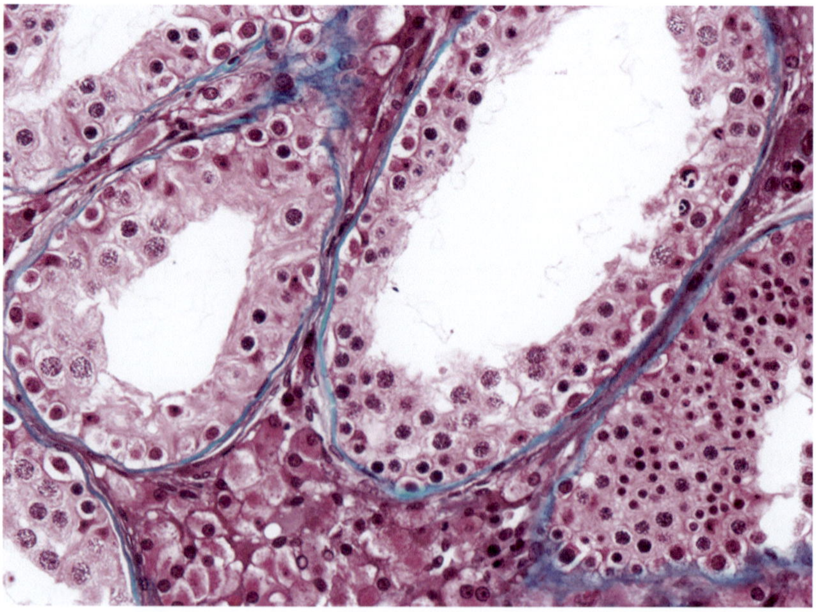

Fig. 12.5 Late first-order spermatocyte. Seminiferous tubules with dilated lumen. Germ cells are represented by a normal number of spermatogonia and spermatocytes of the first order. The number of spermatids is very low

extent. Histological lesions were mixed atrophy in nine cases with spermatogenesis in more than 50 % of the tubules, late spermatocyte sloughing in seven cases, one case of early first-order spermatocyte sloughing, and one case of Sertoli cell-only.

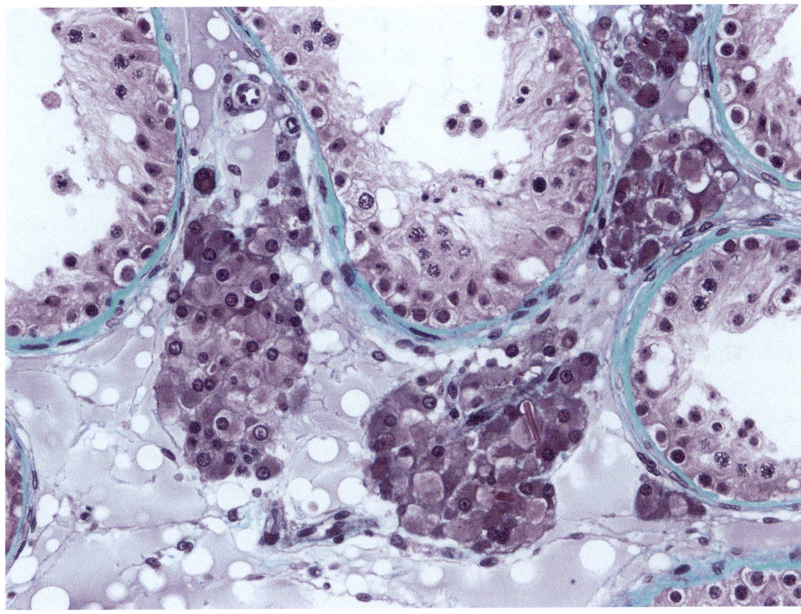

Fig. 12.6 Early first-order spermatocyte sloughing. Tubular sections with numerous spermatogonia, small number of first-order spermatocytes, and isolated spermatids are observed. The interstitium shows nodular Leydig cell hyperplasia

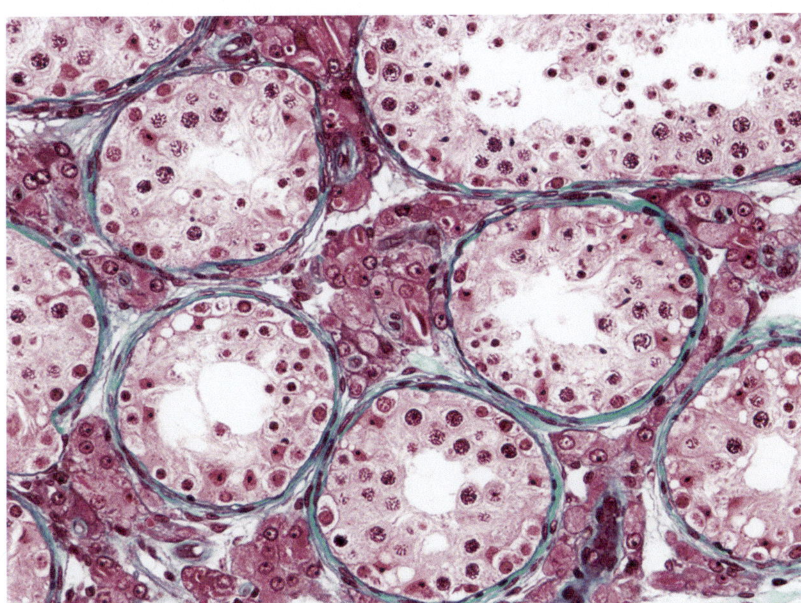

Fig. 12.7 Seminiferous tubes with hypospermatogenesis. The seminiferous tubules are small. All types of germ cells are present in proportionally decreased number. The interstitium showed diffuse Leydig cell hyperplasia

12.2 Correlation Between Pre- and Postpubertal Biopsies

In patients of group B, the lesions found in prepubertal biopsy were compared with the biopsy performed in adulthood. The lesions of the first biopsy (biopsy at the time of orchiopexy) of 25 patients with undescended testes were classified according to previous studies [13–15] already discussed in Chap. 11, in normal or type I (testes with slight alterations), 3 cases; type II (testes with marked germinal cell hypoplasia), 4 cases; and type III (testes with severe germinal cell hypoplasia), 18 testes. As for the contralateral testes (15 testes), 11 had minimal alterations or type I lesions, 2 had type II lesions, 2 had type III lesions, and 1 testis was not found.

Patients with type I lesions or minimal alterations developed diffuse spermatogenesis in more than two thirds of cases and a pattern of mixed atrophy in the remaining cases, but complete spermatogenesis was quantitatively abnormal. All patients with type II lesions and 85 % of patients with type III lesions develop mixed atrophy, which makes the mixed atrophy the most common lesion in adult's testes that were descended in childhood (68 %). These data confirm that the number of germ cells [16],and the presence of Ad spermatogonia type [17, 18] are the two most important data for the prognostic assessment of testicular biopsy.

While mixed atrophy is defined as the presence of tubules with Sertoli cell-only side by side with spermatogenesis, several details of this lesion should be specified; some are related to tubules with Sertoli cell-only and others with tubules with spermatogenesis. With respect to the tubules with Sertoli cell-only, it is necessary to evaluate (a) the number of tubules with Sertoli cell-only in relation to the tubules with spermatogenesis. In cryptorchidic testes the number of seminiferous tubules with Sertoli cell-only is greater than 50 %, while in the contralateral scrotal, it is less than 50 %; (b) Sertoli cell type. In the tubules with Sertoli cell-only in cryptorchidic testes, Sertoli cells are preferably dysgenetic, while they are the adult type in descended testes. With respect to the tubules with spermatogenesis, the most common lesions are located in the adluminal compartment (late first-order spermatocyte sloughing and early first-order spermatocyte sloughing). Hypospermatogenesis cases are rare and arrested maturation of spermatocytes or spermatogonia was not observed.

12.3 Associated Secondary Testicular Lesions in Adult Testes

12.3.1 Obstruction

Three parameters were applied to assess the possibility of an obstruction. One was a histological parameter (set of tubular lesions secondary to increased hydrostatic pressure that form a pattern [see Chap. 17, Lesions of the Obstructive Mechanism Simulating Primary Testicular Lesions]) (Fig. 12.8). Another parameter was quantitative: the number of adult spermatids higher than the number of young spermatids in

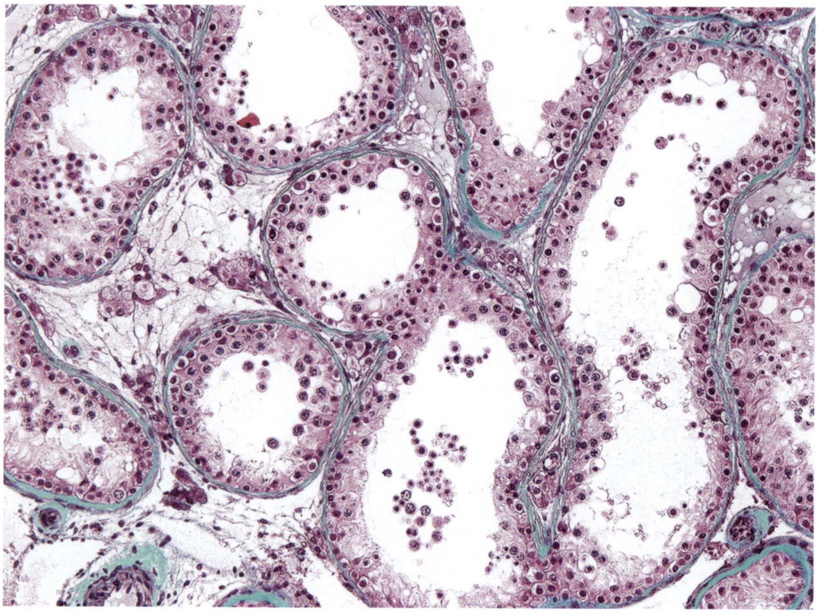

Fig. 12.8 Seminiferous tubules showing marked lumen dilatation and atrophy of the seminiferous epithelium characteristic of obstructive patterns

the cross tubular section of the seminiferous tubules [19]. In the B and C groups, a third parameter applied was the correlation between the number of adult spermatids per tubular section in the biopsy and the number of sperm in the semen per ml [20]. Signs of partial or total obstruction in the spermatic pathway were observed in four testes in group A, in nine ex-cryptorchidic and six contralateral testes of group B, and in five contralateral testes of group C. These findings were surprising but they could be expected if we consider the frequent anomalies described in the epididymis [21, 22]. In group B, deferential absence of the ipsilateral testicle to the surgically descended one was expressly confirmed in the clinical history in one case and herniorrhaphy in another case. Concerning the epididymis two cases had epididymis-testicular dissociation and ten cases an elongated epididymis.

12.3.2 Varicocele

In a total of 21 patients studied for infertility with a clinical history of surgically descended cryptorchidism in childhood (group B), varicocele was observed in three patients, ipsilateral with a surgically descended testis in childhood in one case. Varicocele was also observed in three patients of group C, one in the ex-cryptorchidic testicle and two in the contralateral one.

12.4 Summary of the Nature of Testicular Lesions

The following facts are noteworthy:

1. Elevated temperature exerts a less important effect on the testicle than has conventionally been claimed in the literature. Lesions in scrotal contralateral testes are very similar to those of the ex-cryptorchidic testes.
2. The most common lesion in both undescended and contralateral scrotal testes is mixed atrophy. They differ in the percentage of tubules with Sertoli cell-only and the severity of lesions of the tubules with germ cells.
3. The patchy distribution of the groups of seminiferous tubules with Sertoli cell-only observed, both in children testes (testicles with type II and type III lesions) and in second biopsies of these same patients in adulthood, suggests on the one hand that tubules with Sertoli cell-only belong to the same lobule and on the other hand that they never possessed these germ cells or they disappeared during fetal life.
4. The presence and number of Ad spermatogonia type is much higher in children's testes with type I lesions than in those showing type II and III lesions, which is related to a more careful observation of spermatogenesis of these patients in the second biopsy.
5. In a significant number of adult testes, both ex-cryptorchidic and contralateral, there are obstructive lesions associated with either organic or functional nature. These lesions are focal and multiple; they affect the seminiferous tubules with spermatogenesis and may be secondary to dysgenesis of the rete testis and epididymis or deferential anomalies.
6. Lesions in the undescended testes, both caused by hypogonadism and secondary to temperature or obstruction of the spermatic ducts, are progressive and lead not only to the loss of all germ cells but also to the disappearance of Sertoli cells thus causing a diffuse tubular hyalinization
7. A significant percentage of cryptorchidic patients with azoospermia show groups of seminiferous tubules with spermatogenesis that, although quantitatively abnormal, may be sufficient to provide sperm for assisted reproduction techniques.
8. Although the beneficial effects of hormonal treatments on semen at the time of surgical descent are known, larger studies are needed that allow (a) to know the diminution of infertility consults of ex-cryptorchidic patients; (b) to compare in infertile patients who have been given supplemental hormonal treatment at the time of surgical descent, the biopsies practiced in childhood, and those made when consulting for infertility; and (c) to identify lesions secondary to obstruction that aggravate and blur preexisting lesions.

References

1. Jeong SC, Lee S, Ku JY, Lee SD. Clinical characteristics and treatment of cryptorchidism in adults: a single center experience. World J Mens Health. 2014;32:110–5.
2. Nistal M, Paniagua R, Abaurrea MA, Santamaría L. Hyperplasia and the immature appearance of Sertoli cells in primary testicular disorders. Hum Pathol. 1982;13:3–12.
3. Rogatsch H, Jezek D, Hittmair A, Mikuz G, Feichtinger H. Expression of vimentin, cytokeratin, and desmin in Sertoli cells of human fetal, cryptorchid, and tumour-adjacent testicular tissue. Virchows Arch. 1996;427:497–502.
4. Kruse R, Eigelshoven S, Kaiser A, Ruzicka T, Neumann NJ. Cytokeratin 18 expression in immature Sertoli cells: co-localization with interstitial lymphocytic infiltrates. Folia Histochem Cytobiol. 2009;47: 127–30.
5. Nistal M, Pastrián LG, González-Peramato P, De Miguel MP. Inhibin bodies: a new marker for immature Sertoli cells. Histopathology. 2011;58:1019–27.
6. Regadera J, Martínez-García F, González-Peramato P, Serrano A, Nistal M, Suárez-Quian C. Androgen receptor expression in sertoli cells as a function of seminiferous tubule maturation in the human cryptorchid testis. J Clin Endocrinol Metab. 2001;86:413–21.
7. Gotoh M, Miyake K, Mitsuya H. Elastic fibers in tunica propria of undescended and contralateral scrotal testes from cryptorchid patients. Urology. 1987;30:359–63.
8. Santamaria L, Martinez-Onsurbe P, Paniagua R, Nistal M. Laminin, type IV collagen, and fibronectin in normal and cryptorchid human testes. An immunohistochemical study. Int J Androl. 1990;13:135–46.
9. Paniagua R, Martinez-Onsurbe P, Santamaria L, Saez FJ, Amat P, Nistal M. Quantitative and ultrastructural alterations in the lamina propria and Sertoli cells in human cryptorchid testes. Int J Androl. 1990;13: 470–87.
10. Welter H, Kampfer C, Lauf S, Feil R, Schwarzer JU, Köhn FM, Mayerhofer A. Partial loss of contractile marker proteins in human testicular peritubular cells in infertility patients. Andrology. 2013;1:318–24.
11. Nistal M, Paniagua R, Abaurrea MA. Multivacuolated Leydig cells in human adult cryptorchid testes. Andrologia. 1981;13:436–9.
12. Nistal M, Jimenez-Hefferman JA. Rete testis dysgenesis: a characteristic lesion of undescended testes. Arch Pathol Lab Med. 1997;121:1259–64.
13. Nistal M, Riestra ML, Paniagua R. Correlation between testicular biopsies (prepubertal and postpubertal) and spermiogram in cryptorchid men. Hum Pathol. 2000;31:1022–30.
14. Nistal M, Paniagua R, Díez-Pardo JA. Histologic classification of undescended testes. Hum Pathol. 1980;11:666–74.
15. Nistal M, Paniagua R, Riestra ML, Reyes-Múgica M, Cajaiba MM. Bilateral prepubertal testicular biopsies predict significance of cryptorchidism-associated mixed testicular atrophy, and allow assessment of fertility. Am J Surg Pathol. 2007;1:1269–76.
16. Cortes D, Thorup JM, Lindenberg S. Fertility potential after unilateral orchiopexy: simultaneous testicular biopsy and orchiopexy in a cohort of 87 patients. J Urol. 1996;155:1061–5.
17. Hadziselimovic F, Hoecht B. Testicular histology related to fertility outcome and postpubertal hormone status in cryptorchidism. Klin Padiatr. 2008;220:302–7.
18. Thorup J, Kvist K, Clasen-Linde E, Petersen BL, Cortes D. The relation between adult dark spermatogonia and other parameters of fertility potential in cryptorchid testes. J Urol. 2013;190(4 Suppl): 1566–71.
19. Nistal M, Riestra ML, Galmés-Belmonte I, Paniagua R. Testicular biopsy in patients with obstructive azoospermia. Am J Surg Pathol. 1999;3:1546–54.
20. Nistal M, Codesal J, Santamarıa L, Paniagua R. Correlation between spermatozoon numbers in spermiogram and seminiferous epithelium histology in testicular biopsies from subfertile men. Fertil Steril. 1987;48:507–9.
21. DePalma L, Carter D, Weiss RM. Epididymal and vas deferens immaturity in cryptorchidism. J Urol. 1988;140:1194–6.
22. Mollaeian M, Mehrabi V, Elahi B. Significance of epididymal and ductal anomalies associated with undescended testis: study in 652 cases. Urology. 1994;43: 857–60.

Testicular Dysgenesis Syndrome (TDS)

13

Manuel Nistal, Pilar González-Peramato, and
Álvaro Serrano

13.1 Concept of Testicular Dysgenesis Syndrome

The term "testicular dysgenesis syndrome" was forged in 1992 following a study carried out by Danish researchers who communicated a 50 % decrease in the sperm count during the period 1938–1992 [1, 2]. The term was introduced to try to explain under only one umbrella the different disorders of the male reproductive apparatus that had the distinction of having experienced – although this was not accepted by all authors [3] – a rise in recent decades and had two peculiarities: that the increase of one of them was a risk factor for the other and also suspicion that they are secondary to human exposure to hormonally active chemicals. The TDS includes cryptorchidism, testicular cancer, hypospadias, and infertility [4].

13.1.1 Testicular Germ Cell Tumors

The increase in testicular germ cell tumors (TGCT) began to be observed in countries with Northern European ancestry, including Denmark, Norway, and New Zealand. Large increases were also observed between descendants of Europeans in the USA and more recently in countries traditionally with low rates of TGCT as Italy, Spain, and Finland. Overall it is estimated that the incidence of TGCT is 2–3 times higher than 30–40 years ago [5] with the exception of African-Americans, among whom it remains very low. Less than 25 % of cases are considered secondary to genetic factors, although 19 genetic polymorphisms associated with TGCT have been identified. The remaining TGCTs seem to be more related to environmental factors acting during the fetal life [6].

Patients with germ cell neoplasia in situ (GCNIS) and testicular cancer often have impaired spermatogenesis in the contralateral testicle. They also often have elevated levels of FSH and LH and low serum testosterone rates [7]. Most TGCTs originate in a cell originally called carcinoma in situ (CIS). These cells are derived from gonocytes that are unable to differentiate into spermatogonia *in the uterus*. This failure in differentiation probably depends on inappropriate age signaling from Sertoli (mainly growth factor GDNF and platelet-derived growth factor (PDGF) and Leydig cells, secondary to androgen/estrogen imbalance during fetal life [8].

13.1.2 Cryptorchidism

The assessment of the incidence of cryptorchidism among different countries is subjected to variations in approach, diagnosis, and registration. Congenital cryptorchidism affects 2–9 % of all newborn boys and 1–3 % of boys at 3 months of age, decreasing further to 0.7–1 % at the age

M. Nistal et al., *Clues in the Diagnosis of Non-tumoral Testicular Pathology*,
DOI 10.1007/978-3-319-49364-0_13

of 1. The incidence of acquired cryptorchidism is estimated between 1.5 and 2 % and justifies the higher prevalence of cryptorchidism between 5 and 11 years of age compared to its prevalence at birth. The incidence of undescended testes has increased in several countries such as Denmark from 1.8 % in 1959–1961 to 8.5 % in 1997–2001 [9]; in the UK a significant overall increase in the incidence of cryptorchidism at the age of three in children over 2500 g at birth has been observed, from 0.9 % in the 1950s to 1.6 % in the late 1980s and 4.0–5.4 % when including all newborn babies [10]. The risk of developing cancer for an undescended testicle is 5–10 times higher than in the general population [11]. The risk of testicular cancer is also increased in the contralateral testis [12].

13.1.3 Hypospadias

An increased incidence of hypospadias was noticed in many countries. In 1997, the Centers for Disease Control and Prevention (CDC) in the USA reported an increase from 20.2 per 10,000 live births in 1970 to 39.7 per 10,000 live births in 1993 ($p < 10^{-6}$) [13]. Denmark, Sweden, England and Wales, Hungary, Italy, and France also reported an increase in the rates of hypospadias during the 1960s, 1970s, and 1980s according to the International Clearinghouse for Birth Defects Monitoring Systems [14]. Recent studies also show a significant increase in Australia and New Zealand.

The etiology of hypospadias is multifactorial in which genetic factors and environment are somehow involved. Increasing rates of hypospadias have been linked to the increase in other pathologies of the male reproductive tract such as testicular cancer [15], cryptorchidism, and decreased sperm and sperm quality [16]. The association of hypospadias and cryptorchidism is reported in 4–20 % of cases [17]. A congenital deficiency of the Leydig cells would determine a decrease in testosterone production and INSL3, and in consequence both the masculinization of the external genitalia and testicular descent would be affected [18].

13.1.4 Infertility

The prevalence of infertility is estimated to affect 16 % of couples. The male is responsible for 20–30 % of infertility cases and contributes to 50 % of cases overall. There are significant geographic differences in sperm parameters between and within countries. A meta-analysis of 63 studies, mainly from the USA and from Western Europe, showed a reduction of nearly 50 % in mean sperm concentration, during the period 1940–1990 [1]. The conclusion was that there was a significant time-related negative trend in sperm concentration both in North America (0.8 % per year) and in Western Europe (2.4 % per year) during this period.

A significant decrease in sperm concentration and morphology has recently been observed in other countries (Finland, Israel, Spain, Tunisia, Scotland) and in sperm donors in France [19]. Fertility is decreased in patients with cryptorchidism and in those patients that will subsequently develop testicular cancer.

Fifty percent of masculine infertility cases cannot be explained by chromosomal abnormalities or acquired diseases such as orchitis, mumps, testicular torsion, varicocele, trauma, drugs, or irradiation. The cause of reduced spermatogenesis could be the exposure to environmental chemicals during fetal life and lifestyle factors throughout life [20]. The severity of male infertility seems to be directly related to the rate of hypospadias and undescended testicles during childhood [21]. The incidence of GCNIS in infertile men has been estimated between 1.1 and 4 %, so infertile men are at risk of developing testicular cancer [4].

13.2 Etiology of TDS

Endocrine disruptors are emerging as possible etiologic agents. They are exogenous chemical substances that once introduced in our organism modify the function of the endocrine system. Chemical components are not rapidly biodegradable but are bioaccumulative. The human embryo and fetus are exposed to endocrine disruptors through the placenta from conception to birth.

Lesions in the fetus and embryo are related, on the one hand with maternal exposure time and concentration and on the other hand with the time of development of the fetus.

Pesticides, concentrated food products containing natural plants estrogens, and by-products and final products of modern technology are outstanding among chemical disruptors. Endocrine disruptors may have either estrogenic or androgenic activity, or even both activities. Among those with estrogenic activity, the actions of bisphenol A and diethystilbestrol are well known [22]. The use of the estrogenic compound DES from the 1940s to 1971 produced in exposed boys an increased risk of cryptorchidism and epididymal cysts.

The most widely studied chemical components with both antiestrogenic and antiandrogenic action are phthalates. Phthalates are used as plasticizers in soft polyvinyl chloride (PVC). It is estimated that one trillion pounds of phthalates are produced every year. They are virtually ubiquitous. The routes by which man can contact them are manifold. They are in the air, dust, food and beverages, cleaning products, packages, toys, cosmetics, and construction materials, among others. Experimentally, phthalates produced lesions initially in Sertoli cells and Leydig cells through their metabolites, which have an antiandrogenic action.

Estrogens inhibit the proliferation of Sertoli cells, cause gonocyte multinucleation, and block gonocyte emigration from the central part of the seminiferous tubule to its basal part, thus preventing their transformation into spermatogonia. The consequence of the persistence of gonocytes is their eventual transformation into GCNIS and a low number of Ad spermatogonia, and in the long term, they cause a defect in spermatogenesis. Other functions, dependent largely on Sertoli cells, which are affected, are to maintain the phenotype of myoid peritubular cells and the Leydig cell population [23]. Exposure to phthalates was reported to be associated with deterioration of classical sperm parameters and sperm DNA integrity [24].

Aggregation of fetal Leydig cells not associated with increased Leydig cell number or volume [25], reduction of INSL3 [26], decreased production of testosterone, as well as gene expressions for androgen biosynthesis have been described in experimental models [27, 28]. A subtle reduction in the production of testosterone can cause not only alterations in fetal life but also in adult life. Fetal reduction in androgen production leads to reduced Leydig cell stem numbers after birth and concomitant failure of Leydig cells in the adult [29].

Other frequently used endocrine disruptors are pain relievers such as acetaminophen, which has been associated with congenital cryptorchidism in boys. These drugs inhibit testosterone synthesis. Due to its antiandrogenic effect, tobacco brings about a 30 % reduction of sperm number and a reduction of the seminal volume between 10 and 30 % [30]. In humans, exposure to estrogens and antiandrogens in the treatment of patients undergoing change gender causes dedifferentiation of Sertoli cells, disappearance of spermatogenesis, and atrophy of Leydig cells in the testis, lesions that have a strong resemblance with those observed in undescended testes [31].

13.3 Histological Findings in TDS

The lesions most frequently observed in testicular biopsies of patients with cryptorchidism, infertility, and parenchyma peripheral to the germ cell tumors and patients with hypospadias are mixed atrophy, hypoplastic tubules, Sertoli cell nodules, granular changes in Sertoli cells, tubules with germ cell hypoplasia, microlithiasis, focal Leydig cell hyperplasia, and GCNIS.

Mixed Atrophy (Focal Sertoli Cell-Only Tubules)

Mixed atrophy is defined by the presence of seminiferous tubules with Sertoli cell-only side by side with other tubules with spermatogenesis (Fig. 13.1). The number of tubules with Sertoli cell-only can vary from isolated tubules to constitute the majority of the biopsy. The degree of dysgenesis is related to the number of Sertoli cell-only tubules. The morphology of the nuclei of Sertoli cells of the tubules with Sertoli cell-only can be of three types: dysgenetic Sertoli cells (cells with central spherical or elongated nuclei), adult Sertoli cells (triangular nuclei with large

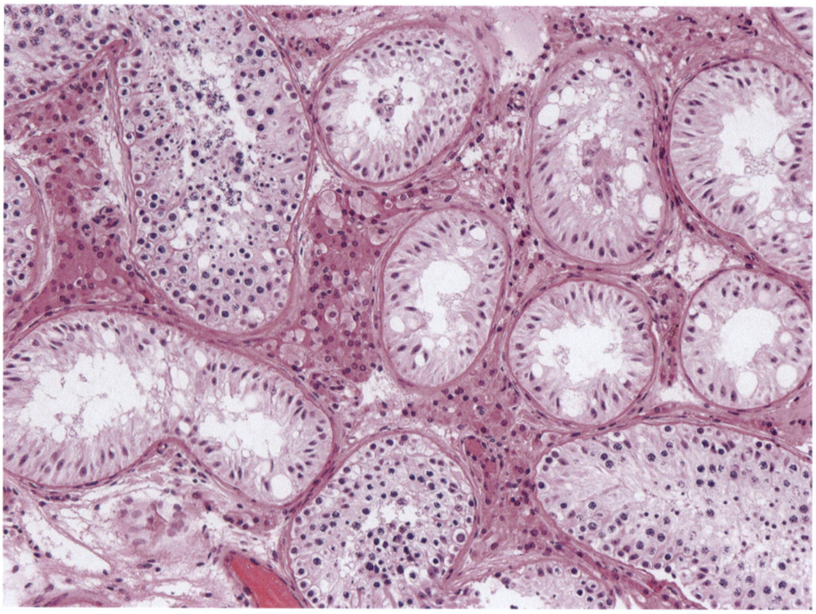

Fig. 13.1 Mixed atrophy. Among the seminiferous tubules with complete spermatogenesis, there are half a dozen tubes with Sertoli cell-only. Diffuse Leydig cell hyperplasia is also shown

central nucleoli), and involutive Sertoli cells (lobulated nuclei and central nucleoli). Tubules with dysgenetic Sertoli cell-only typically have a large number of cells by cross section and lack of lumen. The tubular wall has reduced elastic fibers. Most times tubules with spermatogenesis also show alterations either in the adluminal or the basal compartment.

Hypoplastic Tubules

They are seminiferous tubules with Sertoli cell-only that preferably appear isolated from others with germline. They have a very small diameter and a thickened wall. Sertoli cells are of immature characteristics, and the nuclei are small, spherical, hyperchromatic, and located at different heights, which gives the epithelium a pseudostratified appearance. In the apical cytoplasm, inhibin bodies stand out. Many cells lack androgen receptors. Sometimes the tubules have GCNIS and germ microliths.

Sertoli Cell Nodules (Hypoplastic Zones)

They are clusters of immature seminiferous tubules, small, well defined but not encapsulated (Fig. 13.2). The size varies from microscopic to several millimeters. The tubules have a variable wall thickening due to the accumulation of laminin and collagen IV. These thickenings cause protrusions into the tubule. Sertoli cells are similar to those of hypoplastic tubules. The microliths are frequent. Hypoplastic tubules located in the peripheral parenchyma may contain GCNIS cells (Fig. 13.3).

Granular Changes in Sertoli Cells

Sertoli cells, in tubules devoid of germ cells, show an enlarged cytoplasm filled with numerous eosinophilic granulations (Fig. 13.4). Granulations correspond to lysosomes (positive for CD68 and alpha-1 antitrypsin). These changes can affect isolated Sertoli cells, but more frequently they affect all the cells of several seminiferous tubules. The proximity of the affected tubules suggests that all of them belong to the same lobule. Sertoli cells with granular changes are observed in decreasing order of frequency in cryptorchidism, CAIS patients, and infertile patients with Sertoli cell-only and in the peripheral parenchyma of germ cell tumors [32, 33].

Germ Cell Hypoplasia

This term refers to the presence of abnormal spermatogenesis in adult seminiferous tubules (Fig. 13.5). The lesions may be diffuse or focal. They are usually associated with an increase in the number of Sertoli cells by tubular section and

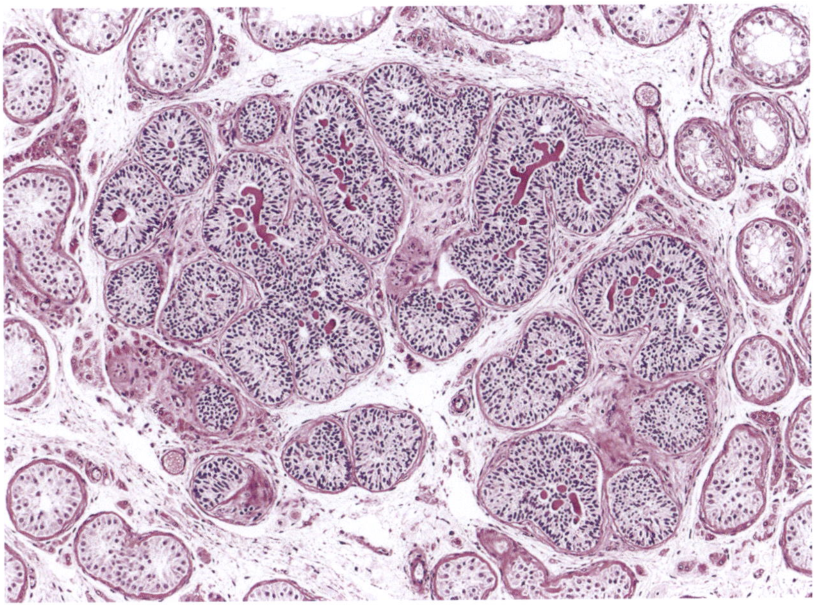

Fig. 13.2 Sertoli cell nodule that consists of small adjacent seminiferous tubules lacking of lumen. The lesion is well demarcated from the rest of the testicular parenchyma

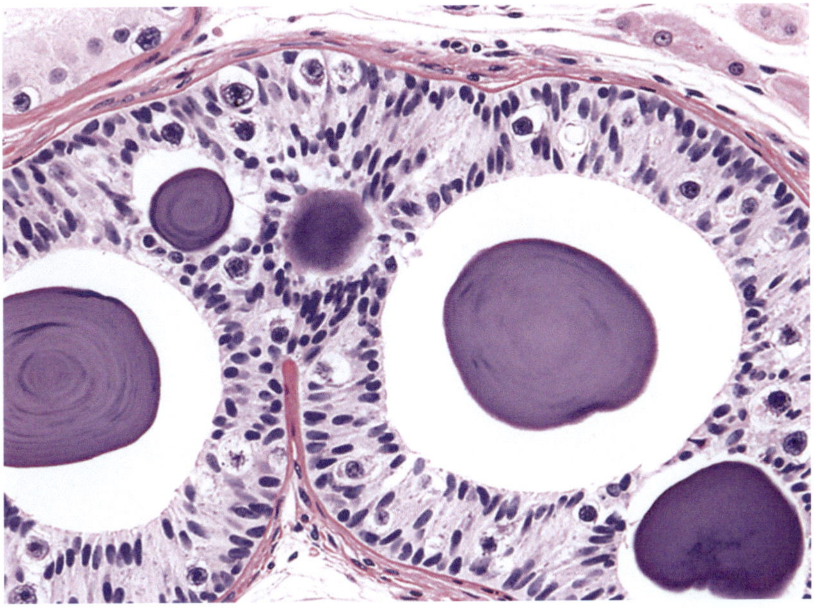

Fig. 13.3 Seminiferous tubules of a Sertoli cell nodule with microlithiasis and GCNIS. Tumor cells are located both on the basement membrane and among Sertoli cells

a certain degree of immaturity in them (few nuclei with triangular morphology, the absence of folds in the karyotheca, and persistence of heterochromatin granulations).

Microlithiasis

The presence of microlithiasis is estimated at 2.4–5.6 % of the general population, and the figure rises to 20 % of subfertile patients. It is observed in 9.52 % of ex-cryptorchidic testis and half of patients with testicular germ cell tumors. The microliths develop in the tubular wall and probably represent a local anomaly in the cells in the involved basal membrane (Sertoli cells) and tubular wall (myoid cells) formation. Most microliths are removed from the seminiferous tubules.

Focal Leydig Cell Hyperplasia

In testicular biopsies from infertile patients, where the impairment of spermatogenesis is

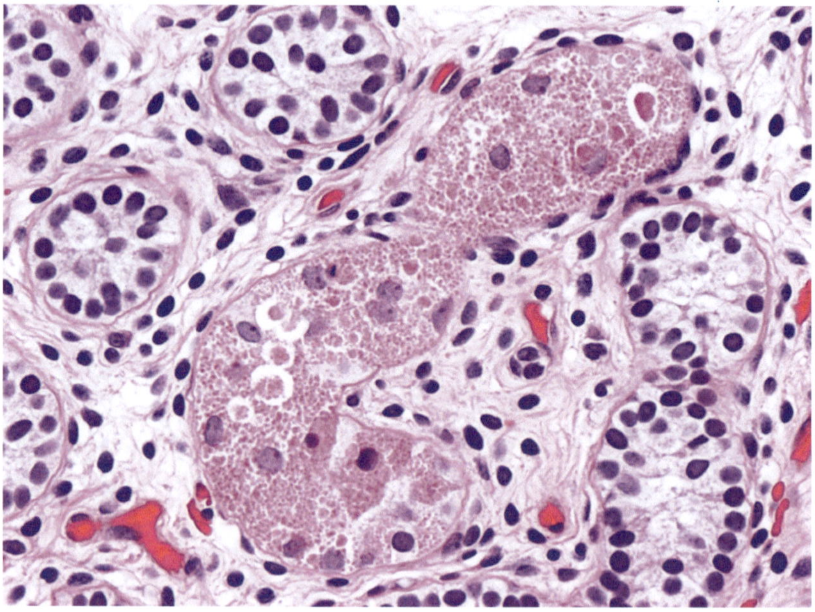

Fig. 13.4 Granular changes in Sertoli cells in prepubertal testis. In the central tubule, a few Sertoli cells with large full eosinophilic cytoplasms granulations are observed

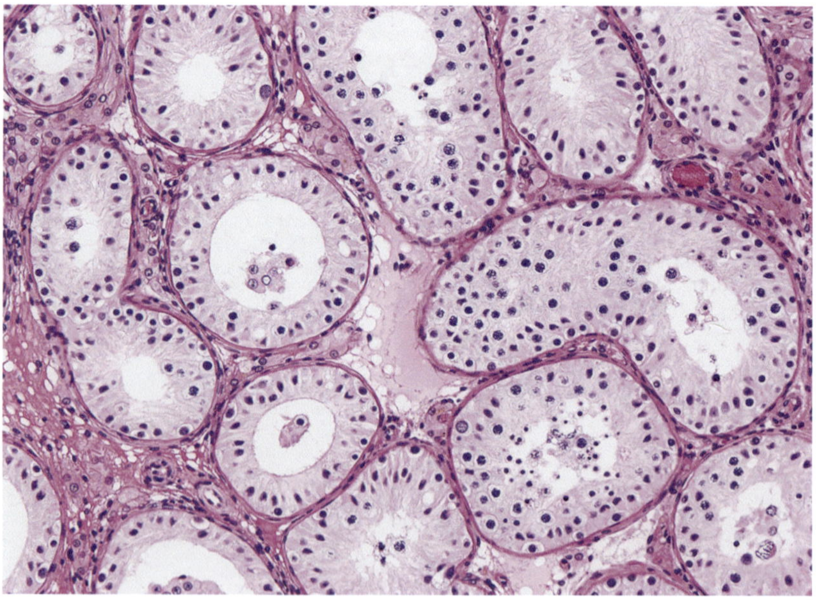

Fig. 13.5 Hypospermatogenesis. The provision of germ cells is variable from one tubule to another, but overall quantitative studies show that there is a proportional reduction in all germ cell types

important, Leydig cells, without being increased in number, are grouped giving the appearance of Leydig cell hyperplasia (Fig. 13.6). Patients often have decreased testosterone/LH ratio [34] and testosterone/estradiol ratio [35]. In adulthood this is probably the consequence of a defect in the number of Leydig stem cell during fetal life, a defect that could be mediated by Sertoli cells [36].

GCNIS

Tubules with GCNIS, also known as carcinoma in situ (CIS), are characterized by their smaller size and the relative uniformity of their cells in contrast to the pleomorphism of tubules with spermatogenesis. GCNIS cells are large, with spherical nucleus with abundant granulations of heterochromatin, one or two nucleoli, and abundant pale cytoplasm. They are arranged over the

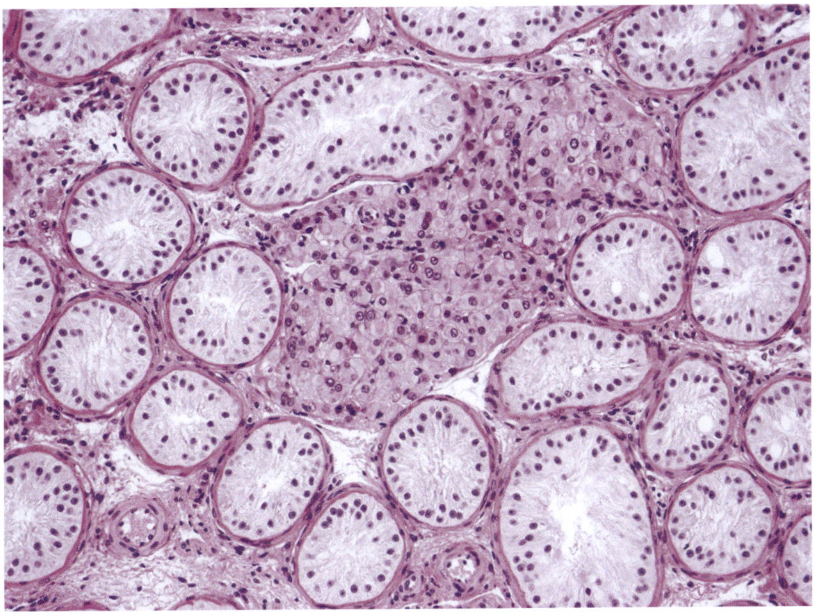

Fig. 13.6 Nodular Leydig cell hyperplasia in a testis with small seminiferous tubules and Sertoli cell-only

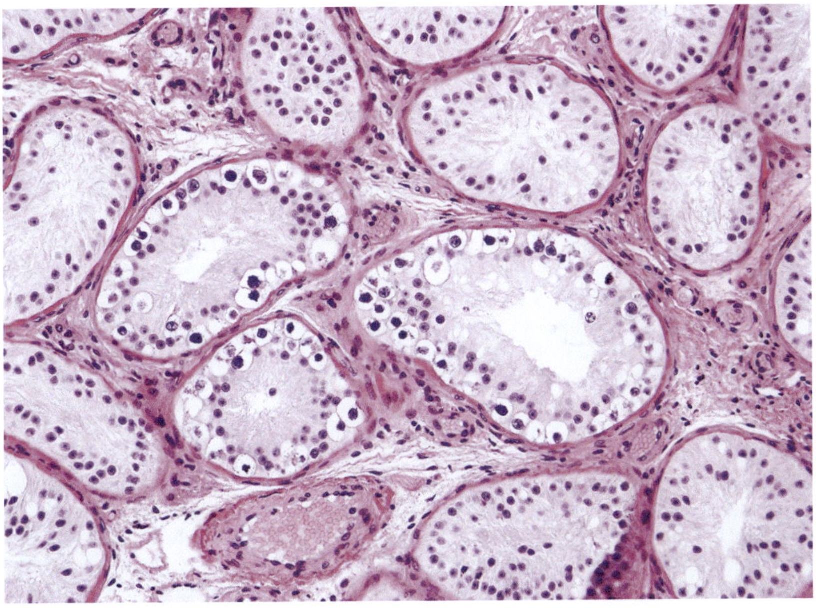

Fig. 13.7 GCNIS in a testicular biopsy of an ex-cryptorchidic infertile patient. Neoplasia affects only the three central tubules. The remaining Sertoli cell-only tubules show dysgenetic Sertoli cells

basement membrane moving Sertoli cells into the lumen (Fig. 13.7). They are positive for the following antibodies: PLAP, c-kit, D2-40, and OCT3/4 (Fig. 13.8). The nuclei of Sertoli cells become smaller and arranged as a spherical crown on a floor above the tumor cells.

The incidence of these lesions in the parenchyma peripheral to germ cell tumors is mixed atrophy 55 %, Sertoli cell nodules 25 %, microlithiasis 47 %, and GCNIS either focal (51 %) or diffuse (38 %) [37]. In the contralateral testis to the one bearer of a germ cell tumor, the incidence of these lesions is mixed atrophy 13.8 %, hypoplastic tubules and Sertoli cell nodules 4.6 %, microlithiasis 6 %, and GCNIS 8.7 %. The cumulative incidence of at least one sign of dysgenesis is 25.2 % [38].

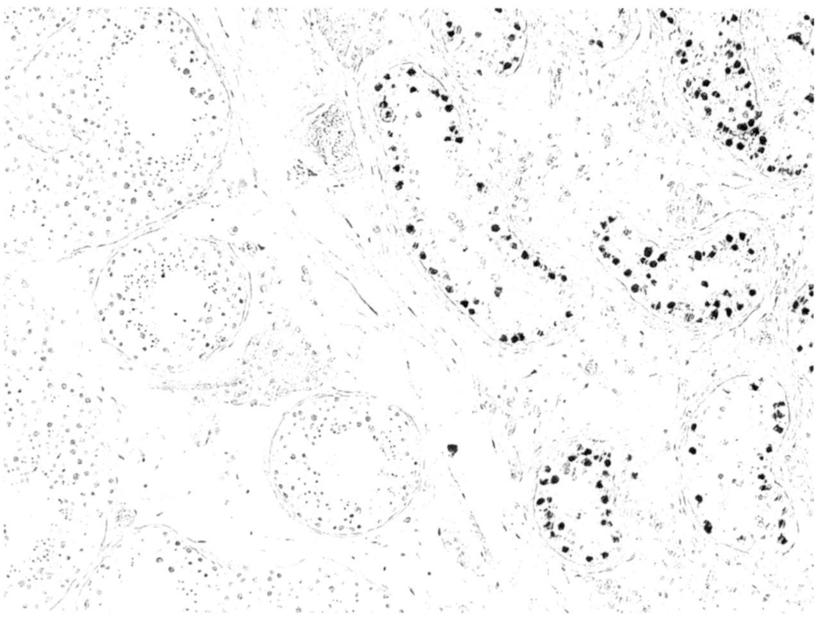

Fig. 13.8 Infertile patient with oligozoospermia. Next to a lobule with spermatogenesis, there are others with GCNIS. Immunostaining for OCT3/4

References

1. Carlsen E, Giwercman A, Keiding N, Skakkebaek NE. Evidence for decreasing quality of semen during past 50 years. BMJ. 1992;305:609–13.
2. Jouannet P, Wang C, Eustache F, Kold-Jensen T, Auger J. Semen quality and male reproductive health: the controversy about human sperm concentration decline. APMIS. 2001;109:333–44.
3. Nohynek GJ, Borgert CJ, Dietrich D, Rozman KK. Endocrine disruption: fact or urban legend? Toxicol Lett. 2013;223:295–305.
4. Skakkebaek NE, Rajpert-De Meyts E, Main KM. Testicular dysgenesis syndrome: an increasingly common developmental disorder with environmental aspects. Hum Reprod. 2001;6:972–8.
5. Rosen A, Jayram G, Drazer M, Eggener SE. Global trends in testicular cancer incidence and mortality. Eur Urol. 2011;60:374–9.
6. Skakkebaek NE, Rajpert-De Meyts E, Buck Louis GM, Toppari J, Andersson AM, Eisenberg ML, Jensen TK, Jørgensen N, Swan SH, Sapra KJ, Ziebe S, Priskorn L, Juul A. Male reproductive disorders and fertility trends: influences of environment and genetic susceptibility. Physiol Rev. 2016;96:55–97.
7. Petersen PM, Giwercman A, Hansen SW, Berthelsen JG, Daugaard G, Rørth M, Skakkebaek NE. Impaired testicular function in patients with carcinoma-in-situ of the testis. J Clin Oncol. 1999;17:173–9.
8. Rajpert-De Meyts E. Developmental model for the pathogenesis of testicular carcinoma in situ: genetic and environmental aspects. Hum Reprod Update. 2006;12:303–23.
9. Boisen KA, Kaleva M, Main KM, Virtanen HE, Haavisto AM, Schmidt IM, Chellakooty M, Damgaard IN, Mau C, Reunanen M, Skakkebæk NE, Toppari J. Difference in prevalence of congenital cryptorchidism in infants between two Nordic countries. Lancet. 2004;363:1264–9.
10. Ward B, Hunter WM. The absent testicle, a report on a survey carried outamong schoolboys in Nottingham. Br Med J. 1960;1:1110.
11. Pettersson A, Richiardi L, Nordenskjold A, Kaijser M, Akre O. Age at surgery for undescended testis and risk of testicular cancer. N Engl J Med. 2007;356:1835–41.
12. Dieckmann KP, Pichlmeier U. Clinical epidemiology of testicular germ cell tumors. World J Urol. 2004;22:2–14.
13. Paulozzi LJ, Erickson JD, Jackson RJ. Hypospadias trends in two US surveillance systems. Pediatrics. 1997;100:831–4.
14. Paulozzi LJ. International trends in rates of hypospadias and cryptorchidism. Environ Health Perspect. 1999;107:297–302.
15. Bergström R, Adami HO, Möhner M, Zatonski W, Storm H, Ekbom A, Tretli S, Teppo L, Akre O, Hakulinen T. Increase in testicular cancer incidence in six European countries: a birth cohort phenomenon. J Natl Cancer Inst. 1996;88:727–33.
16. Carlsen E, Giwercman A, Keiding N, Skakkebaek NE. Declining semen quality and increasing incidence of testicular cancer: is there a common cause? Environ Health Perspect. 1995;103(Suppl 7):137–9.
17. Khuri FJ, Hardy BE, Churchill BM. Urologic anomalies associated with hypospadias. Urol Clin North Am. 1981;8:565–71.

18. Ge RS, Chen GR, Tanrikut C, Hardy MP. Phthalate ester toxicity in Leydig cells: developmental timing and dosage considerations. Reprod Toxicol. 2007;23:366–73.
19. Splingart C, Frapsauce C, Veau S, Barthélémy C, Royère D, Guérif F. Semen variation in a population of fertile donors: evaluation in a French centre over a 34-year period. Int J Androl. 2012;35:467–74.
20. Sharpe RM. The 'oestrogen hypothesis'- where do we stand now? Int J Androl. 2003;26:2–15.
21. Dallinga JW, Moonen EJ, Dumoulin JC, Evers JL, Geraedts JP, Kleinjans JC. Decreased human semen quality and organochlorine compounds in blood. Hum Reprod. 2002;17:1973–9.
22. Palmer JR, Herbst AL, Noller KL, Boggs DA, Troisi R, Titus-Ernstoff L, Hatch EE, Wise LA, Strohsnitter WC, Hoover RN. Urogenital abnormalities in men exposed to diethylstilbestrol in utero: a cohort study. Environ Health. 2009;8:37.
23. Rebourcet D, O'Shaughnessy PJ, Monteiro A, Milne L, Cruickshanks L, Jeffrey N, Guillou F, Freeman TC, Mitchell RT, Smith LB. Sertoli cells maintain Leydig cell number and peritubular myoid cell activity in the adult mouse testis. PLoS One. 2014;9:e105687.
24. Petersen JH, Breindahl T. Plasticizers in total diet samples, baby food and infant formulae. Food Addit Contam. 2000;17:133–41.
25. Parks LG, Ostby JS, Lambright CR, Abbott BD, Klinefelter GR, Barlow NJ, Gray Jr LE. The plasticizer diethylhexyl phthalate induces malformations by decreasing fetal testosterone synthesis during sexual differentiation in the male rat. Toxicol Sci. 2000;58:339–49.
26. Adham IM, Emmen JM, Engel W. The role of the testicular factor INSL3 in establishing the gonadal position. Mol Cell Endocrinol. 2000;160:11–6.
27. Scott HM, Hutchison GR, Jobling MS, McKinnell C, Drake AJ, Sharpe RM. Relationship between androgen action in the "male programming window", fetal Sertoli cell number, and adult testis size in the rat. Endocrinology. 2008;149:5280–7.
28. Li L, Bu T, Su H, Chen Z, Liang Y, Zhang G, Zhu D, Shan Y, Xu R, Hu Y, Li J, Hu G, Lian Q, Ge RS. Inutero exposure to diisononyl phthalate caused testicular dysgenesis of rat fetal testis. Toxicol Lett. 2015;232:466–74.
29. Kilcoyne KR, Smith LB, Atanassova N, Macpherson S, McKinnell C, van den Driesche S, Jobling MS, Chambers TJ, De Gendt K, Verhoeven G, O'Hara L, Platts S, Renato de Franca L, Lara NL, Anderson RA, Sharpe RM. Fetal programming of adult Leydig cell function by androgenic effects on stem/progenitor cells. Proc Natl Acad Sci U S A. 2014;111:E1924–32.
30. Brouwers MM, Feitz WF, Roelofs LA, Kiemeney LA, de Gier RP, Roeleveld N. Hypospadias: a transgenerational effect of diethylstilbestrol? Hum Reprod. 2006; 21:666–9.
31. Nistal M, Gonzalez-Peramato P, De Miguel MP. Sertoli cell dedifferentiation in human cryptorchidism and gender reassignment shows similarities between fetal environmental and adult medical treatment estrogen and antiandrogen exposure. Reprod Toxicol. 2013;42:172–9.
32. Nistal M, Garcia-Rodeja E, Paniagua R. Granular transformation of Sertoli cells in testicular disorders. Hum Pathol. 1991;22:131–7.
33. Nistal M, Regadera J, Winitzky P, Tejerina E, Chemes H. Granular changes in Sertoli cells in children and pubertal patients. Fertil Steril. 2005;83:1489–99.
34. Holm M, Rajpert-De Meyts E, Andersson AM, Skakkebaek NE. Leydig cell micronodules are a common finding in testicular biopsies from men with impaired spermatogenesis and are associated with decreased testosterone/LH ratio. J Pathol. 2003;199: 378–86.
35. Andersson AM, Jørgensen N, Frydelund-Larsen L, Rajpert-De Meyts E, Skakkebaek NE. Impaired Leydig cell function in infertile men: a study of 357 idiopathic infertile men and 318 proven fertile controls. J Clin Endocrinol Metab. 2004;89:3161–7.
36. Juul A, Almstrup K, Andersson AM, Jensen TK, Jørgensen N, Main KM, Rajpert-De Meyts E, Toppari J, Skakkebæk NE. Possible fetal determinants of male infertility. Nat Rev Endocrinol. 2014;10:553–62.
37. Nistal M, Gonzalez-Peramato P, Regadera J, Serrano A, Tarin V, De Miguel MP. Primary testicular lesions are associated with testicular germ cell tumors of adult men. Am J Surg Pathol. 2006;30:1260–8.
38. Hoei-Hansen CE, Holm M, Rajpert-De Meyts E, Skakkebaek NE. Histological evidence of testicular dysgenesis in contralateral biopsies from 218 patients with testicular germ cell cancer. J Pathol. 2003;200:370–4.

14 Differential Diagnosis of Macroorchidism

Manuel Nistal, Pilar González-Peramato, and Álvaro Serrano

14.1 Asymmetric Testicular Size: Compensating Hypertrophy

Testicular hypertrophy is a physiological response to the absence of functional sufficiency of the contralateral testicle. Compensatory testicular hypertrophy was first reported by Laron and Zilka in 1969 [1] in unilateral cryptorchidic patients. The disorder is defined during childhood by an increased volume of the descended testis, higher than 2 ml [2] and a testicular volume higher than 25 ml in adulthood. The compensatory hypertrophy occurs by pituitary FSH stimulation. Experimentally, when FSH is added to a culture of Sertoli cells, their proliferative activity increases. When hemicastration of immature rats is done, there is an increased mitotic activity in the contralateral testicle. A fall in the production of inhibin by the Sertoli cells occurs after castration. Pituitary feedback to a negative lower production increases FSH that stimulates the division of Sertoli cells [3]. The conditions for a compensatory hyperplasia to occur are the following [4]:

- That the descended testicle is normal
- Absence of contralateral testis or testicular atrophy greater than 50 %
- Age between birth and 3 years [5]

A compensatory hypertrophy is observed in monorchisms and in descended testis of patients with cryptorchidism. The hypertrophy is larger in the first. The degree of hypertrophy maintains along infancy and puberty and ceases when puberty is completed. The size of the compensated testis at adulthood is normal or slightly increased [6]. The future of testicular function in patients with compensatory hypertrophy is probably not optimal since levels of inhibin B are low during childhood and FSH levels are high, so it is advisable to perform a sperm analysis at the start of adulthood [7].

14.2 Non-tumoral Macroorchidism

14.2.1 Early Harmonious Development of the Testis: Gonadotropin-Dependent Precocious Puberty – Central Precocious Puberty (CPP)

When development of the testis, which simulates the changes that normally occur at puberty, occurs at an early age, most likely the patient has a gonadotropin-dependent precocious puberty. Although the sequence in which these changes occur is accelerated, it can start by testicular enlargement. Early activation of the hypothalamic-pituitary-gonadal axis initiates the changes [8]. The proliferation of Sertoli cells followed by their maturation is controlled by a complex multitude of endocrine (FSH and TH),

M. Nistal et al., *Clues in the Diagnosis of Non-tumoral Testicular Pathology*,
DOI 10.1007/978-3-319-49364-0_14

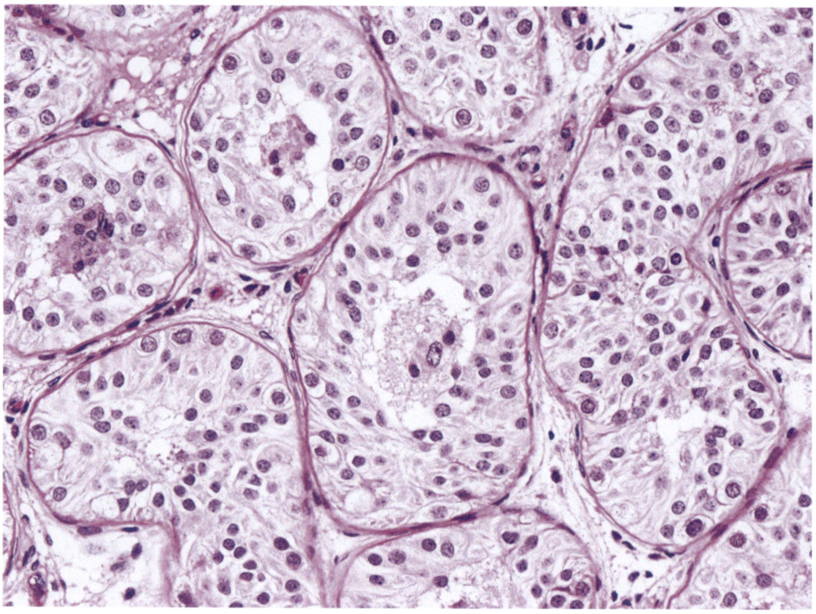

Fig. 14.1 Precocious puberty. Six-year-old boy who presented with rapid enlargement of both testicles secondary to a pineal gland tumor. The seminiferous tubules show increased size and cellularity affecting both germ cells and Sertoli cells

paracrine (androgen-transforming grow factor), beta family (TGF-beta and glial-derived neurotrophic factor), and autocrine factor (endotoxins and post-inflammatory cytokines) [9]. Maturation of Sertoli cells is revealed by significant nuclear and cytoplasmic changes, the blood-testis barrier formation, and the appearance of tubular light and the start of spermatogenesis (Fig. 14.1). The rapid testicular enlargement continues with the development of axillary and pubic hair, increase of the penis size, and acceleration of body growth and bone maturation. The most common age of onset is between 4 and 8 years. In 50 % of men with symptoms of precocious puberty, testicular hypertrophy is secondary to the excessive production of FSH and LH.

The causes of CPP, thanks to the widespread use of CT scan and magnetic resonance techniques [10], are known in 60 % of cases, and 2/3of them are caused by lesions of the central nervous system. The remaining 40 % are considered idiopathic.

Injuries of the central nervous system preferentially affect the posterior hypothalamus (medial eminence and tuber cinereum), mammillary bodies, the third ventricle bottom, or the pineal gland [11, 12]. The most frequent causes are the following: tumors (hypothalamic tumors, pineal cysts, hamartomas, tumors of the pineal gland), brain traumas, infections, cerebral malformations, and hereditary diseases such as neurofibromatosis and tuberous sclerosis and cerebral irradiation.

The most frequent genetic causes of familial CPP are MKRN3 defects [13].

Idiopathic central precocious puberty has been related to genetic factors, ethnic factors, pediatric obesity, family history, psychosocial stress, adoption [14], and DDT degradation products [15]. The presentation of idiopathic precocious puberty is familial in nearly half of cases, and puberty starts after 7 years in most of the boys. The inheritance can be either autosomal recessive or sex linked with variable penetrance [16]. The treatment of choice is gonadotropin-releasing hormone agonists [17].

14.2.2 Dissociation of Tubular and Interstitial Development

14.2.2.1 Sertoli Cell Hyperplasia

An increased number of Sertoli cells are the common finding in macroorchidisms observed in the following pathologies: Fra X syndrome, hypothyroidism, FSH-secreting adenoma, Russell-Silver's syndrome, and idiopathic benign macroorchidism.

Fragile X-Chromosome Syndrome

The fragile X-chromosome syndrome (FXS), also known as Martin Bell syndrome [18], is a genetic disease caused by an expansion of trinucleotide CGG named full mutation (more than 200 repeats of CGG) in the *FMR1* gene on the Xp27.3 locus. This mutation produces a hypermethylation of the promoter region of the gene silencing and decreasing the expression levels of the FMRP protein linked to neuronal plasticity and maturation. The normal individuals have between 6 and 54 repeats with 29 or 30 repeats being the most common allele [19]. When the number of repeats expands to between 60 and 200, it is referred to as permutation carriers. About 32.4 % of males with permutation carriers have macroorchidism and a significant number lower verbal and full scale IQ [20]. The classic diagnosis was made with karyotype in a special culture medium. Today more sensitive and specific molecular tests are used including PCR and Southern blot [21]. The worldwide prevalence is estimated at 1 per 5000 men and one per 4000 to 6000 women [22].

Clinical Features Patients show a slight to moderate mental retardation and autism with hyperkinetic behavior [23]. The physical characteristics of affected patients include macrocephaly (prominent forehead and ears, long face, prognathism), macroorchidism, and multiple connective tissue abnormalities (hypotonia, flat feet, mitral valve prolapse, soft skin, hyperextensible finger joints, and high arched palate). Males with full fragile X mutation also present intellectual disability, low IQ, and symptoms in common with autism spectrum disorder such as delays in speech and language development, impaired theory of mind and impaired social and emotional processing, irritability, hyperactivity, and attention deficits [24]. The prevalence and severity of FXS in females is more attenuated because of X-inactivation.

Histopathology The most important findings occur in those tissues with a higher expression of FMRP, such as the neuronal cells in the hippocampus and cerebellum, and the testes [25]. Macroorchidism is present in more than 75 % of adult affected patients. The average testicular volume in these patients is 70 ml. Testicular enlargement probably begins during fetal life [26]. In infancy, the testes are enlarged, the scrotal pouches are more developed than normal, and genital pigmentation appears earlier. This genital development is difficult to explain, because the

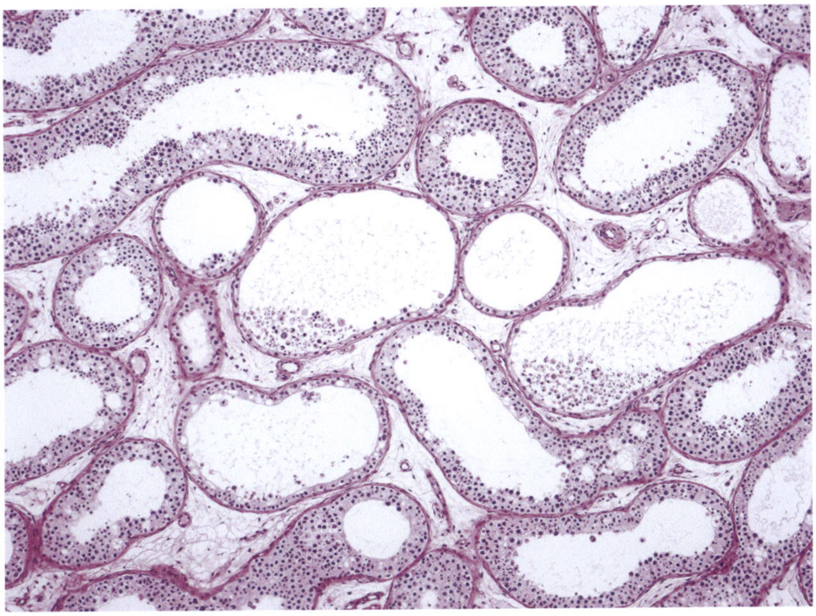

Fig. 14.2 Fragile X-chromosome syndrome. The seminiferous tubules show marked tubular ectasia and atrophy of the seminiferous epithelium caused by compression of the epithelium against the tubular wall by the intratubular fluid

function of the hypothalamic-pituitary-gonadal axis is completely normal; however, some patients show slightly increased FSH levels, suggesting an abnormally high receptivity to this hormone [27].

Testicular biopsies in adult patients show severe pathological changes. There have been reported marked tubular ectasia and atrophy of the seminiferous epithelium, mixed atrophy with or without Sertoli cell hyperplasia, Sertoli cell nodules, and granular changes in Sertoli cells (Figs. 14.2, 14.3, 14.4, and 14.5). An apparent low number of Leydig cells are observed in the interstitium, probably masked by large tubular development and groups of fully hyalinized seminiferous tubules. Other facts secondary to ectasia are seminiferous tubules full of spermatozoa and tubulitis. The rete testis is enlarged, and in

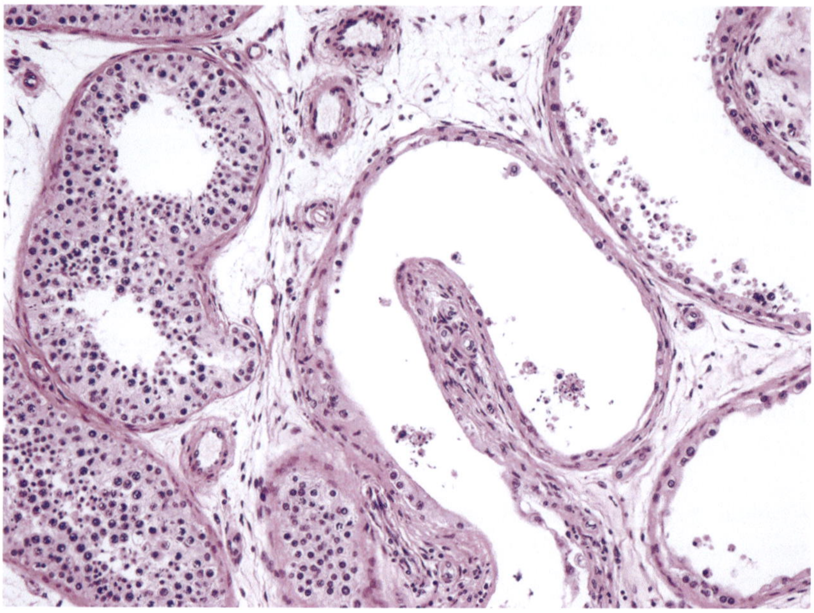

Fig. 14.3 Fragile X-chromosome syndrome. Ectasic seminiferous tubules are next to other tubules with normal spermatogenesis

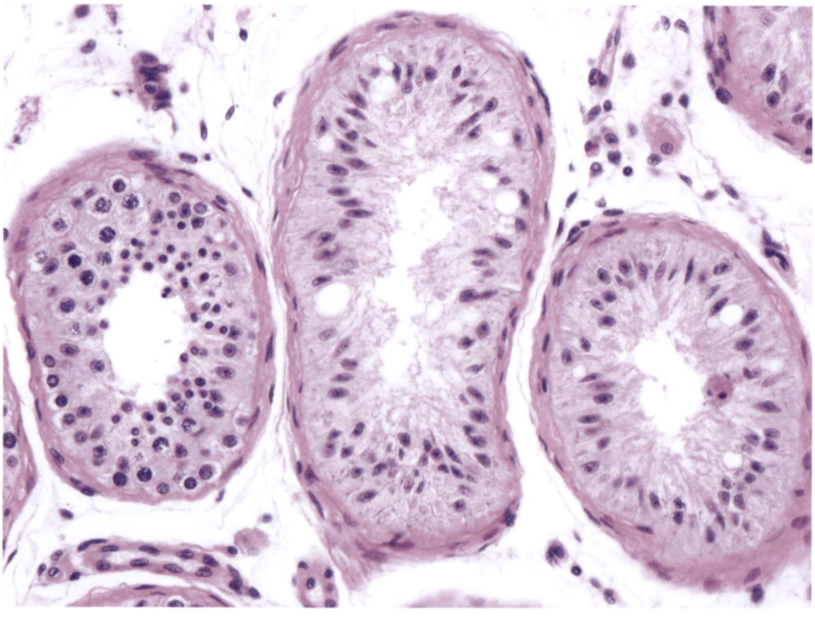

Fig. 14.4 Fragile X-chromosome syndrome. Sertoli cell-only tubules with dysgenetic Sertoli cells are side by side with other tubules showing marked hypospermatogenesis

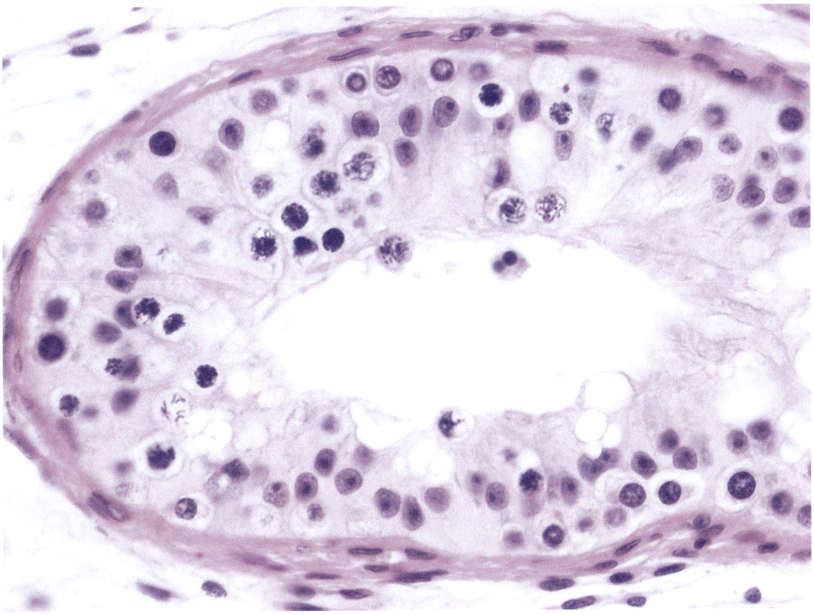

Fig. 14.5 Fragile X-chromosome syndrome. Seminiferous tubule with large number of Sertoli cells, normal number of spermatogonia, a few first-order spermatocytes, and absence of spermatids

its cavities both germ cells and sloughed epithelial cells are observed. The epididymis does not show alterations. The cause determining the increase in testicular size seems to be an excessive Sertoli cell proliferation which determines an abnormal growth in length of the seminiferous tubules [27]. This effect has been experimentally checked in FMR1 knockout mice [28]. The repeatedly observed low spermatozoon numbers in spermiogram might be explained by an abnormal Sertoli cell maturation leading to deficient spermatogenesis.

Macroorchidism Associated with Hypothyroidism

Children with hypothyroidism frequently show testicular enlargement without virilization, delayed bone age [29], and a macroorchidism of about 80 % [30]. When hypothyroidism is primary, the macroorchidism is earlier than in secondary hypothyroidism. The longer the hypothyroidism, the more severe is the degree of testicular changes. Most patients with primary hypothyroidism show elevated FSH serum levels and prepubertal LH serum levels [31]. Serum testosterone levels are within normal infantile values, the response to FSH and LH stimulation is altered, and no pulsatile LH is released [32].

Histopathology Testicular biopsies in infancy show an accelerated growth of the testis, increased diameter of the seminiferous tubules with a larger number of Sertoli cells, minimal changes in spermatogenesis, and absence of Leydig cell development (Fig. 14.6). Testicular biopsies in adults with untreated juvenile hypothyroidism show hyalinized tubules, peritubular and interstitial fibrosis, and scanty Leydig cells [33, 34]. Pubertal and adult patients with chronic untreated hypothyroidism usually show alterations in the testicular biopsies and the spermiogram [35].

Pathogenesis Macroorchidism in hypothyroidism has been the object of different hypotheses related to the different causes of hypothyroidism:

In primary hypothyroidism:

(a) The decrease of T3 and T4 induces increased thyrotropin-releasing hormone (TRH) secretion, and as a consequence, the levels of TSH, prolactin, and gonadotropins would increase. The elevation of FSH found in some cases would induce the testicular hypertrophy [36]; when the FSH is normal, hyperfunction of the FSH receptor could be called upon [37].

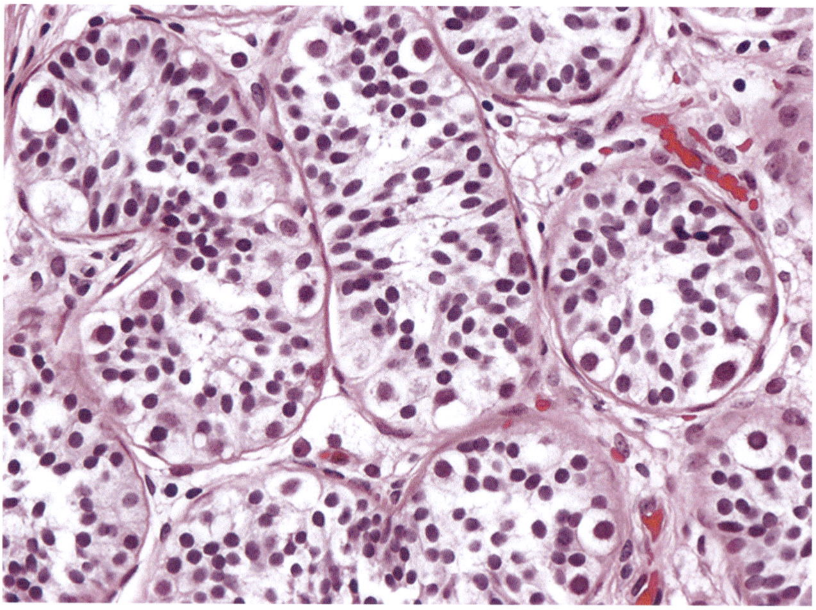

Fig. 14.6 Three-year-old patient with hypothyroidism and macroorchidism. The seminiferous tubules have an increased diameter secondary to larger number of Sertoli cells. The number of spermatogonia is preserved. In the interstitium, Leydig cells not recognized

(b) Direct action of TSH on the testis, mediated by the FSH receptors of testicular cells due to the similar structure of the glycoprotein hormone receptors [38].
(c) The decrease of thyroid hormones lengthens the period of proliferation of Sertoli cells resulting in an increase in their number and macroorchidism [39].

In secondary hypothyroidism:

(a) Loss-of-function mutations in *IGSF1* (immunoglobulin superfamily member that causes an X-linked syndrome of central hypothyroidism, *IGSG1*-deficiency syndrome). *IGSF1* is expressed in the testis and plays a role in testicular development and maturation from childhood to adult. In patients whose *IGSF1* is mutated, testicular volume starts to increase in adolescence although the mechanism is unknown [40, 41].
(b) Other hypotheses include hyperprolactinemia and alterations of the steroid metabolism of testicular cells [42].

Testicular size in macroorchidism is reduced as soon as the substitutive treatment is administered [43].

Macroorchidism in FSH-Secreting Adenoma

Immunohistochemical studies in most (80–90 %) of pituitary adenomas, clinically nonfunctioning, are seen expressing intact gonadotropins or gonadotropin subunits. Either because the serum levels of intact FSH and LH or the alpha and beta subunits of these hormones are biologically inert, no testicular changes are observed or there even is testicular atrophy. Exceptionally a bilateral macroorchidism develops [44]. An increased FSH is associated with normal serum levels of inhibin B, subnormal serum testosterone, and LH in the low normal range. The complaint of some patients is infertility [45]. Histological studies suggest that macroorchidism is the consequence of an increased length of the seminiferous tubules by Sertoli cell hyperplasia [46]. After pituitary surgery, the serum FSH is normalized, and the testicular volume decreases [47].

Russell-Silver Syndrome

Russell-Silver syndrome is a clinically and genetically heterogeneous syndrome characterized by severe intrauterine and postnatal growth retardation and a characteristic small, triangular face, with a prominent forehead and micrognathia, downturned corners of the mouth, and ear anomalies [48]. Other associated dysmorphic anomalies are fifth finger clinodactyly and limb and body asymmetry [49]. The original description already included precocious puberty. The cause of precocious puberty lies in Sertoli cells hyperplasia that aromatizes the estrogens. High levels of estrone are responsible for advanced bone age and gynecomastia. Treatment with aromatase inhibitors associated with GnRH agonist slows bone growth and lowers the estradiol levels [50].

Benign Idiopathic Macroorchidism

The diagnosis of benign idiopathic macroorchidism is made by exclusion once bilateral testicular tumor (germ cell, stromal tumors, leukemia, or lymphoma), adrenal rest tumors, X-linked mental retardation, hypothyroidism, FSH-secreting adenomas, and idiopathic or cerebral precocious puberty have been ruled out. Some prepubertal and pubertal males show a pronounced bilateral asymptomatic [51, 52] or unilateral [53] testicular hypertrophy.

Morphometric studies have shown that the main histological findings are Sertoli cell hyperplasia and a deficient spermatogenesis. The cause would be the serum FSH elevation observed in some cases that cause excessive Sertoli cell proliferation [27, 54]. In other cases, where levels of FSH are normal, overactivity of the receptor is suggested [55]. This disorder has been considered the morphological expression of particular testicular parenchyma receptivity to hormonal stimulation. Unilateral presentations seem to be the evidence of a well-known feature: the pubertal development of both testes can be asynchronous.

A peculiar situation of testicular enlargement was observed in a 14-year-old boy. The patient was asymptomatic and only showed bilateral testicular enlargement. The sonogram disclosed a testicular parenchyma with diffuse conspicuous lobulations that seemed to separate testicular lobules, giving a picture similar to fetal kidney lobulations in newborn children [56].

14.2.2.2 Leydig Cell Hyperplasia

Congenital Leydig Cell Hyperplasia

Congenital Leydig cell hyperplasia is observed in pathologies with a marked placental edema such as diabetes, triploid fetuses, Beckwith-Wiedemann syndrome, leprechaunism, nonimmune hydrops fetalis, Rh isoimmunization, and several complications of pregnancy [57]. Under these circumstances large amounts of hCG enter the fetal circulation producing Leydig cell hyperplasia.

Histopathology The Leydig cell proliferation can be diffuse or nodular. The seminiferous tubules show little changes (Fig. 14.7). When cell proliferation is nodular, the clusters of Leydig cells are preferably located near the mediastinum testis. In these cases, it may pose a differential diagnosis with intratesticular adrenal remnants and bilateral Leydig cell tumors. Congenital Leydig cell hyperplasia regresses in the first weeks of postnatal life.

Familial Testotoxicosis (Gonadotropin-Independent Precocious Puberty (GIPP) or Familial Male Limited Precocious Puberty (FMPP))

This disorder is a form of male precocious puberty, characterized by the early maturation of Leydig cells in absence of pituitary gonadotropic stimulation. The cause is a constitutive-activating mutation of LH/CGR gene [58] mapped in 2p21 [59].

Histological studies reveal an adult development of Leydig cells. The hyperplasia can be diffuse or nodular [60]. Seminiferous tubules can show complete spermatogenesis, although with many morphological spermatid anomalies [61] (Fig. 14.8).

Clinical Features The patients, usually from 1 to 4 years of age, present signs of pubertal development including rapid virilization, acceleration of growth with eventual closure of epiphyses, and short stature at adulthood. Although the testes are enlarged, their size is not correlated to virilization.

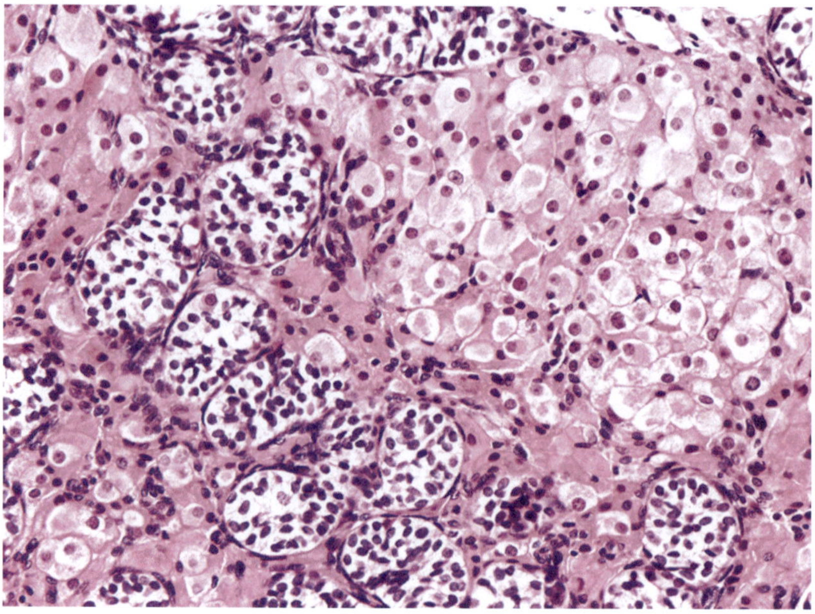

Fig. 14.7 Congenital Leydig cell hyperplasia in a newborn child of diabetic mother

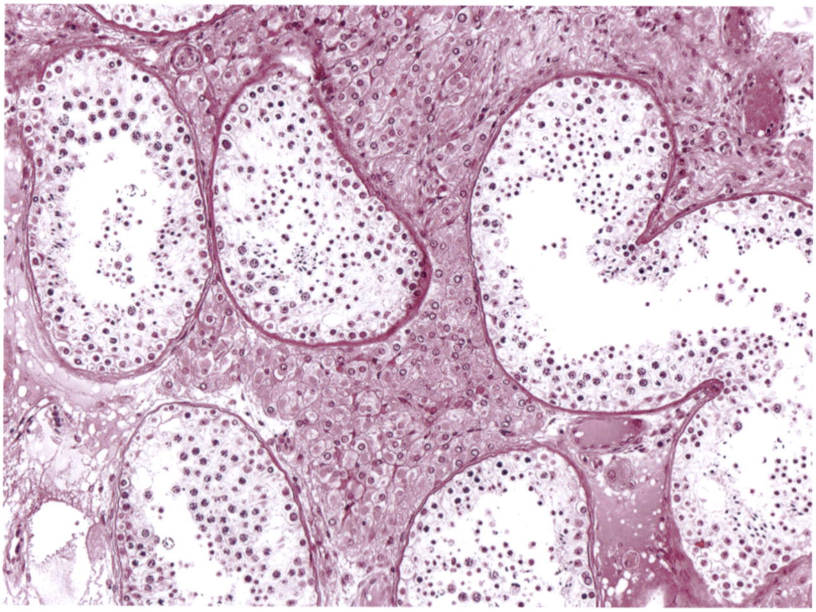

Fig. 14.8 Testotoxicosis. Seven-year-old patient showing virilization associated with rapid acceleration of growth. A focus of Leydig cell hyperplasia surrounded by seminiferous tubules with complete spermatogenesis was observed in the testicular biopsy

Hormonal assays show elevated serum testosterone levels, low levels of dehydroepiandrostenedione (DHAS), androstenedione, 17-hydroxyprogesterone, GnRH, and LH; absence of pubertal LH pulsatile pattern [58]; and elevated levels of inhibin B before the normal age of puberty [62]. The response of gonadotropins to GnRH stimulation is negative.

14.2.2.3 Sertoli Cell and/or Leydig Cell Hyperplasia

McCune-Albright Syndrome

There are clinical syndromes, of which McCune-Albright syndrome (MAS) is the prototype, where the cause of macroorchidism has been described associated with both activation of Sertoli cells and Leydig cell hyperplasia.

MAS is characterized by polyostotic fibrous dysplasia, "cafe au lait" skin pigmentation, and autonomous endocrine hyperfunction. Precocious puberty is present in 15 % of males. Male patients show testicular enlargement, prepubertal penile size, and absence of axillary and pubic hair. This syndrome is originated by a post-zygotic gain of function mutation at codon 201 in the guanine-nucleotide binding protein α-subunit (*GNAS1*) genes that encode the GS-α protein [63]. The anomaly is followed by inactivation of both LHR and FSHR [64].

Macroorchidism due to autonomous Sertoli cell hyperfunction shows abnormally elevated serum levels of inhibin B and AMH in correlation to decreased serum levels of both FSH and testosterone. Therefore, a pubertal inhibin B serum level would suggest a Sertoli cell hyperfunction that would cause a negative feedback on FSH secretion.

The testes show focus of uniformly enlarged seminiferous tubules arranged in groups that are not mixed with the normal-for-age seminiferous tubules with child development. The enlarged seminiferous tubules show Sertoli cell hyperplasia and absence of spermatogenesis. The interstitium lacks Leydig cells [65]. In 62 % of the cases, testicular microlithiasis is associated [66]. The absence of Leydig cells has been related to the presence of the somatic mutation in *GNAS1* gene in Sertoli cells [67], but not in Leydig cells. The different early embryologic origin of precursor cells that contribute to Sertoli cell and Leydig cell lineages might underlie the differential occurrence of the mutated *GNAS1* gene.

MAS mechanism associated with Leydig cell hyperplasia is presumably related to excess of cAMP signaling [68]. GS-α mutation in MAS triggers differentiation of immature Leydig cells present in childhood, which in some patients causes the autonomous maturation of Leydig cells that causes a precocious puberty secondary to excess testosterone [69].

There are a number of data supporting the idea that gonadotropin-independent precocious puberty could begin with early activation of Sertoli cells followed by the activation of Leydig cells. In the same patient, Sertoli cell hyperplasia in the first biopsy and Leydig cell hyperplasia in the surgical specimen have been observed with a difference of years [70]. Macroorchidisms secondary to Sertoli cells hyperplasia have been observed in childhood [65], and in a Leydig cell hyperplasia, the subjects are older children and pubertal and adult patients [71].

Macroorchidism is not always bilateral, and unilateral macroorchidism may be its first manifestation [72, 73].

References

1. Laron Z, Zilka E. Compensatory hypertrophy of testicle in unilateral cryptorchidism. J Clin Endocrinol Metabol. 1969;29:1409–13.
2. Hodhod A, Capolicchio JP, Jednak R, El-Sherbiny M. Testicular hypertrophy as a predictor for contralateral monorchism: Retrospective review of prospectively recorded data. J Pediatr Urol. 2016;12:34. e1–5.
3. Moon JH, Yoo DY, Jo YK, Kim GA, Jung HY, Choi JH, Hwang IK, Jang G. Unilateral cryptorchidism induces morphological changes of testes and hyperplasia of Sertoli cells in a dog. Lab Anim Res. 2014;30:185–9.
4. Koff SA. Does compensatory testicular enlargement predict monorchism? J Urol. 1991;146:632–3.
5. Huff DS, Snyder 3rd HM, Hadziselimovic F, Blyth B, Duckett JW. An absent testis is associated with contralateral testicular hypertrophy. J Urol. 1992;148:627–8.
6. Laron Z, Dickerman Z, Ritterman I, Kaufman H. Follow-up of boys with unilateral compensatory testicular hypertrophy. Fertil Steril. 1980;33:297–301.
7. Gaudino R, Cavarzere P, Camilot M, Teofoli F, Zampieri N, Tatò L. Prepubertal serum inhibin B in cryptorchid infants and in monorchid boys with compensatory testicular hypertrophy. Fertil Steril. 2008;90:2217–21.
8. Chirico V, Lacquaniti A, Salpietro V, Buemi M, Salpietro C, Arrigo T. Central precocious puberty: from physiopathological mechanisms to treatment. J Biol Regul Homeost Agents. 2014;28:367–75.
9. Tarulli GA, Stanton PG, Loveland KL, Rajpert-De Meyts E, McLachlan RI, Meachem SJ. A survey of Sertoli cell differentiation in men after gonadotropin suppression and in testicular cancer. Spermatogenesis. 2013;3(1):e24014.

10. Faizah M, Zuhanis A, Rahmah R, Raja A, Wu L, Dayang A, Zulfiqar M. Precocious puberty in children: a review of imaging findings. Biomed Imaging Interv J. 2012;8(1):e6.
11. Cloutier MD, Hayles AB. Precocious puberty. Adv Pediatr. 1970;17:125–38.
12. Bierich JR. Sexual precocity. Clin Endocrinol Metab. 1975;4:107–42.
13. Bulcao Macedo D, Nahime Brito V, Latronico AC. New causes of central precocious puberty: the role of genetic factors. Neuroendocrinology. 2014;100:1–8.
14. Soriano-Guillén L, Corripio R, Labarta JI, Cañete R, Castro-Feijóo L, Espino R, Argente J. Central precocious puberty in children living in Spain: incidence, prevalence, and influence of adoption and immigration. J Clin Endocrinol Metab. 2010;95:4305–13.
15. Deng F, Tao FB, Liu DY, Xu YY, Hao JH, Sun Y, Su PY. Effects of growth environments and two environmental endocrine disruptors on children with idiopathic precocious puberty. Eur J Endocrinol. 2012;166:803–9.
16. De Vries L, Kauschansky A, Shohat M, Phillip M. Familial central precocious puberty suggests autosomal dominant inheritance. J Clin Endocrinol Metab. 2004;89:1794–800.
17. Krysiak R, Marek B, Okopień B. Central precocious puberty. Endokrynol Pol. 2008;59:530–40.
18. Martin JP, Bell J. A pedigree of mental defect showing sex-linkage. J Neurol Psychiatry. 1943;6:154–7.
19. Yu S, Pritchard M, Kremer EJ, Lynch M, Nancarrow J, Baker E, Holman K, Mulley JC, Warren ST, Schlessinger D, Sutherland GR, Richards RI. Fragile X genotype characterized by an unstable region of DNA. Science. 1991;252:1179–81.
20. Lozano R, Summers S, Lozano C, Mu Y, Hessl D, Nguyen D, Tassone F, Hagerman R. Association between macroorchidism and intelligence in FMR1 premutation carriers. Am J Med Genet A. 2014;164A:2206–11.
21. Sofocleous C, Kolialexi A, Mavrou A. Molecular diagnosis of Fragile X syndrome. Expert Rev Mol Diagn. 2009;9:23–30.
22. Coffee B, Keith K, Albizua I, Malone T, Mowrey J, Sherman SL, Warren ST. Incidence of fragile X syndrome by newborn screening for methylated FMR1 DNA. Am J Hum Genet. 2009;85:503–14.
23. Hessl D, Rivera SM, Reiss AL. The neuroanatomy and neuroendocrinology of fragile X syndrome. Ment Retard Dev Disabil Res Rev. 2004;10:17–24.
24. Garber KB, Visootsak J, Warren ST. Fragile X syndrome. Eur J Hum Genet. 2008;16:666–72.
25. Zhang M, Wang Q, Huang Y. Fragile X mental retardation protein FMRP and the RNA export factor NXF2 associate with and destabilize Nxf1 mRNA in neuronal cells. Proc Natl Acad Sci U S A. 2007;104:10057–62.
26. Rudelli RD, Jenkins EC, Wisniewski K, Moretz R, Byrne J, Brown WT. Testicular size in fetal fragile X syndrome. Lancet. 1983;1:1221–2.
27. Nistal M, Martínez-García F, Regadera J, Cobo P, Paniagua R. Macro-orchidism: light and electron microscopic study of four cases. Hum Pathol. 1992;23:1011–8.
28. Slegtenhorst-Eegdeman KE, de Rooij DG, Verhoef-Post M, van de Kant HJ, Bakker CE, Oostra BA, Grootegoed JA, Themmen AP. Macroorchidism in FMR1 knockout mice is caused by increased Sertoli cell proliferation during testicular development. Endocrinology. 1998;139:156–62.
29. Laron Z, Karp M, Dolberg L. Juvenile hypothyroidism with testicular enlargement. Acta Paediatr Scand. 1970;59:317–22.
30. Jannini EA, Ulisse S, D'Armiento M. Thyroid hormone and male gonadal function. Endocr Rev. 1995;16:443–59.
31. Castro-Magana M, Angulo M, Canas A, Sharp A, Fuentes B. Hypothalamic-pituitary gonadal axis in boys with primary hypothyroidism and macroorchidism. J Pediatr. 1988;112:397–402.
32. Cordero GL, Gracia R, Nistal M, Lledo G, Peralta A. Hypothyroidism and precocious testicular maturation. Report of a case and review of the literature. Rev Clin Esp. 1973;128:83–8.
33. De La Balze F, Arrillaga F, Mancini RE, Janches M, Davidson OW, Gurtman AI. Male hypogonadism in hypothyroidism: a study of six cases. J Clin Endocrinol Metabol. 1962;22:212–22.
34. Hoffman WH, Kovacs KT, Gala RR, Keel BA, Jarrell TS, Ellegood JO, Burek CL. Macroorchidism and testicular fibrosis associated with autoimmune thyroiditis. J Endocrinol Invest. 1991;14:609–16.
35. Mendis-Handagama SM, SirilAriyaratne HB. Leydig cells, thyroid hormones and steroidogenesis. Indian J Exp Biol. 2005;43:939–62.
36. Bruder JM, Samuels MH, Bremner WJ, Ridgway EC, Wierman ME. Hypothyroidism-induced macroorchidism: use of a gonadotropin-hormone agonist to understand its mechanism and augment adult stature. J Clin Endocrinol Metab. 1995;80:11–6.
37. Alvarez-Acevedo García M, Molina Rodríguez MA, González Casado I, Nistal Martín de Serrano M, Gracia Bouthelier R. Macroorchidism: a case report. An Pediatr (Barc). 2006;64:89–92.
38. Suarez EA, D'alva CB, Campbell A, Miller-Horn J, Dever M, Faerber E, Medonca BB, Latronico AC, De Luca F. Absence of mutation in the follicle-stimulating hormone receptor gene in severe primary hypothyroidism associated with gonadal hyperstimulation. J Pediatr Endocrinol Metab. 2007;20:923–31.
39. De Franca LR, Hess RA, Cooke PS, Russell LD. Neonatal hypothyroidism causes delayed Sertoli cell maturation in rats treated with propylthiouracil: evidence that the Sertoli cell controls testis growth. Anat Rec. 1995;242:57–69.
40. Sun Y, Bak B, Schoenmakers N, van Trotsenburg AS, Oostdijk W, Voshol P, et al. Loss-of-function mutations in IGSF1 cause an X-linked syndrome of central hypothyroidism and testicular enlargement. Nat Genet. 2012;44:1375–81.

41. Joustra SD, Andela CD, Oostdijk W, van Trotsenburg AS, Fliers E, Wit JM, Pereira AM, Middelkoop HA, Biermasz NR. Mild deficits in attentional control in patients with the IGSF1 deficiency syndrome. Clin Endocrinol (Oxf). 2016;84:896–903.
42. Ruvalcaba RH, Castro-Magana M, Angulo M. Macrotestes associated with hyperprolactinemia. J Pediatr Endocrinol Metab. 1996;9:617–22.
43. Esen I, Demirel F. Hypothyroidism-associated testicular enlargement: is it a form of precocious puberty or not? A case report. Turk J Pediatr. 2011;53:210–2.
44. Hanson PL, Aylwin SJ, Monson JP, Burrin JM. FSH secretion predominates in vivo and in vitro in patients with non-functioning pituitary adenomas. Eur J Endocrinol. 2005;52:363–70.
45. Wang X, Ge L, Cui Y, Lang C, Hao C. A FSH-secreting pituitary macroadenoma causing A testosterone deficiency syndrome. Int J Fertil Steril. 2014;8:99–104.
46. Heseltine D, White MC, Kendall-Taylor P, De Kretser DM, Kelly W. Testicular enlargement and elevated serum inhibin concentrations occur in patients with pituitary macroadenomas secreting follicle stimulating hormone. Clin Endocrinol (Oxf). 1989;31:411–23.
47. Dahlqvist P, Koskinen LO, Brännström T, Hägg E. Testicular enlargement in a patient with a FSH-secreting pituitary adenoma. Endocrine. 2010;37:289–93.
48. Silver HK, Kiyasu W, George J, Deamer WC. Syndrome of congenital hemihypertrophy, shortness of stature, and elevated urinary gonadotropins. Pediatrics. 1953;12:368–76.
49. Russell A. A syndrome of intra-uterine dwarfism recognizable at birth with cranio-facial dysostosis, disproportionately short arms, and other anomalies (5 examples). Proc R Soc Med. 1954;47:1040–4.
50. Lodish MB, Gartner LA, Albini P, Sabnis G, Brodie A, Meck JM, Meloni-Ehrig AM, Hill S, Tsilou E, Valera VA, Walter BA, Merino MJ, Stratakis CA. Intrauterine growth retardation associated with precocious puberty and sertoli cell hyperplasia. Horm Metab Res. 2010;42:682–8.
51. Nisula BC, Loriaux DL, Sherins RJ, Kulin HE. Benign bilateral testicular enlargement. J Clin Endocrinol Metabol. 1974;38:440–5.
52. Breen DH, Braunstein GD, Neufeld N, Kudish H. Benign macro-orchidism in a pubescent boy. J Urol. 1981;125:589–91.
53. Lee PA, Marshall FF, Greco JM, Jeffs RD. Unilateral testicular hypertrophy: an apparently benign occurrence without cryptorchidism. J Urol. 1982;127:329–31.
54. Somuncu S, Cakmak M, Caglayan F, Akman H, Ulusoy S, Kaya M. Idiopathic benign bilateral testicular enlargement in a pubertal boy: a case report and review of literature. J Pediatr Surg. 2005;40:23–5.
55. Alvarez-Acevedo Garcia M, Molina Rodriguez MA, Gonzalez Casado I, Nistal M, Gracia Bouthelier R. Macrorchidism: a case report. An Pediatr. 2006;64:89–92.
56. Adeb M, Darge K, Snyder H. Idiopathic macroorchidism with testicular lobulation in an adolescent. J Pediatr Urol. 2012;8:e10–2.
57. Nistal M, González-Peramato P, Paniagua R. Congenital Leydig cell hyperplasia. Histopathology. 1988;12:307–17.
58. Shenker A, Laue L, Kosugi S, Merendino Jr JJ, Minegishi T, Cutler Jr CB. A constitutively activating mutation of the luteinizing hormone receptor in familial male precocious puberty. Nature. 1993;365:652–4.
59. Rousseau-Merck MF, Misrahi M, Atger M, Loosfelt H, Milgrom E, Berger R. Localization of the human luteinizing hormone/choriogonadotropin receptor gene (LHCGR) to chromosome 2p21. Cytogenet Cell Genet. 1990;54:77–9.
60. Piolat C, Dyon JF, Chavanis N, Jacquier C, Durand C, Pasquier D. Testicular Leydig cell hyperplasia in children. Prog Urol. 2003;13:110–4.
61. Gondos B, Egli CA, Rosenthal SM, Grumbach MM. Testicular changes in gonadotropin-independent familial male sexual precocity. Familial testotoxicosis. Arch Pathol Lab Med. 1985;109:990–5.
62. Soriano-Guillen L, Mitchell V, Carel JC, Barbet P, Roger M, Lahlou N. Activating mutations in the LH receptor gene: a human model of non FSH-dependent inhibin production and germ cell maturation. J Clin Endocrinol Metab. 2006;91:3041–7.
63. Weinstein LS, Shenker A, Gejman PV, Merino MJ, Friedman E, Spiegel AM. Activating mutations of the stimulatory G protein in the McCune-Albright syndrome. N Engl J Med. 1991;325:1688–95.
64. Latronico AC, Segaloff DL. Naturally occurring mutations of the luteinizing-hormone receptor: lessons learned about reproductive physiology and G protein-coupled receptors. Am J Hum Genet. 1999;65:949–58.
65. Coutant R, Lumbroso S, Rey R, Lahlou N, Venara M, Rouleau S, Sultan C, Limal JM. Macroorchidism due to autonomous hyperfunction of Sertoli cells and G(s) alpha gene mutation: an unusual expression of McCune-Albright syndrome in a prepubertal boy. J Clin Endocrinol Metabol. 2001;86:1778–81.
66. Wasniewska M, De Luca F, Bertelloni S, Matarazzo P, Weber G, Crisafulli G, Valenzise M, Lala R. Testicular microlithiasis: an unreported feature of McCune-Albright syndrome in males. J Pediatr. 2004;145:670–2.
67. Rey RA, Venara M, Coutant R, Trabut JB, Rouleau S, Lahlou N, Sultan C, Limal JM, Picard JY, Lumbroso S. Unexpected mosaicism of R201H-GNAS1 mutant-bearing cells in the testes underlie macro-orchidism without sexual precocity in McCune-Albright syndrome. Hum Mol Genet. 2006;15:3538–43.
68. Colecchia M, Nistal M, Gonzalez-Peramato P, Carmignani L, Salvioni R, Nicolai N, Regadera J. Leydig cell tumor and hyperplasia: a review. Anal Quant Cytol Histol. 2007;29:139–47.
69. Svechnikov K, Landreh L, Weisser J, Izzo G, Colón E, Svechnikova I, Söder O. Origin, development and regulation of human Leydig cells. Horm Res Paediatr. 2010;73:93–101.

70. Rustagi VT, Khadilkar VV, Khadilkar AV, Kinare AS. Macroorchidism in an Indian boy with McCune-Albright syndrome. Indian J Pediatr. 2011;78: 1145–7.
71. Boyce AM, Chong WH, Shawker TH, Pinto PA, Linehan WM, Bhattacharryya N, Merino MJ, Singer FR, Collins MT. Characterization and management of testicular pathology in McCune-Albright syndrome. J Clin Endocrinol Metab. 2012;97:E1782–90.
72. Arrigo T, Pirazzoli P, De Sanctis L, Leone O, Wasniewska M, Messina MF, De Luca F. McCune-Albright syndrome in a boy may present with a monolateral macroorchidism as an early and isolated clinical manifestation. Horm Res. 2006;65:114–9.
73. Khanna G, Kantawala K, Shinawi M, Sarwate S, Dehner LP. McCune-Albright syndrome presenting with unilateral macroorchidism and bilateral testicular masses. Pediatr Radiol. 2010;40(Suppl 1):S16–20.

15 Macroorchidisms Secondary to Functioning Tumors during Childhood

Manuel Nistal, Pilar González-Peramato, and Álvaro Serrano

15.1 Introduction

The presence of Leydig cells in the testis of children is not easy to detect with standard histological techniques. The use of electron microscopy has shown that the population of fetal Leydig cells disappears in early infancy and a new differentiation of adult cells starts from peritubular and perivascular cells with fibroblast appearance. But there are several entities that are characterized sometimes by hyperplasia or hypertrophy of the Leydig cells and others by tumor formation during childhood. Among the first ones, the most frequent are diffuse and nodular hyperplasia of Leydig cells in newborn infants of diabetic mothers [1]; hypertrophy of Leydig cells due to fat accumulation in the androgen insensitivity syndrome, a defect in 5-alpha-reductase, defects in AMH, and mutations of the steroidogenic factor-1 (SF-1/NR5A1) [2]; and focal or diffuse hyperplasia associated with activating mutations of the luteinizing hormone receptor (LHR) [3]. The Leydig cell tumors can be found among the latter [4]. Both diffuse and focal hyperplasia and Leydig cell tumors may present with a picture of androgen hyperfunction causing gonadotropin-independent sexual precocity in boys.

15.2 Leydig Cell Tumors

The Leydig cell tumors represent only 4–9 % of all testicular tumors in prepubertal age [5]. The clinical presentation in childhood is mainly dependant on the endocrine effects of the endocrine neoplasia causing premature isosexual pseudopuberty and macrogenitosomia [6]. Leydig cell tumors are responsible for 10 % of all cases of early pseudopuberty in children. The presentation of the precocious pseudopuberty symptoms is variable – in most cases they start in the first 5 years of life [7]. In some cases, probably because of an early diagnosis, tumors only cause increased testicular size secondary to precocious tubular maturation, and the precocious pseudopuberty symptomatology is absent [8]. The contralateral testis is rarely enlarged.

Histopathology The testicle is enlarged in most patients due to the tumor size and also because of the accelerated maturation of the testicular parenchyma. In most cases there is a palpable nodule, but some cases have been reported in which the diagnosis, in the absence of a palpable mass, was made by ultrasound. They are not encapsulated tumors (Fig. 15.1); the color varies from yellow to brown. Tumor cells are arranged in sheet or trabeculae separated by a rich vascular network. Other patterns observed in the adult such as spindle cells, microcystic, pseudoglandular, lipid-rich cells, and tumors with osseous and adipose metaplasia are rare in childhood. In childhood, the tumor margins are not sharp due to the absence of a capsule, and the tumor often includes some seminiferous tubules peripherally.

Tumor cells are polyhedral, with eosinophilic cytoplasm and eccentric nucleus; spherical; or

M. Nistal et al., *Clues in the Diagnosis of Non-tumoral Testicular Pathology*,
DOI 10.1007/978-3-319-49364-0_15

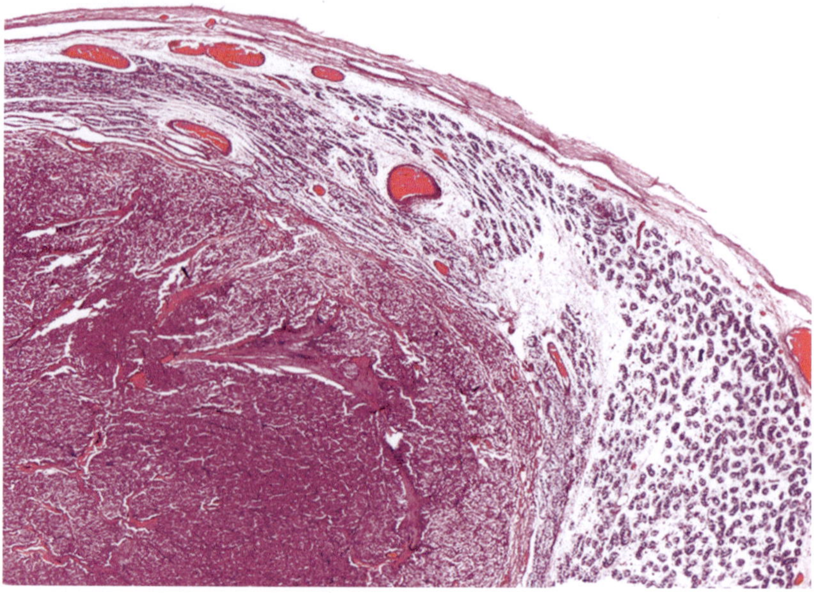

Fig. 15.1 Leydig cell tumor and precocious pseudopuberty. A well-defined but not encapsulated tumor present in a child

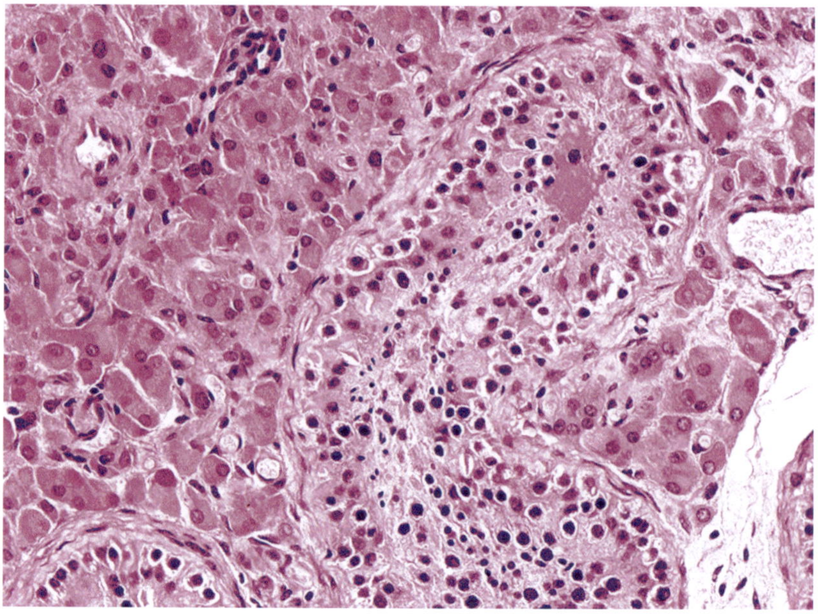

Fig. 15.2 Complete spermatogenesis is shown in a seminiferous tubule trapped by a Leydig cell tumor in a child

ovoid, with central nucleolus. Small vacuoles and lipofuscins can be observed in the cytoplasm. There are no Reinke crystals. All functioning tumors studied under electron microscopy have the following organelles and inclusions in common: tubular cristae mitochondria, great development of the smooth endoplasmic reticulum, lysosomes, lipofuscins, and lipid droplets. Areas of hemorrhage and necrosis are absent.

In all functioning tumors, the peritumoral parenchyma shows an advanced tubular maturation with the presence, even in infancy, of complete spermatogenesis [9] (Fig. 15.2). This maturation is limited to the seminiferous tubules encompassed by the tumor or in its immediate neighborhood (Fig. 15.3). The maturation is secondary to the high rate of androgens that tumor cells are capable of producing. The seminiferous

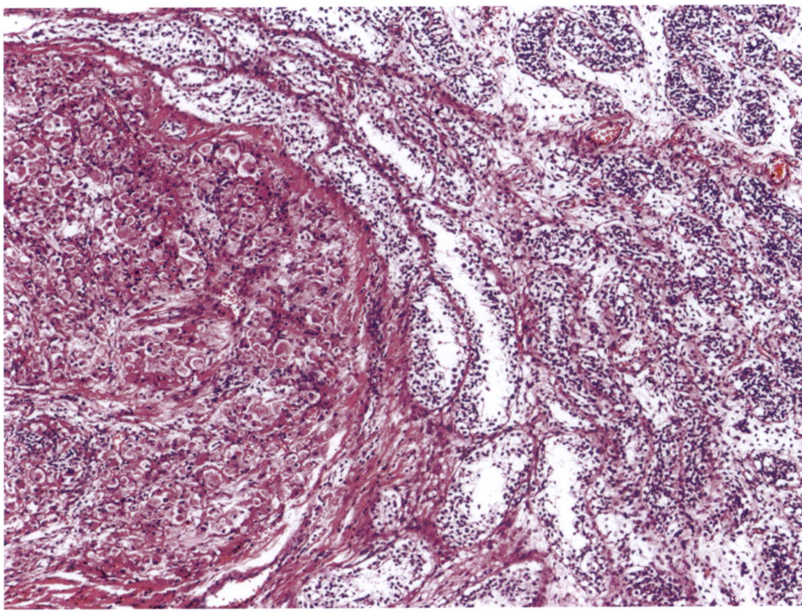

Fig. 15.3 Leydig cell tumor in a child surrounded by seminiferous tubules with lumen and more externally tubules with prepubertal maturation

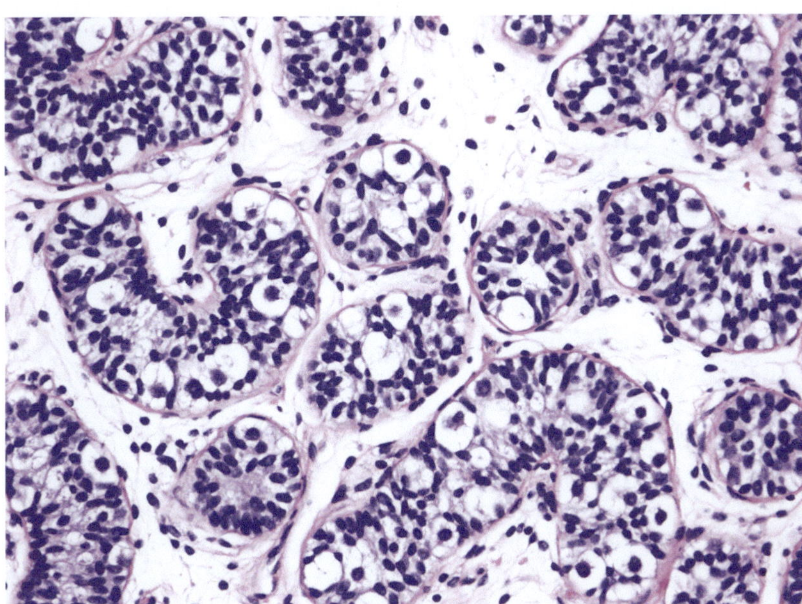

Fig. 15.4 Infantile appearance of the testicular parenchyma far from the Leydig cell tumor shown in the figure above

tubules located far from the tumor, with decreasing concentration of androgens, scarcely show any change (Fig. 15.4). In some tumors androgen production is sufficient to induce tubular maturation and therefore an enlarged size, but insufficient to rise testis serum testosterone levels and produce a premature isosexual pseudopuberty. Ultrasound scanning, selective venous sampling, and the hCG stimulation test help diagnose the tumor [10].

The *clinical differential diagnosis* arises with other forms of precocious pseudopuberty such as virilizing forms of adrenal hyperplasia, adrenal tumors that produce chorionic gonadotropin, male-limited precocious puberty, and the McCune-Albright syndrome. Prepubertal patients virilized by a Leydig cell tumor have low or normal serum levels of gonadotropins, with high levels of testosterone, androstenediol, 17-hydroxyprogesterone, and 17-ketosteroids.

The *histologic differential diagnosis* in childhood covers Leydig cell hyperplasia in patients with gonadotropin-independent male-limited precocious puberty, the "tumors" of the adrenogenital syndrome (TTAGS) (see Chap. 7), and large cell calcifying Sertoli cell tumor.

Since the clinical picture and proliferating cell type in gonadotropin-independent male-limited precocious puberty and functioning Leydig cell tumors are similar, it would seem logic that some relationship should exist between these two pathologies. The fact that symptoms of sexual development appear in Leydig cell tumors preferably between 5 and 9 years [11] while in male-limited precocious puberty they appear before 4 years [3] might suggest as much. Most authors, however, are inclined to think that there is no relationship between them and that they are different pathologies altogether [12]. Patients with precocious puberty due to activating mutations in the gene for the luteinizing hormone receptor do not have an increased risk of Leydig cell tumors [4]. However, there are at least five cases of functioning tumors of Leydig cells with somatic activating mutation (Asp578His) of the LHR gene which reopens the relationship between the two entities, and those somatic activating mutations of gonadotropin receptors are involved in testicular tumorigenesis [13, 14].

The differential diagnosis between Leydig cell hyperplasia and Leydig cell tumors developing precocious pseudopuberty is not easy. Histological studies of patients with this type of testicular Leydig cell hyperplasia, except for the nodule size, number, and the presence therein of seminiferous tubules with spermatogenesis, do not differ from those of Leydig cell tumors. An open excision testicular biopsy has been recommended. If the sample allows the diagnosis of a Leydig cell tumor, enucleation of the tumor mass is advisable [15, 16].

Leydig cell tumors differ from large cell calcifying Sertoli cell tumors by the absence in the tumor of Leydig cells of multifocal, bilateral, intratubular calcifications, by a stroma rich in polymorphonuclear leukocytes, laminated calcifications, and the tendency of cells to be arranged in a pseudoacinar pattern. The absence of a hyalinizing intratubular Sertoli cell neoplasia is another fact of importance in the differential diagnosis. Immunohistochemically, both tumors share the expression of several antibodies even though some differences in the expression of Melan A, CD10, mitochondria, and S100 protein beta have been observed [17].

Prognosis and Treatment The vast majority of Leydig cell tumors in children are benign in contrast to the 10 % rate observed in malignant tumors of adults [7]. Malignancy has only been reported in some bilateral tumors [18]. The criteria for malignancy, as occurs in adult tumors, are not well established. The presence of necrosis, the high cellular pleomorphism, the high number of mitoses, the atypical mitoses, and both vascular and the tunica albuginea infiltration can issue an alert for aggressive behavior. Since the vast majority of tumors have a benign biological behavior, their treatment is enucleation [19, 20].

15.3 Sex Cord Tumors

Large cell hyalinizing Sertoli cell neoplasia (Figs.15.5 and 15.6) and the large cell calcifying Sertoli cell tumor can induce bilateral testicular enlargement (caused by the tumor and the precocious tubular maturation) and a precocious pseudopuberty, which is isosexual (development of musculature, appearance of axillary and pubic hair) and heterosexual (gynecomastia). Tumor cells have been suggested to stimulate the Leydig cells to synthesize androgens. Tumor cells themselves would aromatize these androgens into estrogens, and both steroid hormones would be responsible for the clinical symptoms [21, 22]. These tumors are frequently observed in the Peutz-Jeghers syndrome [23–25] and the Carney complex [26].

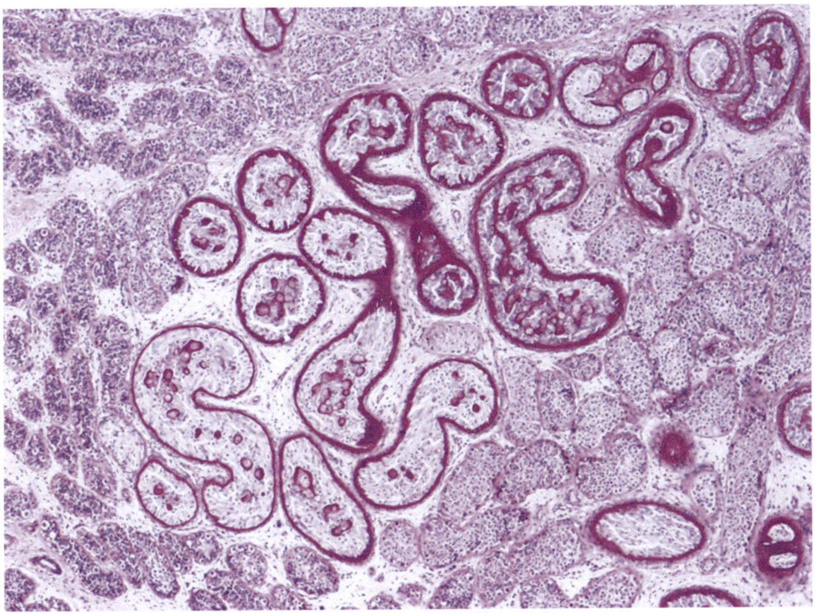

Fig. 15.5 Large cell hyalinizing Sertoli cell neoplasia in a prepubertal patient. The tumoral tubules show basement membrane thickening and protrusions inward (immunostaining with collagen IV)

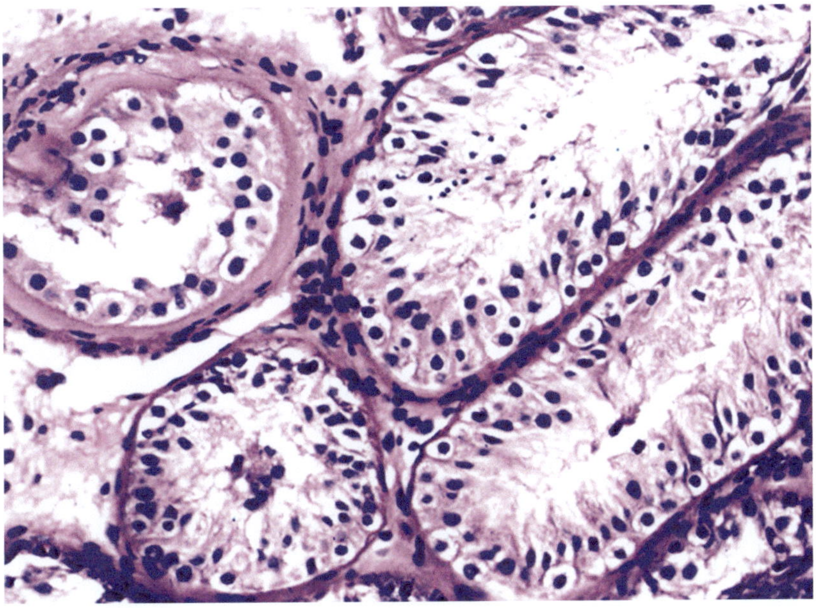

Fig. 15.6 Initial spermatogenesis is shown in the seminiferous tubules peripheral to a large cell hyalinizing Sertoli cell neoplasia (same case of the previous figure)

15.4 Adrenocortical Tumors

Adrenocortical tumors are rare in childhood and account for less than 0.2 % of all pediatric tumors [27]. There are two peaks of higher incidence, before age four and in the fourth decade. Several congenital malformations such as the Beckwith-Wiedemann's syndrome and the Li-Fraumeni's syndrome may be associated with this tumor [28].

In childhood, most patients with virilizing tumors of the adrenal cortex show small testes, but boys with testicular hypertrophy have exceptionally been observed [29]. It has been suggested that, in these cases, the seminiferous tubules could be developed under the adrenal androgenic action [30]. Other patients with virilizing adrenocortical carcinoma after removal of the adrenal tumor develop a central precocious puberty requiring treatment to delay pubertal progression with a gonadotropin-releasing hormone agonist [31]. In the untreated or inadequately treated congenital adrenal hyperplasia, both tests can reach a big size because of the "tumoral" growth of cells that are similar to the cells of the adrenal cortex [32]. A similar condition can be observed in Nelson's syndrome patients (see Chap. 7)..

15.5 Extratesticular HCG-Secreting Tumors

In patients with hCG-secreting germ cell tumors, complete suppression of plasma LH and FSH with increased plasma concentrations of both testosterone and estradiol is often discovered [33]. The increased testicular size observed in patients with paraneoplastic precocious pseudopuberty secondary to hepatoblastoma [34–37] and extratesticular (retroperitoneum, mediastinum, basal ganglia, pineal, or suprasellar region) hCG-secreting germ cell tumors are very mild [38–43]. However, some patients show a precocious pubertal maturation that can be either diffuse or nodular. These nodules consist of hyperplastic Leydig cells and seminiferous tubules that can show complete spermatogenesis. Outside the nodule, the seminiferous tubules maintain their prepubertal pattern. In some cases, only Leydig cell hyperplasia is diffusely observed [44].

15.6 Other Tumors

We recently had the opportunity to study an 11-year-old patient with unilateral macroorchidism not associated with any of the situations discussed above. Hormonal determinations were normal for his age. The sonographic diagnosis was a 1 cm intraparenchymal tumor. Orchiectomy was performed. The histological examination disclosed a focally advanced maturation of the spermatogenesis responsible for the patient's testicular enlargement. Only the study of serial sections highlighted in the central part of this lesion is a microscopic capillary angioma. Our interpretation was that local maturation was produced by the larger hormonal inflow provided by the angioma vessels (Figs. 15.7 and 15.8).

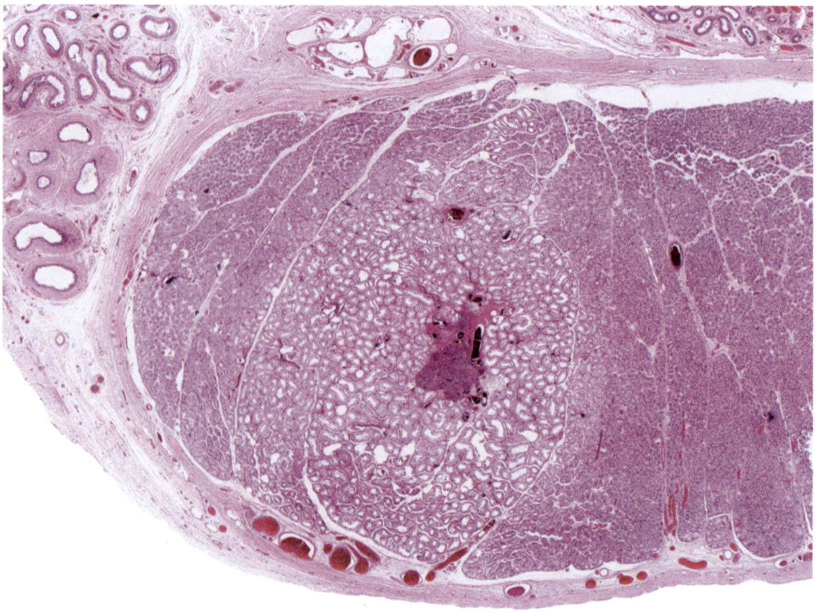

Fig. 15.7 Macroorchidism secondary to maturation of seminiferous tubules located in the vicinity of a microscopic hemangioma in a prepubertal child

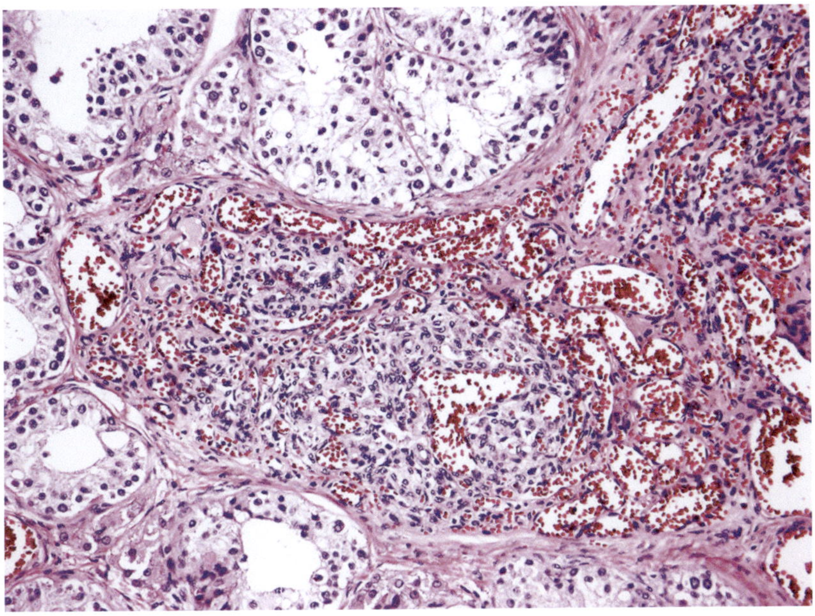

Fig. 15.8 Capillary hemangioma is surrounded by seminiferous tubules with spermatogenesis in a child (same case of the previous figure)

References

1. Nistal M, González-Peramato P, Paniagua R. Congenital Leydig cell hyperplasia. Histopathology. 1988;12:307–17.
2. Camats N, Pandey AV, Fernández-Cancio M, Andaluz P, Janner M, Torán N, Moreno F, Bereket A, Akcay T, García-García E, Muñoz MT, Gracia R, Nistal M, Castaño L, Mullis PE, Carrascosa A, Audí L, Flück CE. Ten novel mutations in the NR5A1 gene cause disordered sex development in 46,XY and ovarian insufficiency in 46,XX individuals. J Clin Endocrinol Metab. 2012;97:E1294–306.
3. Holland FJ. Gonadotropin-independent precocious puberty. Endocrinol Metab Clin North Am. 1991;20: 191–210.
4. Wilson BE, Netzloff ML. Primary testicular abnormalities causing precocious puberty Leydig cell tumor, Leydig cell hyperplasia, and adrenal rest tumor. Ann Clin Lab Sci. 1983;13:315–20.
5. Pohl HG, Shukla AR, Metcalf PD, Cilento BG, Retik AB, Bagli DJ, Huff DS, Rushton HG. Prepubertal testis tumors: actual prevalence rate of histological types. J Urol. 2004;172:2370–2.
6. Gracia R, Nistal M, Gallego ME, Lledo G, Oliver A, Utrilla J, Gancedo P. Tumor de células de Leydig con pseudopubertad precoz. An Esp Pediatr. 1980;13: 593–8.
7. Kim I, Young RH, Scully RE. Leydig cell tumors of the testis: a clinico-pathological analysis of 40 cases and review of the literature. Am J Surg Pathol. 1985;9: 177–92.
8. Polepalle SK, Shabaik A, Alagiri M. Leydig cell tumor in a child with spermatocyte maturation and no pseudoprecocious puberty. Urology. 2003;62:551vi–551vii.
9. O'Grady MJ, McGrath N, Quinn FM, Capra ML, McDermott MB, Murphy NP. Spermatogenesis in a prepubertal boy. J Pediatr. 2012;161:369–369.e1.
10. Alonso Domínguez FJ, Osorio Acosta VA. Leydig cell tumor presenting as precocious pseudopuberty in a 4-year-old boy. Arch Esp Urol. 2004;57:426–8.
11. Scully RE. Testicular tumors with endocrine manifestations. In: De Groot LJ, editor. Endocrinology. Philadelphia: Saunders WB; 1995. p. 2442–8.
12. Naughton CK, Nadler RB, Basler JW, Humphrey PA. Leydig cell hyperplasia. Br J Urol. 1998;81:282–9.
13. Liu G, Duranteau L, Carel JC, Monroe J, Doyle DA, Shenker A. Leydig-cell tumors caused by an activating mutation of the gene encoding the luteinizing hormone receptor. N Engl J Med. 1999;341:1731–6.
14. Canto P, Söderlund D, Ramón G, Nishimura E, Méndez JP. Mutational analysis of the luteinizing hormone receptor gene in two individuals with Leydig cell tumors. Am J Med Genet. 2002;108:148–52.
15. Leung AC, Kogan SJ. Focal lobular spermatogenesis and pubertal acceleration associated with ipsilateral Leydig cell hyperplasia. Urology. 2000;56:508–9.
16. Tazi MF, Mellas S, El Fassi MJ, Farih MH. Leydig cell hyperplasia revealed by gynecomastia. Rev Urol. 2008;10:164–7.
17. Sato K, Ueda Y, Sakurai A, Ishikawa Y, Okamoto SY, Ikawa H, Katsuda S. Large cell calcifying Sertoli cell tumor of the testis: comparative immunohistochemical study with Leydig cell tumor. Pathol Int. 2005;55: 366–71.
18. Slama A, Elleuch A, Yacoubi MT, Ben Sorba N, Mosbah AT. Bilateral Leydig cell tumor of the test: a case report. Ann Urol (Paris). 2003;37:213–6.
19. Konrad D, Schoenle EJ. Ten-year follow-up in a boy with Leydig cell tumor after selective surgery. Horm Res. 1999;51:96–100.

20. Henderson CG, Ahmed AA, Sesterhenn I, Belman AB, Rushton HG. Enucleation for prepubertal Leydig cell tumor. J Urol. 2006;176:703–5.
21. Berensztein E, Belgorosky A, De Davila MTG, Rivarola MA. Testicular steroid biosynthesis in a boy with a large cell calcifying Sertoli cell tumor producing prepubertal gynecomastia. Steroids. 1995;60:220–5.
22. Diamond Jr FB, Root AW, Hoover DL, Monteforte H. Hetero- and isosexual pseudoprecocity associated with testicular sex-cord tumors in an 8 year-old male. J Pediatr Endocrinol Metab. 1996;9:407–14.
23. Coen P, Kulin H, Ballantine T, Zaino R, Frauenhoffer E, Boal D, Inkster S, Brodie A, Santen R. An aromatase-producing sex-cord tumor resulting in prepubertal gynecomastia. N Engl J Med. 1991;324:317–22.
24. Ros P, Nistal M, Alonso M, Calvo de Mora J, Yturriaga R, Barrio R. Sertoli cell tumour in a boy with Peutz-Jeghers syndrome. Histopathology. 1999;34:84–6.
25. Ulbright TM, Amin MB, Young RH. Intratubular large cell hyalinizing Sertoli cell neoplasia of the testis: a report of 8 cases of a distinctive lesion of the Peutz-Jeghers syndrome. Am J Surg Pathol. 2007;31:827–35.
26. Carney JA. Carney complex: the complex of mixomas, spotty pigmentation, endocrine overactivity, and Schwanomas. Semin Dermatol. 1995;14:90–8.
27. Sipayya V, Yadav YK, Arora R, Sharma U, Gupta K. Virilizing adrenocortical carcinoma in a child: a rare enigma. Indian J Endocrinol Metab. 2012;16:621–3.
28. Wieneke JA, Thompson LD, Heffess CS. Adrenal cortical neoplasms in the pediatric population: a clinicopathologic and immunophenotypic analysis of 83 patients. Am J Surg Pathol. 2003;27:867–81.
29. Bonfig W, Bittmann I, Bechtold S, Kammer B, Noelle V, Arleth S, Raile K. Virilising adrenocortical tumours in children. Eur J Pediatr. 2003;162:623–8.
30. Drago JR, Olstein JS, Tesluk H, Sheikholislam B, Palmer JM, Link D. Virilizing adrenal cortical carcinoma with hypertrophy of spermatic tubules in childhood. Urology. 1979;14:70–5.
31. Kim MS, Yang EJ, Cho DH, Hwang PH, Lee DY. Virilizing adrenocortical carcinoma advancing to central precocious puberty after surgery. Korean J Fam Med. 2015;36:150–3.
32. Cunnanh D, Perry L, Dacie JA, Grant DB, Lowe DG, Savage MO, Besser GM. Bilateral testicular tumours in congenital adrenal hyperplasia: a continuing diagnostic and therapeutic dilemma. Clin Endocrinol (Oxf). 1989;30:141–7.
33. Reznik Y, Rieu M, Kuhn JM, Mandard JC, Bottet P, Lemonnier D, Bekka S, Mahoudeau J. Luteinizing hormone regulation by sex steroids in men with germinal and Leydig cell tumours. Clin Endocrinol (Oxf). 1993;38:487–93.
34. Bode HH, Schimana W, Swai B, Bode U. Sexual precocity associated with an abdominal tumor in an African boy. J Pediatr Endocrinol Metab. 2008;21:275–7.
35. Eren E, Demirkaya M, Çakır ED, Sevinir B, Sağlam H, Tarım Ö. A rare cause of precocious puberty: hepatoblastoma. J Clin Res Pediatr Endocrinol. 2009;1:281–3.
36. Al-Jumaily U, Sammour I, Al-Muhaisen F, Ajlouni F, Sultan I. Precocious puberty in an infant with hepatoblastoma: a case report. J Med Case Reports. 2011;5: 422.
37. Marino S, Caruso M, Magro G, D'Amico S, La Spina M, Moscheo C, Russo G, Di Cataldo A. Hepatoblastoma presenting as precocious puberty: a case report. J Pediatr Endocrinol Metab. 2015;28: 429–32.
38. Bowden SA, Germak JA. Klinefelter syndrome presenting with precocious puberty due to a human chorionic gonadotropin (hCG)-producing mediastinal germinoma. J Pediatr Endocrinol Metab. 2006;19: 1371.
39. Marshall GA, McMahon SK, Nicholls W, Pretorius CJ, Ungerer JP. Gonadotrophin-independent precocious puberty in an eight-year-old boy due to ectopic human chorionic gonadotrophin from the central nervous system. Ann Clin Biochem. 2010;47:271–4.
40. Nascimento DJ, Leães CG, Pereira-Lima JF, Oliveira MC. Precocious puberty due to human chorionic gonadotropin secreting germinoma. J Pediatr Neurosci. 2012;7:202–4.
41. Nair M, Kusumakumary P, Ninan A. Precocious puberty as initial presentation in mediastinal tumour. Indian Pediatr. 2013;50:424–6.
42. Wendt S, Shelso J, Wright K, Furman W. Neoplastic causes of abnormal puberty. Pediatr Blood Cancer. 2014;61:664–71.
43. Goswami S, Chakraborty PP, Bhattacharjee R, Roy A, Thukral A, Selvan C, Ghosh S, Mukhopadhyay S, Chowdhury S. Precocious puberty: a blessing in disguise! Indian J Endocrinol Metab. 2013;17(Suppl 1):S111–3.
44. Cohgen AR, Wilson JA, Sadeghi-Nejad A. Gonadotropin-secreting pineal teratoma causing prcocious puberty. Neurosurgery. 1991;28:597–602.

16 Value of Testicular Biopsy in Nonobstructive Azoospermia

Manuel Nistal, Pilar González-Peramato, and Álvaro Serrano

16.1 Tubular Hyalinization

A small percentage of infertile patients (8 %) show an image of diffuse tubular hyalinization in the testicular biopsy. Hyalinization of the seminiferous tubules is a terminal atrophy lesion that includes not only the loss of germ cells and Sertoli cells but also changes in the tunica propria and in the Leydig cells. As a consequence the testicular size is very small. Given a series of histological details and clinical data, specify injury mechanisms can be specified in most cases. The most frequent causes of tubular hyalinization are dysgenetic, hormone deprivation, an ischemic mechanism, post-obstructive, post-inflammatory, and tubular hyalinization secondary to physical and chemical agents.

Dysgenetic Tubular Hyalinization

It is a diffuse lesion; most of the seminiferous tubules are in the same developmental stage. The few preserved seminiferous tubules more often show only dysgenetic Sertoli cells and spermatogenesis only in exceptional cases. Atrophic tubules have absent or decreased elastic fibers. The most common entities that can occur with this image are the Klinefelter's syndrome (see Chap. 18) and most undescended testes that were not descended before puberty. This lesion can be seen in patients with focal mixed atrophy.

Tubular Hyalinization by Hormone Deprivation

The tubular hyalinization by hormone deprivation is a diffuse process. It is the manifestation of a postpubertal onset hypogonadotropic hypogonadism (see Chap. 19).

Tubular Hyalinization by an Ischemic Mechanism

The more frequent testicular atrophies secondary to ischemia are caused by torsion of the spermatic cord, by iatrogenic injury of the testicular artery or its branches during interventions on the inguinal region, and by the involvement of the nodose panarteritis or intense arteriosclerosis (see Chaps. 24 and 25).

Post-obstructive Tubular Hyalinization

Obstruction of the spermatic ducts can lead to atrophy of the seminiferous tubules. However, for the obstruction to originate tubular hyalinization, the obstruction is required to be located very close to the testicle, e.g., at the head of the epididymis, and specifically the efferent ducts that act as shock absorbers to absorb 90 % of the testicular fluid (see Chap. 17).

Post-inflammatory Tubular Hyalinization

Virus infections often affect the testicle, and what is more important, in many cases they do so without any symptoms or subclinical manifestations (see Chap. 26). An immunologically based tubular

M. Nistal et al., *Clues in the Diagnosis of Non-tumoral Testicular Pathology*, DOI 10.1007/978-3-319-49364-0_16

atrophy is observed in peripheral seminiferous tubules with germ cell tumors or in carriers of a "burned" tumor [1].

Tubular Hyalinization Secondary to Physical and Chemical Agents

The range of agents capable of producing a tubular hyalinization is very broad. Radiation and chemotherapy are among the main ones (see Chap. 40).

16.2 Sertoli Cell-Only Syndrome (SCOS)

This term groups all scenarios of secretory azoospermia in which the seminiferous tubules show only Sertoli cells. They represent 13 % of biopsies of infertile patients who present with azoospermia [2]. The presence of both mature and functional Sertoli cells is the basic requirement for germ cell survival. The morphology of Sertoli cells allows to distinguish three types of Sertoli cell-only syndromes in infertile patients: dysgenetic Sertoli cell-only, adult or mature Sertoli cell-only, and atrophic or involutive Sertoli cell-only.

Dysgenetic Sertoli Cell-Only Syndrome

Dysgenetic Sertoli cells are cells that during puberty acquire a morphology different from that of the normal adult cells. There are basically two types of tubules with dysgenetic Sertoli cells. One in which Sertoli cells predominate whose nuclei are reminiscent of adult cells due to their large size, lax chromatin, and well-developed central nucleolus. But contrary to normal adult cells, the nuclear membrane does not show any folds or these are minimal [3]. The configuration of the nuclei is spherical or ovoid rather than triangular, and there are small aggregates of heterochromatin irregularly dispersed in the nucleoplasm. Another configuration in which Sertoli cells showing elongated nuclei with generally well-developed nucleolus and several irregularly arranged granulations of heterochromatin is observed [4, 5] (Fig. 16.1). Immunohistochemically, in addition to vimentin, dysgenetic Sertoli cells express antimüllerian hormone (AMH) and cytokeratin 18. The presence of AMH immunoreactivity [6] and cytokeratin 18 [7] is considered an evidence of immaturity, like the absence of elastic fibers in the tubular wall [8].

Mature or Adult Sertoli Cell-Only Syndrome

In this syndrome most seminiferous tubules are lined with Sertoli cells with nuclear characteristics

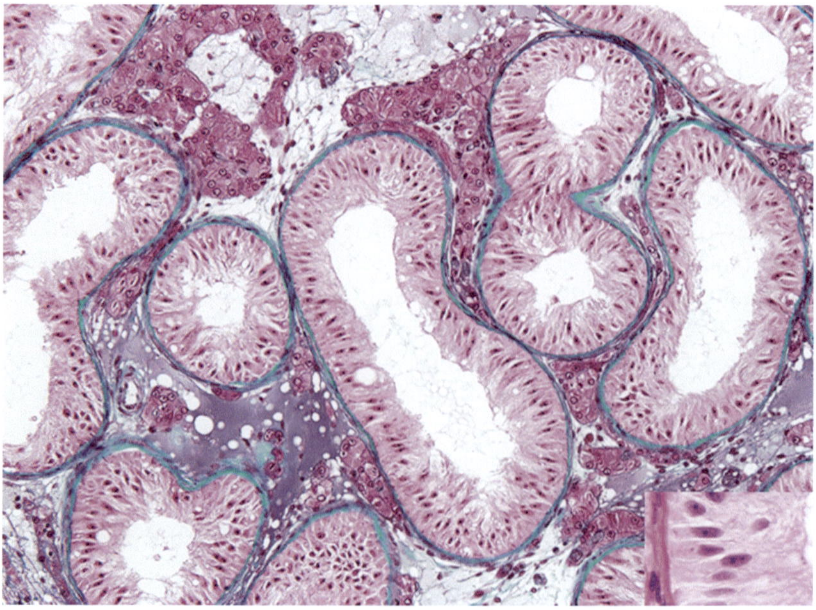

Fig. 16.1 Dysgenetic Sertoli cell-only syndrome. Seminiferous tubules are lined by Sertoli cells with high cylindrical cytoplasm. Inset: Sertoli cells show elongated nuclei with central nucleolus. In the interstitium there is mild Leydig cell hyperplasia

similar to normal adult cells (Fig. 16.2). The only disagreeing datum is a large number of Sertoli cells by transverse tubular section (14 + 0.89). Similarly to other types of tubules with Sertoli cell-only syndromes, the lamina propria often is thickened with increased collagen type IV and the beta2 chain of laminin [9].

Involutive or Atrophic Sertoli Cell-Only Syndrome

There are testicles that may have had a germline for some time, but due to a series of circumstances, they have suffered an involution that affected not only the germline but also the Sertoli cells, leaving in them morphological consequences at both the cytoplasm and nuclei. Seminiferous tubules with Sertoli cell-only with irregular nucleus with multiple and deep folds predominate, giving them a lobed appearance rather than the characteristic triangular nuclei of adult Sertoli cells. The nucleolus can be of normal size. The number of Sertoli cells by transverse tubular section is not as increased as in the preceding syndromes [10]. The seminiferous tubules retain the lumen and have a reduced size, varying degrees of thickening of the tunica propria, and persistence of elastic fibers.

Etiology SCOS may be caused by epigenetic and/or genetic factors. The patient's pathology may be ascertained depending on the type of the Sertoli cells. Dysgenetic Sertoli cell-only syndrome can be seen in undescended adult testes, whether they have been descended in childhood or not [11, 12]; in patients with chromosomal abnormalities such as 45,X, 48,XYYY, and 46,XX and Y chromosome deletions [13]; and in patients with idiopathic infertility and scrotal testes (TERADA 1991). Except for cases with a history of cryptorchidism, in which injuries can be both uni- and bilateral, the other lesions are bilateral.

When Del Castillo described the adult Sertoli cell-only syndrome in 1947 [14], he suggested that the failure would lie in the absence of migration of germ cells from the wall of the yolk sac to the genital ridges. Experimentally, the development of seminiferous tubules with Sertoli cell-only with both cold testicular ischemia [15] and blocking migration of germ cells has been achieved with busulfan [16]. A mutation of the c-KIT gene or its ligands could cause an anomaly in the migration, proliferation, and survival of primordial germ cells. [17]. *PLK4* mutations, a protein that plays a critical role in centriole dupli-

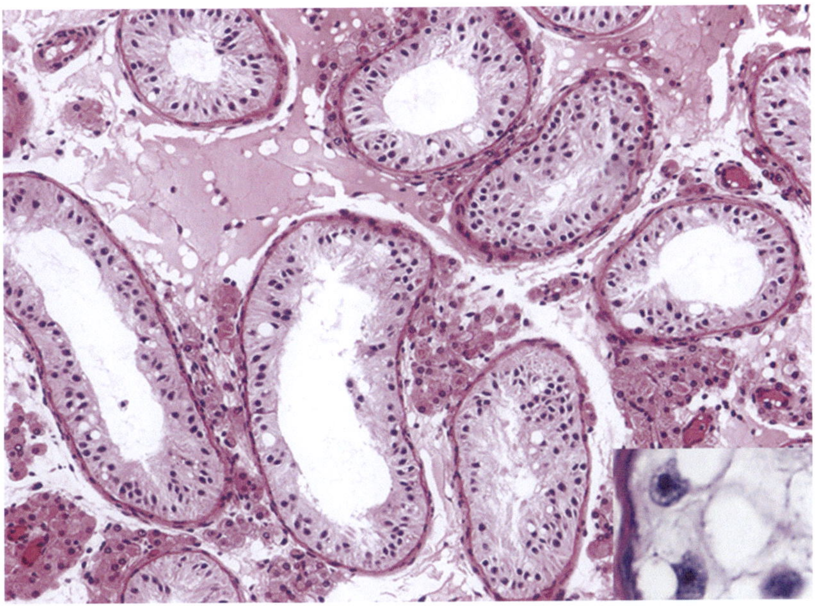

Fig. 16.2 Adult Sertoli cell-only syndrome. Seminiferous tubules are lined by Sertoli cells with low cylindrical cytoplasm. Inset: triangular-folded nuclei and voluminous nucleolus

cation and nuclei formation, cause impaired spermatogenesis and Sertoli cell-only in humans [18]. The analysis of genes whose expression occurs only in germ cells during spermatogenesis may be of prognostic value as it allows to discard the presence of Sertoli cell-only tubules in other areas of the parenchyma.

Other genetic risk factors that have been associated with SCOS are SEPTIN12 and the genotype and allele frequencies in SNP3, SNP4, and SNP6 which are higher than in controls [19]. In studies of human *LRWD1* gene, the allele frequencies of two of the three SNPs (SNP1 and SNP2) are also more frequent than in controls [20]. In evaluations of copy number variants (CNVs), sex chromosomal CNVs have been observed to be overexpressed in SCOS patients [21].

Involutive Sertoli cell-only syndrome is related to treatment with physical agents such as ionizing radiation or chemical agents such as corticosteroids or treatments used in antitumor chemotherapy and nephrotic syndromes. There is also the possibility that these alterations are a manifestation of early aging of a dysgenetic testis (see Chap. 40).

There is a small group of patients showing dysgenetic Sertoli cell-only or adult Sertoli cell-only in the testicular biopsy who have sperm in the ejaculates. This apparent disagreement between the testicular biopsy and the spermiogram is due to the existence of mixed atrophy in the testicles, in these cases the biopsy being unrepresentative of the testicular pathology. The search for meiotic (lactate dehydrogenase C4) and post-meiotic (transition protein 1 and protamine 1 and 2) germ cell gene products ensures the presence of germ cells [22].

16.3 Mixed Atrophy

Mixed atrophy is a descriptive term that refers to the presence of a group or groups of seminiferous tubules with Sertoli cell-only in the same testicle, side by side with other tubules with germline [23] (Fig. 16.3). The extension of tubules with Sertoli cell-only is very variable, from a few to most tubules in the biopsy. Tubules with spermatogenesis may be normal or show any type of lesion in the germline. Sometimes associated with these lesions, there are some tubules with complete hyalinization. The testicles are usually small. The lesions may be unilateral or bilateral.

This lesion is more common than that expressed by the literature, and many cases could have been included in other lesional patterns. Thus, it is said that in some cases of hyposper-

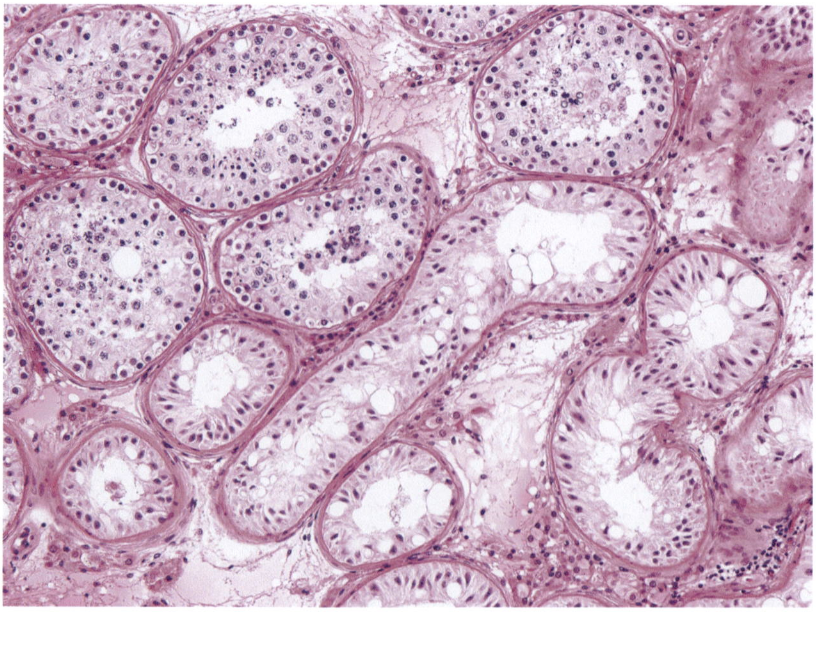

Fig. 16.3 Mixed atrophy. Group of seminiferous tubules with Sertoli cell-only side by side to larger tubules with complete spermatogenesis

matogenesis, decreased germ cells can become so important that they appear in Sertoli cell-only tubules, or otherwise, in some Sertoli cell-only syndromes, focal hypospermatogenesis can be observed [24]. Once the lesion is detected, it is necessary to quantify the number of tubules with spermatogenesis and to perform a quantitative study of the seminiferous epithelium to assess the quality of spermatogenesis.

This type of testicular atrophy is observed in patients with idiopathic infertility and a history of cryptorchidism, even if it was properly corrected in childhood. This lesion may appear in the testis that was undescended and also in the contralateral scrotal testis. Mixed atrophy can also be seen in patients with retractile testes, patients with macroorchidism [25], patients with intravaginal spermatic cord torsion, both in the twisted testis and in the contralateral one [26], in patients with chromosomal abnormalities such as Down's syndrome, in 47,XYY and 46,XX individuals, in some Klinefelter's syndromes, microdeletion of the Y chromosome, and giant Y chromosome. It has also been reported in patients with incomplete androgen insensitivity [27, 28], in patients who were undergoing chemotherapy or corticosteroid therapy when spermatogenesis [29] is retrieved, and in patients with a history of viral orchitis.

16.4 Lesions of Basal and Adluminal Compartment

16.4.1 Hypospermatogenesis

Hypospermatogenesis is defined as a lesion characterized by the presence of a number of spermatogonia and first-order spermatocytes lower than normal, but with a preserved ratio between these two cell types. Most seminiferous tubules have a small number of spermatids (Fig. 16.4). There is a tubular focal hyalinization in 8 % of the patients [23]. Most patients have severe oligozoospermia. Inhibin B is the most sensitive and specific endocrine marker of hypospermatogenesis [30].

We can distinguish two different forms of hypospermatogenesis: pure hypospermatogenesis and hypospermatogenesis associated with sloughing of first-order spermatocytes. Pure hypospermatogenesis is characterized by maintaining cell proliferation and differentiation at levels lower than normal, but keeping the same proportionality between germ cells. In the hypospermatogenesis associated with sloughing of the first-order spermatocytes, we observe (a) a low number of spermatogonia and first-order spermatocytes, the number of first-order sper-

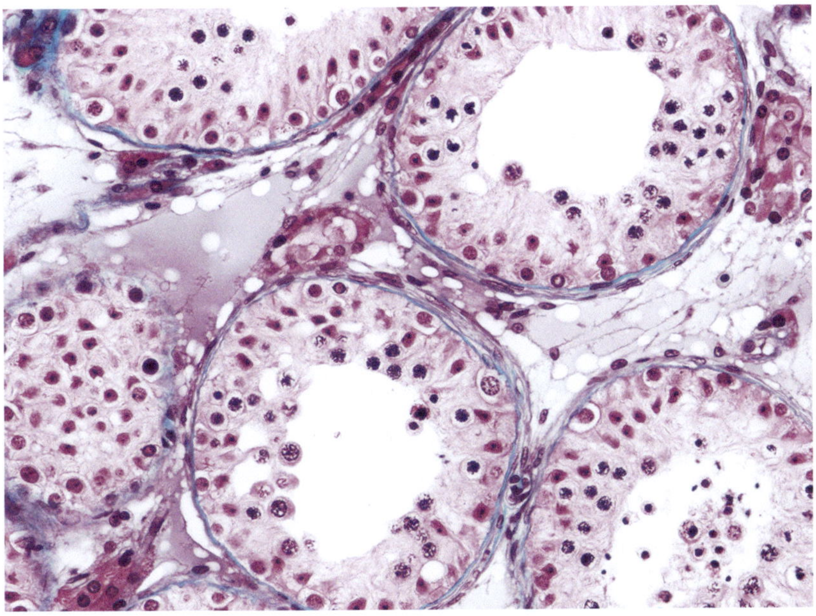

Fig. 16.4 Hypospermatogenesis. Transverse tubular sections of several seminiferous tubules. The count of all germ cells shows a marked decrease in both spermatogonia and spermatocytes and spermatids. The variable number of germ cells in each tubular section is characteristic

matocytes always being higher than the number of spermatogonia, which is consistent with the definition of hypospermatogenesis, and (b) a loss of most spermatocytes by degeneration, leading the remaining ones to be isolated spermatids.

The etiology of pure hypospermatogenesis has been linked in the past with the following situations: hormonal dysregulation, congenital deficiency of germ cells, Sertoli cell deficit [31], dysfunction of Leydig cells [32], androgen insensitivity [33], and exposure to physical and chemical agents [34].

Quantitative and qualitative studies of the seminiferous epithelium in hypospermatogenesis associated with sloughing of first-order spermatocytes allow to distinguish at least three situations:

- Seminiferous tubules with adult Sertoli cells with increased apical cytoplasmic vacuoles, associated with spermatogenesis with a low number of maturational abnormalities and tubular ectasia. These changes suggest a lesion of the seminiferous epithelium secondary to an obstructive mechanism, which in many cases is associated with an ipsilateral varicocele.
- Seminiferous tubules with involutive Sertoli cells (nuclei with excessively folded contours and hyperchromatism), with or without morphological abnormalities of the germ cells. These changes suggest a primary or secondary Sertoli cell alteration and secondary abnormalities of the germ cells. It is observed in cases of idiopathic infertility.
- Seminiferous tubes with normal adult Sertoli cells and germ cell abnormalities that preferentially affect first-order spermatocytes and spermatids. It is observed in anomalies of meiosis.

16.4.2 Maturation Arrest

Spermatogonial Maturation Arrest

This situation is found when the following two factors are present in the testicular biopsy: a number of spermatogonia less than 17 by cross tubular section and a number of first-order spermatocytes lower than the number of spermatogonia. Spermatids are generally absent (Fig. 16.5). This situation is the result of an insufficient proliferation of spermatogonia. Bearing in mind that Sertoli cells are directly involved in the regulation of spermatogonia proliferation, an

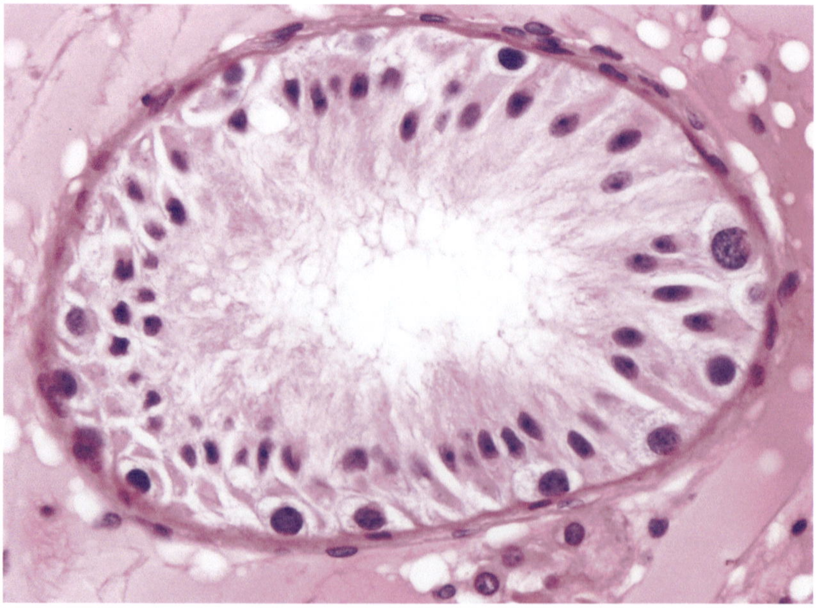

Fig. 16.5 Infertile patients with spermatogonial maturation arrest. The number of Sertoli cells is increased

approach to the etiology of spermatogonia maturation arrest has been attempted by assessing the characteristics of companion Sertoli cells [35]. In this way, we can distinguish the following maturation arrests:

- Maturation arrest with *immature Sertoli cells*, which is a bilateral lesion typical of primary hypogonadotropic hypogonadisms.
- Maturation arrest with *adult Sertoli cells*. Testicular involvement may be unilateral or bilateral. In unilateral cases it is associated with ipsilateral varicocele, epididymitis, and testicular trauma, situations that may injure the testicle through an obstructive mechanism. The current knowledge considers the bilateral cases to be idiopathic.
- Maturation arrest with *involutive Sertoli cells*. In most cases the lesions are bilateral and caused by the action of physical and chemical agents [36].
- Maturation arrest with *dedifferentiated Sertoli cells*. The seminiferous tubules show a great thickening of the tunica propria. Spermatogonia present are mostly Ad type and Sertoli cells, increased in number by cross tubular section, and have spherical nuclei with a small central nucleolus. The cytoplasm is rich in vacuoles and lipid inclusions. Leydig cells are decreased in number and show signs of atrophy. The lesion is bilateral and occurs in treatments with estrogen, GnRH agonists, and antiandrogens [37].
- Maturation arrest with *dysgenetic Sertoli cells*. The seminiferous tubules are similar to those of dysgenetic Sertoli cell-only syndrome, but all tubules have several spermatogonia. Half of the patients have a history of cryptorchidism.

Spermatocyte Maturation Arrest

Some patients with first-order spermatocytes sloughing are carriers of abnormalities in meiosis [38, 39]. This anomaly may be simply suggested by the histological pattern when the arrest in maturation occurs in the preleptotene and leptotene spermatocytes, which is infrequent [40], or in pachytene spermatocytes, which is much more common [41]. The lesion is bilateral. The anomaly in meiosis determines two facts, the practical absence of spermatids and a large accumulation of first-order spermatocytes in the seminiferous tubules (Fig. 16.6). It has been reported in association with trisomies, microdeletions of the Y chromosome, and balanced autosomal anomalies. In patients with abnormal chromosomal con-

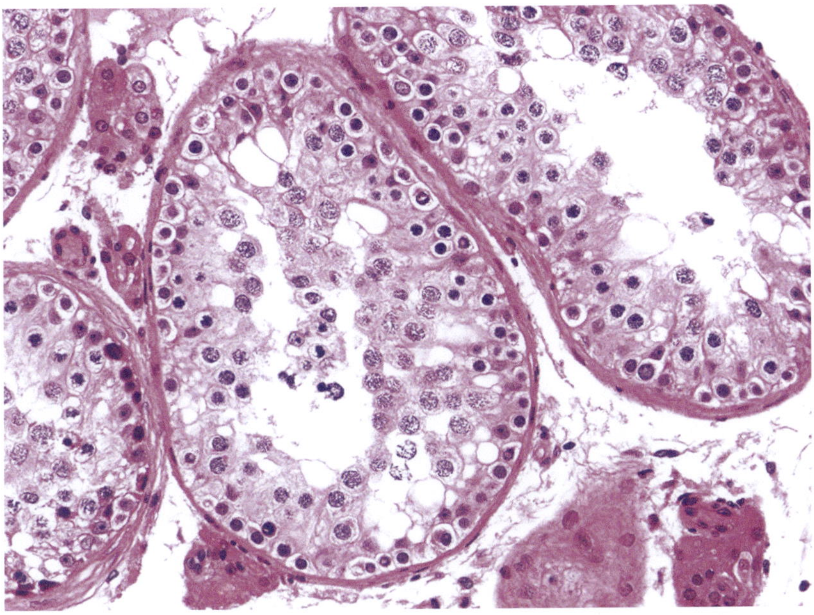

Fig. 16.6 Spermatocyte maturation arrest. Azoospermic patient with sudden arrest of spermatogenesis in first-order spermatocyte. These cells show degenerative signs and sloughing in the lumen

stitutions, this may affect some spermatocytes and not others, producing a greater number of spermatids [42]. In patients with spermatocyte arrest in which the number of spermatocytes is not increased, the etiology may be of an obstructive nature (see Chap. 17). When these two situations are not separated, as occurs in most series, the poor prognosis of an abnormality in meiosis is not adequately evaluated [43].

Meiotic arrest has been linked to the lack of expression of several genes such as the absence of BOULE protein expression [44]; altered expression of heat shock transcription factor; Y chromosome (HSFY) [45], HSPA2, that is involved in DNA mismatch repair [46]; downregulation of microRNA-383 [47]; lack of expression of survivin, an inhibitor of apoptosis [48]; and lack of expression of BET genes [49]. Meiotic arrest is also associated with copy number variations (CNVs) [50] and with TEX11 deletions and mutations [51]. Comparing patients with maturation arrest with controls, a high methylation in specific CpG island of the promoter region of MTHFR [52] that contains tissue-specific differentially methylated regions (TDMRs) in the VASA gene [53] and inactivation of the PIWI pathway genes [54] were observed.

Spermatid Maturation Arrest

The absence of adult spermatids in relation to a normal number of round spermatids is rare. There are two intrinsic histological patterns: spermatic arrest secondary to abnormality in meiosis and spermatic arrest by defects in spermatogenesis. There is also a pattern related to cell ageing, age, and spermatic duct obstruction, syncytia formation of round spermatids.

- Testes with *spermatic maturation arrest secondary to abnormality in meiosis* usually display a normal number of spermatogonia and first-order spermatocytes; frequent multinucleation of Sa + b spermatids (Fig. 16.7); the presence of Sa + b spermatids with large, hyperchromatic, probably polyploid nuclei; and the presence of adult binucleate spermatids sharing the acrosome. All these data suggest that the defect in meiosis manifests very differently, either as the absence of cytokinesis at the end of meiosis with diploid spermatids formation or by dissociation between cytokinesis and spermatogenesis.
- *Spermatic arrest by defects in spermiogenesis.* Some patients have a good number of Sa + b spermatids and intense decrease or absence of Sc + d spermatids (Fig. 16.8). There is an inability

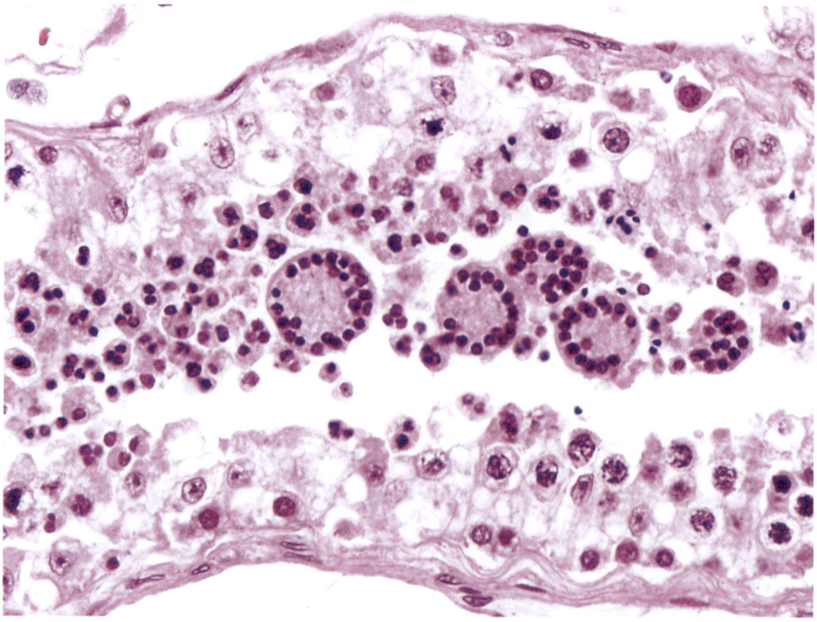

Fig. 16.7 Spermatid maturation arrest. Abundant multinucleated spermatids forming syncytia

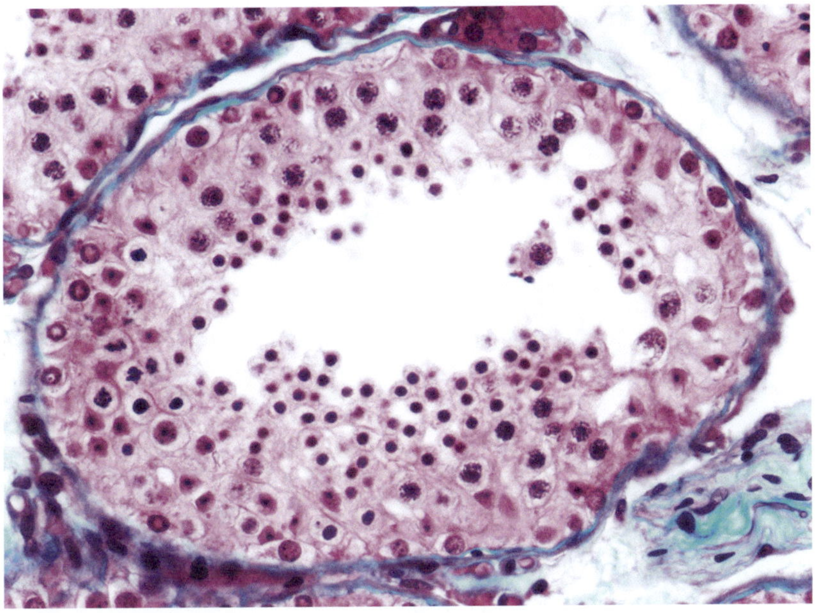

Fig. 16.8 Spermatid arrest caused by spermatogenesis default. Plentiful of round nuclei spermatids with highly condensed chromatin

to transform young into adult spermatids. This fact has been related to specific structural defects of the proteins that form microtubules and microfilaments [55] and defects in spermatogenesis-linked Krüppel-like factor 4 (KLF4), or cAMP-responsive element modulator (CREM) [56], or aberrant mRNA expression of chromatin remodeling factors [57]. Patients show only round spermatids in the ejaculates. It is a pattern that can appear in a familial manner.

16.5 Potentially Predictive Factors

Numerous attempts have been made to predict spermatogenesis in patients with NOA using noninvasive techniques, with limited success. The most studied clinical data are testicular size and hormone levels. The testicular volume has no effect on successful sperm retrieval [58]. Small testes associated with high levels of FSH may have foci of spermatogenesis. Patients with normal volumes and FSH hormone levels between 10–15 mU/mL are less likely to have sperm than those with higher or lower figures [59]. Serum LH, testosterone, and inhibin B rates have no predictive value.

The only reliable predictor of successful TESE is the testicular histology [60]. But we need to keep in mind that only a small portion of the testicle is explored with a biopsy. The study must be maximized, particularly in patients with tubular hyalinization or SCOS to try to find a tubule with spermatogenesis in which sperm may be retrieved from testicular biopsies (TESE, micro-TESE) and achieve pregnancy with ICSI. Histopathological findings are the most useful predictive factors for successful TESE. However, it is questionable whether a biopsy should be done before scheduling TESE [61]. Sperm retrieval rates with micro-TESE in patients with Sertoli cell-only in the biopsy range from 22.5 % [62] to 44.5 % [59], maturation arrest in 44 % [63] to 75 % [64]. Sperm retrieval rate was significantly higher in the hypospermatogenesis group compared with that in SCOS and maturation arrest groups [65], with rates ranging from 81 % [66] to 100 % [63].

References

1. Azzopardi JG, Mostofi FK, Theiss EA. Lesions of testes observed in certain patients with widespread choriocarcinoma and related tumors. The significance and genesis of hematoxylin-staining bodies in the human testis. Am J Pathol. 1961;38:207–25.
2. Turek PJ, Kim M, Gilbaugh 3rd JH, Lipshultz LI. The clinical characteristics of 82 patients with Sertoli cell-only testis histology. Fertil Steril. 1995;64:1197–200.

3. Bruning G, Dierichs R, Stümpel C, Bergmann M. Sertoli cell nuclear changes in human testicular biopsies as revealed by three dimensional reconstruction. Andrologia. 1993;25:311–6.
4. Nistal M, Paniagua R, Abaurrea MA, Santamaría L. Hyperplasia and the immature appearance of Sertoli cells in primary testicular disorders. Hum Pathol. 1982;13:3–12.
5. Terada T, Hatakeyama S. Morphological evidence for two types of idiopathic 'Sertoli-cell-only' syndrome. Int J Androl. 1991;14:117–26.
6. Steger K, Rey R, Kliesch S, Louis F, Schleicher G, Bergmann M. Immunohistochemical detection of immature Sertoli cell markers in testicular tissue of infertile adult men: a preliminary study. Int J Androl. 1996;19:122–8.
7. Bar-Shira Maymon B, Paz G, Elliott DJ, Hammel I, Kleiman SE, Yogev L, Hauser R, Botchan A, Yavetz H. Maturation phenotype of Sertoli cells in testicular biopsies of azoospermic men. Hum Reprod. 2000;15:1537–42.
8. Gotoh M, Miyake K, Mitsuya H. Elastic fibers in tunica propria of undescended and contralateral scrotal testes from cryptorchid patients. Urology. 1987;30:359–63.
9. Ooba T, Ishikawa T, Yamaguchi K, Kondo Y, Sakamoto Y, Fujisawa M. Expression and distribution of laminin chains in the testis for patients with azoospermia. J Androl. 2008;29:147–52.
10. Schulze C, Holstein AF, Schirren C, Körner F. On the morphology of the human Sertoli cells under normal conditions and in patients with impaired fertility. Andrologia. 1976;8:167–78.
11. Leeson CR. An electron microscopic study of cryptorchid and scrotal human testes, with special reference to pubertal maturation. Invest Urol. 1966;3:498–511.
12. Schulze C. Sertoli cells and Leydig cells in man. Adv Anat Embryol Cell Biol. 1984;88:1–104.
13. Taniuchi I, Mizutani S, Namiki M, Okuyama A, Kodama M. Short arm dicentric Y chromosome in a sterile man: a case report. J Urol. 1991;146:415–6.
14. Del Castillo EB, Trabucco A, de la Balze FA. Syndrome produced by absence of the germinal epithelium without impairment of the Sertoli or Leydig cells. J Clin Endocrinol Metab. 1947;7:493–502.
15. Young GP, Goldstein M, Phillips DM, Sundaram K, Gunsalus GL, Bardin CW. Sertoli cell-only syndrome produced by cold testicular ischemia. Endocrinology. 1988;122:1074–82.
16. Viguier-Martinez MC, Hochereau-de Reviers MT, Barenton B, Perreau C. Effect of prenatal treatment with busulfan on the hypothalamo-pituitary axis, genital tract and testicular histology of prepubertal male rats. J Reprod Fertil. 1984;70:67–73.
17. Loveland KL, Schlatt S. Stem cell factor and c-kit in the mammalian testis: lessons originating from Mother Nature's gene knockouts. J Endocrinol. 1997;153:337–44.
18. Miyamoto T, Bando Y, Koh E, Tsujimura A, Miyagawa Y, Iijima M, Namiki M, Shiina M, Ogata K, Matsumoto N, Sengoku K. A PLK4 mutation causing azoospermia in a man with Sertoli cell-only syndrome. Andrology. 2016;4:75–81.
19. Miyakawa H, Miyamoto T, Koh E, Tsujimura A, Miyagawa Y, Saijo Y, Namiki M, Sengoku K. Single-nucleotide polymorphisms in the SEPTIN12 gene may be a genetic risk factor for Japanese patients with Sertoli cell-only syndrome. J Androl. 2012;33:483–7.
20. Miyamoto T, Koh E, Tsujimura A, Miyagawa Y, Saijo Y, Namiki M, Sengoku K. Single-nucleotide polymorphisms in the LRWD1 gene may be a genetic risk factor for Japanese patients with Sertoli cell-only syndrome. Andrologia. 2014;46:273–6.
21. Tüttelmann F, Simoni M, Kliesch S, Ledig S, Dworniczak B, Wieacker P, Röpke A. Copy number variants in patients with severe oligozoospermia and Sertoli-cell-only syndrome. PLoS One. 2011;6:e19426.
22. Patrizio P, Ricci SM, Tomaszewski JE, Hecht NB. Identification of meiotic and postmeiotic gene expression in testicular tissue of patients histologically classified as Sertoli cell only. Fertil Steril. 2000;74:785–90.
23. Sigg C. Classification of tubular testicular atrophies in the diagnosis of sterility. Significance of the so-called "bunteAtrophie". Schweiz Med Wochenschr. 1979;109:1284–93.
24. Sigg C, Hedinger C. Quantitative and ultrastructural study of germinal epithelium in testicular biopsies with "mixed atrophy". Andrologia. 1981;13:412–24.
25. Nistal M, Martínez-García F, Regadera J, Cobo P, Paniagua R. Macro-orchidism: light and electron microscopic study of four cases. Hum Pathol. 1992;23:1011–8.
26. Nistal M, Martínez C, Paniagua R. Primary testicular lesions in the twisted testis. Fertil Steril. 1992;57:381–6.
27. Akin JW, Behzadian A, Tho SP, McDonough PG. Evidence for a partial deletion in the androgen receptor gene in a phenotypic male with azoospermia. Am J Obstet Gynecol. 1991;165:1891–4.
28. Akin JW. The use of clomiphene citrate in the treatment of azoospermia secondary to incomplete androgen resistance. Fertil Steril. 1993;59:223–4.
29. Buchanan JD, Fairley KF, Barrie JU. Return of spermatogenesis after stopping cyclophosphamide therapy. Lancet. 1975;2:156–7.
30. Kumanov P, Nandipati KC, Tomova A, Robeva R, Agarwal A. Significance of inhibin in reproductive pathophysiology and current clinical applications. Reprod Biomed Online. 2005;10:786–812.
31. Sharpe RM, McKinnell C, Kivlin C, Fisher JS. Proliferation and functional maturation of Sertoli cells, and their relevance to disorders of testis function in adulthood. Reproduction. 2003;125:769–84.
32. Andersson AM, Jørgensen N, Frydelund-Larsen L, Rajpert-De Meyts E, Skakkebaek NE. Impaired Leydig cell function in infertile men: a study of 357 idiopathic infertile men and 318 proven fertile controls. J Clin Endocrinol Metab. 2004;89:3161–7.

33. Hiort O, Holterhus PM. Androgen insensitivity and male infertility. Int J Androl. 2003;26:16–20.
34. Schrag SD, Dixon RL. Occupational exposures associated with male reproductive dysfunction. Annu Rev Pharmacol Toxicol. 1985;25:567–92.
35. Nistal M, De Mora JC, Paniagua R. Classification of several types of maturational arrest of spermatogonia according to Sertoli cell morphology: an approach to aetiology. Int J Androl. 1998;21:317–26.
36. Pajarinen JT, Karhunen PJ. Spermatogenic arrest and 'Sertoli cell-only' syndrome–common alcohol-induced disorders of the human testis. Int J Androl. 1994;17:292–9.
37. Nistal M, Gonzalez-Peramato P, De Miguel MP. Sertoli cell dedifferentiation in human cryptorchidism and gender reassignment shows similarities between fetal environmental and adult medical treatment estrogen and antiandrogen exposure. Reprod Toxicol. 2013;42:172–9.
38. Guichaoua MR, Perrin J, Metzler-Guillemain C, Saias-Magnan J, Giorgi R, Grillo JM. Meiotic anomalies in infertile men with severe spermatogenic defects. Hum Reprod. 2005;20:1897–902.
39. North MO, Lellei I, Erdei E, Barbet JP, Tritto J. Meiotic studies of infertile men in case of non-obstructive azoospermia with normal karyotype and no microdeleted Y-chromosome precise the clinical couple management. Ann Genet. 2004;47:113–23.
40. Breucker H, Hofmann N, Holstein AF. Transformed spermatocytes constituting the ejaculate of an infertile man. Andrologia. 1988;20:526–35.
41. Soderström KO, Suominen J. Histopathology and ultrastructure of meiotic arrest in human spermatogenesis. Arch Pathol Lab Med. 1980;104:476–82.
42. Matsuda T, Horii Y, Hayashi K, Yoshida O. Quantitative analysis of seminiferous epithelium in subfertile carriers of chromosomal translocations. Int J Fertil. 1991;36:344–51.
43. Foresta C, Ferlin A, Moro E. Deletion and expression analysis of AZFa genes on the human Y chromosome revealed a major role for DBY in male infertility. Hum Mol Genet. 2000;9:1161–9.
44. Luetjens CM, Xu EY, Rejo Pera RA, Kamischke A, Nieschlag E, Gromoll J. Association of meiotic arrest with lack of BOULE protein expression in infertile men. J Clin Endocrinol Metab. 2004;89:1926–33.
45. Sato Y, Yoshida K, Shinka T, Nozawa S, Nakahori Y, Iwamoto T. Altered expression pattern of heat shock transcription factor, Y chromosome (HSFY) may be related to altered differentiation of spermatogenic cells in testes with deteriorated spermatogenesis. Fertil Steril. 2006;86:612–8.
46. Terribas E, Bonache S, García-Arévalo M, Sánchez J, Franco E, Bassas L, Larriba S. Changes in the expression profile of the meiosis-involved mismatch repair genes in impaired human spermatogenesis. J Androl. 2010;31:346–57.
47. Lian J, Tian H, Liu L, Zhang XS, Li WQ, Deng YM, Yao GD, Yin MM, Sun F. Downregulation of microRNA-383 is associated with male infertility and promotes testicular embryonal carcinoma cell proliferation by targeting IRF1. Cell Death Dis. 2010;1:e94.
48. Weikert S, Schrader M, Krause H, Schulze W, Müller M, Miller K. The inhibitor of apoptosis (IAP) survivin is expressed in human testicular germ cell tumors and normal testes. Cancer Lett. 2005;223:331–7.
49. Barda S, Paz G, Yogev L, Yavetz H, Lehavi O, Hauser R, Botchan A, Breitbart H, Kleiman SE. Expression of BET genes in testis of men with different spermatogenic impairments. Fertil Steril. 2012;97:46–52.e5.
50. Eggers S, DeBoer KD, van den Bergen J, Gordon L, White SJ, Jamsai D, McLachlan RI, Sinclair AH, O'Bryan MK. Copy number variation associated with meiotic arrest in idiopathic male infertility. Fertil Steril. 2015;103:214–9.
51. Yatsenko AN, Georgiadis AP, Röpke A, Berman AJ, Jaffe T, Olszewska M, Westernströer B, Sanfilippo J, Kurpisz M, Rajkovic A, Yatsenko SA, Kliesch S, Schlatt S, Tüttelmann F. X-linked TEX11 mutations, meiotic arrest, and azoospermia in infertile men. N Engl J Med. 2015;372:2097–107.
52. Khazamipour N, Noruzinia M, Fatehmanesh P, Keyhanee M, Pujol P. MTHFR promoter hypermethylation in testicular biopsies of patients with non-obstructive azoospermia: the role of epigenetics in male infertility. Hum Reprod. 2009;24:2361–4.
53. Sugimoto K, Koh E, Sin HS, Maeda Y, Narimoto K, Izumi K, Kobori Y, Kitamura E, Nagase H, Yoshida A, Namiki M. Tissue-specific differentially methylated regions of the human VASA gene are potentially associated with maturation arrest phenotype in the testis. J Hum Genet. 2009;54:450–6.
54. Heyn H, Ferreira HJ, Bassas L, Bonache S, Sayols S, Sandoval J, Esteller M, Larriba S. Epigenetic disruption of the PIWI pathway in human spermatogenic disorders. PLoS One. 2012;7:e47892.
55. Aumüller G, Fuhrmann W, Krause W. Spermatogenetic arrest with inhibition of acrosome and sperm tail development. Andrologia. 1987;19:9–17.
56. Weinbauer GF, Behr R, Bergmann M, Nieschlag E. Testicular cAMP responsive element modulator (CREM) protein is expressed in round spermatids but is absent or reduced in men with round spermatid maturation arrest. Mol Hum Reprod. 1998;4:9–15.
57. Steilmann C, Cavalcanti MC, Bergmann M, Kliesch S, Weidner W, Steger K. Aberrant mRNA expression of chromatin remodelling factors in round spermatid maturation arrest compared with normal human spermatogenesis. Mol Hum Reprod. 2010;16:726–33.
58. Bryson CF, Ramasamy R, Sheehan M, Palermo GD, Rosenwaks Z, Schlegel PN. Severe testicular atrophy does not affect the success of microdissection testicular sperm extraction. J Urol. 2014;191:175–8.
59. Berookhim BM, Palermo GD, Zaninovic N, Rosenwaks Z, Schlegel PN. Microdissection testicular sperm extraction in men with Sertoli cell-only testicular histology. Fertil Steril. 2014;102:1282–6.
60. Ezeh UI, Taub NA, Moore HD, Cooke ID. Establishment of predictive variables associated with testicular sperm

retrieval in men with non-obstructive azoospermia. Hum Reprod. 1999;14:1005–12.
61. Abdel Raheem A, Garaffa G, Rushwan N, De Luca F, Zacharakis E, Abdel Raheem T, Freeman A, Serhal P, Harper JC, Ralph D. Testicular histopathology as a predictor of a positive sperm retrieval in men with non-obstructive azoospermia. BJU Int. 2013;111:492–9.
62. Gul U, Turunc T, Haydardedeoglu B, Yaycioglu O, Kuzgunbay B, Ozkardes H. Sperm retrieval and live birth rates in presumed Sertoli-cell-only syndrome in testis biopsy: a single centre experience. Andrology. 2013;1:47–51.
63. Tsujimura A, Matsumiya K, Miyagawa Y, Tohda A, Miura H, Nishimura K, Koga M, Takeyama M, Fujioka H, Okuyama A. Conventional multiple or microdissection testicular sperm extraction: a comparative study. Hum Reprod. 2002;17:2924–9.
64. Okada H, Dobashi M, Yamazaki T, Hara I, Fujisawa M, Arakawa S, Kamidono S. Conventional versus microdissection testicular sperm extraction for nonobstructive azoospermia. J Urol. 2002;168:1063–7.
65. Aydin T, Sofikerim M, Yucel B, Karadag M, Tokat F. Effects of testicular histopathology on sperm retrieval rates and ICSI results in non-obstructive azoospermia. J Obstet Gynaecol. 2015;35:829–31.
66. Ramasamy R, Yagan N, Schlegel PN. Structural and functional changes to the testis after conventional versus microdissection testicular sperm extraction. Urology. 2005;65:1190–4.

Obstructive Mechanism Lesions Simulating Primary Testicular Lesions

17

Manuel Nistal, Pilar González-Peramato, and Álvaro Serrano

17.1 Histological Characteristics of the Obstructive Mechanism Lesions

Identification of an obstructive mechanism can be quickly done by comparing the number of adult spermatids by seminiferous tubule with the number of sperm per ml, according to a power curve [1]. This allows not only to state that the azoospermia is obstructive but to identify a significant number of patients with obstructive oligozoospermias. For a more complete assessment of the degree of damage to the seminiferous epithelium, a qualitative and quantitative study of all cross tubular sections of the sample is required.

17.1.1 Qualitative Data

Seminiferous epithelium lesions vary from one area to another in the biopsy, adopting a mosaic pattern that correlates with a different involvement of the adjoining lobules. In some cases, it is possible to see a lobule that shows a sequence of images ranging from slightly dilated tubes with normal spermatogenesis to small tubes with seminiferous epithelium formed by Sertoli cells and some spermatogonia and dilated tubes exhibiting different lesions of the seminiferous epithelium. Two or more of the following findings are always present [2]:

- *Ductal ectasia*. The tubular diameter, the tubular lumen, and the number of tubular diverticula are increased. The seminiferous tubules are frequently larger than 200 microns in diameter. The tubular lumen, which normally does not exceed the height of the seminiferous epithelium, can be two to three times higher (Figs. 17.1 and 17.2). The tubular diverticula are not only more numerous but their size is larger [3] (Fig. 17.3).
- The *seminiferous epithelium of some seminiferous tubules is irregular in height,* which presents a serrated appearance as a result of the separation in the adluminal compartment of Sertoli cell cytoplasm (Fig. 17.4).
- In many tubules the inner contour of the seminiferous epithelium of the dilated tubules is linear, which highlights the apposition of an eosinophilic PAS-slightly positive material.
- A higher number of adult spermatids (Sc + Sd) than young spermatids (Sa + Sb) or seminiferous tubules with varying degrees of atrophy and a large number of spermatozoa in their lumen (microspermatoceles) [4] (Fig. 17.5).
- Vacuolization the apical pole of Sertoli cells.
- Presence of lymphoid infiltrates around isolated atrophic tubes (Fig. 17.6).

17.1.2 Quantitative Data

It is confirmed that most of the lesions affect the adluminal compartment. Depending on the type of germ cell from which all others are reduced in number or sloughed in the lumen, the following

M. Nistal et al., *Clues in the Diagnosis of Non-tumoral Testicular Pathology*, DOI 10.1007/978-3-319-49364-0_17

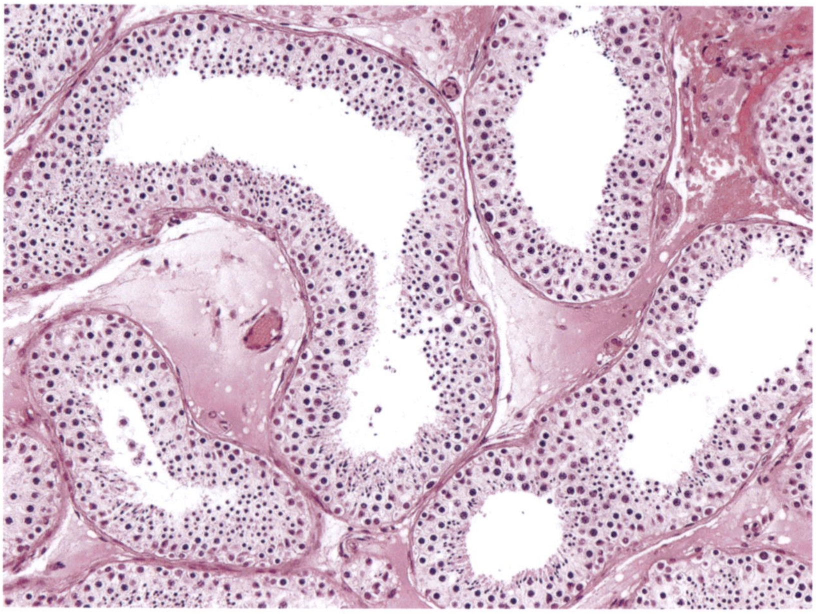

Fig. 17.1 Seminiferous tubules only differ from normal by the marked dilatation of the lumen. The height of the seminiferous epithelium and the different cell types are well preserved

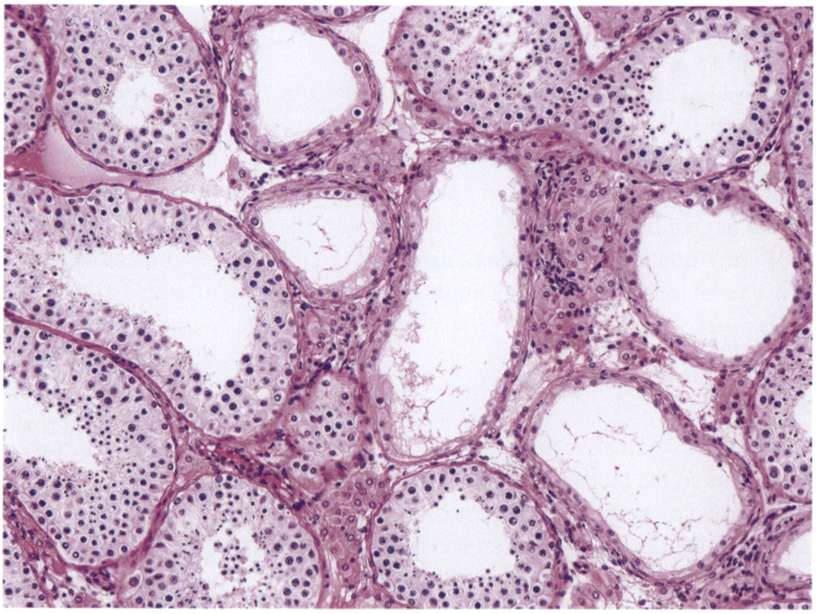

Fig. 17.2 All seminiferous tubules show tubular ectasia. Five of them, probably part of the same lobule, show higher dilation of the lumen and atrophy of the seminiferous epithelium which is reduced to Sertoli cells and spermatogonia

variants of testicular lesion with severity ranging from lower to higher are distinguished: young spermatid sloughing, late primary spermatocyte sloughing, early primary spermatocyte sloughing, and hypospermatogenesis associated with primary spermatocyte sloughing.

- *Young spermatid sloughing*. Seminiferous tubules have a normal number of spermatogonia (>17), primary spermatocytes (>25), and round spermatids (>30) and a marked reduction in the number of adult spermatids. In the wide tubular lumen, some round spermatids and elongated spermatids can be observed (Fig. 17.7).
- *Late primary spermatocyte sloughing*. Spermatogenesis usually progresses to first-order spermatocytes, whose number (most are in the pachytene stage) is also normal.

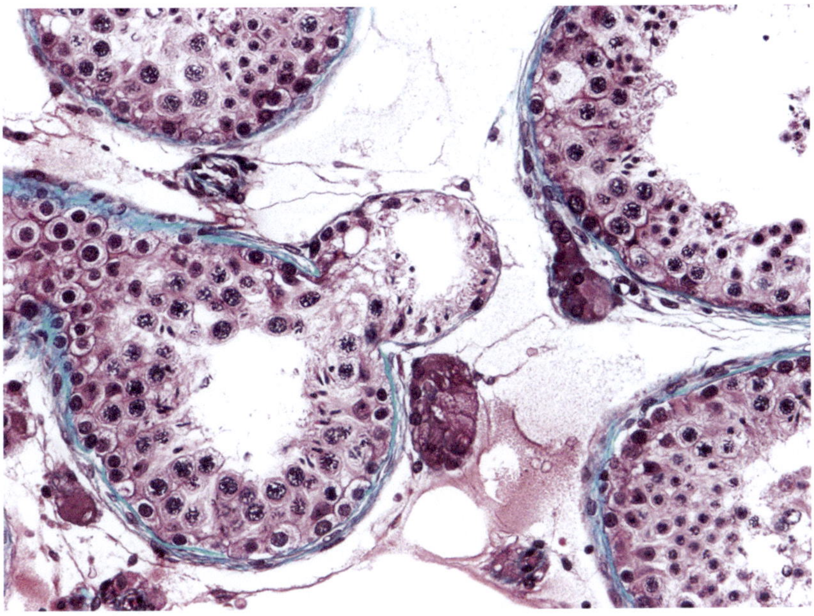

Fig. 17.3 A protrusion of a seminiferous tubule (diverticulum) stands out in the middle of the figure. Diverticulum wall is thin and lacks of several layers of myoid cells. The seminiferous epithelium is reduced to Sertoli cells and isolated spermatogonia

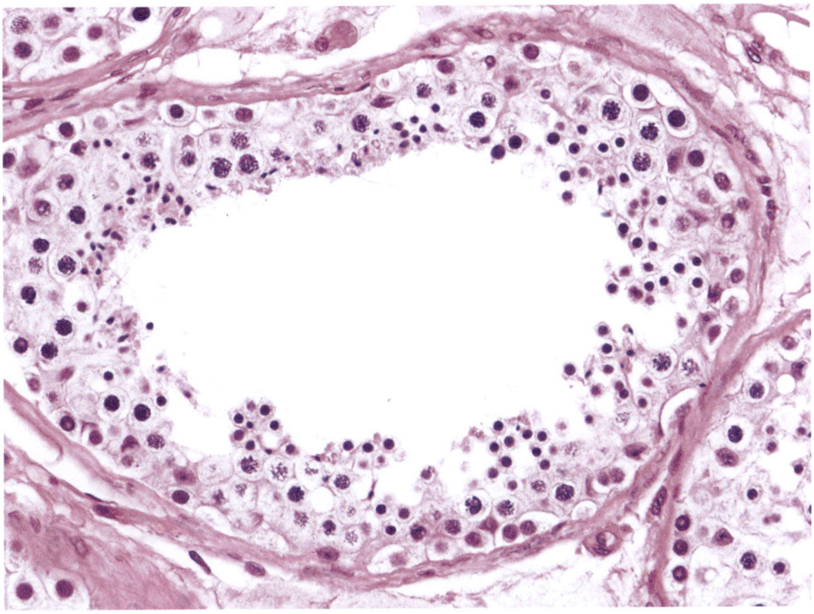

Fig. 17.4 Serrated appearance of the inner contour of a seminiferous tubule showing dilated lumen. The separation of the apical pole of Sertoli cell cytoplasm allows to appreciate the germ cells dependent on each Sertoli cell

Many spermatocytes degenerate without completing meiosis and slough in the lumen. Consequently the number of young spermatids is lower than expected. The number of adult spermatids can be increased.

- *Early primary spermatocyte sloughing*. Cell counts show a normal number of spermatogonia and a number of spermatocytes less than 25 per tubular cross section, which represents the lower limit of a normal number of primary spermatocytes. The seminiferous tubules may contain some spermatids or lack of them. Most first-order spermatocytes reach the pachytene stage before degenerating and sloughing. The histological pattern is similar to that observed experimentally after efferent duct ligation. It highlights the intense vacuolization of the apical pole of Sertoli cells as an

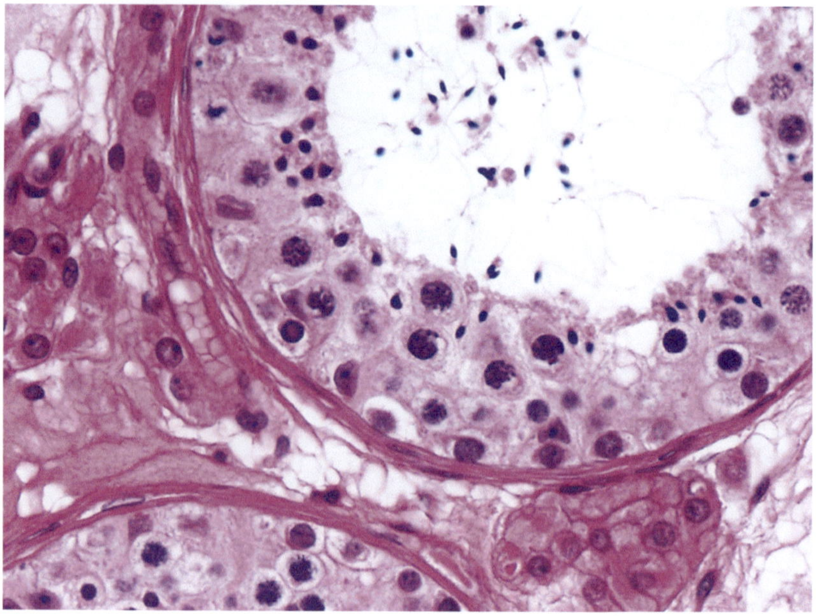

Fig. 17.5 Adult spermatids accumulate in the lumen of a dilated seminiferous tubule

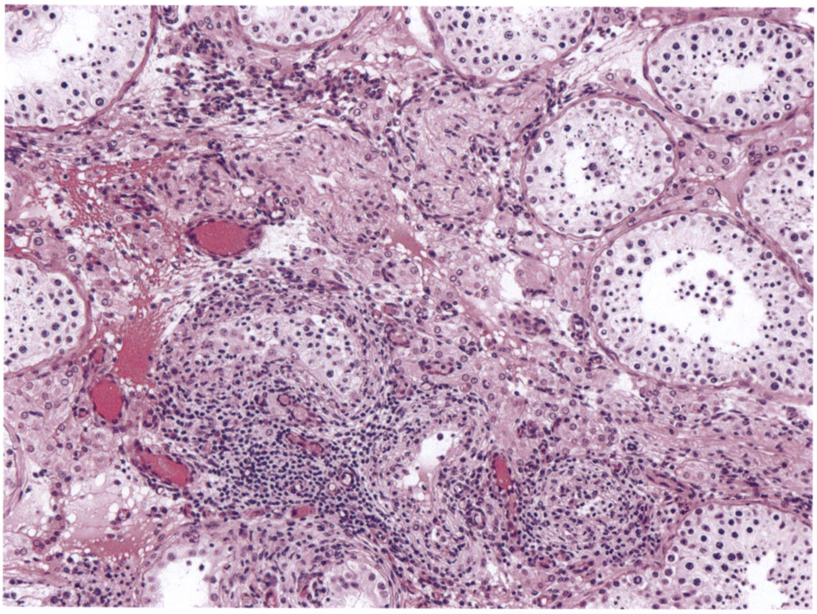

Fig. 17.6 Focal lymphoid infiltrates around several small seminiferous tubules with seminiferous epithelium atrophy

expression of the germinal loss and occasionally the presence of Sertoli cells with hyperchromatic nuclei.

- *Hypospermatogenesis associated with primary spermatocyte sloughing*. This lesion is characterized by (a) a low number of spermatogonia and first-order spermatocytes, the number of spermatocytes being always higher than the number of spermatogonia and (b) a loss from degeneration of most of the spermatocytes, leading to isolated remaining spermatids. Of the three types of hypospermatogenesis associated with primary spermatocyte sloughing described in the previous chapter about this topic, one has an obstructive pattern and signs of severe oligozoospermia and varicocele [5].

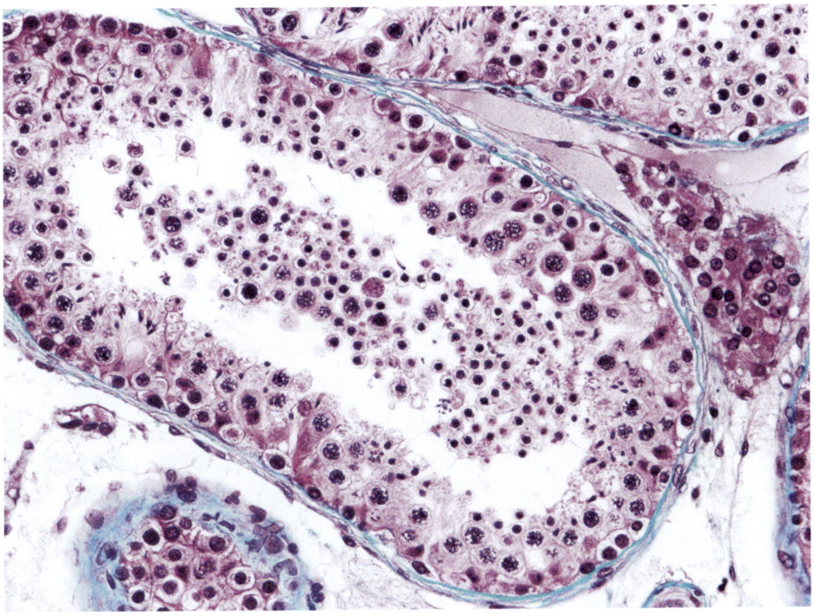

Fig. 17.7 Seminiferous tube with plenty of germ cell sloughing. Although some primary spermatocytes are observed, most cells are young spermatids

17.2 Mechanism of the Testicular Lesions

The intimate mechanism by which an obstructive process of the spermatic ducts determines germ cell sloughing is not entirely known. The trigger of impaired spermatogenesis is the high hydrostatic pressure caused by obstruction of the seminiferous tubules. The fact that Sertoli cells are responsible for the maintenance of all germ cells in the adluminal compartment suggests that the Sertoli cells are the target cell. The latter undergoes major ultrastructural changes, especially in the apical pole [6–8].

Under normal conditions Sertoli cells carry fluids and different substances from the basal pole to the tubule lumen, and their secretory functions are regionalized. When the blockage of the spermatic ducts determines an increase in intraluminal pressure, the adluminal cytoplasm is selectively damaged, leaving the functions performed there blocked. Among these functions are those related to the adhesion between Sertoli cells and germ cells. Normally in the cytoplasm of Sertoli cells, there is an accumulation of actin filaments that are attached to the plasma membrane by an adhesive protein, vinculin. A defect in the vinculin synthesis or action alters intercellular adhesion and could release immature germ cells [9].

17.3 Factors Affecting the Development of Testicular Lesions

The severity of lesions secondary to obstruction depends on three factors: location of the obstruction, congenital or acquired nature of the obstruction, and evolution time [10–12].

- *Location of the obstruction:* Distal obstructions, defined as those affecting the ampulla deferens, the seminal vesicles, and the ejaculatory ducts, cause just mild alterations in the testis and the epididymis. Proximal obstructions, i.e., those affecting the vas deferens, the epididymis, or the epididymal-testicular union, in all cases cause more or less severe changes not only to the backward spermatic ducts but to the testicular parenchyma.
- The *nature of the obstruction* also conditions the lesions. In *congenital bilateral absence of the vas deferens* (BAVD) (with or without cystic fibrosis), the increased hydrostatic pressure has been observed to be well tolerated.

Quantitative studies of testicular biopsies have shown that 42.8 % have a normal germ cell count. Twenty-one point 4 % of the testicles show late primary spermatocyte sloughing. This injury may be related to the fact that a number of patients associate a partial agenesis of the body and cauda epididymis with BAVD. Thirty-two point 14 % of the testes have lesions in the two compartments, basal and adluminal (mild hypospermatogenesis and hypospermatogenesis-associated primary spermatocyte sloughing). In the remaining cases, there are different associated pathologies such as tubular hyalinization, Sertoli cell-only, and spermatogenetic arrest.

All *vasectomized patients* were observed to have qualitative alterations of the seminiferous epithelium with the presence of an obstructive pattern similar to those observed in experimental animals [13]. In the quantitative study, the germ cell count was normal in 29.1 %, and 70.8 % had primary spermatocytes sloughing.

In blockages of the spermatic pathway secondary to *herniorrhaphy in childhood*, quantitative studies showed that the germline depletion was even more important than that of patients. All testicles had an adluminal compartment pathology compared to 29.1 % of the testicles that were quantitatively normal in vasectomized patients. The largest number of lesions observed in this group can perhaps be correlated to a longer obstruction [14, 15] (Fig. 17.8).

In obstructive azoospermias *secondary to hydrocelectomy*, it is more frequent to observe small seminiferous ducts, severe vacuolization of the apical pole of Sertoli cells, and early primary spermatocyte sloughing, i.e., lesions very similar to those experimentally observed by ligation of efferent ducts [16, 17]. The lesions are related to the damage able to suffer by the epididymis during hydrocelectomy.

In our experience, when the etiology is *inflammatory*, the most common testicular lesions are located in the adluminal compartment and are late primary spermatocyte sloughing (38.8 %) followed by early primary spermatocyte sloughing (16, 6 %). In the remaining cases, there are lesions of both compartments with the presence of groups of hyalinized tubules. Late atrophy of the testis is a not uncommon complication of acute epididymitis. The cause, probably ischemic, would lie in the compression of the testicular blood vessels by an edematous epididymis, tension or constrictive funiculitis secondary to inflammatory involvement of the cord [18], or

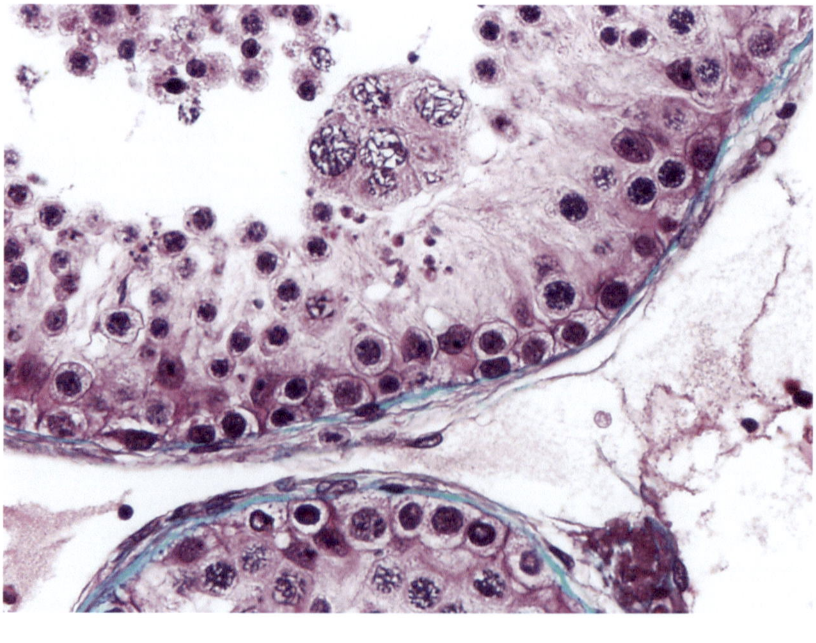

Fig. 17.8 Late primary spermatocyte sloughing. Germ cell maturation arrest in first-order spermatocytes is seen most seminiferous tubules. Note a cluster of megalospermatocytes

development of thrombophlebitis or endoarteritis of the testicular vessels.

- The *time of evolution* affects negatively all obstructions. The shorter the evolution time, the better the prognosis [11, 14]. In vasectomized patients, it has been said that the testicular changes are not so much in relation to the duration of the obstruction, as the initial insult until the intraductal pressure is balanced [19]. But as time passes, the chances of having a normal semen analysis when reanastomosis is performed decrease considerably [20].

17.4 Differential Diagnosis Between Obstructive Mechanism Lesions and Primary Testicular Lesions

Oligozoospermia can be observed both in patients with AO and with NOA [21]. The first step is to identify whether there is an obstructive process because testicular lesions have different mechanisms, different prognoses, and different treatments [22]. The differentiation between the two processes is easy when the average number of adult spermatids per cross section of the seminiferous tubules is compared with the sperm count in millions per milliliter using the power curve [1].

Once known whether or not an obstructive component exists, another problem arises. There are a number of lesions seen in obstructive azoospermia and oligozoospermias with some histological resemblance to some lesions observed in the NOA. The most common problems arise when it comes to differentiating between spermatids and spermatocyte sloughing observed in obstructive azoospermia and different signs of maturation arrest (spermatid arrest, spermatocyte arrest, and between different types of hypospermatogenesis).

Young spermatid sloughing versus spermatid arrest. The quantitative study shows that in both situations, the number of spermatogonia, primary spermatocytes, and round spermatids (Sa + Sb) is normal. They differ in the following:

- The elongated spermatids (Sc + Sd) are absent or very rare in the testes with spermatic arrest, and, although diminished in number, they are present in most tubules with young spermatid sloughing of the AO.
- The round spermatids in the testes with spermatic arrest often have large hyperchromatic nuclei and multinucleation.

Late primary spermatocyte sloughing versus spermatocyte arrest. The basal compartment is normal in both of them. They differ in:

- The number of primary spermatocytes of the testicles with spermatocyte arrest is very high as a result of abnormalities in meiosis, compared with a normal number in late primary spermatocyte sloughing.
- In the testis with spermatocyte arrest, spermatids are either not observed or very rare. In the testes with late primary spermatocyte sloughing, the number of round spermatids may be slightly decreased, but it is accompanied by an increase in the number of spermatids (Sc + Sd) as a result of the blockage.

Hypospermatogenesis associated with primary spermatocyte sloughing versus spermatogonial arrest. In both cases the tubules contain a low number of spermatogonia and spermatocytes. While in spermatogonial arrest, the presence of spermatocytes is rare; these are present in most hypospermatogenesis tubules associated with primary spermatocyte sloughing, and often their number is greater than that of spermatogonia. In the testes with spermatogonial arrest, no changes suggestive of an obstructive pattern are observed.

References

1. Nistal M, Codesal J, Santamaría L, Paniagua R. Correlation between spermatozoon numbers in spermiogram and seminiferous epithelium histology in testicular biopsies from subfertile men. Fertil Steril. 1987;48:507–9.
2. Nistal M, Riestra ML, Galmés-Belmonte I, Paniagua R. Testicular biopsy in patients with obstructive azoospermia. Am J Surg Pathol. 1999;23:1546–1554.5.

3. Nistal M, Santamaria L, Regadera J, Paniagua R. Diverticula of human seminiferous tubules in the normal and pathologic testis. J Androl. 1988;9:55–61.
4. Nistal M, Gonzalez-Peramato P, Paniagua R. Diagnostic value of differential quantification of spermatids in obstructive azoospermia. J Androl. 2003;24:721–6.
5. Nistal M, Paniagua R, Gonzalez-Peramato P. Non-neoplastic diseases of the testis. In: Bostwick DG, Cheng JN, editors. Urological surgical pathology. Philadelphia: Saunders; 2014. p. 652–720.
6. Cameron DF, Snydle FE, Ross MH, Drylie DM. Ultrastructural alterations in the adluminal testicular compartment in men with varicocele. Fertil Steril. 1980;33:526–33.
7. Baccetti B, Burrini AG, Capitani S, Collodel G, Di Cairano G, Piomboni P, Renieri T, Setacci C. Studies on varicocele. 1. Submicroscopical and endocrinological features. J Submicrosc Cytol Pathol. 1991;23:659–65.
8. Meyer JM, Maetz JL, Rumpler Y. Cellular relationship impairment in maturation arrest of human spermatogenesis: an ultrastructural study. Histopathology. 1992;21:25–33.
9. Grove BD, Vogl AW. Sertoli cell ectoplasmic specializations: a type of actin-associated adhesion junction? J Cell Sci. 1989;93:309–23.
10. Niederberger C, Ross LS. Microsurgical epididymovasostomy: predictors of success. J Urol. 1993;149:1364–7.
11. Matsuda T, Horii Y, Muguruma K, Komatz Y, Yoshida O. Microsurgical epididymovasostomy for obstructive azoospermia: factors affecting postoperative fertility. Eur Urol. 1994;26:322–6.
12. Pasqualotto FF, Agarwal A, Srivastava M, Nelson DR, Thomas Jr AJ. Fertility outcome after repeat vasoepididymostomy. J Urol. 1999;162:1626–8.
13. Kong LS, Huang AP, Deng XZ, Yang ZW. Quantitative (stereological) study of the effects of vasectomy on spermatogenesis in rabbits. J Anat. 2004;205:147–56.
14. Matsuda T, Hiura Y, Muguruma K, Okuno H, Horii Y, Yoshida O. Quantitative analysis of testicular histology in patients with vas deferens obstruction caused by childhood inguinal herniorrhaphy: comparison to vasectomized men. J Urol. 1996;155:564–7.
15. Khodari M, Ouzzane A, Marcelli F, Yakoubi R, Mitchell V, Zerbib P, Rigot JM. Azoospermia and a history of inguinal hernia repair in adult. Prog Urol. 2015;25:692–7.
16. Dixit VP, Lohiya NK, Arya M, Agrawal M. The effects of chemical occlusion of vas deferens on the testicular function of dog: a preliminary study. Acta Eur Fertil. 1975;6:348–53.
17. Anton E. Early ultrastructural changes in the rat testis after ductuliefferentes ligation. Fertil Steril. 1979;31:187–94.
18. Desai KM, Gingell JC, Haworth JM. Fate of the testis following epididymitis: a clinical and ultrasound study. J R Soc Med. 1986;79:515–9.
19. Jenkins IL, Muir VY, Blacklock NJ, Turk JL, Hanley HG. Consequences of vasectomy: an immunological and histological study related to subsequent fertility. Br J Urol. 1979;51:406–10.
20. Belker AM, Thomas Jr AJ, Fuchs EF, Konnak JW, Sharlip ID. Results of 1,469 microsurgical vasectomy reversals by the Vasovasostomy Study Group. J Urol. 1991;145:505–11.
21. Wosnitzer M, Goldstein M, Hardy MP. Review of azoospermia. Spermatogenesis. 2014;4:e28218. eCollection 2014.
22. Galmés-Belmonte I, Nistal M. Partial obstruction of the seminal path, a frequent cause of oligozoospermia in men. Hum Reprod. 1998;13:3402–5.

18 Fertility in Patients with Chromosome Abnormalities

Manuel Nistal, Pilar González-Peramato, and Álvaro Serrano

18.1 Numerical Chromosome Aberrations

18.1.1 Klinefelter's Syndrome

Clinical Data

Klinefelter's syndrome (KS) is a clinical condition that starts by a primary testicular failure associated with a karyotype 47,XXY. Patients have small testicles, azoospermia, eunuchoidism, gynecomastia, mental retardation, and increased serum gonadotropin [1].

This syndrome is the most common genetic cause of infertility. Its prevalence is estimated at 1 in every 500–600 phenotypic males, 1 % of adults in institutions for mentally retarded patients, 3.4 % of infertile patients, 15 % of azoospermic males, 0.7 % of oligozoospermic patients [2], and 10 % of patients with NOA [3].

The karyotype in 85 % of KS is 47,XXY, and the remaining are mosaicisms, most of them with two cell lines 47,XXY and 46,XY [4]. The classic form is caused by a meiotic nondisjunction of X chromosome in meiotic cells of either parent (spermatocytes or ovocytes). Mosaicisms arise from either nondisjunction in a mitotic division of the zygote after fertilization or from loss of one of the X chromosomes of 47,XXY conception due to anaphase lagging [5].

Histology

During fetal life (studies in abortions between 18 and 22 weeks), a loss of germ cells is detected [6]. During the first month of life, cell proliferation and differentiation characteristics of the mini-puberty are not observed. Consequently, the enlargement of both testes, dependent on the Sertoli cells, and the establishment of an optimal number of Ad spermatogonia do not occur [7]. In adolescence the testicular size increases parallel to the activation of the hypothalamic-pituitary-testicular axis, but spermatogenesis only develops in some tubes and not in all cases [8].

Alterations in virtually all cells and testicular structures have been reported in adulthood. Most seminiferous tubules become hyalinized and are transformed into phantom tubes. Those who remain may show Sertoli cell-only and, less frequently, spermatogenesis [9]. Most Sertoli cells are dysgenetic, lack expression of the androgen receptor [8], and are unable to produce normal amounts of inhibin B [10] and collagen type IV. Myoid peritubular cells are unable to form elastic fibers [11]. Leydig cells, despite taking an adenomatous aspect, have shown in quantitative studies that their number is not increased and testis testosterone production is low [12, 13] (Fig. 18.1).

A focal spermatogenesis is present in about 50 % of KS. Cytogenetic studies show 46,XY spermatogonia and spermatocytes. 47,XXY spermatogonia could lose the extra X chromosome

M. Nistal et al., *Clues in the Diagnosis of Non-tumoral Testicular Pathology*,
DOI 10.1007/978-3-319-49364-0_18

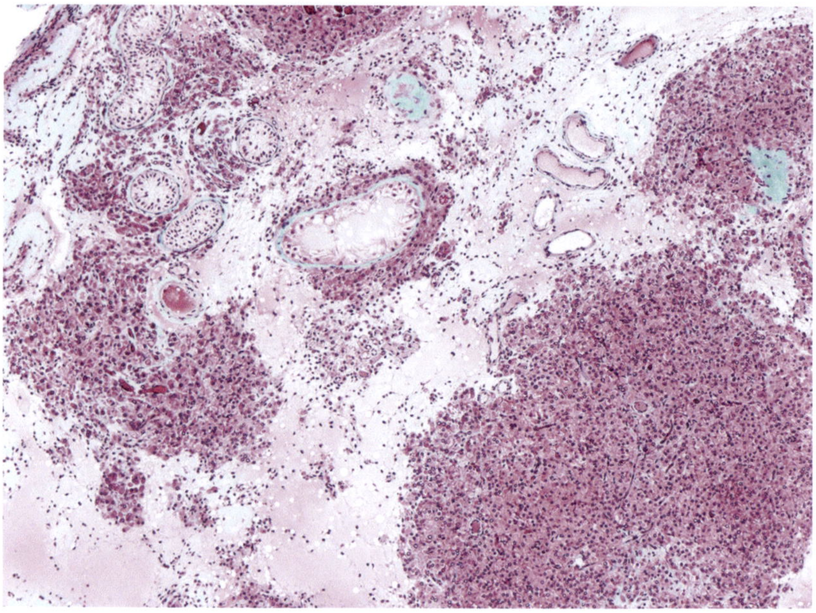

Fig. 18.1 Klinefelter syndrome 47,XXY. Nodular Leydig cell hyperplasia and diffuse tubular hyalinization with persistence of isolated Sertoli cell-only tubules is shown

during mitosis, forming clones of spermatogonia 46,XY, capable of a normal spermatogenesis [14].

Fertility Potential of KS Patients

Two decades ago, 47,XXY patients were considered sterile. Only 8 % of KS patients have sperm in the ejaculates. They have severe oligozoospermia with sperm concentration lower than 1 million/mL, with altered morphology and motility [15]. With the advancement of assisted reproduction techniques, especially with the combined practice of micro-testicular sperm extraction (micro-TESE) and intracytoplasmic sperm injection (ICSI), a significant number of patients are able to be biological fathers.

The first case of high rates of fertilization with ICSI using sperm from patients with KS was published in 1995 by Harari [16]. Tournaye in 1996 [17] achieved the first successful sperm recovery by TESE in a KS with azoospermia. Hinney [18] and Bourne [19] in 1997 achieved the first pregnancies with ejaculated sperm and ICSI. Palermo in 1998 [20] reported the first births after TESE combined with ICSI. Testicular biopsies performed during TESE show tubules with spermatogenesis form small groups isolated among other completely hyalinized tubules.

The pregnancy rates combining TESE with ICSI per embryo transfer vary from 27.25 % [21] to 50 % [22] and do not differ from those obtained in other patients with NOA. Of the 150 born children of KS patients, the risk of aneuploidy, if any, is very low, similar to the group of patients with NOA. Only one fetus of a triple pregnancy had the 47,XXY karyotype. Sperm in KS come from spermatogonia with a normal karyotype 46,XY [23].

Prediction Factors of Sperm Retrieval and Pregnancy

The most studied clinical data are hormonal rates, patient age, history of cryptorchidism, testicular volume, previous hormone treatment, and sperm retrieval method used.

Serum FSH rates, inhibin B and inhibin B/FSH ratio, INSL3, estradiol and AMH, useful for predicting fertility in normal karyotype males, are of no use in patients with KS. Normal serum testosterone levels do have positive predictive value of sperm retrieval [24].

The patient's age is one of the most important data. Since testicular lesions in KS patients are progressive, sperm extraction should be performed as early as possible [25]. There are patients who in just 2 years happen to go from severe oligozoospermia to azoospermia. In normal conditions, sperm can be found in the ejaculates of many adolescents aged 13 and in all 15-year-old adolescents. Spermatogenesis quality progressively improves until 17 years of age at which it is completely normal. Fifteen years of age could be established as the lower age limit. The preservation of fertility through sperm banking in mid-puberty is under study. Currently, a major problem is the frequent delay in the diagnosis of KS patients, usually postponed until the couple consults for infertility. Thirty-five years old looks like a critical age for sperm extraction [26].

Patients with cryptorchidism have a worse prognosis, even if the testis has been descended early during childhood.

The testicular volume generally reflects the histology and the testicular function. It might be a valuable datum, but it is difficult to assess, given the small size of many testes of patients with KS [26].

An important group of patients undergoes testosterone treatment for their hypogonadism. It is recommended that treatment be interrupted for several months prior to testicular sperm extraction since it carries a risk of decreasing focal spermatogenesis by lowering gonadotropins [27]. HCG treatment may be useful as it seeks to increase intra-testicular testosterone concentration that would improve spermatogenesis. The best results are being achieved with the use of aromatase inhibitors [28].

The two methods used for sperm retrieval are TESE and micro-TESE. It is estimated that, as happens in other patients with NOA, the best results are achieved with micro-TESE. The rates of successful sperm recovery in two series confirm this: 42 % by TESE and 57 % by micro-TESE [23], and 47 % by TESE and 61 % by micro-TESE [29]. One important thing worth being planned is that patients who have undergone micro-TESE, probably due to iatrogenic injuries in the testicular parenchyma during sperm extraction, typically show severe decrease in testosterone levels that require a hormone supplementation treatment [30].

Variants of the Klinefelter's Syndrome

In 46,XY/47,XXY patients, azoospermia is only observed in 50 % of cases. The testicles are larger, and spermatogenesis is best preserved by the high number of spermatogonia with normal chromosomal constitution.

Patients with 48,XXYY, 48,XXXY and 49,XXXXY constitutions are rare, and their problem is not infertility, which is present in most cases, but multiple congenital malformations, a variety of clinical symptoms, and the need for individualized therapy for their problems [31].

18.1.2 The XX Male Syndrome

The XX-male syndrome was described by De la Chapelle in 1964 [32]. The combination of a normal male phenotype, male external genitalia, testicular differentiation of gonads, and 46,XX karyotype in the conventional cytogenetic analysis is characteristic of these patients. In 80 % of patient fluorescence, in situ hybridization or molecular methods can show the presence of Y-chromosome translocated material onto the tip of one X chromosome [33]. Translocated DNA material containing the *SRY* gene is required to initiate testicular differentiation. The *SRY* translocation occurs during paternal meiosis [34]. Ten percent of the remaining patients may have 46,XX/47,XXY mosaicism, and in the remaining 10 %, autosomal genes would be involved.

The prevalence of 46,XX males is estimated at 1:10,000–1:25,000 [35], representing 0.2 % of infertile patients. These patients differ clinically from KS patients in that they have normal intelligence, shorter height, and increased incidence of cryptorchidism. They have in common hypergonadotropic hypogonadism with gynecomastia, small testes, and azoospermia [36].

In adults the testicular biopsy can show from a pattern similar to the classic Klinefelter's syndrome (diffuse tubular hyalinization and adenomatous hyperplasia of Leydig cells) to a Sertoli cell-only syndrome with varying degrees of tubular hyalinization (Fig. 18.2). Infertility is the rule [37].

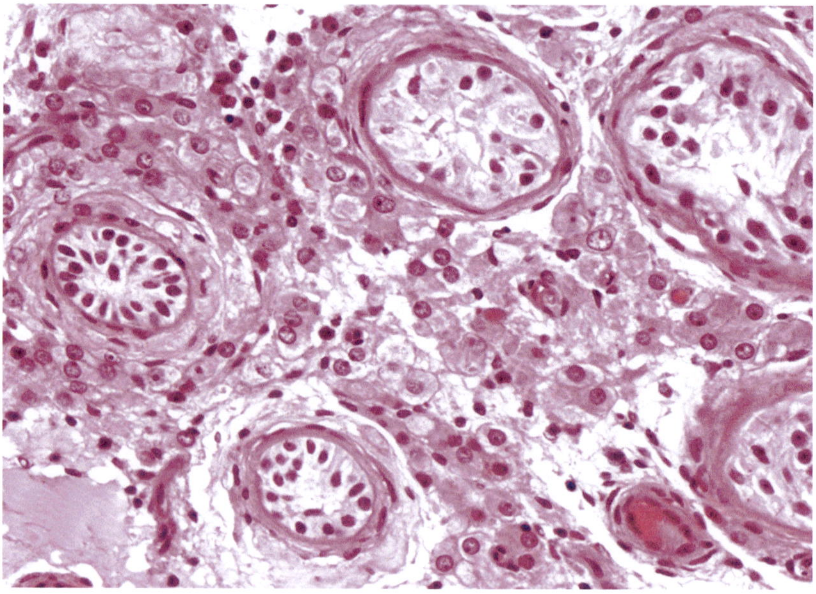

Fig. 18.2 46,XX patient who consulted for infertility. Seminiferous tubes of small diameter, no lumen, and scarce Sertoli cells with dysgenetic features are observed. Wide interstitium with Leydig cell hyperplasia

18.1.3 The XYY Syndrome

The XYY syndrome is an aneuploidy first reported in 1961 by SANDBERG in a phenotypically normal man, father of a mongoloid child, to whom karyotyping was performed [38]. It is a relatively common syndrome with an incidence of 1 in 1000 live male births [39]. The extra Y chromosome appears by one of two mechanisms: (a) paternal nondisjunction at meiosis II after a normal chiasmate meiosis I (84 %) and (b) a post-zygotic mitotic error (16 %) [40].

Most patients are tall. The XYY syndrome is detected from 6 years. It is associated with macrocephaly, hypertelorism, hypotonia, and tremor. Asthma and dental problems are more common than in the general population. The patients' weight increases with age with a trend toward central adiposity. The intellectual development is normal, and most people show no aggressive behavior [41]. The testicular size is normal in childhood, and most patients acquire a standard testicular size in puberty.

Markers of testicular function in childhood (AMH and inhibin B) are normal in most patients. At puberty 5 % of them have low levels of inhibin and high levels of FSH, reflecting an altered function of the Sertoli cells [42]. At puberty testosterone levels are normal except for isolated cases in which it is increased. Most patients have normal spermatogenesis. A small group of patients consult by oligozoospermia and NOA [43].

It has been suggested that the presence of an extra Y chromosome in the pachytene state is associated with a high degeneration of pachytene spermatocytes by apoptosis and a low rate of aneuploid spermatozoa. If the loss of supernumerary Y chromosome occurs before meiosis, the spermatogenesis can be normal [44].

In histology normal spermatogenesis has been reported in some cases and a combination of different lesions (normal spermatogenesis, maturation arrest of primary spermatocytes, and Sertoli cell-only tubules) in other cases [45].

Patients with 48,XYYY karyotype have a normal phenotype, mild mental retardation, frequent infections of the upper respiratory tract, and azoospermia [46]. The testes show Sertoli cell-only tubules, basement membrane hyalinization, and Leydig cell hyperplasia. Patients with 49,XYYYY karyotype have a number of facial and skeletal abnormalities, mild mental retardation, antisocial behavior, and azoospermia [47].

18.2 Structural Chromosome Aberrations

18.2.1 Structural Aberrations of the Autosomes

Structural aberrations of the autosomes that appear most often in infertile patients are Robertsonian translocations, reciprocal translocations, inversions, and small supernumerary marker chromosomes. Somatic chromosomal rearrangements are seen in infertile patients 10 times more than in the general population [48]. The prevalence of autosomal balanced translocations in infertile men is estimated at between 1.6 and 6.6 % [49]. Most patients are likely fertile. Any carrier of any of these aberrations who wants to be a father should receive genetic counseling.

Robertsonian Translocations

They are observed in approximately 1:1000 newborn babies. The incidence in infertile patients is 0.7 %. While this type of rearrangement is rare in azoospermic patients (0.09 %), the rate rises to 1.6 % in the oligozoospermic ones. They are considered the most common balanced structural chromosomal rearrangements. The most frequent balanced Robertsonian translocations are 13:14 and 14:21, and the most frequent unbalanced one is 21:21. About 25.7 % of patients with Robertsonian translocations have sperm parameters within the normal ranges [50]. The histological pattern is not characteristic, ranging from severe impairment of spermatogenesis to about almost normal testis [51].

Reciprocal Translocations

The incidence of reciprocal translocations in infertile patients is 1 % compared with 0.1 % in the general population. They are more common among azoospermic than among oligozoospermic patients [52]. Reciprocal translocations frequently are 11:22 [53] and 17:21 [54]. A histological pattern of Sertoli cell-only in patients with unbalanced chromosomal translocation has been observed [55].

Inversions

Inversions are structural chromosome abnormalities that may be associated with infertility, multiple miscarriage, and chromosomally unbalanced offspring. The most common one is the pericentric inversion inv. (9) (p11q13), with an incidence of 1–4 % in the general population. It is not considered relevant to the field of infertility [56]. Paracentric and pericentric inversions (excluding pericentric inversion of the heterochromatic region of chromosome 9) are eight times higher in the series of infertile patients (0.16 %) than in the general population (0.02 %) [57]. The chromosomes most often affected are 1, 5, 7, 9, and 21. The increased risk of infertility has been detected in patients with pericentric inversion of chromosome 1 [58].

Small Supernumerary Marker Chromosomes (SSMC)

Small supernumerary marker chromosomes are structurally abnormal chromosomes that cannot be unambiguously identified by banding cytogenetics. The incidence in infertile patients is 0.125 %, while in the general population, it is 0.043 % [59]. Seventy-two percent (SSMC) detected in infertile patients derived from an acrocentric chromosome. Infertility could be due to the partial trisomy of some genes but also to mechanical effects that perturb meiosis [60].

18.2.2 Structural Aberrations of the Sex Chromosomes

Structural Abnormalities of Chromosome Y

The following are included among the most frequent structural Y-chromosome abnormalities: monocentric deleted Yq-chromosomes, dicentric Yp-isochromosomes, ring Y chromosomes, Y/Y translocation chromosomes, translocation from Y chromosome to X chromosome, and autosomal translocation of Y chromosome. Other Y-chromosome structural anomalies are pericentric and paracentric inversions.

Monocentric Deleted Yq-Chromosomes
Patients show only small testes and elevated serum FSH with normal rates of LH and testosterone. The most common testicular lesion is Sertoli cell-only, consistent with the loss of AZF [61].

Dicentric Yp-Isochromosomes
It is the most frequent structural abnormality of the Y chromosome. The karyotype is associated, in most cases, with 45,X0 cell line. The phenotype can be male, female, or ambiguous genitalia. Patients with male phenotype are usually infertile. Testicular lesions are similar to those observed in monocentric Yq-chromosome patients, which consist of dysgenetic Sertoli cell-only with Leydig cell hyperplasia [62]. In those patients with mosaicisms, primary spermatocyte maturation arrest has been reported [63].

Ring Y Chromosomes
The phenotype of these patients varies from ambiguous genitalia, hypospadias, and sexual infantilism to a normal male phenotype with azoospermia. Some patients have mosaicism with a 45,X0 line [64]. The testicular histological pattern is similar to that of dicentric Yp-isochromosomes patients.

Y/Y Translocation Chromosomes
Patients may show mosaicism with a 45,X0 cell line [65]. They have azoospermia and maturation arrest of primary spermatocytes.

Translocation from Y Chromosome to X Chromosome
Both in patients in which the translocation is non-visible in cytogenetical studies and in those with visible X-Y translocation, infertility is the rule. They are azoospermic patients. In the first ones, the phenotype is similar to patients 46,XX, and their testicular histology is a picture of Sertoli cell-only [66]. In the latter, the phenotype is reminiscent of KS, and the histology is diffuse hyalinization of the seminiferous tubules associated with Leydig cell hyperplasia.

Autosomal Translocation of Y Chromosome
Translocations of the Y-chromosome distal heterochromatic region to the short arm of an acrocentric chromosome are not infrequent. Patients may be fertile or infertile depending on the point of rupture. Their testicular histology is very varied, from Sertoli cell-only to testes with minimal alterations [67].

Structural Abnormalities of Chromosome X
The following abnormalities are associated with infertility: translocation of the X chromosome to an autosome, distal duplication of Xp, inversions, and 47,XXX males.

Patients with X chromosome translocation of autosomal are generally subfertile or infertile [68]. Patients 46,XY with distal duplication of Xp can show female, male, or ambiguous phenotype regarding the genetic content of the duplicated segment [69]. Patients with male external genitalia have low testosterone levels associated with multiple congenital anomalies. Male patients with 47 XXX have a hypoplastic scrotum, small testes, gynecomastia and mental retardation, low rates of serum testosterone, and hyalinization of the seminiferous tubules [70].

18.3 Y-Chromosome Microdeletions

Most patients with Y-chromosome microdeletions have azoospermia or severe oligozoospermia. The Y chromosome plays an essential role in the genetic regulation of spermatogenesis [71]. The long arm of the Y chromosome contains three subregions located in intervals 5 and 6 designated as AZFa, AZFb, and AZFc. The loss can be of the AZF entire region or only of one or two subregions. In most cases, it leads to infertility.

The incidence of Y-chromosome microdeletions varies by geographic region or ethnicity studied. It is generally estimated at 13–18 % of patients with idiopathic infertility, in 5–10 % of patients with azoospermia, and 2–5 % of the oligozoospermic patients. The incidence is much higher in several Asian countries [72] and in Iran [73].

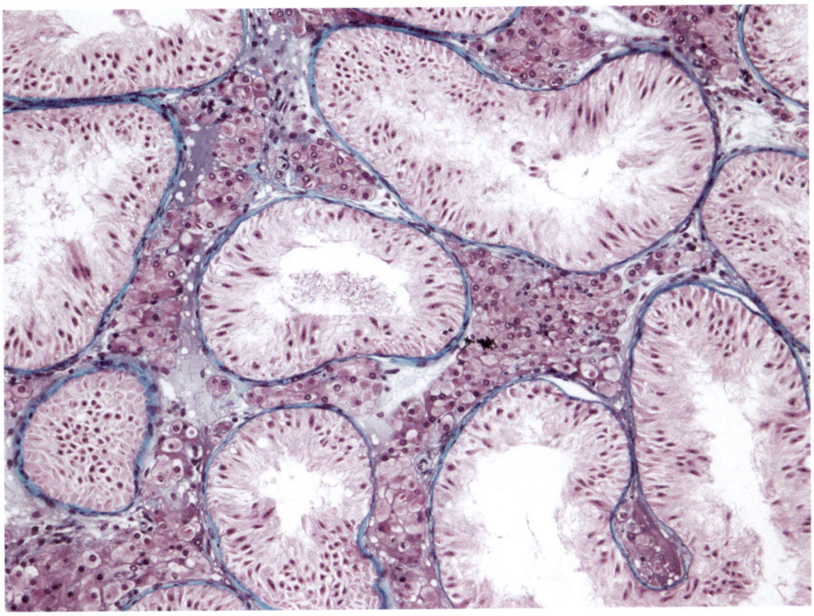

Fig. 18.3 Infertile patient with microdeletion of the AZFb subregion. The seminiferous tubules are lined only by Sertoli cells. The interstitium has diffuse Leydig cell hyperplasia

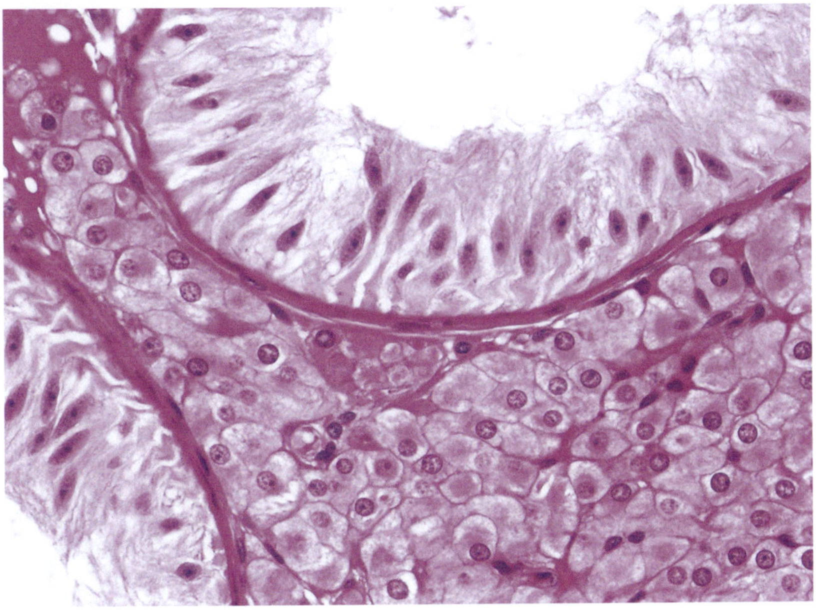

Fig. 18.4 The seminiferous epithelium consists of Sertoli cells of elongated nuclei and high and eosinophilic cytoplasms. Diffuse Leydig cell hyperplasia (same case of the previous figure)

Microdeletions of the AZFa Subregion Represent 5 % of the AZF deletions. Complete deletions occur in most cases; they have a histological pattern of Sertoli cell-only [74] and focal spermatogenesis in the remaining cases. Partial microdeletions are rare, and the impact on spermatogenesis is minimal [75].

Microdeletions of the AZFb Subregion Represent 10–16 % of Y-chromosome microdeletions. When the deletion is complete, patients are azoospermic, and histologically they show either just Sertoli cells or maturation arrest [76]. They are exceptionally oligozoospermic [77]. When the deletion is incomplete, 50 % of patients have sperm in the ejaculates [77] (Figs. 18.3 and 18.4).

Microdeletions of the AZFc Subregion Represent 80 % of all deletions of AZF [78]. When the deletion is complete, 50 % of patients are oligozoosper-

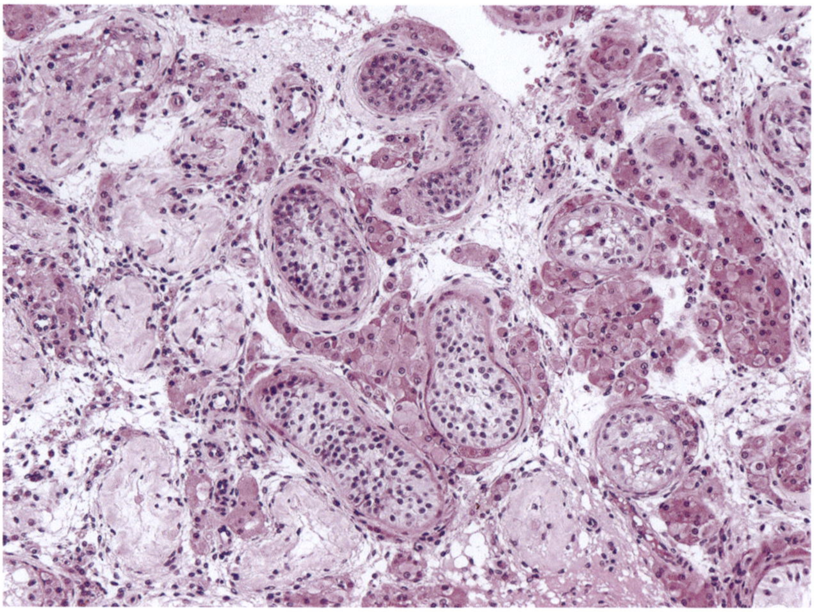

Fig. 18.5 Infertile patient with microdeletion of the AZFc subregion. Variegated histological pattern by the presence of hyalinized seminiferous tubules, dysgenetic Sertoli cell-only tubules, and focal Leydig cell hyperplasia

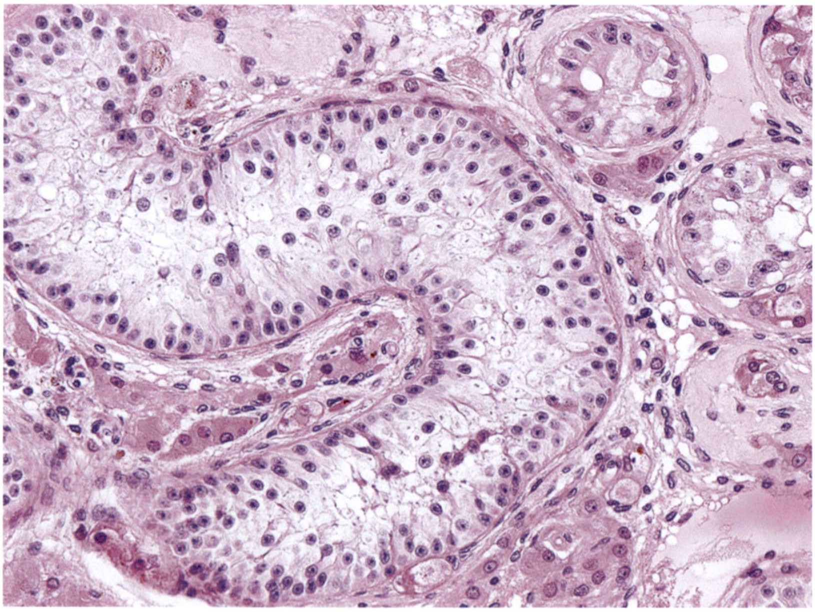

Fig. 18.6 Seminiferous tubes with Sertoli cell-only. In the central tubule, the high number of Sertoli cells, the sphericity of the nuclei, and the absence of lumen can be appreciated (same case of the previous figure)

mic. In half of the remaining cases (azoospermic patients), sperm can be extracted with TESE [79] (Figs. 18.5, 18.6, and 18.7).

Testicular damage is in relation with lost copies of DAZ (deleted in azoospermia). DAZ1/DAZ2 deletion is associated with incomplete maturation arrest of primary spermatocytes [80], maturation arrest of spermatids [81], or mixed atrophy [82], while DAZ3/DAZ4 deletion can be observed both in fertile and infertile patients. Partial deletions that remove only part of the subregion AZFc known as "gr/gr deletion rearrangements" may also cause subfertility. They were observed in 3.9 % of controls and in 6.8 % of infertile patients [83].

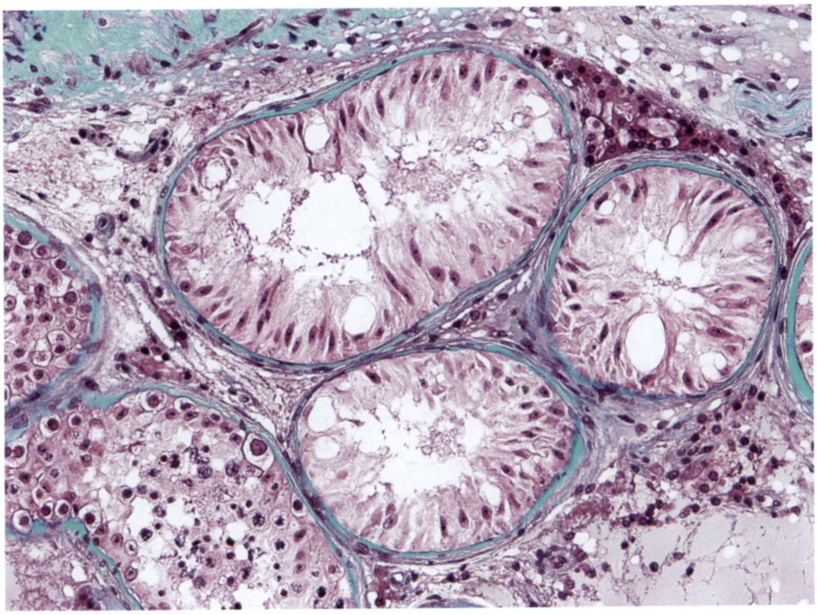

Fig. 18.7 Azoospermic patient with microdeletion of chromosome Y. The testis shows an image of mixed atrophy. The three central tubules have a Sertoli cell-only pattern, and the two in the periphery show complete spermatogenesis

References

1. Klinefelter HF, Reifenstein EC, Albright F. Syndrome characterized by gynecomastia, aspermatogenesis without A Leydigism, and increased excretion of follicle-stimulating hormone. J Clin Endocrinol. 1942;2:615–27.
2. Anawalt BD. Approach to male infertility and induction of spermatogenesis. J Clin Endocrinol Metab. 2013;98:3532–42.
3. Mau-Holzmann UA. Somatic chromosomal abnormalities in infertile men and women. Cytogenet Genome Res. 2005;111:317–36.
4. Karimi H, Sabbaghian M, Haratian K, Vaziri Nasab H, Farrahi F, Moradi SZ, Tavakolzadeh T, Beheshti Z, Gourabi H, Meybodi AM. A rare case of Klinefelter syndrome patient with quintuple mosaic karyotype, diagnosed by GTG-banding and FISH. Int J Fertil Steril. 2014;8:221–4.
5. Maiburg M, Repping S, Giltay J. The genetic origin of Klinefelter syndrome and its effect on spermatogenesis. Fertil Steril. 2012;98:253–60.
6. Coerdt W, Rehder H, Gausmann I, Johannisson R, Gropp A. Quantitative histology of human fetal testes in chromosomal disease. Pediatr Pathol. 1985;3:245–59.
7. Gracia R, Martín Alvarez L, Figols J, Lledó G, Nistal M, Barreiro E. Klinefelter's syndrome in prepubertal age. An Esp Pediatr. 1974;7:510–23.
8. Wikström AM, Hoei-Hansen CE, Dunkel L, Rajpert-De Meyts E. Immunoexpression of androgen receptor and nine markers of maturation in the testes of adolescent boys with Klinefelter syndrome: evidence for degeneration of germ cells at the onset of meiosis. J Clin Endocrinol Metab. 2007;92:714–9.
9. Skakkebaek NE. Two types of tubules containing only Sertoli cells in adults with Klinefelter's syndrome. Nature. 1969;223:643–5.
10. Dunkel L, Siimes MA, Bremner WJ. Reduced inhibin and elevated gonadotropin levels in early pubertal boys with testicular defects. Pediatr Res. 1993;33:514–8.
11. Martin R, Santamaría L, Nistal M, Fraile B, Paniagua R. The peritubular myofibroblasts in the testes from normal men and men with Klinefelter's syndrome. A quantitative, ultrastructural, and immunohistochemical study. J Pathol. 1992;168:59–66.
12. Regadera J, Codesal J, Paniagua R, Gonzalez-Peramato P, Nistal M. Immunohistochemical and quantitative study of interstitial and intratubular Leydig cells in normal men, cryptorchidism, and Klinefelter's syndrome. J Pathol. 1991;164:299–306.
13. Nistal M, Santamaria L, Paniagua R. Quantitative and ultrastructural study of Leydig cells in Klinefelter's syndrome. J Pathol. 1985;146:323–31.
14. Lejeune H, Brosse A, Groupe Fertipreserve, Plotton I. Fertility in Klinefelter syndrome. Presse Med. 2014;43:162–70.
15. Selice R, Di Mambro A, Garolla A, Ficarra V, Iafrate M, Ferlin A, Foresta C. Spermatogenesis in Klinefelter syndrome. J Endocrinol Invest. 2010;33:789–93.
16. Harari O, Bourne H, Baker G, Gronow M, Johnston I. High fertilization rate with intracytoplasmic sperm injection in mosaic Klinefelter's syndrome. Fertil Steril. 1995;63:182–4.
17. Tournaye H, Staessen C, Liebaers I, Van Assche E, Devroey P, Bonduelle M, Van Steirteghem A. Testicular

sperm recovery in nine 47 XXY Klinefelter patients. Hum Reprod. 1996;11:1644–9.
18. Hinney B, Guttenbach M, Schmid M, Engel W, Michelmann HW. Pregnancy after intracytoplasmic sperm injection with sperm from a man with a 47 XXY Klinefelter's karyotype. Fertil Steril. 1997;68:718–20.
19. Bourne H, Stern K, Clarke G, Pertile M, Speirs A, Baker HW. Delivery of normal twins following the intracytoplasmic injection of spermatozoa from a patient with 47 XXY Klinefelter's syndrome. Hum Reprod. 1997;12:2447–50.
20. Palermo GD, Schlegel PN, Sills ES, Veeck LL, Zaninovic N, Menendez S, Rosenwaks Z. Births after intracytoplasmic injection of sperm obtained by testicular extraction from men with nonmosaic Klinefelter's syndrome. N Engl J Med. 1998;338:588–90.
21. Ulug U, Bener F, Akman MA, Bahceci M. Partners of men with Klinefelter syndrome can benefit from assisted reproductive technologies. Fertil Steril. 2003;80:903–6.
22. Kahraman S, Ozgür S, Alataş C, Aksoy S, Taşdemir M, Nuhoğlu A, Taşdemir I, Balaban B, Biberoğlu K, Schoysman R, Nijs M, Vanderzwalmen P. Fertility with testicular sperm extraction and intracytoplasmic sperm injection in non-obstructive azoospermic men. Hum Reprod. 1996;11:756–60.
23. Aksglaede L, Juul A. Testicular function and fertility in men with Klinefelter syndrome: a review. Eur J Endocrinol. 2013;168:R67–76.
24. Rohayem J, Fricke R, Czeloth K, Mallidis C, Wistuba J, Krallmann C, Zitzmann M, Kliesch S. Age and markers of Leydig cell function, but not of Sertoli cell function predict the success of sperm retrieval in adolescents and adults with Klinefelter's syndrome. Andrology. 2015;3:868–75.
25. Ichioka K, Utsunomiya N, Kohei N, Ueda N, Inoue K, Terai A. Adult onset of declining spermatogenesis in a man with nonmosaic Klinefelter's syndrome. Fertil Steril. 2006;85:1511. e1–2.
26. Ramasamy R, Ricci JA, Palermo GD, Gosden LV, Rosenwaks Z, Schlegel PN. Successful fertility treatment for Klinefelter's syndrome. J Urol. 2009;182:1108–13.
27. Plotton I, Brosse A, Cuzin B, Lejeune H. Klinefelter syndrome and TESE-ICSI. Ann Endocrinol (Paris). 2014;75:118–25.
28. Majzoub A, Arafa M, Al Said S, Agarwal A, Seif A, Al Naimi A, El Bardisi H. Outcome of testicular sperm extraction in nonmosaic Klinefelter syndrome patients: what is the best approach? Andrologia. 2016;48:171–6.
29. Mehta A, Paduch DA. Klinefelter syndrome: an argument for early aggressive hormonal and fertility management. Fertil Steril. 2012;98:274–83.
30. Ozveri H, Kayabasoglu F, Demirel C, Donmez E. Outcomes of micro-dissection TESE in patients with non-mosaic Klinefelter's syndrome without hormonal treatment. Int J Fertil Steril. 2015;8:421–8.
31. Roche C, Sonigo C, Benmiloud-Tandjaoui N, Boujenah J, Benzacken B, Poncelet C, Hugues JN. 48,XXYY men with azoospermia: how to manage infertility? Gynecol Obstet Fertil. 2014;42:528–32.
32. De la Chapelle A, Hortling H, Niemi M, Wennstrom J. XX sex chromosomes in a human male: first case. Acta Med Scand Suppl. 1964;412:25–38.
33. Pastor Guzmán JM, Pastor Navarro H, Quintanilla Mata ML, Carrión López P, Martínez Ruíz J, Martínez Sanchiz C, Perán Teruel M, Virseda Rodríguez JA. 46,XX testicular disorder of sex development Case report. Arch Esp Urol. 2011;64:468–73.
34. Fechner PY, Marcantonio SM, Jaswaney V, Stetten G, Goodfellow PN, Migeon CJ, Smith KD, Berkovitz GD, Amrhein JA, Bard PA, et al. The role of the sex-determining region Y gene in the etiology of 46 XX maleness. J Clin Endocrinol Metab. 1993;76:690–5.
35. De la Chapelle A, Hästbacka J, Korhonen T, Mäenpää J. The etiology of XX sex reversal. Reprod Nutr Dev. 1990;Suppl 1(30):39s–49s.
36. Vorona E, Zitzmann M, Gromoll J, Schüring AN, Nieschlag E. Clinical, endocrinological, and epigenetic features of the 46,XX male syndrome, compared with 47,XXY Klinefelter patients. J Clin Endocrinol Metab. 2007;92:3458–65.
37. Nistal M, Paniagua R. Ultrastructure of testicular biopsy from an XX male. Virchows Arch B Cell Pathol Incl Mol Pathol. 1979;31:45–55.
38. Sandberg AA, Koepf GF, Ishihara T, Hauschka TS. An XYY human male. Lancet. 1961;2:488–9.
39. Geerts M, Steyaert J, Fryns JP. The XYY syndrome: a follow-up study on 38 boys. Genet Couns. 2003;14:267–79.
40. Robinson DO, Jacobs PA. The origin of the extra Y chromosome in males with a 47, XYY karyotype. Hum Mol Genet. 1999;8:2205–9.
41. Götz MJ, Johnstone EC, Ratcliffe SG. Criminality and antisocial behaviour in unselected men with sex chromosome abnormalities. Psychol Med. 1999;29:953–62.
42. Bardsley MZ, Kowal K, Levy C, Gosek A, Ayari N, Tartaglia N, Lahlou N, Winder B, Grimes S, Ross JL. 47,XYY syndrome: clinical phenotype and timing of ascertainment. J Pediatr. 2013;163:1085–94.
43. Abdel-Razic MM, Abdel-Hamid IA, ElSobky ES. Nonmosaic 47,XYY syndrome presenting with male infertility: case series. Andrologia. 2012;44:200–4.
44. Wong EC, Ferguson KA, Chow V, Ma S. Sperm aneuploidy and meiotic sex chromosome configurations in an infertile XYY male. Hum Reprod. 2008;23:374–8.
45. Moretti E, Anichini C, Sartini B, Collodel G. Sperm ultrastructure and meiotic segregation in an infertile 47, XYY man. Andrologia. 2007;39:229–34.
46. Hori N, Kato T, Sugimura Y, Tajima K, Tochigi H, Kawamura J. A male subject with 3 Y chromosomes (48, XYYY): a case report. J Urol. 1988;139:1059–61.
47. Shanske A, Sachmechi I, Patel DK, Bishnoi A, Rosner F. An adult with 49,XYYYY karyotype: case report and endocrine studies. Am J Med Genet. 1998;80:103–6.

48. Ceylan GG, Ceylan C, Elyas H. Genetic anomalies in patients with severe oligozoospermia and azoospermia in eastern Turkey: a prospective study. Genet Mol Res. 2009;8:915–22.
49. Dul EC, van Ravenswaaij-Arts CM, Groen H, van Echten-Arends J, Land JA. Who should be screened for chromosomal abnormalities before ICSI treatment? Hum Reprod. 2010;25:2673–7.
50. Pastuszek E, Kiewisz J, Kulwikowska PM, Lukaszuk M, Lukaszuk K. Sperm parameters and DNA fragmentation of balanced chromosomal rearrangements carriers. Folia Histochem Cytobiol. 2015;53:314–21.
51. Chandley AC, Edmond P, Christie S, Gowans L, Fletcher J, Frackiewicz A, Newton M. Cytogenetics and infertility in man. I. Karyotype and seminal analysis: results of a five-year survey of men attending a subfertility clinic. Ann Hum Genet. 1975;39:231–54.
52. Van Assche E, Bonduelle M, Tournaye H, Joris H, Verheyen G, Devroey P, Van Steirteghem A, Liebaers I. Cytogenetics of infertile men. Hum Reprod. 1996;11:1–24.
53. Brandriff B, Gordon L, Ashworth LK, Littman V, Watchmaker G, Carrano AV. Cytogenetics of human sperm: meiotic segregation in two translocation carriers. Am J Hum Genet. 1986;38:197–208.
54. Luciani JM, Guichaoua MR, Delafontaine D, North MO, Gabriel-Robez O, Rumpler Y. Pachytene analysis in a 17;21 reciprocal translocation carrier: role of the acrocentric chromosomes in male sterility. Hum Genet. 1987;77:246–50.
55. Shapiro CE. Unbalanced chromosomal translocation associated with Sertoli-cell-only histology. J Urol. 1991;145:563–4.
56. Colls P, Blanco J, Martínez-Pasarell O, Vidal F, Egozcue J, Márquez C, Guitart M, Templado C. Chromosome segregation in a man heterozygous for a pericentric inversion, inv(9)(p11q13), analyzed by using sperm karyotyping and two-color fluorescence in situ hybridization on sperm nuclei. Hum Genet. 1997;99:761–5.
57. Anton E, Blanco J, Egozcue J, Vidal F. Sperm studies in heterozygote inversion carriers: a review. Cytogenet Genome Res. 2005;111:297–304.
58. Bache I, Assche EV, Cingoz S, et al. An excess of chromosome 1 breakpoints in male infertility. Eur J Hum Genet. 2004;2:993–1000.
59. Liehr T, Ewers E, Hamid AB, Kosyakova N, Voigt M, Weise A, Manvelyan M. Small supernumerary marker chromosomes and uniparental disomy have a story to tell. J Histochem Cytochem. 2011;59:842–8.
60. Armanet N, Tosca L, Brisset S, Liehr T, Tachdjian G. Small Supernumerary Marker Chromosomes in Human Infertility. Cytogenet Genome Res. 2015;146:100–8.
61. Reijo R, Alagappan RK, Patrizio P, Page DC. Severe oligozoospermia resulting from deletions of azoospermia factor gene on Y chromosome. Lancet. 1996;347:1290–3.
62. Kalantari H, Asia S, Totonchi M, Vazirinasab H, Mansouri Z, Zarei Moradi S, Haratian K, Gourabi H, Mohseni Meybodi A. Delineating the association between isodicentric chromosome Y and infertility: a retrospective study. Fertil Steril. 2014;101:1091–6.
63. Yoshida A, Nakahori Y, Kuroki Y, Miura K, Shirai M. An azoospermic male with an unbalanced autosomal-Y translocation. Jpn J Hum Genet. 1997;42:451–5.
64. Dong Y, Yu XW, Wang RX, Li LL, Jiang YT, Liu RZ. 45,X/46,X,r(Y)/46,X,dic r(Y) karyotype in an azoospermic male: a case report. Cytogenet Genome Res. 2014;142:140–4.
65. Wahlström J, Kyllerman M, Hansson A, Taranger J. Unequal mitotic sister chromatid exchange and different length of Y chromosomes. Hum Genet. 1985;70:186–8.
66. Petit C, de la Chapelle A, Levilliers J, Castillo S, Noël B, Weissenbach J. An abnormal terminal X-Y interchange accounts for most but not all cases of human XX maleness. Cell. 1987;49:595–602.
67. Pinho MJ, Neves R, Costa P, Ferrás C, Sousa M, Alves C, Almeida C, Fernandes S, Silva J, Ferrás L, Barros A. Unique t(Y;1)(q12;q12) reciprocal translocation with loss of the heterochromatic region of chromosome 1 in a male with azoospermia due to meiotic arrest: a case report. Hum Reprod. 2005;20:689–96.
68. Karaer K, Ergun MA, Weise A, Ewers E, Liehr T, Kosyakova N, Mkrtchyan H. The case of an infertile male with an uncommon reciprocal X-autosomal translocation: how does this affect male fertility? Genet Couns. 2010;21:397–404.
69. Sanlaville D, Schluth-Bolard C, Turleau C. Distal Xq duplication and functional Xq disomy. Orphanet J Rare Dis. 2009;4:4.
70. Ogata T, Matsuo M, Muroya K, Koyama Y, Fukutani K. 47,XXX male: a clinical and molecular study. Am J Med Genet. 2001;98:353–6.
71. Tiepolo L, Zuffardi O. Localization of factors controlling spermatogenesis in the nonfluorescent portion of the human Y chromosome long arm. Hum Genet. 1976;34:119–24.
72. Chiang HS, Wei HJ, Chen YT. Genetic screening for patients with azoospermia and severe oligoasthenospermia. Int J Androl. 2000;23(Suppl 2):20–5.
73. Malekasgar AM, Mombaini H. Screening of 'Y' chromosome microdeletions in Iranian infertile males. J Hum Reprod Sci. 2008;1:2–9.
74. Krausz C, McElreavey K. Y chromosome and male infertility. Front Biosci. 1999;4:E1–8.
75. Kleiman SE, Yogev L, Hauser R, Botchan A, Maymon BB, Paz G, Yavetz H. Expression profile of AZF genes in testicular biopsies of azoospermic men. Hum Reprod. 2007;22:151–8.
76. Mirfakhraie R, Mirzajani F, Kalantar SM, Montazeri M, Salsabili N, Pourmand GR, Houshmand M. High prevalence of AZFb microdeletion in Iranian patients with idiopathic non-obstructive azoospermia. Indian J Med Res. 2010;132:265–70.
77. Soares AR, Costa P, Silva J, Sousa M, Barros A, Fernandes S. AZFb microdeletions and oligozoospermia – which mechanisms? Fertil Steril. 2012;97:858–63.

78. Simoni M, Tüttelmann F, Gromoll J, Nieschlag E. Clinical consequences of microdeletions of the Y chromosome: the extended Münster experience. Reprod Biomed Online. 2008;16:289–303.
79. Krausz C, Forti G, McElreavey K. The Y chromosome and male fertility and infertility. Int J Androl. 2003;26:70–5.
80. Reijo R, Lee TY, Salo P, Alagappan R, Brown LG, Rosenberg M, Rozen S, Jaffe T, Straus D, Hovatta O, et al. Diverse spermatogenic defects in humans caused by Y chromosome deletions encompassing a novel RNA-binding protein gene. Nat Genet. 1995;10:383–93.
81. Vogt PH, Edelmann A, Kirsch S, Henegariu O, Hirschmann P, Kiesewetter F, Köhn FM, Schill WB, Farah S, Ramos C, Hartmann M, Hartschuh W, Meschede D, Behre HM, Castel A, Nieschlag E, Weidner W, Gröne HJ, Jung A, Engel W, Haidl G. Human Y chromosome azoospermia factors (AZF) mapped to different subregions in Yq11. Hum Mol Genet. 1996;5:933–43.
82. Mulhall JP, Reijo R, Alagappan R, Brown L, Page D, Carson R, Oates RD. Azoospermic men with deletion of the DAZ gene cluster are capable of completing spermatogenesis: fertilization, normal embryonic development and pregnancy occur when retrieved testicular spermatozoa are used for intracytoplasmic sperm injection. Hum Reprod. 1997;12:503–8.
83. Stouffs K, Lissens W, Tournaye H, Haentjens P. What about gr/gr deletions and male infertility? Systematic review and meta-analysis. Hum Reprod Update. 2011;17:197–209.

19 Fertility Potential of Patients with Hypogonadotropic Hypogonadism

Manuel Nistal, Pilar González-Peramato, and Álvaro Serrano

19.1 The Male Reproductive Axis

The male reproductive axis starts with GnRH neurons. They are cells that are present in the olfactory placode in 6-week-old fetuses. They migrate with olfactory axons and vessels through the cribriform plate to the brain where they arrive at weeks 9–10. On reaching the hypothalamus, GnRH neurons detach from their axonal guides and distribute in the medial basal hypothalamus and the arcuate nucleus. At the end of fetal life, their axons project to the median eminence, and their secretion is released into the hypophyseal portal system. Decapeptide GnRH acts through a specific receptor for gonadotropic cells of the anterior pituitary, and these cells control the synthesis and release of the follicle-stimulating hormone (FSH) and the luteinizing hormone (LH) [1].

The following genes, among other, are involved in the migration of GnRH neurons: Genes encoding fibroblast growth factor 8 (*FGF8*) signaling pathway proteins, chromodomain helicase DNA-binding protein 7 (*CHD7*), and sex-determining region Y Box 10 (*SOX10*) affect the neurogenic niche in the nasal area and craniofacial development. The migration of GnRH neurons is also influenced by Kallmann syndrome protein (anosmin 1 encoded by *ANOS1*), prokineticin-2 and prokineticin receptor 2 (encoded by *PROK2* and *PROKR2*, respectively), WD repeat domain 11 (encoded by *WDR11*), semaphorin 3A (encoded by *SEMA3A*), and FEZ family zinc finger 1 (encoded by *FEZF1*) [2, 3].

Among the afferents receiving GnRH neurons, kisspeptin-producing neurons, the inactivating mutations in the genes encoding kisspeptin-1 (*KISS1*), and its receptor (*KISS1R*) that halt pubertal development can be found. The same applies to mutations in *TAC3* (encoding tachykinin-3) and *TACR3* (encoding tachykinin receptor 3). Modulation of the GnRH secretion is also dependent on genes encoding leptin (*LEP*) or its receptor (*LEPR*). Patients with inactivating mutations of these genes have no pubertal development, and they have hypogonadotropic hypogonadism.

Pubertal development begins with the activation of the pulsatile secretion of GnRH. This discharge produces an LH elevation that stimulates differentiation of Leydig cells and testosterone secretion. FSH stimulates the first proliferation of the Sertoli cells and then, along with other factors, their maturation. As puberty progresses, the levels of inhibin B increase and AMH decrease. Parallel to the Sertoli cell maturation, proliferation of germ cells occurs.

19.2 Classification of Hypogonadotropic Hypogonadism

Hypogonadotropic hypogonadism can be classified in (1) congenital hypogonadotropic hypogonadism (CHH) and (2) acquired hypogonadotropic hypogonadism (AHH).

M. Nistal et al., *Clues in the Diagnosis of Non-tumoral Testicular Pathology*,
DOI 10.1007/978-3-319-49364-0_19

CHH is caused by a deficiency in GnRH production, secretion, or action. Depending on the severity of the deficit, it may appear during the neonatal period or in childhood, puberty as delayed puberty, or in adulthood as a lack of gonadal development and infertility. It can appear as isolated GnRH or associated with anosmia or hyposmia; in the latter case, the CHH is termed Kallmann's syndrome. Other associated anomalies may be cleft lip or palate, dental agenesis, ear anomalies, congenital hearing impairment, renal agenesis, bimanual synkinesis, and skeletal anomalies.

AHH can be caused by acquired lesions such as intrasellar and extrasellar tumors such as astrocytoma, craniopharyngioma, germinoma, and glioma and also, systemic diseases such as hemochromatosis, sarcoidosis and histiocytosis X, infections, vascular disorders, head injuries, hypophysitis, syndrome of the empty sella, brain irradiation, and hydrocephalus. Other causes are functional: drugs (e.g., sex steroids and gonadotropin-releasing hormone analogues), exhausting exercise, excessive alcohol consumption or illicit drug intake, fasting, and serious illnesses such as sepsis and severe stress. Finally, chronic diseases such as liver diseases, celiac disease, inflammatory bowel disease, beta thalassemia, Cushing's syndrome, obesity, and hypothyroidism can also cause AHH [4].

19.2.1 Congenital Hypogonadotropic Hypogonadism (CHH)

Most CHH cases are sporadic. One third of them constitute a familial pattern. Cases with autosomal-recessive, dominant, or X chromosome-linked recessive as well as oligogenic forms of inheritance have been reported [5].

Neonatal and Childhood CHH Should be suspected in children with small testes (FSH deficit), undescended testes (androgen and INSL3 insufficiency secondary to LH defect), and micropenis (hypoandrogenism secondary to LH defect). A family history of anosmia or hyposmia and malformations in the cerebral pituitary and hypothalamic regions reinforces the diagnosis. The absence of increase of FSH, LH, and testosterone levels during minipuberty (around 2–3 months) and the absence of LH elevation in an intravenous GnRH test complete the diagnosis [6, 7]. The neonatal hypotonia and the developmental delay are characteristic of the Prader-Willi syndrome [8, 9]. The association with primary adrenal failure is characteristic of congenital adrenal hypoplasia due to *DAX1* mutation [10].

In Adolescence Patients with CHH lack pubertal activation of the hypothalamus-pituitary-gonadal axis (HPG). They do not experience testicular enlargement at the age of 14. In most patients, puberty never occurs (absent puberty), and less commonly puberty starts but is not fully developed (partial puberty). Adolescents with CHH exhibit a steady linear growth and thus lack the growth spurts. They have delayed epiphysis closure and eunuchoid proportions. Patients consult for absent or minimal virilization, low libido, and lack of sexual function. The differential diagnosis during adolescence has to be made through constitutional delay of growth and puberty (CDGP). This is favored by the association with short height, low growth rate, and delayed skeletal maturation. The presence of cryptorchidism, micropenis, poor sense of smell, and cleft lip/palate, suggesting a Kallmann's syndrome, oppose the CDGP diagnosis. GnRH testing in combination with a 3-day and 19-day hCG test may help the differential diagnosis [11].

Idiopathic Hypogonadotropic Hypogonadism There are three clinical variants: hypogonadotropic hypogonadism with anosmia or Kallmann's syndrome, idiopathic normosmic hypogonadotropic hypogonadism, and hypogonadotropic hypogonadism by LH deficit or fertile eunuch syndrome [12].

Hypogonadotropic Hypogonadism with Anosmia It is also known as *Kallmann's syndrome* [13]. This syndrome results from mutations in the genes involved in the development and migration of

GnRH neurons from the olfactory placode to the hypothalamus. The deficit of GnRH production is associated with hypoplasia or aplasia of the olfactory bulbs. The genes most frequently involved are *KAL1*, *FGF8* and its receptor *FGFR1*, *PROK2* and its receptor *PROKR2, CHD7, NELF, HS6ST1, WDR11, SEMA3A* [2]. It represents about two thirds of all idiopathic hypogonadotropic hypogonadisms. The first case was described by Maestre de San Juan in 1856 [14].

In childhood and puberty, the most important data to make us suspect a diagnosis of Kallmann's syndrome are anosmia or hyposmia, hypoplasia of the penis and cryptorchidism, as well as hearing loss, renal agenesis, and/or synkinesis [15]. The diagnosis is confirmed by the absence of olfactory bulbs and olfactory tract on nuclear magnetic resonance.

Normosmic Isolated Hypogonadotropic Hypogonadism (NIHH) It is caused by a defect in the genes involved in the regulation and function of GnRH neurons via kisspeptin, neurokinin, or leptin signaling or their respective receptors. GnRHR gene mutations are responsible for an impaired pituitary response to GnRH. The secretion of FSH and LH is affected in all cases except by deficits in the neurokinin system.

Isolated LH Deficit The patients with LH deficiency and normal or higher serum FSH levels are the consequence of mutations in the *LHb* gene, encoding the b subunit of LH, and neurokinin system defects responsible for the regulation of GnRH pulses. From the clinical viewpoint, micropenis and cryptorchidism can observed, as a consequence of the fetal hypoandrogenism during the second and third quarters. The testicular volume in the newborn baby and in childhood remains preserved given normal FSH secretion. Hypoandrogenism signs are observed in the adult, such as the presence of eunuchoid proportions. The testes can reach a normal size and produce sperm (Fig. 19.1). This situation is also known by the name of *fertile eunuch syndrome*.

CHH Histology

The testicular morphology is different depending on the severity of the GnRH defect and the presence or absence of cryptorchidism. We can distinguish various patterns.

(a) Incomplete and delayed childhood testicular development when compared even in childhood with children of their own age. The average tubular diameter is decreased (<60

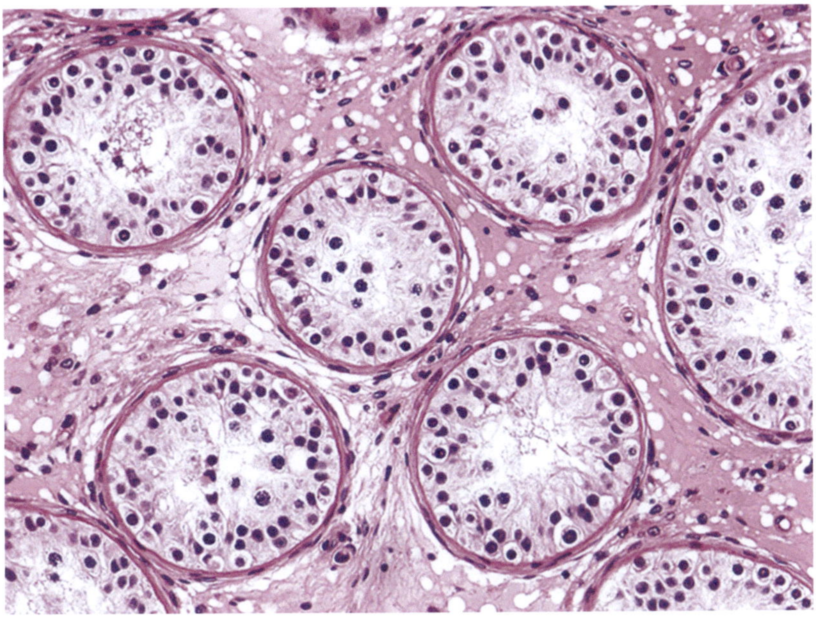

Fig. 19.1 Hypogonadotropic hypogonadism due to LH congenital deficit. The seminiferous tubules show advanced pubertal development with poor spermatogenesis. The interstitium lacks Leydig cells

microns), the number of Sertoli cells by tubular section is low (14–16), and there is a decrease of spermatogonia, while there are tubular sections devoid of all germ cells [16, 17]. The number of Ad spermatogonia is low or they are absent. The tubular wall is slightly thickened (Fig. 19.2). This is observed in patients with absence of minipuberty, small testes, or a history of cryptorchidism (GnRH serious defects).

(b) Infantile testes. The development is similar to that of a child of 4–5 years. The tubular diameter is 60–80 microns, the number of Sertoli cells by tubular section is 16–18, and spermatogonia are observed in all the tubular sections including Ad spermatogonia [18–20]. It is observed in patients with a defect in GnRH with undescended testes and absence of micropenis with normal testes for the age during childhood or over 4 ml in adults.

(c) Pubertal and adult testes. In adult patients with testicular sizes above 4 ml, it can be seen from the beginning of the pubertal development to full spermatogenesis. In the first case, an increased number of Sertoli cells by tubular section (18–20) stands out. Sertoli cells still show no signs of pubertal maturation. The tubular diameter varies from 80 to 100 microns. The presence of several spermatogonia per tubular section, and even isolated first-order spermatocytes, is a sign of the onset of puberty. In the second case, there is a dissociation of the tubular development that presents complete maturation of the Sertoli cells, tubular lumen and complete but quantitatively very poor spermatogenesis, and an interstitium devoid of Leydig cells (Fig. 19.3). The image is characteristic of a fertile eunuch patient [21].

19.2.2 Acquired Hypogonadotropic Hypogonadism (AHH)

In recent decades, there has been an increase of hypogonadism among the population of adult patients. Three to eight percent of adults between 20 and 45 years have hypogonadism. The prevalence of hypogonadism in men over 45 years in the USA is estimated at 13.8 million [22]. Acquired hypogonadism hypogonadism is very common in pathology of other glands and chronic diseases. This type of hypogonadism is not included in this text. The most disturbing causes nowadays are:

(a) Exogenous testosterone supplementation therapy to combat symptoms of hypogonadism such as decreased libido, erectile dysfunction, fatigue, and depression.

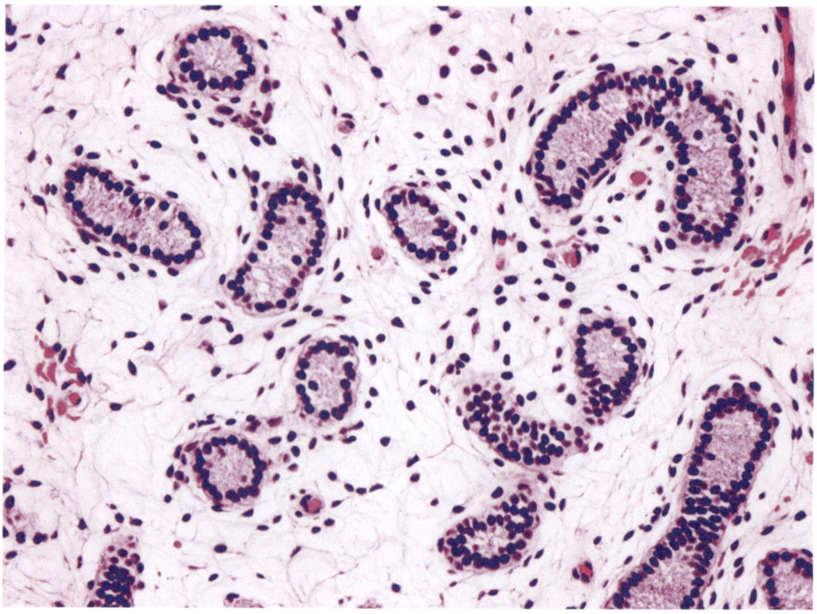

Fig. 19.2 Congenital hypogonadotropic hypogonadism. Child with Prader-Willi syndrome. Seminiferous tubes with small diameter, absence of germ cells, and wide interstitium

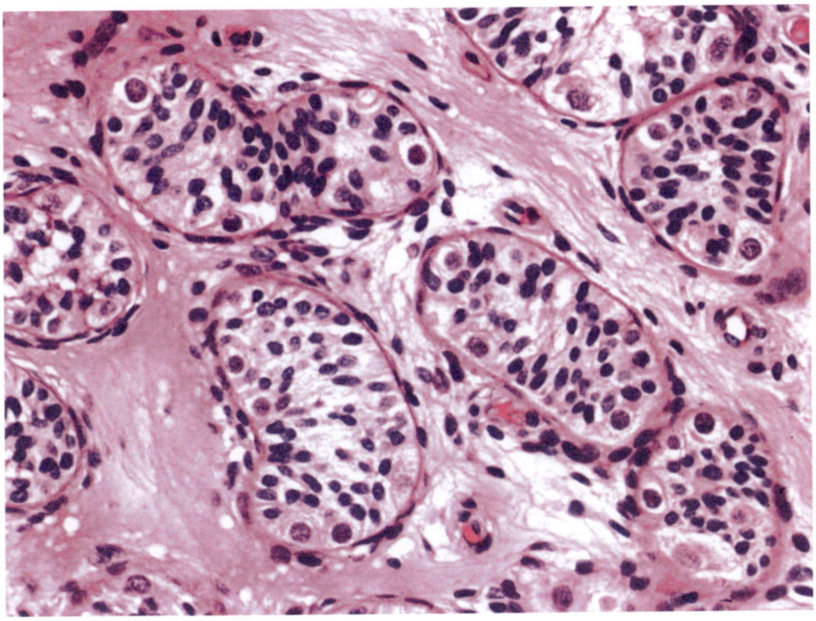

Fig. 19.3 Hypogonadotropic hypogonadism due to GnRh congenital deficit in 18-year-old patient. The seminiferous tubules show infantile development. Spermatogonia in all tubular sections are observed although there are no signs of maturation. The interstitium lacks Leydig cells and shows an important collagenization

(b) Use of anabolic steroids in the USA is estimated at 1–3 million of individuals, mostly young athletes. Not less than 6.6 % of high school seniors use or have used them [23].

In healthy adult males, GnRH leads to the release of LH from the anterior pituitary, which then stimulates Leydig cells in the testes to produce testosterone. As testosterone levels increase, negative feedback occurs on both the hypothalamus and the anterior pituitary. Exogenous testosterone use, therefore, results in both impaired endocrine regulation of GnRH and LH release and subsequent decrease of endogenous testosterone.

The use of testosterone supplementation in reproductive age males leads to the atrophy of the seminiferous epithelium, suppressing spermatogenesis and reaching azoospermia after 10 weeks of use [24].

Histology In pediatric patients with space-occupying or destructive lesions of the hypothalamic-pituitary axis or chronic diseases, the testes are small. The seminiferous tubules can be reduced to large epithelial cords with an important thickening of the tubular wall and decreased number of Sertoli cells. Sertoli cells show spherical hyperchromatic nuclei and scant cytoplasm. The interstitium, which may seem enlarged, lacks Leydig cells [25] (Fig. 19.4).

Adult patients who develop pituitary or hypothalamic lesions present an involution of the adult testicular development, which can even lead to the disappearance of spermatogenesis, involution of differentiation of Sertoli cells, hyalinization of the tubular wall, and disappearance of Leydig cells. The seminiferous tubules with this form of atrophy still show elastic fibers as an expression of the adult development they had previously had (Fig. 19.5).

In patients with exogenous testosterone supplementation therapy or who use anabolic steroids and consult for infertility, the lesions are less severe as they do not cause the disappearance of the germ cells.

19.3 Fertility Predictor Data

There are a lot of clinical, hormonal, and histological data that enable to predict the testicular behavior before hypogonadism is treated, in order to inform the couple of the possibility of being fertile.

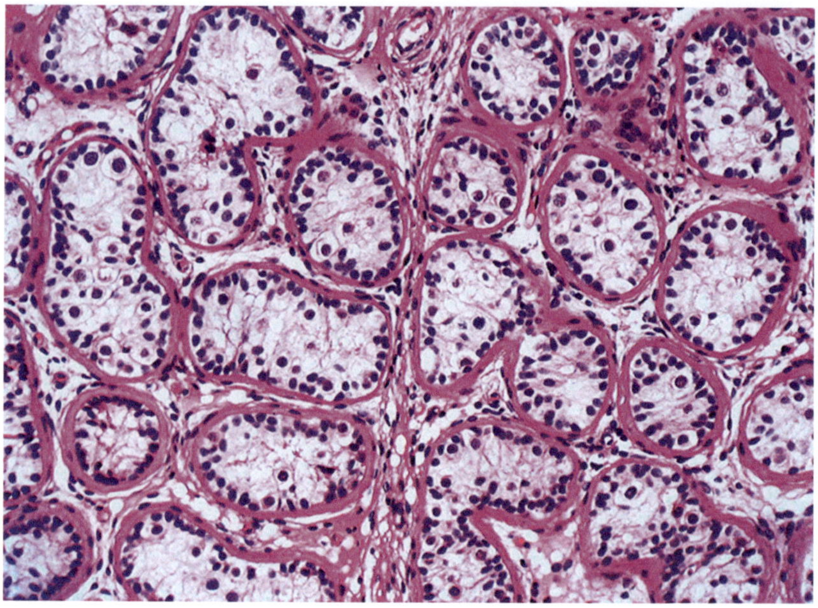

Fig. 19.4 Acquired hypogonadotropic hypogonadism in a patient of 17-year-old patient with craniopharyngioma. There is absence of maturation in both the seminiferous tubules and interstitium

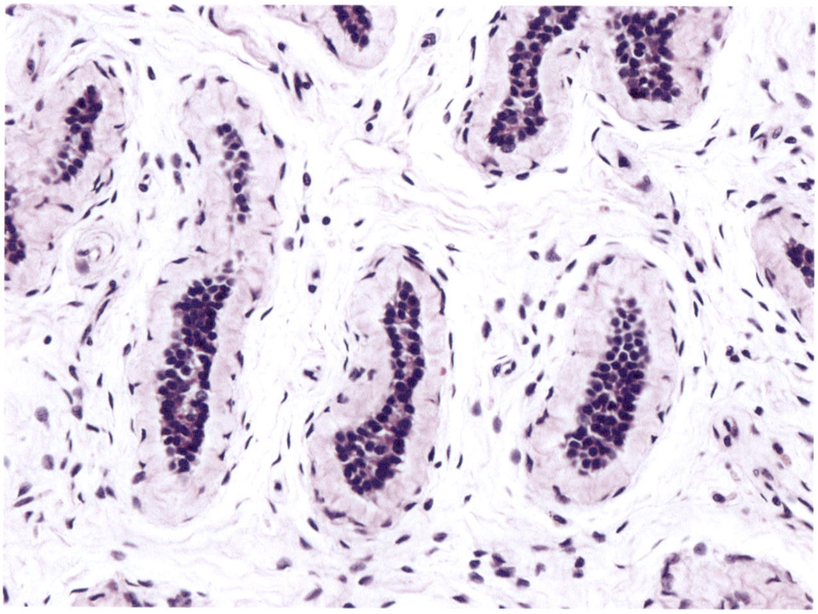

Fig. 19.5 Acquired hypogonadotropic hypogonadism. Tubular and interstitial atrophy in a patient with chronic disease

Clinical Data In CHH the following findings are considered important:

- The presence of testicular maldescent is associated with an unfavorable prognosis for fertility.
- The absence of minipuberty. Minipuberty is a window of time in life of great importance for future fertility, as the HPG axis is transiently activated during the first months of postnatal life. Gonadotropin, testosterone, and inhibin levels increase to pubertal or adult rates at 3 months of age. This activation of the HPG axis is important to increase the mitotic activity of Sertoli cells and germ cells and the increase in length of the seminiferous tubules [26].
- Low inhibin B levels <30 pg/ml, which is in fact related to the number of Sertoli cells.
- Absence of pubertal development. Patients with absent pubertal development have poorer

fertility outcomes [27].

- Prior androgen treatment in adolescence before treatment with gonadotropins in the adult to establish fertility.
- Patients with X-linked form of CHH with the *KAL1* mutation are less responsive to treatment.

Histopathological Data The testicular volume. Approximately 90 % of the testicular volume depends on the seminiferous tubules. In childhood the diameter of the seminiferous tubules depends primarily on the number of Sertoli cells and the length of the seminiferous tubules. The undescended testicles are generally smaller in size [28]. Low testicular volumes are signs of poor prognosis [29].

- The undescended testicles have a decreased germ cell number, which can be associated or not to reduced Sertoli cells. Decreased Ad spermatogonia are also a sign of poor prognosis [30].

19.4 Treatment Methods

In childhood, testicles should be descended between 6 and 12 months of age. Micropenis can be corrected with short-term low-dose testosterone or FSH and LH if there is evidence of absence of minipuberty. The induction of male sexual characteristics can be achieved with the administration of testosterone. The dose and time of administration varies according to the age of the patients – it will be higher in older adolescents or following some physiological steps that start with FSH administration that stimulates Sertoli cells proliferation, inhibin B synthesis and testicular enlargement, followed by administration of hCG.

In adulthood we have to know if what we want is solely to reach sexual development or we wish to achieve further fertility. Classically, in patients with testes >4 ml without a history of cryptorchidism, and in patients with the fertile eunuch syndrome, spermatogenesis can be induced with only hCG. If there are no sperm in the ejaculates, Sertoli cells are stimulated with FSH [3]. When the testicular volume is <4 ml, the treatment is either pulsatile GnRH or combined gonadotropin therapy (hCG + FSH) [4, 31].

Treatment with GnRH has provided new data illuminating CHH related to clinical and histological data. Patients with IHH receiving long-term GnRH normalize FSH and LH levels and serum testosterone levels and show sperm in the ejaculates in 74 %. Twenty-six percent of them consist of patients with three types of different answers:

Patients with the "triple defect": GnRH deficiency, pituitary resistance, and testicular failure (11 %). These are patients who remain with hypogonadotropic hypogonadism (low/normal LH/FSH and testosterone less than 200 ng/dl) and azoospermia:

(a) Patients with the "dual defect," GnRH deficiency, and testicular resistance (9.5 %) are patients with high levels of FSH and normal LH and testosterone levels with sperm in the ejaculates.
(b) Patients with the "dual defect," GnRH deficiency, and azoospermia (5.5 %). Patients acquire normal hormone serum levels but remain with azoospermia [5].
(c) Adult patients of childbearing age receiving testosterone supplementation benefit from the hCG therapy in that it not only maintains optimum intratesticular levels of testosterone but prevents damage to the seminiferous tubules. Azoospermia can also be prevented by testosterone treatment associating selective estrogen receptor modulators such as clomiphene citrate [32].

References

1. Dwyer AA, Raivio T, Pitteloud N. Gonadotrophin replacement for induction of fertility in hypogonadal men. Best Pract Res Clin Endocrinol Metab. 2015;29:91–103.
2. Beate K, Joseph N, Nicolas de R, Wolfram K. Genetics of isolated hypogonadotropic hypogonadism: role of GnRH receptor and other genes. J Endocrinol. 2012;2012:147893.
3. Boehm U, Bouloux PM, Dattani MT, de Roux N, Dodé C, Dunkel L, Dwyer AA, Giacobini P, Hardelin JP, Juul A, Maghnie M, Pitteloud N, Prevot V, Raivio T, Tena-Sempere M, Quinton R, Young J. Expert consensus document: European Consensus Statement on

congenital hypogonadotropic hypogonadism–pathogenesis, diagnosis and treatment. Nat Rev Endocrinol. 2015;11:547–64.
4. Fraietta R, Zylberstejn DS, Esteves SC. Hypogonadotropic hypogonadism revisited. Clinics (Sao Paulo). 2013;68(Suppl 1):81–8.
5. Sykiotis GP, Hoang XH, Avbelj M, Hayes FJ, Thambundit A, Dwyer A, Au M, Plummer L, Crowley Jr WF, Pitteloud N. Congenital idiopathic hypogonadotropic hypogonadism: evidence of defects in the hypothalamus, pituitary, and testes. J Clin Endocrinol Metab. 2010;95:3019–27.
6. Grumbach MM. A window of opportunity: the diagnosis of gonadotropin deficiency in the male infant. J Clin Endocrinol Metab. 2005;90:3122–7.
7. Braslavsky D, Grinspon RP, Ballerini MG, Bedecarrás P, Loreti N, Bastida G, Ropelato MG, Keselman A, Campo S, Rey RA, Bergadá I. Hypogonadotropic hypogonadism in infants with congenital hypopituitarism: a challenge to diagnose at an early stage. Horm Res Paediatr. 2015;84:289–97.
8. Martín Zurro A, Sánchez Franco F, Cerdán Vallejo A, Nistal M. Prader-Willi syndrome. Rev Clin Esp. 1972;125:445–50.
9. Angulo MA, Butler MG, Cataletto ME. Prader-Willi syndrome: a review of clinical, genetic, and endocrine findings. J Endocrinol Invest. 2015;38:1249–63.
10. Suntharalingham JP, Buonocore F, Duncan AJ, Achermann JC. DAX-1 (NR0B1) and steroidogenic factor-1 (SF-1, NR5A1) in human disease. Best Pract Res Clin Endocrinol Metab. 2015;29:607–19.
11. Segal TY, Mehta A, Anazodo A, et al. Role of gonadotropin releasing hormone and human chorionic gonadotropin stimulation tests in differentiating patients with hypogonadotropic hypogonadism from those with constitutional delay of growth and puberty. J Clin Endocrinol Metab. 2009;94:780–5.
12. Pallardo Sanchez LF, Santiago Corchado M, Cerdan Vallejo A, Nistal M. Algunos aspectos del hipogonadismo hipogonadotrópico. Med Clin. 1972;59:390–6.
13. Kallmann FJ, Schoenfeld WA, Barrera SE. The genetic aspects of primary eunuchoidism. Am J Ment Defit. 1944;48:203–36.
14. Maestre De San Juan A. Teratología: falta total de nervios olfatorios con anosmia en un individuo en quien existía una atrofia congénita de los testículos y miembro viril. El Siglo Médico. 1856;131:211–21.
15. Kaplan JD, Bernstein JA, Kwan A, Hudgins L. Clues to an early diagnosis of Kallmann syndrome. Am J Med Genet A. 2010;152A:2796–801.
16. Enríquez L, Díaz-Rubio García M, Zamarrón A, González Paramo P, Nistal M. Hypogonadotropic hypogonadism with anosmia. Rev Clin Esp. 1973;131:383–92.
17. Pervaiz N, Hagedoorn J, Mininberg DT. Electron microscopic studies of testes in Kallmann syndrome. Urology. 1979;14:267–9.
18. de Kretser DM. The fine structure of the immature human testis in hypogonadotrophic hypogonadism. Virchows Arch B Cell Pathol. 1968;1:283–96.
19. Kumar PA, Pitteloud N, Andrews PA, Dwyer A, Hayes F, Crowley Jr WF, Dym M. Testis morphology in patients with idiopathic hypogonadotropic hypogonadism. Hum Reprod. 2006;21:1033–40.
20. Vogels A, Moerman P, Frijns JP, Bogaert GA. Testicular histology in boys with Prader-Willi syndrome: fertile or infertile? J Urol. 2008;180:1800–4.
21. Pasqualini RQ, Bur GE. Síndrome hipoandrogénico con gametogénesis conservada: clasificación de la insuficiencia testicular. Rev Asoc Med Argent. 1950;64:6–9.
22. Mulligan T, Frick MF, Zuraw QC, Stemhagen A, McWhirter C. Prevalence of hypogonadism in males aged at least 45 years: the HIM study. Int J Clin Pract. 2006;60:762–9.
23. Buckley WE, Yesalis 3rd CE, Friedl KE, Anderson WA, Streit AL, Wright JE. Estimated prevalence of anabolic steroid use among male high school seniors. JAMA. 1988;260:3441–5.
24. World Health Organization Task Force on Methods for the Regulation of Male Fertility. Contraceptive efficacy of testosterone-induced azoospermia in normal men. Lancet. 1990;336:955–9.
25. Nistal M. Testículo humano. Hipoplasia túbulo-intersticial difusa (hipogonadismo hipogonadotrópico). Arch Esp Urol. 1973;26:253–80.
26. Rey RA, Grinspon RP, Gottlieb S, Pasqualini T, Knoblovits P, Aszpis S, Pacenza N, Stewart Usher J, Bergadá I, Campo SM. Male hypogonadism: an extended classification based on a developmental, endocrine physiology-based approach. Andrology. 2013;1:3–16.
27. Pitteloud N, Hayes FJ, Dwyer A, Boepple PA, Lee H, Crowley Jr WF. Predictors of outcome of long-term GnRH therapy in men with idiopathic hypogonadotropic hypogonadism. J Clin Endocrinol Metab. 2002;87:4128–36.
28. Liu PY, Baker HW, Jayadev V, Zacharin M, Conway AJ, Handelsman DJ. Induction of spermatogenesis and fertility during gonadotropin treatment of gonadotropin-deficient infertile men: predictors of fertility outcome. J Clin Endocrinol Metab. 2009;94:801–8.
29. Warne DW, Decosterd G, Okada H, Yano Y, Koide N, Howles CM. A combined analysis of data to identify predictive factors for spermatogenesis in men with hypogonadotropic hypogonadism treated with recombinant human follicle-stimulating hormone and human chorionic gonadotropin. Fertil Steril. 2009;92:594–604.
30. Hadziselimovic F, Emmons LR, Buser MW. A diminished postnatal surge of Ad spermatogonia in cryptorchid infants is additional evidence for hypogonadotropic hypogonadism. Swiss Med Wkly. 2004;134:381–4.
31. Dwyer AA, Sykiotis GP, Hayes FJ, Boepple PA, Lee H, Loughlin KR, Dym M, Sluss PM, Crowley Jr WF, Pitteloud N. Trial of recombinant follicle-stimulating hormone pretreatment for GnRH-induced fertility in patients with congenital hypogonadotropic hypogonadism. J Clin Endocrinol Metab. 2013;98:E1790–5.
32. Ramasamy R, Armstrong JM, Lipshultz LI. Preserving fertility in the hypogonadal patient: an update. Asian J Androl. 2015;17:197–200.

20 Ultrastructural Pathology of the Spermatozoa with Genetic Basis

Manuel Nistal, Pilar González-Peramato, and
Álvaro Serrano

20.1 Introduction

For fertilization to take place, the spermatozoa have to undergo a series of events orderly in time including capacitation, the demonstration of hyperactivated mobility, acrosome reaction, penetration of the zona pellucida, and fusion with the vitelline membrane of the oocyte. Only morphologically and functionally normal spermatozoa are able to carry out this task. In the era of assisted reproduction, there are a number of situations where it is necessary to investigate the cause of male infertility through an ultrastructural study of the spermatozoa. The field that requires special attention is that of teratozoospermias (presence of a high percentage of abnormal spermatozoa in the semen) with a systematic and homogenous defect in most spermatozoa and when the phenotype has a familiar appearance [1].

20.2 Microcephalic Spermatozoa

Microcephalic spermatozoa can be of two types, round head (globozoospermia or spermatozoa without acrosome) or irregular head (spermatozoa acrosome hypoplasia).

20.2.1 Globozoospermia: Round-Headed Spermatozoa Syndrome

It is a term that refers to the presence of round-headed spermatozoa. The percentage of round-headed spermatozoa in fertile men is 0.5 % ± 0.1, rising to 2.3 % ± 0.5 in subfertile men [2]. When most or all spermatozoa present with this anomaly, this is a rare congenital disorder whose frequency is estimated at 0.1 % of all andrological patients [3]. These spermatozoa are characterized by the following anomalies: spherical nuclei, low chromatin condensation, failure in histones by protamine replacement, absence of acrosome, absence of postacrosomal sheath, and the nuclear ring (Fig. 20.1). Other abnormalities that can be seen are an abnormal midpiece (mitochondrial disorders) and abnormalities in the nuclear membrane [4–6]. Some patients suffer from complete globozoospermia and some from partial globozoospermia (20–90 % of the spermatozoa having round heads) [7]. The syncytia of adult spermatids with spherical nuclei can be observed in the testicular biopsy, and there may be at least two to dozen nuclei (Figs. 20.2 and 20.3).

Most cases are sporadic, but several pairs of brothers with this syndrome are known [8–10]. Different patterns of inheritance have been

M. Nistal et al., *Clues in the Diagnosis of Non-tumoral Testicular Pathology*,
DOI 10.1007/978-3-319-49364-0_20

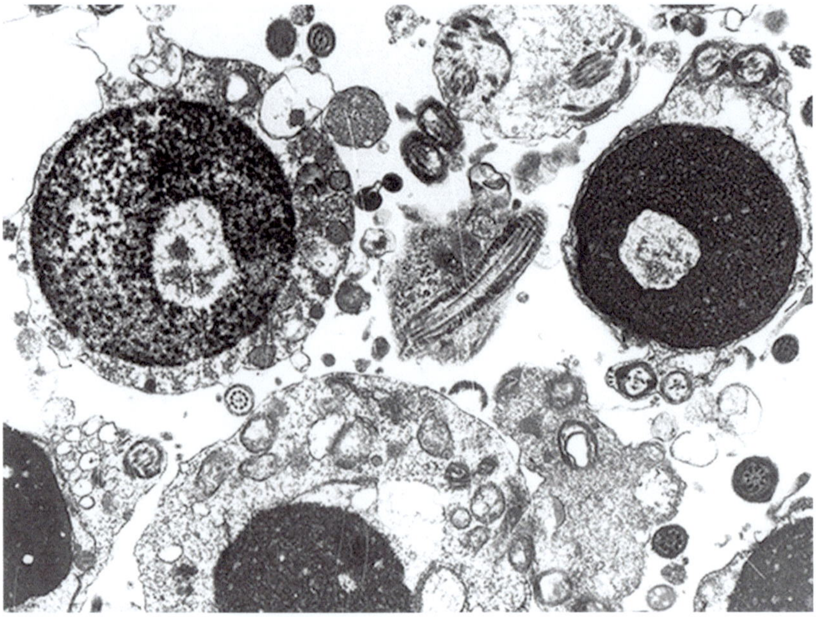

Fig. 20.1 Globozoospermia. Microcephalic spermatozoa with spherical nuclei, poorly condensed chromatin, central vacuole and absence of acrosome (electron microscopy)

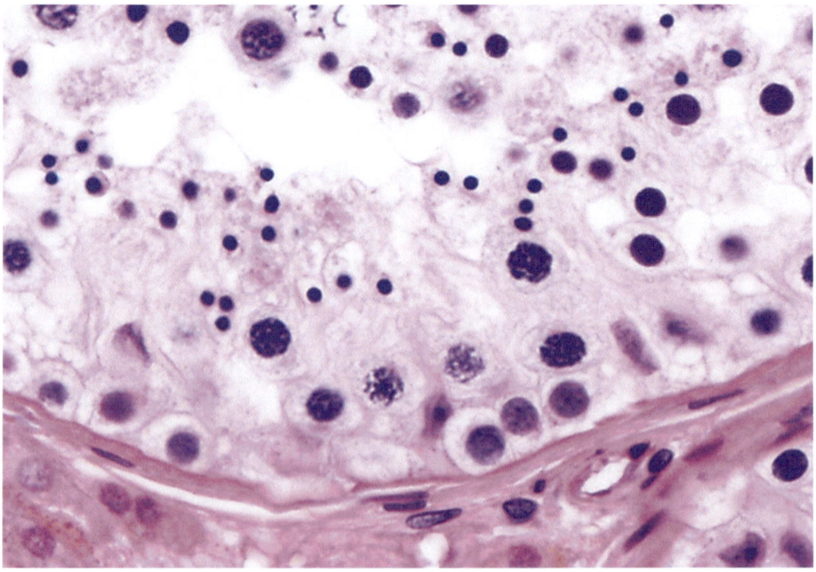

Fig. 20.2 Globozoospermia. In the apical part of the seminiferous epithelium, more than two dozen of adult spermatids with spherical, small, and hyperchromatic nuclei can be seen

suggested: polygenic, X-linked, autosomal dominant, and autosomal recessive. The genetic defect responsible for most cases is a 200 Kb homozygous deletion of DPY19L2 (12q14.2) [11]. DPY19L2 is a transmembrane protein located in the inner nuclear membrane; it is necessary to anchor the acrosome to the nucleus. The absence of the protein leads to the destabilization of both the nuclear dense lamina and the junction between the acroplaxome and the nuclear envelope. As a result, the acrosome and the manchette fail to be linked to the nucleus, which leads to the disruption of vesicular trafficking, failure in nuclear elongation, and unbound acrosomal vesicle. The precursor structures of acrosome or the acrosome itself remain in the cytoplasm of the spermatid and will be phagocytized by the Sertoli cell. Other cases are associated with homozygous missense *PICK1* (protein interacting with C kinase 1) mutation or mutation in a testes-specific gene *SPATA16* (spermatogenesis associated 16) [12].

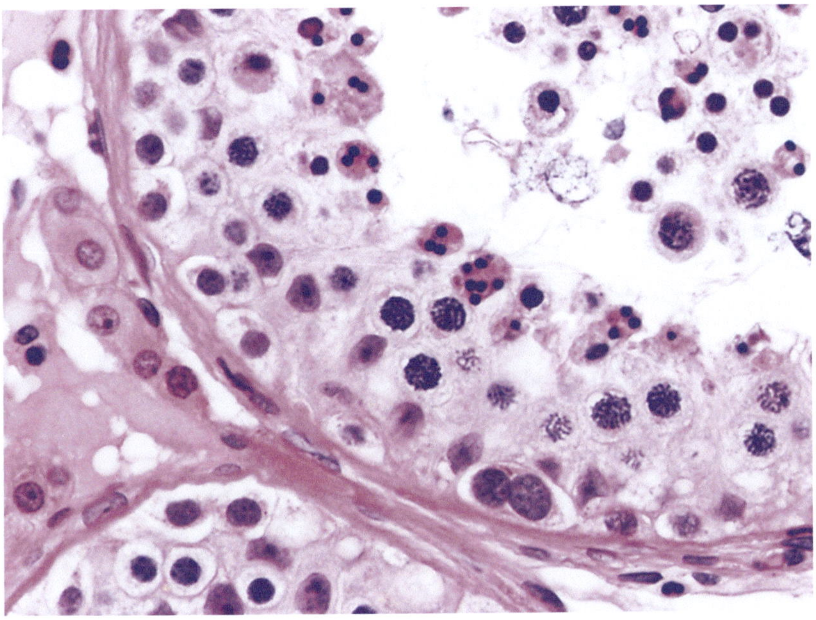

Fig. 20.3 Globozoospermia. Most adult spermatids have small spherical nuclei. Several of them share the same cytoplasm

The number and mobility of round-headed spermatozoa may be normal, but they are not able to penetrate the zona pellucida or merge with the oolemma, and therefore they are unable to fertilize the oocyte. This fact is due to total or partial lack of acrosin [13, 14]. The acrosin is a neutral protein located in the acrosome of spermatozoa in an inactive form (proacrosin). During the acrosome-releasing reaction, the proacrosin becomes acrosin. This acrosin released by exocytosis on the surface of the zona pellucida triggers an interaction spermatozoa-zona which results in the exposure or activation of the binding sites to the egg surface over the postacrosomal head region. ICSI [15] with assisted oocyte activation by calcium ionophore enables a large number of patients to achieve paternity [16, 17].

20.2.2 Microcephalic Spermatozoa with Acrosome Hypoplasia

The microcephalic spermatozoa with acrosome hypoplasia have an irregular and usually small head, and an acrosome separated form the nucleus. Spermatozoa often have excess cytoplasm around the nucleus [18]. In some cases, the anomaly is congenital. A similar acrosome anomaly has been reported in patients with Aarskog syndrome [19].

20.3 Macrocephalic Head Spermatozoa Syndrome: Large-Headed Spermatozoa

The macrocephalic spermatozoa, also known as macronuclear spermatozoa, are characterized by large heads of irregular nuclear contours, defects in the chromatin condensation, and giant cytoplasmic vacuoles and cytoplasmic remnants. They are also carriers of acrosomal abnormalities such as the presence of vacuoles, hypertrophy or hypoplasia, abnormal configuration, and often increased subacrosomal space and absence of postacrosomal sheath. Two variants of macrocephalic spermatozoa have been described: spermatozoa with multiple flagella and spermatozoa without flagellum.

20.3.1 Spermatozoa with Multiple Flagella

This is a rare cause of infertility (prevalence estimated at <1 % in the subfertile population) generally associated to oligozoospermia <2 million/ml [20]. Over a large and irregular nucleus, several flagella with different orientations are implanted. They have frequent anomalies in the intermediate and the principal piece, which contributes to poor mobility of these spermatozoa.

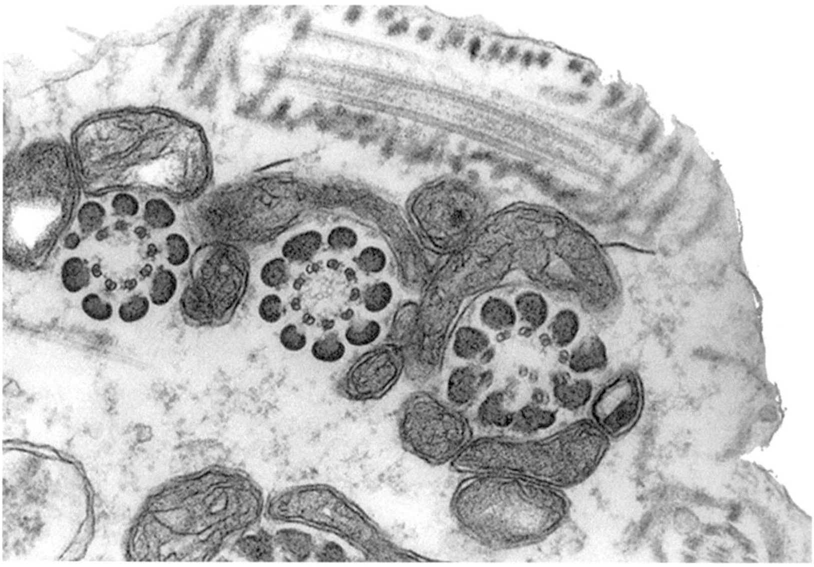

Fig. 20.4 Section at intermediate piece level of a spermatozoon showing cross sections of three flagella and part of a fourth one. Note the absence of the central pair and malformation of the mitochondrial sheath (electron microscopy)

The number of flagella is variable, but spermatozoa with three and four flagella are frequent, and those that show five flagella are unexceptional (Fig. 20.4). The flagella are separated sometimes at the end of the intermediate piece, and the rest remain together along the main piece.

The macrocephalic spermatozoa are tetraploid and represent a failure of meiosis [21]. They originate from first-order spermatocytes with a blockage of organelle displacement at the pachytene stage, which disables the assembly of a bipolar meiotic spindle [22]. The irregular shape of the core is probably related to irregular and unilateral disposition of the microtubular manchette. Most patients display homozygous truncating mutation in the aurora kinase gene (*AURKC*), which is known to play a crucial role in meiotic chromosomal segregation and cytokinesis [23]. It occurs exclusively in people of North African ancestry [24, 25]. Only one case of macrocephalic spermatozoa without mutations in the *AURKC* gene is known [26]. When the defect is not complete, paternity with normal-looking spermatozoa can be achieved [27].

20.3.2 Macrocephalic Spermatozoa Without Flagella

They present in the nucleus with the same morphological abnormalities as multiflagellated spermatozoa.

20.4 Abnormal Head-Tail Attachment

The connecting piece ensures the connection of the flagellum to the nucleus. It is formed by the implantation fossa (a concavity of the nucleus in the area opposite the acrosome) at which level the nuclear membrane lacks pores and the basal plaque or capitellum that adapts to the pit implantation. It is also constituted by a series of nine columns (segmented columns) extending caudally to a distance of 1–5 microns. These columns are followed in its caudal end by nine dense fibers. Inside the connecting piece and immediately distal to the basal plaque lays the proximal centriole transversely oriented, and the distal centriole is aligned inside the segmented columns. The distal centriole may be partially or totally absent in the spermatozoa. Alterations in the connecting piece can lead to separation of heads and flagella [28, 29]. Depending on the severity of the lesion, the seminogram can display these situations: (a) the presence of flagella only. The heads have been phagocytized by Sertoli cells or by macrophages in the epididymis. These spermatozoa are known as acephalic spermatozoa [30]; (b) the presence of spermatozoa with a strangulation at connecting piece level [28] (Fig. 20.5); (c) the presence of heads and flagella separately; and

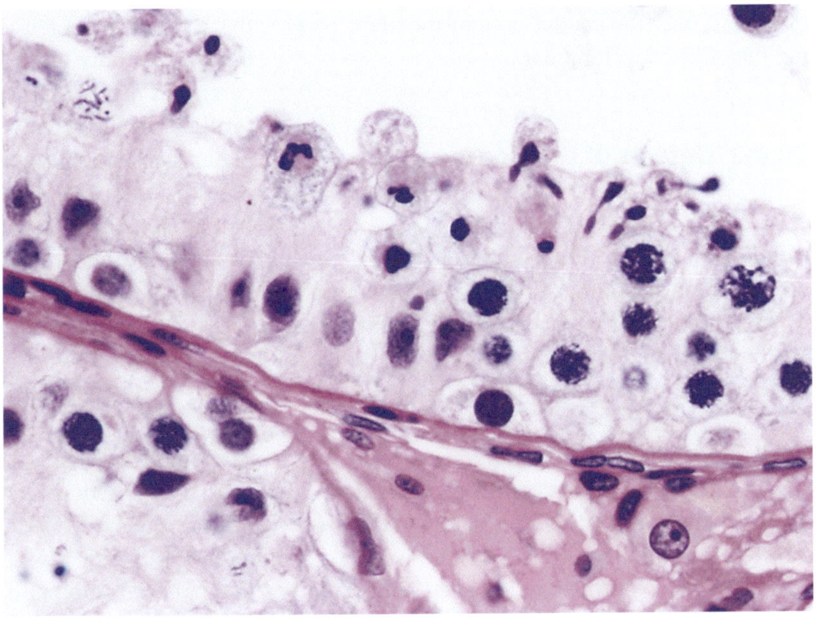

Fig. 20.5 Seminiferous epithelium showing marked reduction in all germ cell types. Spermatids show a strangulation at connecting piece level

(d) "normal" spermatozoa that resulted decapitated when subjected to minimal micromanipulation for ICSI [31].

20.4.1 Decapitated Spermatozoa/Acephalic Spermatozoa

These spermatozoa are known in light microscopy as "pin-headed" spermatozoa, although they do not really have a head [32]. They can be observed in small numbers in the semen of many men, but the anomaly can affect most of the spermatozoa of some patients, which turns it into one of the best studied teratozoospermic syndromes. Most spermatozoa show a small cephalic thickening. This thickening corresponds to a cytoplasmic remnant that encompasses the intermediate piece showing a variable degree of organization of mitochondria. The flagella may show vigorous movements in some patients and lack of mobility in others.

Ultrastructurally two variants have been reported:

- *Type I.* Acephalic spermatozoa with loss of the intermediate piece. The flagellum ends cranially in a cephalic thickening 1–2 microns in diameter. In this cytoplasm, one or both centrioles and some mitochondria without axial organization are observed.
- *Type II.* Sperm-organized intermediate piece. The cephalic end has a 3–5 micron thickening. The connecting piece is better organized, and most of their structures are contained in the apical cytoplasm. The intermediate piece has a high degree of organization.

The acephalic spermatozoa are produced by an early failure in spermatogenesis. In step 1, spermatids have both centrioles away from the nucleus, and the axonema starts from the distal centriole. In step 2, or cap phase, elongation and condensation of the nucleus occurs, the acrosome development continues, but the flagellum approach to the nucleus does not occur, and so the differentiation of both structures continues separately. This syndrome has been described in several members of the same family [30, 32]. In one case, the same patient showed the presence of microcephalic spermatozoa without acrosome and decapitated spermatozoa [33]. The syndrome may result from one of the following hypotheses [34]: (1) a failure to form the basal plaque and the implantation fossa in the post-nuclear region, (2) a chemical abnormality of filamentous material that occupies the space between the capitellum and the basal plaque, and (3) an abnormal position of the tail over the caudal pole of the nuclei during flagellum development.

20.4.2 Defects of the Connecting Piece

Connection defects are evidenced by the presence of strangulation at this level. This anomaly is often associated with loss of alignment of the head and the flagellum axis.

20.4.3 Separated Head and Flagellum: Decapitated and Decaudated Spermatozoa

In most cases, normally elongated nuclei with good development of the acrosome and with no implantation fossa and basal plaque are observed. Flagella are sometimes of the type I and sometimes of the type II. In this variety, exceptionally the heads contain the proximal centriole in the implantation fossa with its basal plaque. Decapitated tails contain the proximal centriole, segmented columns, and most flagellar structures [35, 36]. This anomaly starts during spermiogenesis, but heads and tails separation may occur during spermiation or along the spermatic pathway.

The cause of infertility may lay in a dysfunction of the sperm centrioles that makes them unable to migrate and attach to the caudal pole of the spermatid nucleus and in the decreased proteasome activity that probably prevents normally centriolar release and centrosome formation after fertilization. Most of these patients being amenable to treatment with ICSI, an alteration of the proximal centriole function, could produce insufficient nucleation of the zygote sperm aster, lack of syngamy and embryo cleavage, or defective embryos leading to early abortions [37].

20.5 Fibrous Sheath Dysplasia

The fibrous sheath dysplasia is an autosomal recessive genetic disease. The term refers to the most frequent ultrastructural abnormality of spermatozoa, classically described as short-tail spermatozoa and stump tail syndrome [38, 39]. Under optical microscopy, the spermatozoa have short, thick, and irregularly rigid tails. The intermediate piece is frequently absent. The ultrastructural study shows significant alterations of the fibrous sheath in all the sperm and in the axoneme in more than half of them [40, 41] (Fig. 20.6).

In normal spermatozoa, the fibrous sheath is a cytoskeletal structure formed by two longitudinal columns running along the principal piece and inserted into doublets of microtubules 3 and 8. These columns are connected at regular intervals by transverse semicircular ribs. Spermatozoa with fibrous sheath dysplasia show a distortion of these structures containing a marked hypertrophy

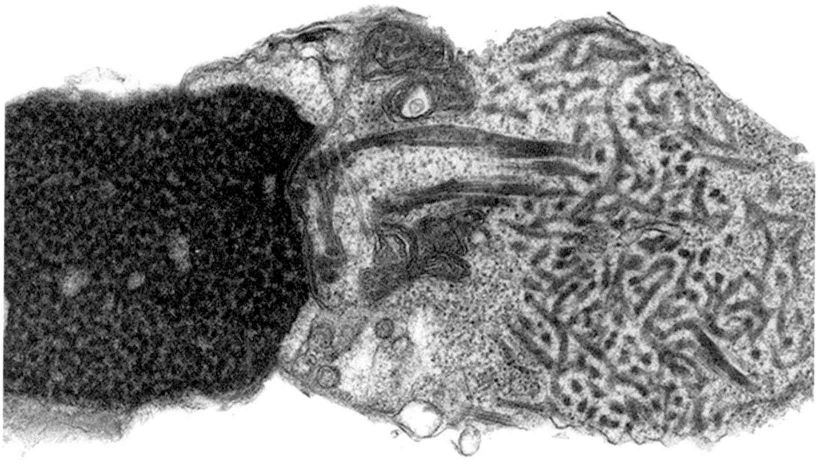

Fig. 20.6 Longitudinal section of a spermatozoon showing intermediate piece hypoplasia and fibrous sheath dysplasia (electron microscopy)

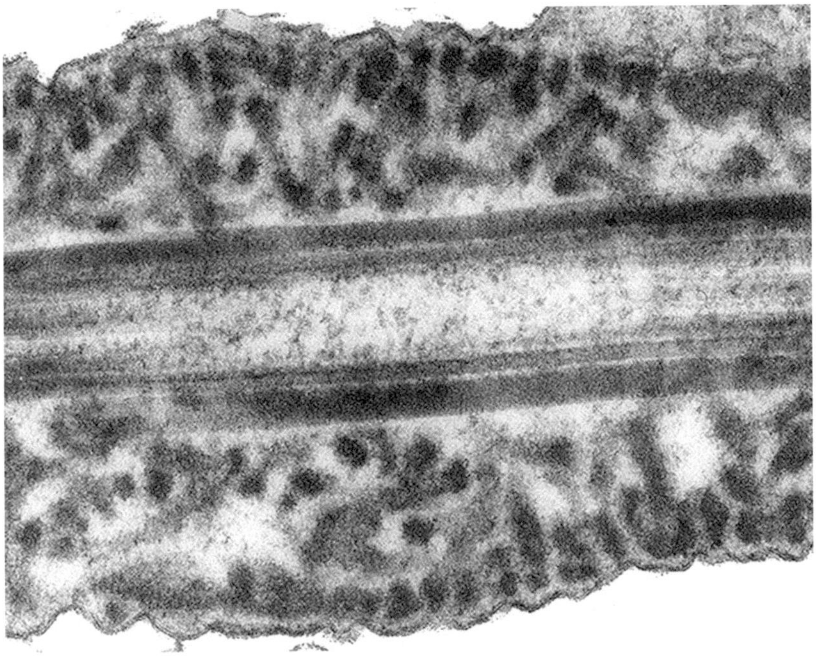

Fig. 20.7 Longitudinal section of a flagellum with fibrous sheath dysplasia (electron microscopy)

and hyperplasia of the fibrous sheath material (Fig. 20.7). The most abundant structural proteins in the fibrous sheath are AKAP3 and 4, members of the A-kinase anchor protein family [42]. The fibrous sheath abnormally associates, in half of the cases, alterations in the axonema such as absence of the central pair and, less frequently, absence of dynein arms.

Other common defects are dense fibers 3 and 8, which are normally only present in the intermediate piece, extending through the principal part; the annulus does not migrate caudally and remains near the connecting piece, as a result of which the intermediate piece is not formed and mitochondria are poorly sorted or absent. A complete form is distinguished when all spermatozoa have fibrous sheath dysplasia and an incomplete form when 20–30 % of the spermatozoa have a normal structure.

Studies of testicular biopsies have shown that these defects originate during late spermatogenesis [43]. The remaining anomalies would accompany secondarily the lack of organization of the fibrous sheath.

Twenty-four percent of patients present with respiratory symptoms such as rhinosinusitis, bronchitis, and bronchiectasis from early childhood. All patients with respiratory symptoms lack dynein arms. Most of them correspond to the complete form of fibrous sheath dysplasia. These patients have been observed to also lack dynein arms in the cilia of the respiratory tree [40, 44], which suggests the existence of an intimate relationship between spermatozoa, fibrous sheath dysplasia, and the immotile cilia syndrome. Offspring has been reported in these patients using ICSI techniques [45].

20.6 Primary Ciliary Dyskinesia (PCD): Immotile Cilia Syndrome

PCD is an autosomal recessive disorder, genetically heterogeneous, secondary to abnormalities of the ciliary mobility. The incidence is 1:20,000 to 1:60,000. The phenotype of patients is very varied: chronic upper and lower respiratory tract infections, situs inversus, heterotaxy with or without congenital heart disease, and male infertility. Clinical manifestations of the immotile cilia syndrome begin in childhood and worsen with age [46]. The cilia are present in numerous epithelia: nasal cavity, paranasal sinuses, middle ear, respiratory tract, fallopian tubes, efferent ducts, and ependymal and embryonic tissues. Spermatozoa flagella are considered to be modified cilia.

Abnormalities in the spermatozoa axoneme have been classified into three groups [34]: numerical aberrations in the normal organization 9 + 2, microtubule ectopia, and structural anomalies.

Numerical Aberrations
The most common numerical aberrations from the functional point of view are the absence of one (9 + 1) or both central microtubules (9 + 0) and the complete absence of axoneme [47]. Sperm 9 + 0 also lack the central sheath, have a normal configuration under optical microscopy, but are immotile. There have been reports of familial presentations [48] and of one patient with autosomal dominant polycystic kidney disease [49]. The absence of axonema in the cilia and flagella has been reported in one patient with Kartagener's syndrome [50].

Microtubules Ectopia
The most frequent abnormality is the presence of supernumerary elements. But there are cases in which one or both central microtubules are located outside the nine doublets.

Structural Anomalies
Men with structural anomalies, except for exceptional cases, are sterile [51, 52]. There is an absence of sperm mobility when both dynein arms are lacking, when there are no peripheral junctions, when the central pair is lacking, and logically in those that lack axonema. Mobility is partially preserved in those cases in which some dynein arms are present [53]. The presence of less than three external dynein arms in each spermatozoon causes dyskinesia and infertility [40].

Kartagener's Syndrome [54] *Kartagener's syndrome* is a subtype of primary ciliary dyskinesia [55]. It is characterized by the classic triad of situs inversus, bronchiectasis, and chronic sinusitis. Its incidence is estimated at 1:40,000 to 1:120,000, and it occurs in about 1 % of cases of bronchiectasis and 20 % of cases of situs inversus [56]. The overall age of onset is 10–19 years. Often patients also show a variety of malformations such as congenital heart disease, hydrocephalus, cleft palate, bilateral cervical ribs, anal atresia, urethral crack, and duplex kidney. It is a genetic defect with autosomal recessive inheritance.

In most patients, spermatozoa lack mobility due to the absence of dynein arms (Fig. 20.8) but are capable of undergoing capacitation, acrosome reaction, and penetration of oocytes in the zona pellucida in free hamsters. With different assisted reproductive techniques such as subzonal insemination [57], intracytoplasmic sperm injection [58], and in vitro fertilization [59], pregnancies have been achieved.

The most common genetic abnormalities found in patients with primary ciliary dyskinesia,

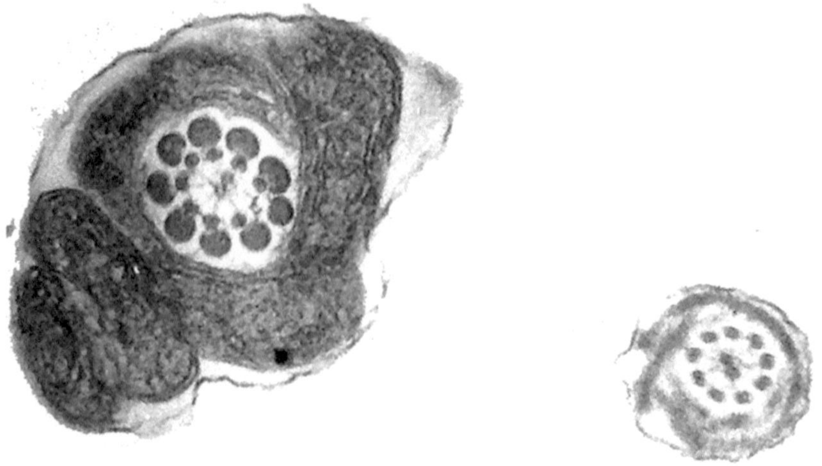

Fig. 20.8 Kartagener syndrome. Cross sections of the intermediate piece and distal end of the principal piece. Note the absence of dynein arms (electron microscopy)

including Kartagener's syndrome, vary depending on the ethnic group or geographic area studied [60]. Among mutations of dynein genes, there are *DNAI1* genes (axonemal dynein intermediate-chain gene 1), *DNAH5* and *DNAH11* [61], and *TXNDC3* [62]. Other mutations associated with cilia disorders are those of *hPF20* gene in patients with abnormalities of the central pair [63]. And that of RPGRIP1L in which primary ciliary dysfunction is associated with a group of autosomal recessive disorders like CORS (Cerebello-oculo-renal) syndrome, also known as Joubert syndrome type B [64].

Some patients with primary ciliary dyskinesia are known to be fertile [65] or else have achieved paternity trough IVF or ICSI [66].

References

1. Baccetti B, Capitani S, Collodel G, Di Cairano G, Gambera L, Moretti E, Piomboni P. Genetic sperm defects and consanguinity. Hum Reprod. 2001;16:1365–71.
2. Kalahanis J, Rousso D, Kourtis A, Mavromatidis G, Makedos G, Panidis D. Round-headed spermatozoa in semen specimens from fertile and subfertile men. J Reprod Med. 2002;47:489–93.
3. Seuanez HN, Carothers AD, Martin DE, Short RV. Morphological abnormalities in spermatozoa of man and great apes. Nature. 1977;270:345–7.
4. Holstein AF, Schirren C, Schirren CG. Human spermatids and spermatozoa lacking acrosomes. J Reprod Fertil. 1973;35:489–91.
5. Vicari E, Perdichizzi A, De Palma A, Burrello N, D'Agata R, Calogero AE. Globozoospermia is associated with chromatin structure abnormalities: case report. Hum Reprod. 2002;17:2128–33.
6. Ricci G, Andolfi L, Zabucchi G, Luppi S, Boscolo R, Martinelli M, Zweyer M, Trevisan E. Ultrastructural morphology of sperm from human globozoospermia. Biomed Res Int. 2015;2015:798754.
7. Dam AH, Ramos L, Dijkman HB, Woestenenk R, Robben H, van den Hoven L, Kremer JA. Morphology of partial globozoospermia. J Androl. 2011;32:199–206.
8. Kullander S, Rausing A. On round-headed human spermatozoa. Int J Fertil. 1975;20:33–40.
9. Nistal M, Paniagua R. Morphogenesis of round-headed human spermatozoa lacking acrosomes in a case of severe teratozoospermia. Andrologia. 1978;10:49–51.
10. Flörke-Gerloff S, Töpfer-Petersen E, Müller-Esterl W, Mansouri A, Schatz R, Schirren C, Schill W, Engel W. Biochemical and genetic investigation of round-headed spermatozoa in infertile men including two brothers and their father. Andrologia. 1984;16:187–202.
11. Koscinski I, Elinati E, Fossard C, Redin C, Muller J, Velez de la Calle J, Schmitt F, Ben Khelifa M, Ray PF, Kilani Z, Barratt CL, Viville S. DPY19L2 deletion as a major cause of globozoospermia. Am J Hum Genet. 2011;88:344–50.
12. Chianese C, Fino MG, Riera Escamilla A, López Rodrigo O, Vinci S, Guarducci E, Daguin F, Muratori M, Tamburrino L, Lo Giacco D, Ars E, Bassas L, Costa M, Pisatauro V, Noci I, Coccia E, Provenzano A, Ruiz-Castañé E, Giglio S, Piomboni P, Krausz C. Comprehensive investigation in patients affected by sperm macrocephaly and globozoospermia. Andrology. 2015;3:203–12.
13. Flörke-Gerloff S, Töpfer-Petersen E, Müller-Esterl W, Schill WB, Engel W. Acrosin and the acrosome in human spermatogenesis. Hum Genet. 1983;65:61–7.
14. Reichart M, Lederman H, Har-Even D, Kedem P, Bartoov B. Human sperm acrosin activity with relation to semen parameters and acrosomal ultrastructure. Andrologia. 1993;25:59–66.
15. Lundin K, Sjögren A, Nilsson L, Hamberger L. Fertilization and pregnancy after intracytoplasmic microinjection of acrosomeless spermatozoa. Fertil Steril. 1994;62:1266–7.
16. Karaca N, Akpak YK, Oral S, Durmus T, Yilmaz R. A successful healthy childbirth in a case of total globozoospermia with oocyte activation by calcium ionophore. J Reprod Infertil. 2015;16:116–20.
17. Chansel-Debordeaux L, Dandieu S, Bechoua S, Jimenez C. Reproductive outcome in globozoospermic men: update and prospects. Andrology. 2015;3:1022–34.
18. Anton-Lamprecht I, Kotzur B, Schopf E. Round-headed human spermatozoa. Fertil Steril. 1976;276:685–93.
19. Meschede D, Rolf C, Neugebauer DC, Horst J, Nieschlag E. Sperm acrosome defects in a patient with Aarskog-Scott syndrome. Am J Med Genet. 1996;66:340–2.
20. Nistal M, Paniagua R, Herruzo A. Multi-tailed spermatozoa in a case with asthenospermia and teratospermia. Virchows Arch B Cell Pathol. 1977;26:111–8.
21. Devillard F, Metzler-Guillemain C, Pelletier R, DeRobertis C, Bergues U, Hennebicq S, Guichaoua M, Sele B, Rousseaux S. Polyploidy in large-headed sperm: FISH study of three cases. Hum Reprod. 2002;17:1292–8.
22. Escalier D. Genetic approach to male meiotic division deficiency: the human macronuclear spermatozoa. Mol Hum Reprod. 2002;8:1–7.
23. Dieterich K, Soto Rifo R, Faure AK, Hennebicq S, Ben Amar B, Zahi M, Perrin J, Martinez D, Sèle B, Jouk PS, Ohlmann T, Rousseaux S, Lunardi J, Ray PF. Homozygous mutation of AURKC yields large-headed polyploid spermatozoa and causes male infertility. Nat Genet. 2007;39:661–5.

24. El Kerch F, Lamzouri A, Laarabi FZ, Zahi M, Ben Amar B, Sefiani A. Confirmation of the high prevalence in Morocco of the homozygous mutation c.144delC in the aurora kinase C gene (AURKC) in the teratozoospermia with large-headed spermatozoa. J Gynecol Obstet Biol Reprod (Paris). 2011;40:329–33.
25. Ounis L, Zoghmar A, Coutton C, Rouabah L, Hachemi M, Martinez D, Martinez G, Bellil I, Khelifi D, Arnoult C, Fauré J, Benbouhedja S, Rouabah A, Ray PF. Mutations of the aurora kinase C gene causing macrozoospermia are the most frequent genetic cause of male infertility in Algerian men. Asian J Androl. 2015;17:68–73.
26. Molinari E, Mirabelli M, Raimondo S, Brussino A, Gennarelli G, Bongioanni F, Revelli A. Sperm macrocephaly syndrome in a patient without AURKC mutations and with a history of recurrent miscarriage. Reprod Biomed Online. 2013;26:148–56.
27. Shimizu Y, Kiumura F, Kaku S, Izuno M, Tomita K, Thumkeo D, Murakami T. Successful delivery following ICSI with macrocephalic sperm head syndrome: a case report. Reprod Biomed Online. 2012;24:603–5.
28. Lüders G. A defect of the head-flagellum-connection of human spermatozoa. Andrologia. 1976;8:365–8.
29. Perotti ME, Giarola A, Gioria M. Ultrastructural study of the decapitated sperm defect in an infertile man. J Reprod Fertil. 1981;63:543–9.
30. Chemes HE, Puigdomenech ET, Carizza C, Olmedo SB, Zanchetti F, Hermes R. Acephalic spermatozoa and abnormal development of the head-neck attachment: a human syndrome of genetic origin. Hum Reprod. 1999;14:1811–8.
31. Kamal A, Mansour R, Fahmy I, Serour G, Rhodes C, Aboulghar M. Easily decapitated spermatozoa defect: a possible cause of unexplained infertility. Hum Reprod. 1999;14:2791–5.
32. Baccetti B, Burrini AG, Collodel G, Magnano AR, Piomboni P, Renieri T, Sensini C. Morphogenesis of the decapitated and decaudated sperm defect in two brothers. Gamete Res. 1989;23:181–8.
33. Aughey E, Orr PS. An unusual abnormality of human spermatozoa. J Reprod Fertil. 1978;53:341–2.
34. Zamboni L. Sperm structure and its relevance to infertility. An electron microscopic study. Arch Pathol Lab Med. 1992;116:325–44.
35. Holstein AF, Schill WB, Breucker H. Dissociated centriole development as a cause of spermatid malformation in man. J Reprod Fertil. 1986;78:719–25.
36. Toyama Y, Iwamoto T, Yajima M, Baba K, Yuasa S. Decapitated and decaudated spermatozoa in man, and pathogenesis based on the ultrastructure. Int J Androl. 2000;23:109–15.
37. Chemes HE, Rawe VY. The making of abnormal spermatozoa: cellular and molecular mechanisms underlying pathological spermiogenesis. Cell Tissue Res. 2010;341:349–57.
38. Nistal M, Paniagua R, Herruzo A. Lack of the central pair of axial filaments in a case of short-tailed spermatozoa human teratospermia. J Gynecol Obstet Biol Reprod (Paris). 1979;8:47–50.
39. Pedersen H, Hammen R. Ultrastructure of human spermatozoa with complete subcellular derangement. Arch Androl. 1982;9:251–9.
40. Escalier D, David G. Pathology of the cytoskeleton of the human sperm flagellum: axonemal and peri-axonemal anomalies. Biol Cell. 1984;50:37–52.
41. Baccetti B, Burrini AG, Capitani S, Collodel G, Moretti E, Piomboni P, Renieri T. Notulae seminologicae. 2. The 'short tail' and 'stump' defect in human spermatozoa. Andrologia. 1993;25:331–5.
42. Eddy EM, Toshimori K, O'Brien DA. Fibrous sheath of mammalian spermatozoa. Microsc Res Tech. 2003;61:103–15.
43. Barthelemy C, Tharanne MJ, Lebos C, Lecomte P, Lansac J. Tail stump spermatozoa: morphogenesis of the defect. An ultrastructural study of sperm and testicular biopsy. Andrologia. 1990;22:417–25.
44. Chemes HE, Morero JL, Lavieri JC. Extreme asthenozoospermia and chronic respiratory disease: a new variant of the immotile cilia syndrome. Int J Androl. 1990;13:216–22.
45. Olmedo SB, Rawe VY, Nodar FN, Galaverna GD, Acosta AA, Chemes HE. Pregnancies established through intracytoplasmic sperm injection (ICSI) using spermatozoa with dysplasia of fibrous sheath. Asian J Androl. 2000;2:125–30.
46. Taylor RE. Abnormal mucociliary transport study in a patient with Kartagener syndrome. Clin Nucl Med. 2006;31:240–2.
47. Baccetti B, Burrini AG, Pallini V. Different axoneme patterns in cilia and flagella of the same animal. J Submicrosc Cytol. 1981;13:479–81.
48. Moryan A, Guay AT, Kurtz S, Nowak PJ. Familial ciliary dyskinesis: a cause of infertility without respiratory disease. Fertil Steril. 1985;44:539–42.
49. Okada H, Fujioka H, Tatsumi N, Fujisawa M, Gohji K, Arakawa S, Kato H, Kobayashi S, Isojima S, Kamidono S. Assisted reproduction for infertile patients with 9 + 0 immotile spermatozoa associated with autosomal dominant polycystic kidney disease. Hum Reprod. 1999;14:110–3.
50. Baccetti B, Burrini AG, Pallini V. Spermatozoa and cilia lacking axoneme in an infertile man. Andrologia. 1980;12:525–32.
51. Afzelius BA, Dallai R, Lanzavecchia S, Bellon PL. Flagellar structure in normal human spermatozoa and in spermatozoa that lack dynein arms. Tissue Cell. 1995;27:241–7.
52. Jonsson MS, McCormick JR, Gillies CG, Gondos B. Kartagener's syndrome with motile spermatozoa. N Engl J Med. 1982;307:1131–3.
53. Schneeberger EE, McCormack J, Issenberg HJ, Schuster SR, Gerald PS. Heterogeneity of ciliary morphology in the immotile-cilia syndrome in man. J Ultrastruct Res. 1980;73:34–43.
54. Kartagener M. Zur Pathogenese der Bronchiektasien. I. Mitteilung: Bronchiektasien bei Situs viscerum inversus. Beitr Klin Tuberk. 1933;83:489–501.
55. Carlen B, Stenram U. Primary ciliary dyskinesia: a review. Ultrastruct Pathol. 2005;29:217–20.

56. Douard R, Feldman A, Bargy F, Loric S, Delmas V. Anomalies of lateralization in man: a case of total situs inversus. Surg Radiol Anat. 2000;22:293–7.
57. Wolf JP, Feneux D, Escalier D, Rodrigues D, Frydman R, Jouannet P. Pregnancy after subzonal insemination with spermatozoa lacking outer dynein arms. J Reprod Fertil. 1993;97:487–92.
58. Chemes HE, Olmedo SB, Carrere C, Oses R, Carizza C, Leisner M, Blaquier J. Ultrastructural pathology of the sperm flagellum: association between flagellar pathology and fertility prognosis in severely asthenozoospermic men. Hum Reprod. 1998;13:2521–6.
59. Kay VJ, Irvine DS. Successful in-vitro fertilization with spermatozoa from a patient with Kartagener's syndrome. Hum Reprod. 2000;15:135–8.
60. Fedick AM, Jalas C, Treff NR, Knowles MR, Zariwala MA. Carrier frequencies of eleven mutations in eight genes associated with primary ciliary dyskinesia in the Ashkenazi Jewish population. Mol Genet Genomic Med. 2015;3:137–42.
61. Schwabe GC, Hoffmann K, Loges NT, Birker D, Rossier C, de Santi MM, Olbrich H, Fliegauf M, Failly M, Liebers U, Collura M, Gaedicke G, Mundlos S, Wahn U, Blouin JL, Niggemann B, Omran H, Antonarakis SE, Bartoloni L. Primary ciliary dyskinesia associated with normal axoneme ultrastructure is caused by DNAH11 mutations. Hum Mutat. 2008;29:289–98.
62. Geremek M, Schoenmaker F, Zietkiewicz E, Pogorzelski A, Diehl S, Wijmenga C, Witt M. Sequence analysis of 21 genes located in the Kartagener syndrome linkage region on chromosome 15q. Eur J Hum Genet. 2008;16:688–95.
63. Pennarun G, Bridoux AM, Escudier E, Dastot-Le Moal F, Cacheux V, Amselem S, Duriez B. Isolation and expression of the human hPF20 gene orthologous to Chlamydomonas PF20: evaluation as a candidate for axonemal defects of respiratory cilia and sperm flagella. Am J Respir Cell Mol Biol. 2002;26:362–70.
64. Devuyst O, Arnould VJ. Mutations in RPGRIP1L: extending the clinical spectrum of ciliopathies. Nephrol Dial Transplant. 2008;23:1500–3.
65. Nowiński A, Hawryłkjewicz I, Sulikowska-Rowińska A, Górecka D. Primary ciliary dyskinesia – Kartagener's syndrome and fertile male. Pneumonol Alergol Pol. 2002;70:312–7.
66. Cayan S, Conaghan J, Schriock ED, Ryan IP, Black LD, Turek PJ. Birth after intracytoplasmic sperm injection with use of testicular sperm from men with Kartagener/immotile cilia syndrome. Fertil Steril. 2001;76:612–4.

21 Spermatic Cord Torsion and Infertility

Manuel Nistal, Pilar González-Peramato, and Álvaro Serrano

21.1 Introduction

The twisting of the spermatic cord causes the sudden interruption of the venous return because the veins collapse, while the blood flow through the spermatic artery is maintained for some time. The result is a hemorrhagic infarction of the testis (Fig. 21.1). Salvage rates of testes with testicular torsion vary from 30 to 50 % [1, 2]. The fertility of patients after unilateral testicular torsion is decreased [3, 4]. Thirty-six percent of patients show sperm counts of less than 20 million/ml [5]. In long-term follow-ups, semen is normal only between 5 and 50 % of patients [1, 3, 6]. Twenty-five percent become infertile [7]. Hormonal values remain within normal limits, and only elevated FSH and LH are observed in some cases of torsions over 8 h or when there is testicular atrophy [8], and decreased inhibin B occurs as a sign of Sertoli cell dysfunction [9].

The diagnosis of testicular torsion is not always easy, especially in young people, and it requires ruling out all pathologies responsible for an acute scrotum such as hydatid of the testis and epididymis torsion, orchioepididymitis, incarcerated inguinal hernia, scrotal trauma, Henoch-Schönlein purpura and bleeding, testicular malignancy, and idiopathic scrotal edema.

The most important factor for salvaging a twisted testicle is the duration of the symptoms. The delay in the nonrecognition of symptoms can lead to orchiectomy. Obstructions are higher in pediatric patients because the clinical presentation may be similar to other nonsurgical entities, such as an epididymal appendix or a testicular appendage torsion [10]. While the adult patient describes the symptoms well (sudden onset of pain, quality of pain, and duration of pain), collection of this data is more difficult in children. The diagnosis is complicated when testicular torsion starts with symptoms such as abdominal pain, nausea, and vomiting. Color Doppler ultrasound scanning is of great usefulness for the evaluation of different pathologies [11].

The twisting of the spermatic cord produces a collapsed veins permeable maintained for some time the blood flow through the spermatic artery.

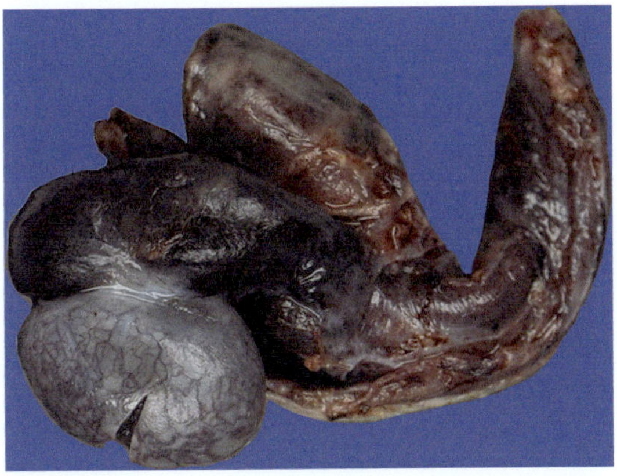

Fig. 21.1 Torsion of the spermatic cord in a 14-year-old boy. High reflection of the tunica vaginalis. Hemorrhagic infarction of the testis and epididymis

M. Nistal et al., *Clues in the Diagnosis of Non-tumoral Testicular Pathology*,
DOI 10.1007/978-3-319-49364-0_21

The result is a hemorrhagic infarction testis. Salvage rates of patients with testicular torsion vary from 30 to 50 % [1, 2]. Fertility patients after unilateral testicular torsion are decreased [3, 4]. Thirty-six percent of patients show less than 20 million sperm/ml [5] counts. In a long-term follow-up, semen is only average between 5 and 50 % [1, 3, 6]. Twenty-five percent become infertile [7]. Serum hormaonal values usually remain within normal limits, and only elevated FSH and LH are observed in some cases in torsions over 8 h or when there is testicular atrophy [8], and decreased inhibin B occurs as a sign of dysfunction of Sertoli cells [9].

21.2 Physiopathology

The initial mechanism that triggers injuries after a testicular torsion is ischemia. The damage caused by ischemia is reinforced by an untwisting-associated secondary damage (reperfusion). Testicular infarction begins before 2 h of onset of symptoms; irreversible damage appears after 6 h and completes infarction after 24 h. During the testicular torsion, a decrease in blood flow to the contralateral testis also occurs, possibly through a reflex arc originating in the neurons of the pelvic area. The unilateral torsion could affect spermatogenesis of the contralateral testis. The contralateral decreased blood flow would result in increased levels of reactive oxygen species that can damage the testicular parenchyma.

Untwisting is not safe and may further damage the testicle. The preservation of twisted testes leads to the ischemic-reperfusion (I/R) damage of both testes [12]. The testicles are very vulnerable to oxidative stress, mainly due to the abundance of unsaturated fatty acids. Oxidative damage is caused by an imbalance between oxidative and antioxidative systems. Many cellular and molecular mechanisms are involved in ischemia-reperfusion injury following testicular torsion. The I/R is associated with overproduction of reactive oxygen species (ROS) such as nitric oxide, hydrogen peroxide, hypochlorous acid, hydroxyl radicals, and superoxide anion [13]. The main source of ROS is leukocytes infiltrating the testicular tissue although they can also be formed from spermatozoa and mitochondria of Leydig cells [14]. Reperfusion is beneficial to the twisted testicle, by preventing ischemia-induced apoptosis and necrosis, but also adversely affects the contralateral testicle. Leaving a severely damaged testis instead of removing it causes more damage in the contralateral testis [3].

21.3 Indicators of Testicular Salvage Ability

Salvage of a testis after torsion is very difficult to predict. There are no other more reliable parameters than the duration of the torsion that can predict what will happen with the testicle.

Duration of Testicular Ischemia Testicular damage is evaluated at three degrees [15].

- *Grade I lesions*: Sloughing of immature germ cells and apical vacuolation in Sertoli cells and spermatogonia are observed at the seminiferous tubule level and edema, vascular congestion, and focal hemorrhages at the interstitial level (Fig. 21.2).
- *Grade II lesions*: The seminiferous epithelium displays sloughing of all germ cell types. Interstitial hemorrhage is important, and Leydig cells show variable degrees of alterations (Figs. 21.3 and 21.4).
- *Grade III lesions*: These lesions are the characteristic lesions of a hemorrhagic infarct with necrosis of the seminiferous epithelium (Fig. 21.5).

Most testicular torsions of less than 4 h have lesions of grade I; if the duration is 4–8 h, the lesions are grade II, and if longer than 12 h, they are grade III. There are a small number of testes with less than 4 h of evolution that may have lesions of grade II and also testes with more than 4 h that can show lesions of grade I [16]. The literature shows exceptions collected as testes salvaged after 3–5 days of torsion. Undescended testes that undergo torsion have even a worse prognosis and between 60–71 % of them end in orchiectomy [17].

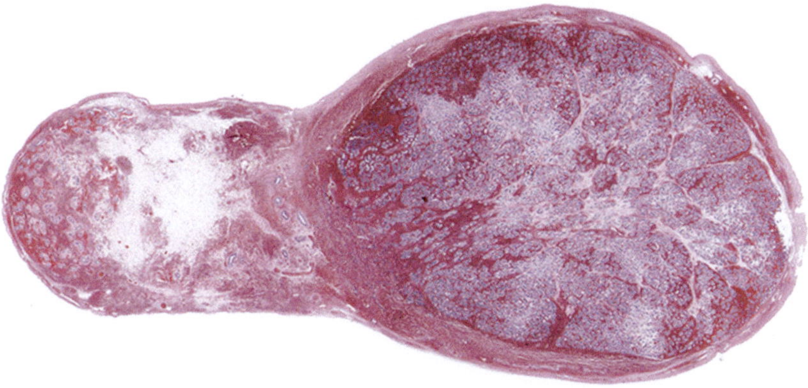

Fig. 21.2 Torsion of the spermatic cord in a 9-year-old child. Interstitial and subalbugineal hemorrhage both in the testis and epididymis

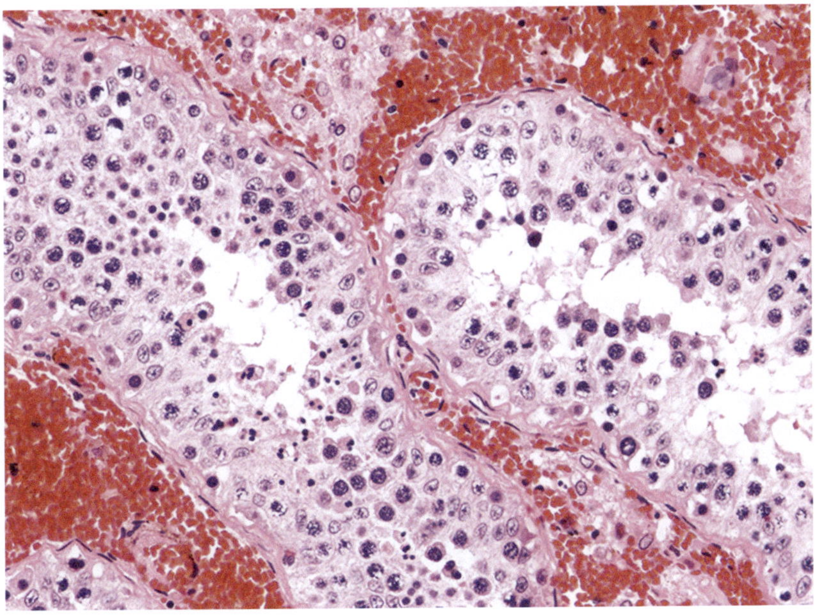

Fig. 21.3 The Torsion of spermatic cord in a pubertal patient. Grade II lesions consist of interstitial hemorrhage and sloughing of inmature germ cells

Within the first 6 h, 93 % of the testes and only 10 % after 24 h are salvaged [18]. Orchiectomy rates are between 39 and 71 % [19]. The risk of orchiectomy is 5 % before 6 h of the onset of pain and rises to 90 % if after 48 h [1].

Color Doppler ultrasound allows to observe the absence of testicular flow. But not in all cases in which flow is not shown testes are unrecoverable [20].

Testicular Echogenicity Two patterns have been described in no-flow twisted testicles in scrotal Doppler ultrasound. In those testes with a hypoechoic and isoechoic homogeneous testicular framework, testicular viability depends on an urgent surgical exploration, while in those testes with dishomogeneous and heterogeneous echotexture (characteristic of testicular necrosis), testicular surgical exploration would not be an emergency [21].

Ultimately the decision to remove or retain the twisted testicle is subjective and primarily based on the appearance of the testicle. After untwisting, if there is bleeding after incision of the tunica albuginea, the testis is fixed to the scrotum, and it is removed only if it appears frankly necrotic. In the best of cases, this only documents that intratesticular flow has been

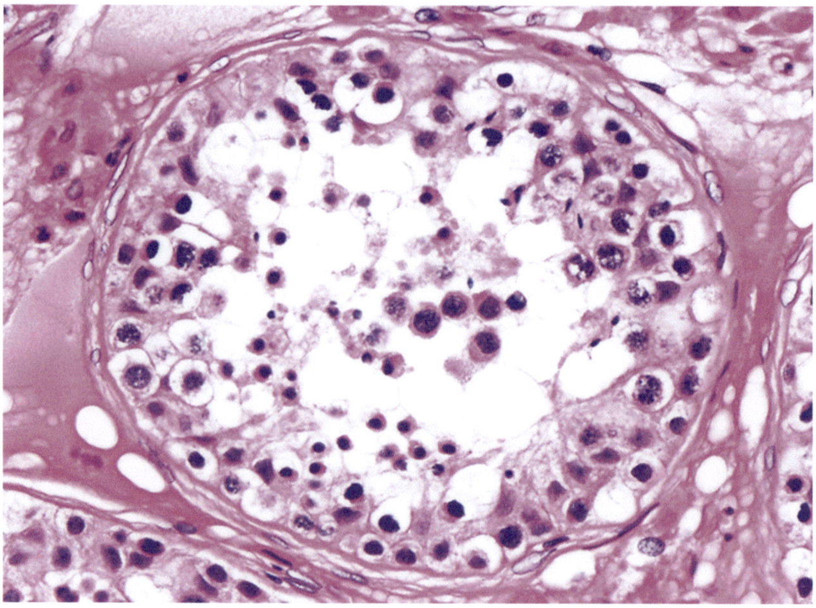

Fig. 21.4 Seminiferous tubule showing apical cytoplasmic vacuolization in both germ cells and Sertoli cells. Separation of some spermatogonia from the basement membrane. Spermatocyte and spermatid sloughing (same case of the previous figure)

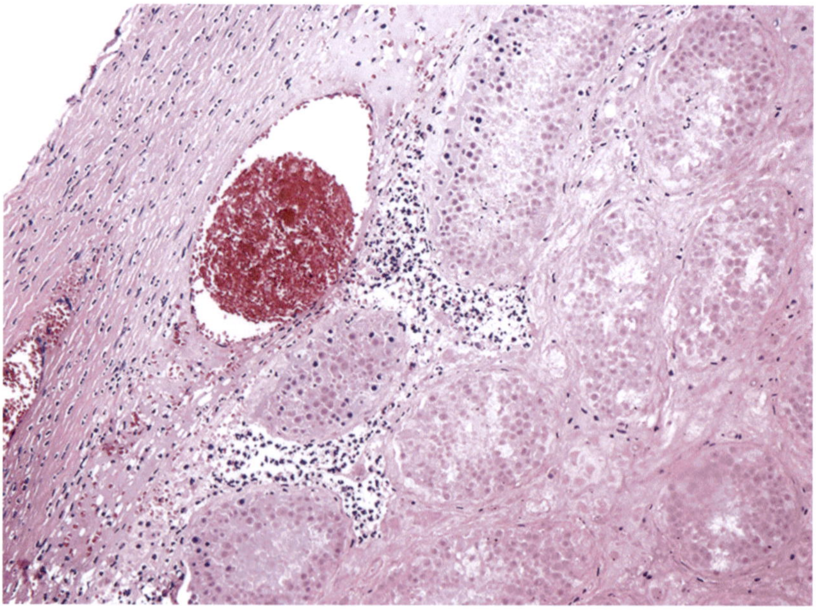

Fig. 21.5 Spermatic cord torsion grade III. Necrosis of testicular parenchyma. Nothing but the silhouettes of the seminiferous tubules can be recognized

restored after untwisting, but it does not confirm its usefulness in predicting the viability of the testicular parenchyma.

Grade of Spermatic Cord Torsion The second important factor in assessing the severity of testicular lesions is the degree of spermatic cord torsion [22, 23]. A high degree of cord twisting causes cellular necrosis within 4 h [24]. Experiments show that if twisting amounts to 180°–360°, recovery of many testes can be expected even after 10 h [25]. Testicular atrophy is always determined by 360° torsions and a 24 h evolution [2].

21.4 Causes of Infertility

Residual Pathology of Twisted Testicle The recovery from the injuries of the preserved testicles may be incomplete, and in the course of time, a certain percentage undergoes atrophy. Histological studies show large areas of fibrosis with microcalcifications (Figs. 21.6 and 21.7). The oligozoospermia could be due to the existence of a previous pathology in both testes. Studies in surgical specimens of twisted testicles with grade II lesions have shown lesions that cannot be attributed to torsion such as mixed atrophy, hypospermatogenesis, and microlithiasis [16] (Fig. 21.8).

Pathology of the Contralateral Testicle The contralateral testis may be carrying primary lesions and develop in addition secondary lesions to I/R. Biopsies performed on the contralateral testis at the time of torsion show that between 57 and 88 % of them are abnormal. The following lesions have been observed: desquamation of the germinative epithelium, atrophy of the Leydig cells, malformation of spermatids, maturation arrest, immature tubules, and tubular hyalinization [26, 27]. There are two possible (nonexclusive) explanations: that they are the result from intermittent episodes of asymptomatic torsion or that they are actually primary lesions themselves. Other lesions attributed to torsion are an important apoptosis of germ cells, a few adult spermatids with frequent malformations, vacuolation of Sertoli cells, and atrophy of Leydig cells [1].

Sympathetic Orchidopathy The testis is an immunologically privileged organ. Ischemia can produce the blood-testis barrier break. Different materials of a twisted testis are exposed to the immune system. The autoantibodies formed could attack the contralateral testis. The presence of immobilizing antibodies has been linked to infertility only [28], so this hypothesis does not have much backing.

Reflex vasoconstriction of contralateral testicular vessels is mediated by sympathetic nerves. The reflex vasoconstriction causes bilateral hypoxia and subsequent testicular damage [29].

21.5 Potential Protective Agents

The damage secondary to reperfusion is even more serious than that caused by ischemia. Several physical and pharmacological agents have been investigated in experimental animals

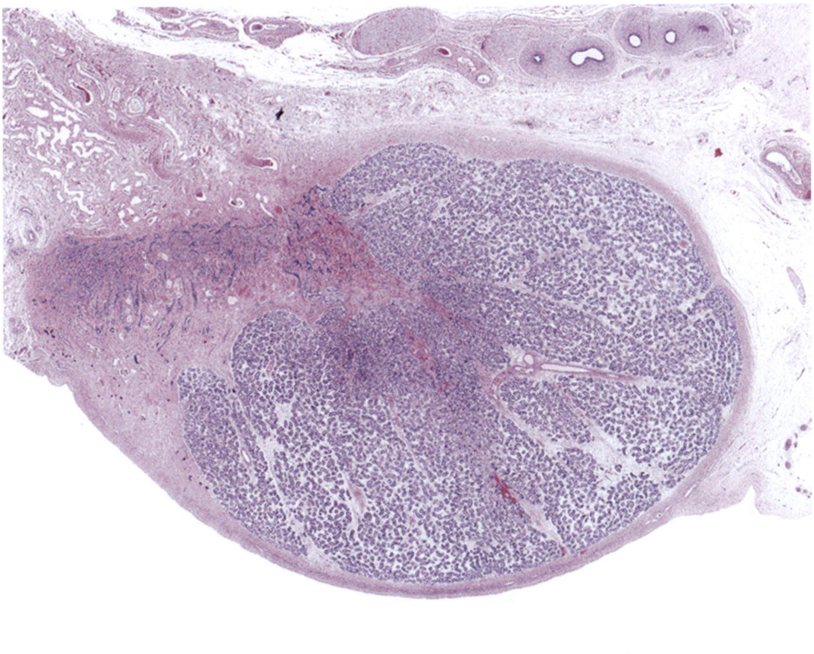

Fig. 21.6 Longitudinal section of a testicle with old spermatic cord torsion after salvage. The testicle was removed by its small size. The upper pole is thinned by extensive fibrosis

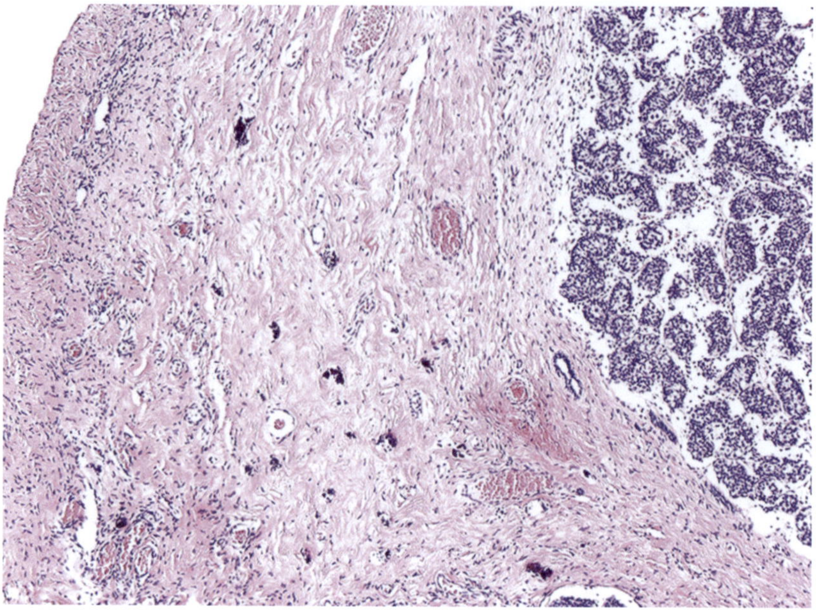

Fig. 21.7 Fibrosis of testicular parenchyma with multiple foci of dystrophic microcalcifications and absence of delimitation of testicular parenchyma from the tunica albuginea (same case of the previous figure)

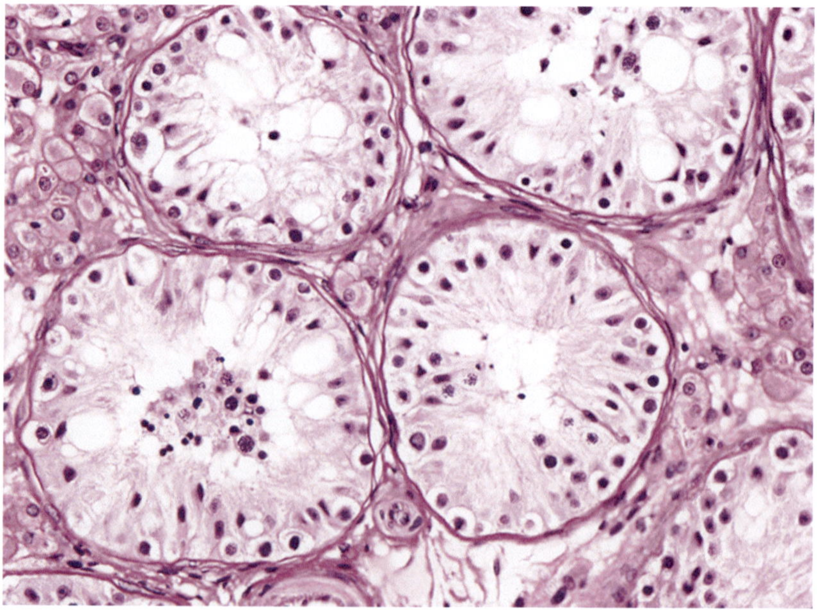

Fig. 21.8 Testicular torsion in 17-year-old patient. Grade I lesions associated with hypospermatogenesis

as supportive therapy of the surgical repair, in order to prevent the effects of ipsilateral and contralateral testicular torsion. These experiments include cooling the testis, limiting the reperfusion injury, suppressing immune-mediated damage, and chemical sympathectomy to prevent contralateral vasoconstriction among others [30].

Physical Therapies Cooling the testis retards the effects of ischemia for some hours. Electroacupuncture increases the testicular blood flow during the time interval that elapses from diagnosis to surgery, contributing to an increased testicular salvage rate [31]. Others are intraperitoneal ozone and/or taurine [32] and hyperbaric oxygen treatment [33].

Antioxidants and Free Radical Scavengers In recent years the use of several antioxidants and free radical scavengers has been proposed to limit the reperfusion injury. The administration of melatonin causes a significant decrease in lipid peroxidation and enzyme activities in the ipsilateral testis [34]. Also administration of N-acetylcysteine [35], vitamin E [36], selenium [37], ebselen [38], ghrelin [39], verapamil platelet-activating surfactant factor inhibitors, sildenafil and undenafil intraperitoneal administration [40], caffeic acid phenethyl ester, resveratrol, arginine [41], and pyrrolidine dithiocarbamate (a low-molecular-weight antioxidant and potent inhibitor of nuclear factor kappa B activation) have an antioxidant effect. [42].

Immunosuppression Immunosuppression with dexamethasone, hydrocortisone, cyclosporine, and azathioprine has been applied to control the potential immunologic effects of torsion. To reduce inflammatory reactions and improve testicular morphology, lipoxin A4 has been used because of its ability to regulate the production of cytokines, oxidative stress, and NF-kB activity [43]; mesenchymal local injections of stem cells have also been used as potent immune modulators [44], as well as caffeic acid phenethyl ester (antioxidant and anti-inflammatory agent). This effect may be due to inhibiting the neutrophil-mediated cellular injury [45].

Chemical sympathectomy is achieved with capsaicin, nitric oxide, 6-hydroxydopamine hydrobromide, and guanethidine monosulphate [1].

Most treatments are not validated, and currently 54 % of the testes undergo atrophy, even though during the intervention they had been considered viable. When the pain lasts more than 1 day and when there is a heterogeneous echogenicity on ultrasound, more than 90 % of the testes suffer atrophy [46].

References

1. Visser AJ, Heyns CF. Testicular function after torsion of the spermatic cord. BJU Int. 2003;92:200–3.
2. Tryfonas G, Violaki A, Tsikopoulos G, Avtzoglou P, Zioutis J, Limas C, Gregoriadis G, Badouraki M. Late postoperative results in males treated for testicular torsion during childhood. J Pediatr Surg. 1994;29:553–6.
3. Bartsch G, Frank S, Marberger H, Mikuz G. Testicular torsion: late results with special regard to fertility and endocrine function. J Urol. 1980;124:375–8.
4. Cuckow PM, Frank JD. Torsion of the testis. BJU Int. 2000;86:349–53.
5. Drlík M, Kočvara R. Torsion of spermatic cord in children: a review. J Pediatr Urol. 2013;9:259–66.
6. Krarup T. The testes after torsion. Br J Urol. 1978;50:43–6.
7. Kapoor S. Testicular torsion: a race against time. Int J Clin Pract. 2008;62:821–7.
8. Brasso K, Andersen L, Kay L, Wille-Jørgensen P, Linnet L, Egense J. Testicular torsion: a follow-up study. Scand J Urol Nephrol. 1993;27:1–6.
9. Romeo C, Impellizzeri P, Arrigo T, Antonuccio P, Valenzise M, Mirabelli S, Borruto FA, Scalfari G, Arena F, De Luca F. Late hormonal function after testicular torsion. J Pediatr Surg. 2010;45:411–3.
10. Ramachandra P, Palazzi KL, Holmes NM, Marietti S. Factors influencing rate of testicular salvage in acute testicular torsion at a tertiary pediatric center. West J Emerg Med. 2015;16:190–4.
11. Remer EM, Casalino DD, Arellano RS, Bishoff JT, Coursey CA, Dighe M, Fulgham P, Israel GM, Lazarus E, Leyendecker JR, Majd M, Nikolaidis P, Papanicolaou N, Prasad S, Ramchandani P, Sheth S, Vikram R, Karmazyn B. ACR Appropriateness Criteria ® acute onset of scrotal pain – without trauma, without antecedent mass. Ultrasound Q. 2012;28:47–51.
12. Filho DW, Torres MA, Bordin AL, Crezcynski-Pasa TB, Boveris A. Spermatic cord torsion, reactive oxygen and nitrogen species and ischemia-reperfusion injury. Mol Aspects Med. 2004;25:199–210.
13. Wei SM, Yan ZZ, Zhou J. Beneficial effect of taurine on testicular ischemia-reperfusion injury in rats. Urology. 2007;70:1237–42.
14. Turner TT, Bang HJ, Lysiak JL. The molecular pathology of experimental testicular torsion suggests adjunct therapy to surgical repair. J Urol. 2004;172:2574–8.
15. Mikuz G. Testicular torsion: simple grading for histological evaluation of tissue damage. Appl Pathol. 1985;3:134–9.
16. Nistal M, Martínez C, Paniagua R. Primary testicular lesions in the twisted testis. Fertil Steril. 1992;57:381–6.
17. Anderson JB, Williamson RC. Testicular torsion in Bristol: a 25-year review. Br J Surg. 1988;75: 988–92.
18. Waldert M, Klatte T, Schmidbauer J, Remzi M, Lackner J, Marberger M. Color Doppler sonography reliably identifies testicular torsion in boys. Urology. 2010;75:1170–4.
19. Baker LA, Sigman D, Mathews RI, Benson J, Docimo SG. An analysis of clinical outcomes using color doppler testicular ultrasound for testicular torsion. Pediatrics. 2000;105:604–7.

20. Woodruff DY, Horwitz G, Weigel J, Nangia AK, et al. Fertil Steril. 2010;94:352.e4-5.
21. Benedetto G, Nigro F, Bratti E, Tasca A. Modifications of echogenicity of the testis during acute torsion may be a predictive factor of organ damage? Arch Ital Urol Androl. 2014;86:371–2.
22. Abuja PM, Albertini R. Methods for monitoring oxidative stress, lipid peroxidation and oxidation resistance of lipoproteins. Clin Chim Acta. 2001;306:1–17.
23. Cummings JM, Boullier JA, Sekhon D, Bose K. Adult testicular torsion. J Urol. 2002;167:2109–10.
24. Mansbach JM, Forbes P, Peters C. Testicular torsion and risk factors for orchiectomy. Arch Pediatr Adolesc Med. 2005;159:1167–71.
25. Thomas WE, Cooper MJ, Crane GA, Lee G, Williamson RC. Testicular exocrine malfunction after torsion. Lancet. 1984;2:1357–60.
26. Anderson JB, Cooper MJ, Thomas WE, Williamson RC. Impaired spermatogenesis in testes at risk of torsion. Br J Surg. 1986;73:847–9.
27. Hagen P, Buchholz MM, Eigenmann J, Bandhauer K. Testicular dysplasia causing disturbance of spermiogenesis in patients with unilateral torsion of the testis. Urol Int. 1992;49:154–7.
28. Mastrogiacomo I, Zanchetta R, Graziotti P, Betterle C, Scrufari P, Lembo A. Immunological and clinical study of patients after spermatic cord torsion. Andrologia. 1982;14:25–30.
29. Kolettis PN, Stowe NT, Inman SR, Thomas Jr AJ. Acute spermatic cord torsion alters the microcirculation of the contralateral testis. J Urol. 1996;155:350–4.
30. Karaguzel E, Kadihasanoglu M, Kutlu O. Mechanisms of testicular torsion and potential protective agents. Nat Rev Urol. 2014;11:391–9.
31. Acar O, Esen T, Colakoglu B, Camli MF, Cakmak YO. Improving testicular blood flow with electroacupuncture-like percutaneous nerve stimulation in an experimental rat model of testicular torsion. Neuromodulation. 2015;18:324–8.
32. Aydos TR, Başar MM, Kul O, Atmaca HT, Uzunalıoğlu T, Kisa Ü, Efe OE. Effects of ozone therapy and taurine on ischemia/reperfusion-induced testicular injury in a rat testicular torsion model. Turk J Med Sci. 2014;44:749–55.
33. Alp BF, Cebi G, Özdemir A, Irkilata HC, Uzun G. Hyperbaric oxygen treatment for unilateral testicular torsion in a child. Diving Hyperb Med. 2014;44:161–2.
34. Parlaktas BS, Atilgan D, Ozyurt H, Gencten Y, Akbas A, Erdemir F, Uluocak N. The biochemical effects of ischemia-reperfusion injury in the ipsilateral and contralateral testes of rats and the protective role of melatonin. Asian J Androl. 2014;16:314–8.
35. Aktaş BK, Bulut S, Bulut S, Baykam MM, Ozden C, Senes M, Yücel D, Memiş A. The effects of N-acetylcysteine on testicular damage in experimental testicular ischemia/reperfusion injury. Pediatr Surg Int. 2010;26:293–8.
36. Ranade AV, Tripathi Y, Rajalakshmi R, Vinodini NA, Soubhagya RN, Nayanatara AK, Rekha DK, Kumari M. Effect of vitamin E administration on histopathological changes in rat testes following torsion and detorsion. Singapore Med J. 2011;52:742–6.
37. Avlan D, Erdouğan K, Cimen B, Düşmez Apa D, Cinel I, Aksöyek S. The protective effect of selenium on ipsilateral and contralateral testes in testicular reperfusion injury. Pediatr Surg Int. 2005;21:274–8.
38. Rifaioglu MM, Motor S, Davarci I, Tuzcu K, Sefil F, Davarci M, Nacar A. Protective effect of ebselen on experimental testicular torsion and detorsion injury. Andrologia. 2014;46:1134–40.
39. Taati M, Moghadasi M, Dezfoulian O, Asadian P. Effects of ghrelin on testicular ischemia/reperfusion-induced Injury. Acta Med Iran. 2016;54:32–8.
40. Ozgür GK, Pişkin B, Sivrikaya A, Gacar N, Erkul S. Effect of testicular torsion on the contralateral testis. Int Urol Nephrol. 1990;22:461–6.
41. Ribeiro CT, Milhomem R, De Souza DB, Costa WS, Sampaio FJ, Pereira-Sampaio MA. Effect of antioxidants on outcome of testicular torsion in rats of different ages. J Urol. 2014;191:1578–84.
42. Kabay S, Ozden H, Guven G, Burukoglu D, Ustuner MC, Topal F, Gunes HV, Ustuner D, Ozbayer C. Protective effects of the nuclear factor kappa B inhibitor pyrrolidine dithiocarbamate on experimental testicular torsion and detorsion injury. Korean J Physiol Pharmacol. 2014;18:321–6.
43. Zhou XL, Yang QS, Ni SZ, Tu XP, Zhao Y, Xu B, Pan ZQ, Shen J. Protective effects of lipoxin A4 in testis injury following testicular torsion and detorsion in rats. Mediators Inflamm. 2014;2014:898056.
44. Hsiao CH, Ji AT, Chang CC, Cheng CJ, Lee LM, Ho JH. Local injection of mesenchymal stem cells protects testicular torsion-induced germ cell injury. Stem Cell Res Ther. 2015;6:113.
45. Atik E, Görür S, Kiper AN. The effect of caffeic acid phenethyl ester (CAPE) on histopathological changes in testicular ischemia-reperfusion injury. Pharmacol Res. 2006;54:293–7.
46. Lian BS, Ong CC, Chiang LW, Rai R, Nah SA. Factors predicting testicular atrophy after testicular salvage following torsion. Eur J Pediatr Surg. 2016;26:17–21.

22 Clues to the Analysis of Testicular Lesions in Infertile Patients with Varicocele

Manuel Nistal, Pilar González-Peramato, and Álvaro Serrano

22.1 Varicocele and Infertility

There is much information regarding varicocele male infertility: (a) the incidence of varicocele in the general population is 4.4–22.6 %, and this figure rises to 21–44 % of the population consulting for infertility; (b) the semen analysis of patients with varicocele shows reduced sperm count, mobility, and morphology [1]; (c) the ipsilateral testis is smaller [2]; (d) the size of the contralateral testicle is diminished; (e) the degree of varicocele is inversely correlated to the testicular size and semen quality [3]; (f) testicular size is also decreased in the so-called subclinical varicoceles [4]; (g) the majority of patients undergoing varicocelectomy have improved semen quality, but the number of spontaneous pregnancies is very low [5, 6]; (h) histological studies show very varied lesions; (i) two thirds of men with varicocele maintain fertility [7, 8]; and (j) the pathogenetic mechanisms discussed over more than 50 years are still controversial [9].

The most common causes of varicocele and preferably involvement of the left side have an anatomical basis. The most frequent are:

- Difficulty in draining the internal spermatic vein that discharges into the renal vein.
- Congenital absence or incompetence of the ostial valves of the internal spermatic vein.
- High hydrostatic pressure in the internal spermatic vein due to its great length (42 cm) and the absence of valves [10].
- The renospermatic reflux could be explained by the condition known as "proximal nutcracker effect" or "compass effect" [11]. This effect consists of compression of the left renal vein between the superior mesenteric artery and the aorta (aortic-mesenteric pincer) or compression of the renal vein that might be exerted by either the Treitz's ligament or an arched testicular "distal" artery [12]. In the iliospermatic refluxes by "distal nutcracker effect," the common right iliac artery goes over the common left iliac vein and can compress it [13, 14].
- Alterations in the fasciomuscular pump of the spermatic cord [15, 16].

22.2 Pathogenetic Mechanism

The pathophysiology of varicocele is multifactorial. A combination of several factors affects spermatogenesis and sperm function. The following possibilities have been proposed: altered testicular thermoregulation, hypoxia, toxic effects of metabolites of renal or adrenal origin, oxidative stress, hormonal imbalances, impaired blood flow, gonadotoxins, apoptosis, alteration of the vascularization of the epididymis and its function, and an effect on the testis contralateral to the varicocele (Fig. 22.1).

M. Nistal et al., *Clues in the Diagnosis of Non-tumoral Testicular Pathology*, DOI 10.1007/978-3-319-49364-0_22

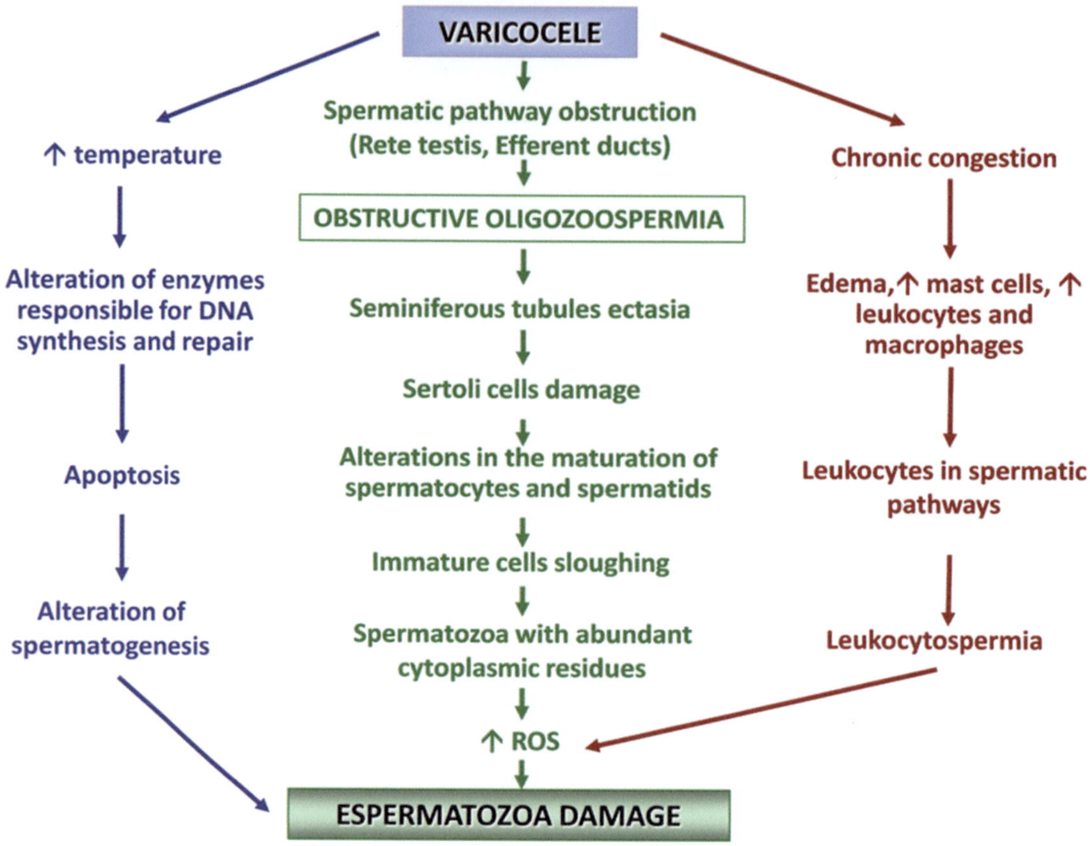

Fig. 22.1 Algorithm that summarizes the mechanisms and factors involved in the pathophysiology of varicocele

Alteration of the Testicular Thermoregulation
The normally functioning testis requires to constantly remain at a temperature lower than other areas of the body. The testis with varicocele has a higher temperature, estimated to be 2.2 °C higher [17]. Experimentally, testicular hyperthermia can destroy the balance between oxidative and antioxidative capacity [18]. Experimentally, testicular hyperthermia promotes apoptosis, thereby affecting mainly primary spermatocytes and round spermatids [19]. Many of the enzymes responsible for DNA synthesis, (such as topoisomerase I and the DNA polymerase), have an optimum activity at temperatures lower than those achieved in the testis with varicocele [20].

Hypoxia
Venous stasis causes vasoconstriction of the precapillary arterioles within the testis as a manner of downregulating the arterial flow and also with the aim to maintain homeostasis. Vasoconstriction leads to hypoperfusion and decrease of both oxygen and other nutrients in the cells and the interstitium [21]. An association between levels of hypoxia-inducible factor 1 alpha (HIF-1 alpha) in testicular veins and germ cell apoptosis has been found in varicocele [22].

Toxic Effects of Metabolites of Renal or Adrenal Origin
Studies are contradictory [23]. Some authors have reported an increase of catecholamine in the spermatic vein, increase that others authors have not confirmed. Also, high levels of PGE, −F, F2alpha, and serotonin have been reported whose meaning remains unclarified [2], as well as increased adrenomedullin (a potent vasodilator peptide), but its function on spermatogenesis is unknown [24].

Oxidative Stress

Spermatozoa normally produce different forms of reactive oxygen species (ROS) involved among others in important functions such as the mechanisms of signal transduction, regulation of spermatic hyperactivation/capacitation, and facilitation of the acrosome reaction and binding of sperm to the oocyte [25, 26]. The seminal plasma contains antioxidant agents that neutralize the excessive production of ROS. In the varicocele there is an excessive production of ROS due to the abundant number of sperm with cytoplasmic residues and increased transepithelial passage of leukocytes and macrophages through the epididymis [27–29].

Excess of free radicals can affect sperm in three different ways [30]: membrane lipid peroxidation, DNA damage, and induction of apoptosis. Cell membranes are very rich in polyunsaturated fatty acids, especially docosahexaenoic acid that confers high sensitivity to oxygen-induced exposure to damage and consequently loss of intracellular adenosine triphosphate, which produces axonemal damage, morphological defects in the midpiece, decreased sperm viability and motility, and decreased ability to fertilize the oocytes [31].

Another effect of free radicals on sperm is DNA damage. Direct attack to the bases of purine and pyrimidine and the phosphodiester backbones destabilizes the DNA molecule and produces abnormalities such as polymorphisms, point mutations, deletions, translocations, and even double-stranded breaks [32]. DNA fragmentation can cause abnormal fertilization, reduced implantation, and poor embryonic development [33, 34].

In the most severe cases, apoptosis of spermatogonia, spermatocytes, and spermatids can be observed, a process that begins with the binding of two members of the tumor necrosis factor family, Fas (a type I transmembrane protein) expressed in spermatogenetic germ cells and FasL (its ligand) in the Sertoli cells [35].

Hormonal Imbalances

There are two cell types that may show a dysfunction in patients with varicocele: Leydig cells and Sertoli cells. Chronic congestion alters hormone levels and other factors involved in endocrine and paracrine regulation of Leydig cells, myoid peritubular cells, and Sertoli cells. Fifty percent of patients with varicocele have an excessive response to stimulation with GnRH. Free testosterone levels are lower than normal, and E2 levels are higher than normal, suggesting an intrinsic defect in testicular steroidogenesis [36]. The following conditions are observed in many patients with varicocele: decreased Sertoli cell responsiveness to FSH and altered serum levels of inhibin [37] and of androgen-binding protein.

Altered Blood Flow

Blood pressure in testicular postcapillary venules and capillaries is very low compared to other tissues. The increase in testicular venous pressure accompanying the varicocele eventually affects the postcapillary venules, resulting in an increased volume of filtration. This excessive interstitial fluid leads to chronic edema and accumulation of testicular catabolites. Among catabolites intermediate products of biosynthesis and catabolism of the androgens are found that can seriously affect the paracrine regulation mechanisms [38–40].

Gonadotoxins

The gonadotoxins act as a cofactor in the pathogenesis of varicocele. In smokers the incidence of varicocele is twice as high, and oligospermia is ten times greater than in nonsmokers [41, 42]. Nicotine would act on the testicle in several ways: by increasing the release of adrenal catecholamines that would reach the testicle through the retrograde flow that there is in the varicocele, by the formation of free radicals, or by the toxic effect of cadmium contained in cigarettes. Cadmium produces a toxic effect on spermatogenesis, increasing apoptosis, provoking endothelial damage, and resulting in edema and increased intratesticular pressure and thickening of the internal spermatic vein wall [43].

Apoptosis

In men with varicocele, the percentage of germ cell apoptosis is increased up to 14.7 % compared with 2 % in normal men; additionally, 10 % of the spermatozoa ejaculated in patients with varicocele show apoptosis as compared to 0.1 % in fertile controls [44]. Apoptosis may be the final common pathway of various pathogenic factors acting in the varicocele, including thermal stress, hypoxia, contact with cadmium and other toxic substances, or an androgen deficiency.

Alteration in the Vascularization of the Epididymis and Its Function
The same disorders that occur in testicular vascularization are applicable to the epididymis; with the peculiarity that since the maturation and the acquisition of progressive mobility of sperm occur at this level, these functions may be affected.

Contralateral Effect
Varicocele is a bilateral vascular disease, and a right-sided venous return is observed in 86 % of infertile patients with clinical varicocele [45]. The contralateral testis has lesions too, although in many cases, they are less important. This testicle could be affected by three mechanisms: direct reflux of the right testicular vein, reflux of the left testicular vein via its communicants, or an increase in temperature by contact with the ipsilateral varicose testis.

22.3 Clues to Interpret Testicular Lesions

The following three situations are observed when analyzing the target cells on which the various mechanisms act: (a) thermal stress and hypoxia result in increased apoptosis preferably acting on the first-order spermatocyte, (b) oxidative stress and vascular changes in the epididymis preferably act on the spermatozoa, and (c) the testicular chronic congestion acts on the interstitium, the Sertoli cells, and the Leydig cells.

The most common lesions described in the testicular biopsies are the following: In the most affected tubules, there is a marked dilatation of the lumen, most times in reverse proportion to atrophy of the seminiferous epithelium [46] (Fig. 22.2). The tubules of smaller caliber have a wall thickening [47, 48] and may have sperm accumulations. Parallel to atrophy there is a progressive thickening of the basement membrane [49] and myoid cells of the tubular wall dedifferentiation [50].

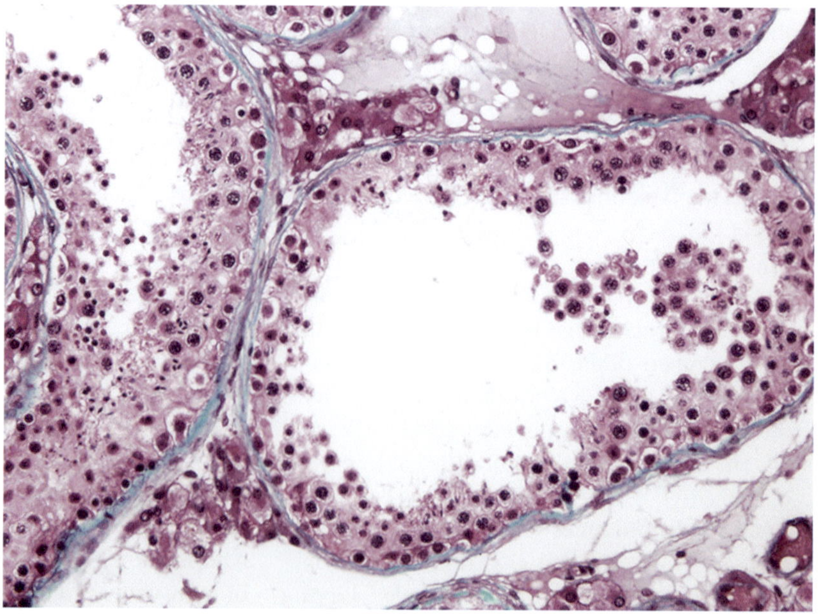

Fig. 22.2 Patient with varicocele and oligozoospermia. Testicular parenchyma showing marked seminiferous tubule ectasia and immature cell sloughing

The seminiferous epithelium may show incomplete spermatogenetic element maturation, hypospermatogenesis, mixed atrophy, Sertoli cell-only, sloughing of immature germ cells (spermatids and even spermatocytes) [51–53], and maturation arrest [47].

Congestion and fibrosis are seen in the interstitium as well as thickening of the vessel wall with narrowing of the lumen and interstitial fibrosis [54–56] (Fig. 22.3). Ectasia of the lymphatic vessels and blood stagnation in the microcirculatory vessels are also present [57]. Leydig cells have been described as atrophic from 4 % [47, 58] to 10 % [48]. Leydig cell hyperplasia has been described in 22 % [59] to 39 % [58] of the testes. In a large number of cases, the contralateral testis shows histological changes similar to those of varicocele, although not as intense [49].

By correlating the lesions produced by different pathogenetic mechanisms, both using data from experimental animals and humans, huge discrepancies with some histological findings become obvious. The first discrepancy is to attribute lesions such as mixed atrophy, Sertoli cell-only syndrome, and severe cases of hypospermatogenesis to proposed pathogenic mechanisms. These lesions are observed both in patients with nonobstructive azoospermia and in patients with abnormal karyotype or cryptorchidic patients. It is very unlikely caused by accepted pathogenetic mechanisms in varicocele, so the first key should be introduced; these are primary lesions of the testis, regardless of whether or not the patient has a varicocele.

The second difficulty is the interpretation of the great variability of lesions affecting both the tubular diameter, the amplitude of the tubular lumen, or the degree of spermatogenesis, lesions that also share the characteristic of being focal. It would be expected that thermal stress or oxidative stress, to name just the most accepted mechanisms, produced diffuse lesions in germline that hardly vary from one to another lobule. This has led us to introduce a second key in interpreting varicocele lesions; in the varicocele there is a partial obstruction of the proximal spermatic pathway [60, 61].

In biopsies and surgical specimens of patients with varicocele, lesions vary from some seminiferous tubules to others, with the peculiarity that, according to the serial studies of samples, those

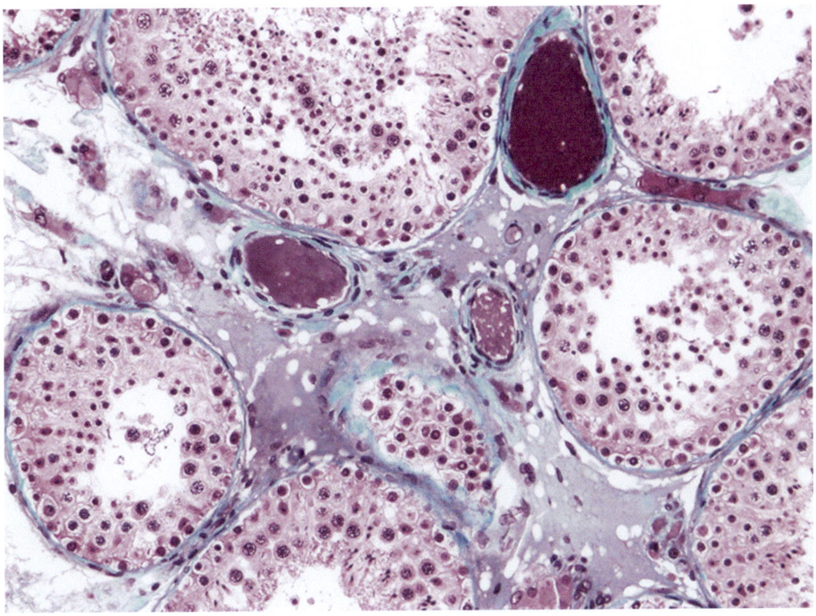

Fig. 22.3 Testicular parenchyma showing dilated veins with fibrous wall and interstitial edema (same patient of the previous figure)

with the same lesion belong to the same lobule. In other words, two adjacent lobules may have lesions in different evolutionary moments. If the lesions are ordered from the lowest to the highest grade of severity, there are tubules with increased diameter and lumen at one end and atrophy of the seminiferous epithelium, disappearance or accumulation of sperm in the lumen, and tubulitis at the other end.

The quantitative study of the seminiferous epithelium shows from an adult spermatid number higher than a young spermatid number, only explainable by an obstruction, to more and more serious lesions of the adluminal compartment, at first the late sloughing of the first-order spermatocytes and then the early sloughing of the first-order spermatocytes. Vacuolation of apical cytoplasm of the Sertoli cells is associated with these lesions in the germ cells. These lesions are similar to those described after blockage of the proximal spermatic ducts, so in a testis with varicocele, there must be a compression in some segment of the spermatic ducts that permits some seminiferous tubules to be even partially obstructed, but not so others.

The logical site of the blockage, probably only partial and only occurring when the patient is standing, is the testicular mediastinum (Fig. 22.4). This densely connective structure houses the first part of the spermatic pathway, septal rete, and mediastinal rete and also the centripetal veins, a group of veins that drain most of the testicular blood [62]. Dilation of these veins (intratesticular varicocele) in an inelastic structure, such as the mediastinum testis, causes stenosis of the intratesticular spermatic pathway (Figs. 22.5 and 22.6).

Studies in testicular autopsies of patients with varicocele have shown that such compression is a reality [60]. The seminiferous tubules, unable to eliminate testicular fluid and sperm through the tubuli recti sometimes stenosed and other times displaced, would suffer an increase in hydrostatic pressure, and the seminiferous epithelium would be compressed by the intratubular fluid against the tunica propria, progressively atrophying the seminiferous epithelium [63] (Fig. 22.7).

In summary, the histological studies of biopsies of infertile patients with varicocele and of surgical specimens of young patients with varicocele are the key to interpret testicular lesions. If the testicles are normal despite the varicocele causing alterations in the testicular parenchyma,

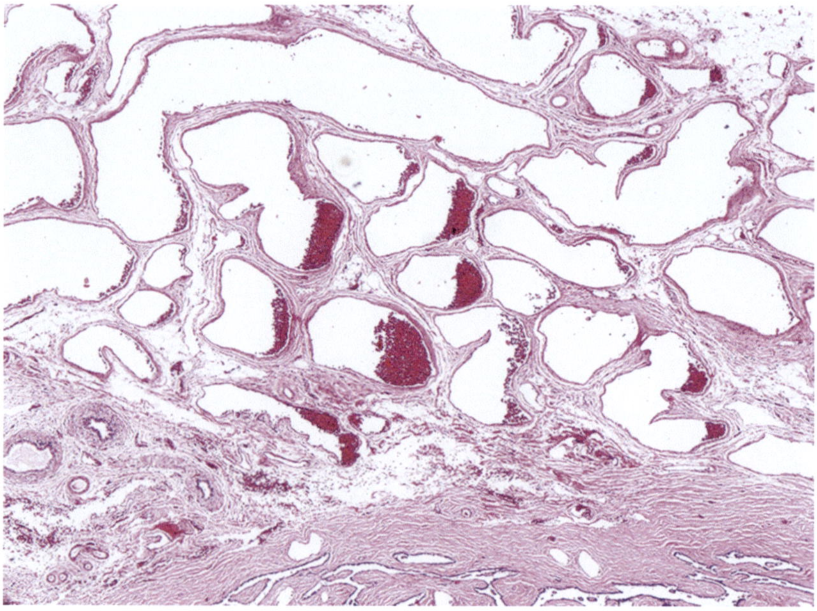

Fig. 22.4 Varicocele. The veins of the pampiniform plexus show marked dilation acquiring an image of cystic transformation without collapsing in the histological section

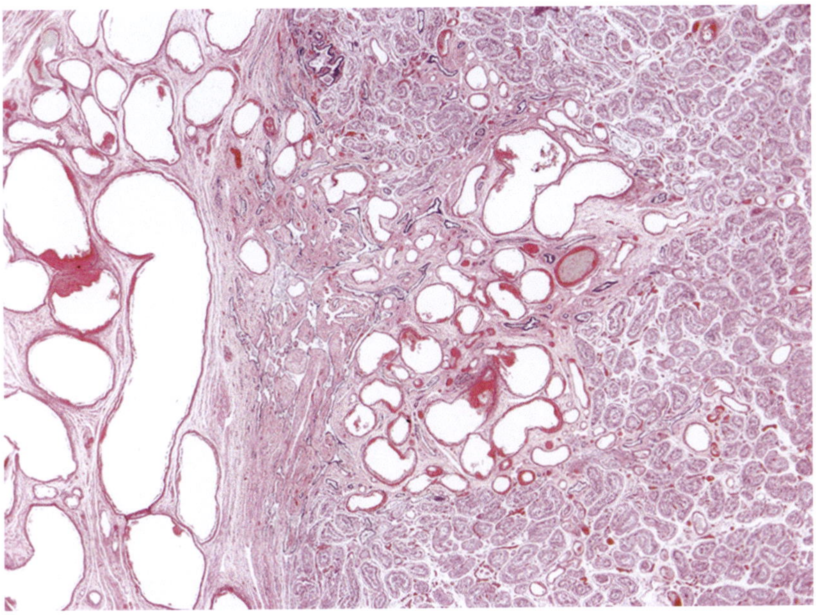

Fig. 22.5 Extra- and intratesticular varicocele. In addition to marked dilation of extratesticular veins, dilation with cystic transformation of the veins located in the mediastinum testis is added

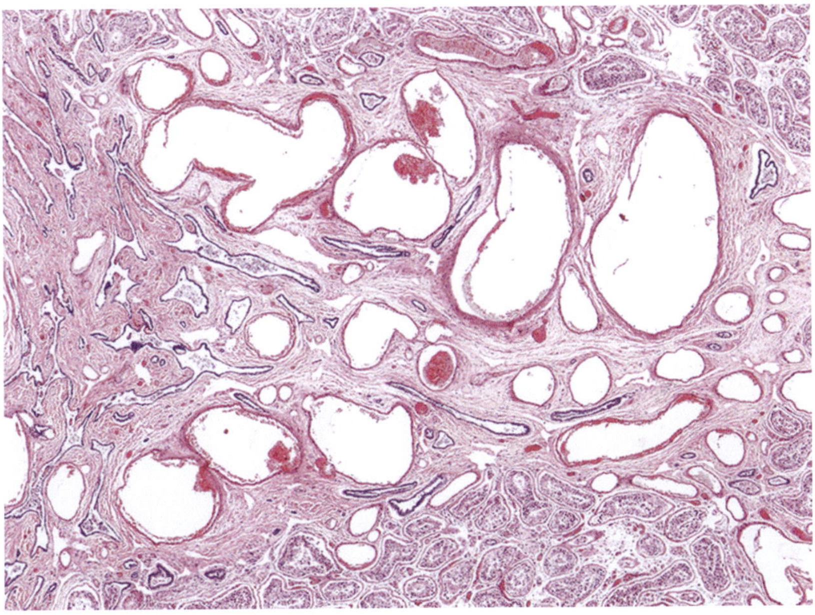

Fig. 22.6 Intratesticular varicocele. The mediastinum testis is occupied by numerous dilated veins

these changes are insufficient for the patient to become infertile. But if the testicle is the bearer of a handicap that in the absence of varicocele would not be a cause of infertility, varicocele altering the parenchyma triggers infertility. Progressivity of lesions may be more related to obstructive phenomena rather than to other pathogenic mechanisms.

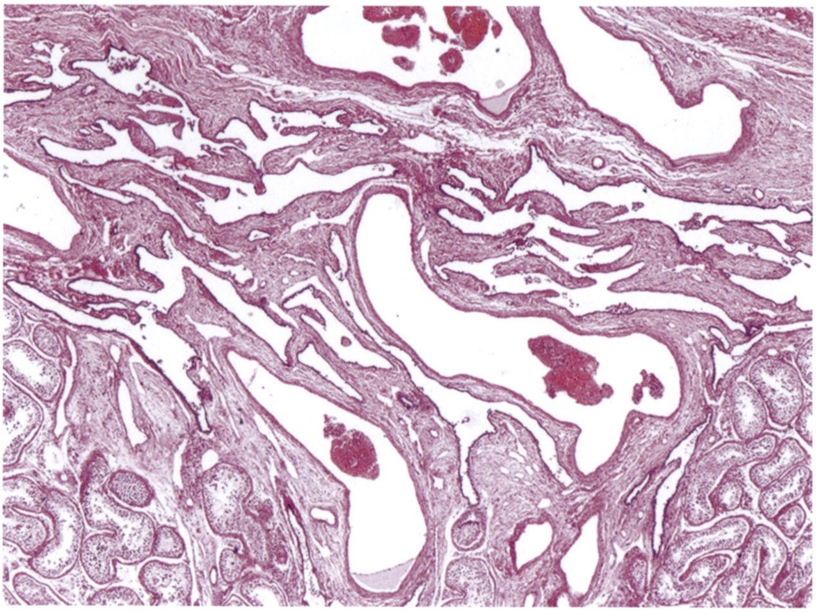

Fig. 22.7 Intratesticular varicocele. Dilated veins disrupt and compress tubuli recti and rete testis cavities

References

1. Agarwal A, Sharma R, Harlev A, Esteves SC. Effect of varicocele on semen characteristics according to the new 2010 World Health Organization criteria: a systematic review and meta-analysis. Asian J Androl. 2016;18:163–70.
2. Cockett AT, Takihara H, Cosentino MJ. The varicocele. Fertil Steril. 1984;41:5–11.
3. Sigman M, Jarow JP. Ipsilateral testicular hypotrophy is associated with decreased sperm counts in infertile men with varicoceles. J Urol. 1997;158:605–7.
4. Zini A, Buckspan M, Berardinucci D, Jarvi K. The influence of clinical and subclinical varicocele on testicular volume. Fertil Steril. 1997;68:671–4.
5. Nieschlag E, Hertle L, Fischedick A, Abshagen K, Behre HM. Update on treatment of varicocele: counselling as effective as occlusion of the vena spermatica. Hum Reprod. 1998;13:2147–50.
6. Redmon JB, Carey P, Pryor JL. Varicocele–the most common cause of male factor infertility? Hum Reprod Update. 2002;8:53–8.
7. Gorelick JI, Goldstein M. Loss of fertility in men with varicocele. Fertil Steril. 1993;59:613–6.
8. Will MA, Swain J, Fode M, Sonksen J, Christman GM, Ohl D. The great debate: varicocele treatment and impact on fertility. Fertil Steril. 2011;95:841–52.
9. Miyaoka R, Esteves SC. A critical appraisal on the role of varicocele in male infertility. Adv Urol. 2012;2012:597495.
10. Turner TT. Varicocele: still an enigma. J Urol. 1983;129:695–9.
11. Sayfan J, Halevy A, Oland J, Nathan H. Varicocele and left renal vein compression. Fertil Steril. 1984; 41:411–7.
12. Notkovich H. Testicular artery arching over renal vein: clinical and pathological considerations with special reference to varicocele. Br J Urol. 1955;27:267–71.
13. Hill JT, Green NA. Varicocele: a review of radiological and anatomical features in relation to surgical treatment. Br J Surg. 1977;64:747–52.
14. Beck EM, Schlegel PN, Goldstein M. Intraoperative varicocele anatomy: a macroscopic and microscopic study. J Urol. 1992;148:1190–4.
15. Shafik A, Khalil AM, Saleh M. The fasciomuscular tube of the spermatic cord. A study of its surgical anatomy and relation to varicocele. A new concept for the pathogenesis of varicocele. Br J Urol. 1972;44:147–51.
16. Shafik A. The cremasteric muscle. Role in varicocelogenesis and in thermoregulatory function of the testicle. Invest Urol. 1973;11:92–7.
17. Wright EJ, Young GP, Goldstein M. Reduction in testicular temperature after varicocelectomy in infertile men. Urology. 1997;50:257–9.
18. Pino JA, Osses N, Oyarzún D, Farías JG, Moreno RD, Reyes JG. Differential effects of temperature on reactive oxygen/nitrogen species production in rat pachytene spermatocytes and round spermatids. Reproduction. 2013;145:203–12.
19. Yin Y, Hawkins KL, DeWolf WC, Morgentaler A. Heat stress causes testicular germ cell apoptosis in adult mice. J Androl. 1997;18:159–65.
20. Fujisawa M, Yoshida S, Matsumoto O, Kojima K, Kamidono S. Decrease of topoisomerase I activity in the testes of infertile men with varicocele. Arch Androl. 1988;21:45–50.
21. Gat Y, Zukerman Z, Chakraborty J, Gornish M. Varicocele, hypoxia and male infertility. Fluid Mechanics analysis of the impaired testicular venous drainage system. Hum Reprod. 2005;20:2614–9.

22. Wang H, Sun Y, Wang L, Xu C, Yang Q, Liu B, Liu Z. Hypoxia-induced apoptosis in the bilateral testes of rats with left-sided varicocele: a new way to think about the varicocele. J Androl. 2010;31:299–305.
23. Steeno O, Koumans J, De Moor P. Adrenal cortical hormones in the spermatic vein of 95 patients with left varicocele. Andrologia. 1976;8:101–4.
24. Ozbek E, Yurekli M, Soylu A, Davarci M, Balbay MD. The role of adrenomedullin in varicocele and impotence. BJU Int. 2000;86:694–8.
25. De Lamirande E, Gagnon C. Human sperm hyperactivation in whole semen and its association with low superoxide scavenging capacity in seminal plasma. Fertil Steril. 1993;59:1291–5.
26. Aitken RJ, Baker MA. Oxidative stress, sperm survival and fertility control. Mol Cell Endocrinol. 2006;250:66–9.
27. Chen SS, Chang LS, Wei YH. Oxidative damage to proteins and decrease of antioxidant capacity in patients with varicocele. Free Radic Biol Med. 2001;30:1328–34.
28. Hendin BN, Kolettis PN, Sharma RK, Thomas Jr AJ, Agarwal A. Varicocele is associated with elevated spermatozoal reactive oxygen species production and diminished seminal plasma antioxidant capacity. J Urol. 1999;161:1831–4.
29. Türkyilmaz Z, Gülen S, Sönmez K, Karabulut R, Dinçer S, Can Başaklar A, Kale N. Increased nitric oxide is accompanied by lipid oxidation in adolescent varicocele. Int J Androl. 2004;27:183–7.
30. Romeo C, Santoro G. Free radicals in adolescent varicocele testis. Oxid Med Cell Longev. 2014;2014: 912878.
31. Agarwal A, Sharma R, Durairajanayagam D, Cui Z, Ayaz A, Gupta S, Willard B, Gopalan B, Sabanegh E. Differential proteomic profiling of spermatozoal proteins of infertile men with unilateral or bilateral varicocele. Urology. 2015;85:580–8.
32. Durairajanayagam D, Agarwal A, Ong C. Causes, effects and molecular mechanisms of testicular heat stress. Reprod Biomed Online. 2015;30:14–27.
33. Zini A, Dohle G. Are varicoceles associated with increased deoxyribonucleic acid fragmentation? Fertil Steril. 2011;96:1283–7.
34. Majzoub A, Esteves SC, Gosálvez J, Agarwal A. Specialized sperm function tests in varicocele and the future of andrology laboratory. Asian J Androl. 2016;18:205–12.
35. Marmar JL. The pathophysiology of varicoceles in the light of current molecular and genetic information. Hum Reprod Update. 2001;7:461–72.
36. Hudson RW. Free sex steroid and sex hormone-binding globulin levels in oligozoospermic men with varicoceles. Fertil Steril. 1996;66:299–304.
37. Plymate SR, Paulsen CA, McLachlan RI. Relationship of serum inhibin levels to serum follicle stimulating hormone and sperm production in normal men and men with varicoceles. J Clin Endocrinol Metab. 1992;74:859–64.
38. Hsu HS, Chang LS, Chen MT, Wei YH. Decreased blood flow and defective energy metabolism in the varicocele-bearing testicles of rats. Eur Urol. 1994;25:71–5.
39. Hsu HS, Wei YH, Li AF, Chen MT, Chang LS. Defective mitochondrial oxidative phosphorylation in varicocele-bearing testicles. Urology. 1995;46: 545–9.
40. Tarhan S, Gümüs B, Gündüz I, Ayyildiz V, Göktan C. Effect of varicocele on testicular artery blood flow in men–color Doppler investigation. Scand J Urol Nephrol. 2003;37:38–42.
41. Klaiber EL, Broverman DM, Vogel W. Increased incidence of testicular varicoceles in cigarette smokers. Fertil Steril. 1980;34:64–5.
42. Klaiber EL, Broverman DM, Pokoly TB, Albert AJ, Howard Jr PJ, Sherer Jr JF. Interrelationships of cigarette smoking, testicular varicoceles, and seminal fluid indexes. Fertil Steril. 1987;47:481–6.
43. Jeng SY, Wu SM, Lee JD. Cadmium accumulation and metallothionein overexpression in internal spermatic vein of patients with varicocele. Urology. 2009;73:1231–5.
44. Baccetti B, Collodel G, Piomboni P. Apoptosis in human ejaculated sperm cells (notulae seminologicae 9). J Submicrosc Cytol Pathol. 1996;28:587–96.
45. Gat Y, Gornish M, Navon U, Chakraborty J, Bachar GN, Ben-Shlomo I. Right varicocele and hypoxia, crucial factors in male infertility: fluid mechanics analysis of the impaired testicular drainage system. Reprod Biomed Online. 2006;13:510–5.
46. Cameron DF, Snydle FE. Ultrastructural surface characteristics of seminiferous tubules from men with varicocele. Andrologia. 1982;14:425–33.
47. Etriby A, Girgis SM, Hefnawy H, Ibrahim AA. Testicular changes in subfertile males with varicocele. Fertil Steril. 1967;18:666–71.
48. Dubin L, Hotchkiss RS. Testis biopsy in subfertile men with varicocele. Fertil Steril. 1969;20:51–7.
49. Spera G, Medolago-Albani L, Coia L, Morgia C, Gonnelli S, Ghilardi C. Histological, histochemical, and ultrastructural aspects of interstitial tissue from the contralateral testis in infertile men with monolateral varicocele. Arch Androl. 1983;10:73–8.
50. Santamaría L, Martín R, Nistal M, Paniagua R. The peritubular myoid cells in the testes from men with varicocele: an ultrastructural, immunohistochemical and quantitative study. Histopathology. 1992;21: 423–33.
51. Ibrahim AA, Awad HA, El-Haggar S, Mitawi BA. Bilateral testicular biopsy in men with varicocele. Fertil Steril. 1977;28:663–7.
52. Cameron DF, Snydle FE, Ross MH, Drylie DM. Ultrastructural alterations in the adluminal testicular compartment in men with varicocele. Fertil Steril. 1980;33:526–33.
53. Wang YX, Lei C, Dong SG, Chandley AC, MacIntyre M, Hargreave TB. Study of bilateral histology and meiotic analysis in men undergoing varicocele ligation. Fertil Steril. 1991;55:152–5.
54. Johnsen SG, Agger P. Quantitative evaluation of testicular biopsies before and after operation for varicocele. Fertil Steril. 1978;29:58–63.

55. Abdelrahim F, Mostafa A, Hamdy A, Mabrouk M, e-Kholy M, Hassan O. Testicular morphology and function in varicocele patients: pre-operative and post-operative histopathology. Br J Urol. 1993; 72:643–7.
56. North MO, Lellei I, Rives N, Erdei E, Dittmar A, Barbet JP, Tritto G. Reversible meiotic abnormalities in azoospermic men with bilateral varicocele after microsurgical correction. Cell Mol Biol (Noisy-le-Grand). 2004;50:281–9.
57. Chakraborty J, Hikim AP, Jhunjhunwala JS. Stagnation of blood in the microcirculatory vessels in the testes of men with varicocele. J Androl. 1985;6:117–26.
58. Agger P, Johnsen SG. Quantitative evaluation of testicular biopsies in varicocele. Fertil Steril. 1978;29:52–7.
59. McFadden MR, Mehan DJ. Testicular biopsies in 101 cases of varicocele. J Urol. 1978;119:372–4.
60. Nistal M, Paniagua R, Regadera J, Santamaria L. Obstruction of the tubuli recti and ductuli efferentes by dilated veins in the testes of men with varicocele and its possible role in causing atrophy of the seminiferous tubules. Int J Androl. 1984;7:309–23.
61. Nistal M, González-Peramato P, Serrano A, Regadera J. Physiopathology of the infertile testicle Etiopathogenesis of varicocele. Arch Esp Urol. 2004;57:883–904.
62. Kormano M, Suoranta H. Microvascular organization of the adult human testis. Anat Rec. 1971;170:31–9.
63. Belmonte IG, Nistal M. Partial obstruction of the seminal path, a frequent cause of oligozoospermia in men. Hum Reprod. 1998;13:3402–5.

23 Surgical Treatment of Varicocele

Manuel Nistal, Pilar González-Peramato, and
Álvaro Serrano

23.1 Indications for Varicocele Surgical Repair

Evaluation of patients with varicocele should be performed to identify potential risk factors associated with long-term subfertility. At present, the points to be considered are the degree of varicocele, testicular size, findings obtained by scrotal Doppler ultrasound (Figs. 23.1 and 23.2), endocrine evaluation, and the results of spermiogram.

The American Urological Association for Male Infertility Best Practice Policy Committee and the American Society for Reproductive Medicine Practice Committee [1] both state that treatment of varicocele in adults should be considered when (1) the varicocele is palpated on physical examination, (2) the couple has known infertility, (3) the woman has a normal fertility study or has a potentially treatable cause of infertility, and (4) the man has altered parameters of sperm with abnormal sperm function tests.

However, surgical treatment in adolescents should be considered when there is objective evidence of reduced ipsilateral testicular size. If there is no objective evidence of decreased testicular size, the committees recommend that adolescents and young adults should be annually evaluated by means of a scrotal Doppler ultrasound and a semen analysis to detect early signs of testicular lesions.

The European Association of Urology [2] has recently released similar guidelines, which state that (1) varicocele treatment is recommended for adolescents with progressive failure of testicular development documented by serial clinical examination, (2) there is no evidence indicating the benefit of varicocele treatment in infertile men who have normal semen analysis or a subclinical varicocele, and (3) varicocele repair should be considered in cases of clinical varicocele, oligospermia, infertility duration greater than 2 years, and otherwise unexplained infertility in the couple.

The key question in varicocele surgery is whether adolescent varicocele repair has any effect on reversal of testicular hypotrophy or improvement in semen parameters. While the ultimate patient goal is paternity, semen analysis is critical to the appropriate treatment of these patients.

23.2 Treatment Options

The objectives pursued in the treatment of varicocele are to improve testicular function, improve sperm parameters in an early stage of development (especially during puberty, onset of spermatogenesis) before noted histological changes to occur, and, finally, to treat pain when it is the symptom that accompanies varicocele, although in adolescents it is infrequent.

M. Nistal et al., *Clues in the Diagnosis of Non-tumoral Testicular Pathology*,
DOI 10.1007/978-3-319-49364-0_23

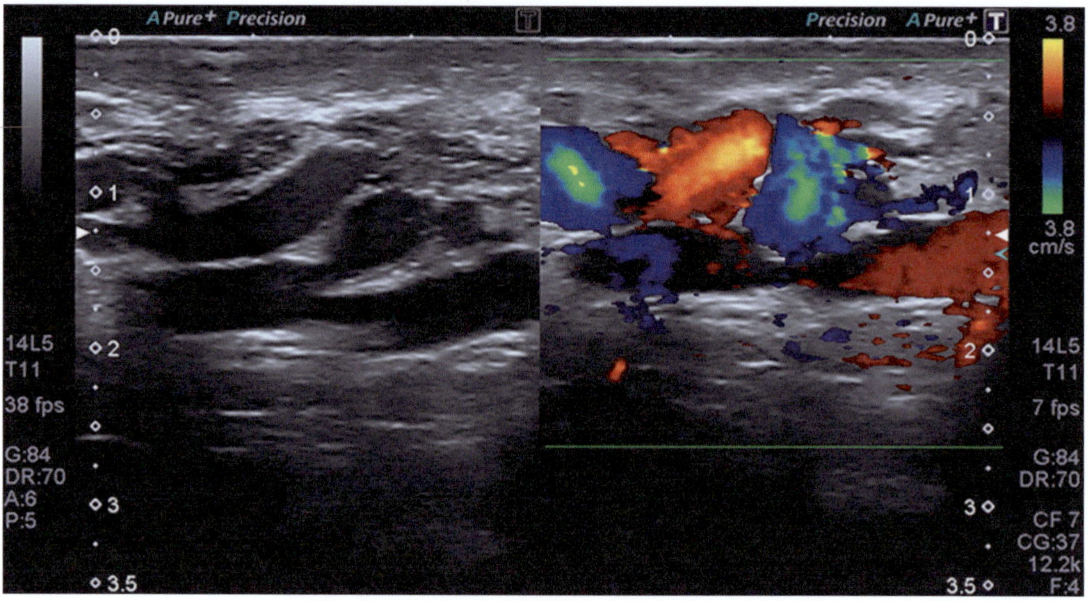

Fig. 23.1 Scrotal ultrasound Doppler shows a marked varicocele

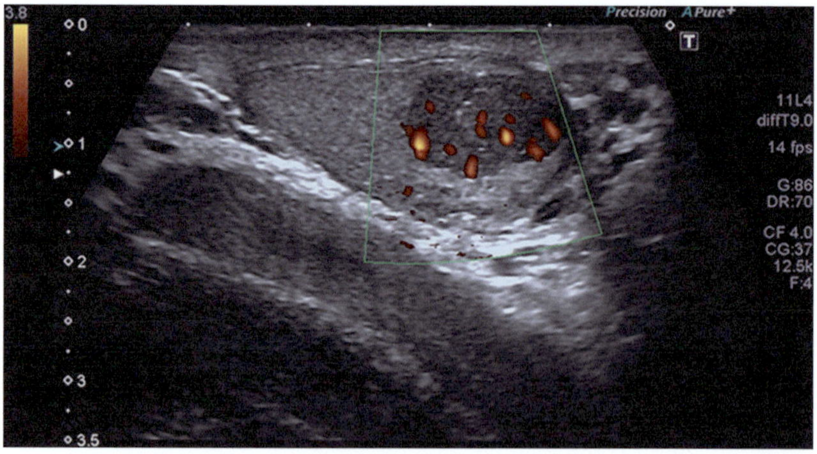

Fig. 23.2 Scrotal ultrasound Doppler evidence a mild left varicocele associated with testicular tumor (*inside green lines*)

There are many possibilities for a surgical treatment of varicocele:

1. Open surgery with three surgical techniques: (a) high retroperitoneal varicocelectomy (Palomo technique with gonadal vein ligation), (b) open inguinal varicocelectomy (Ivanissevich-Buntz technique), and (c) subinguinal microsurgery approach (Marmar technique) (Fig. 23.3)
2. Laparoscopic surgery with a technique similar to Palomo's open surgery
3. Antegrade or retrograde embolization or sclerotherapy of the spermatic veins

23.2.1 Open Surgery

High Retroperitoneal Approach (Palomo Technique) This technique of varicocelectomy was described in 1949 by Palomo [3]. It is a fast technique; it is carried out by means of a transverse incision above the internal inguinal

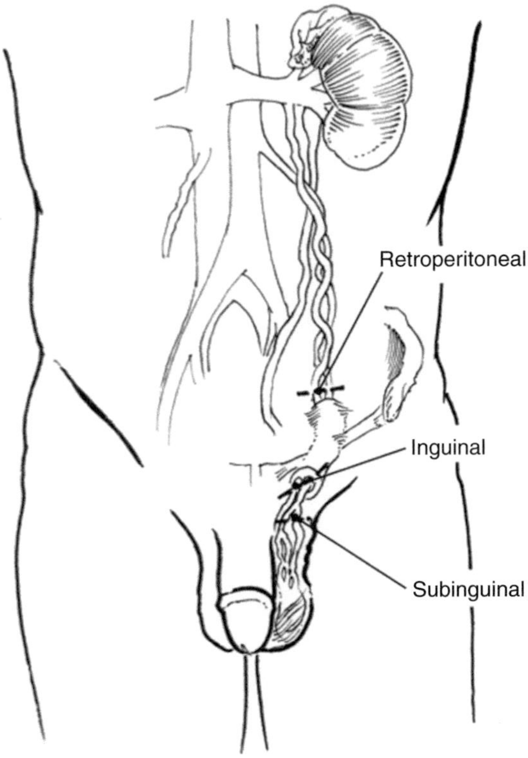

Fig. 23.3 Location of areas of spermatic veins ligation for varicocele treatment

ring, opening of the oblique muscles, and exposure of the testicular artery and the internal spermatic vein near the ureter at the retroperitoneal level. Generally, at this level, the testicular artery has not yet been divided and is clearly different from the neighboring venous trunks, thus avoiding their injury (Fig. 23.4).

The main disadvantage of this technique is its high incidence of recurrence (15 %) and the presence of secondary hydroceles [4]. Fretz et al. [5] reported a higher percentage of recurrences that can reach up to 25 %, also indicated by Pascual et al. [6], compared with rates of varicocele recurrence with the inguinal approach that have been estimated at 5.5 % [6].

Inguinal Approach (Ivanissevich-Buntz Technique) This technique was described by Ivanissevich in 1918 [7]. His experience in 4470 patients was subsequently reported in 1960 [8]. It has the advantage of allowing to pull the spermatic cord out of the inguinal wound, making it easier to identify the testicular artery, the nodes, the internal spermatic vein, and the small periarterial veins (Fig. 23.5).

This open inguinal approach has an incidence of recurrence between 8 and 10 %. The most common complication is the hydrocele with an incidence between 3 and 15 %.

Subinguinal Microsurgery Varicocelectomy (Marmar Technique) This surgical technique was described by Marmar in 1985 [9]. The intervention begins by identifying the external inguinal ring and infiltrating it with lidocaine 1 % and then performing a 2–3 cm incision to expose the spermatic cord, which is taken with a Babcock clamp. The cord is separated and microscopic dissection is performed to preserve the lymphatics vessels and the testicular artery. Papaverine can be used to locate the artery; applying this substance on the surgical field also prevents an arterial spasm. All cord veins exceeding 3 mm in diameter are ligated.

In 466 surgical procedures, Marmar and Kim [10] report an incidence of varicocele recurrence of 2.1 % with this technique. The most frequent complications were epididymal discomfort (5.5 %) and hydrocele (0.8 %).

This subinguinal technique is more thorough and safe in terms of preventing recurrence, and it is less painful when performed below the inguinal ring. Postoperative recurrence is markedly lower as compared with the high ligation and the subinguinal microsurgery techniques (15.51 % vs. 2.11 %), as reported by Cayan et al. [11]. According to Fretz et al., recurrence after the subinguinal approach is only 1 % [5]. Also, in the Cayan et al.'s series [11], the incidence of postoperative hydrocele was significantly lower in the group of patients undergoing microsurgery (9.09 % in the Palomo surgery vs. 0.69 % in the subinguinal microsurgery). If this technique is performed including release of the testis and ligation of the gubernaculum testis veins, the recurrence rate is even lower (0.5 %) [12]. The most frequent complications are epididymis discomfort (5 %) and hydrocele (0.8 %).

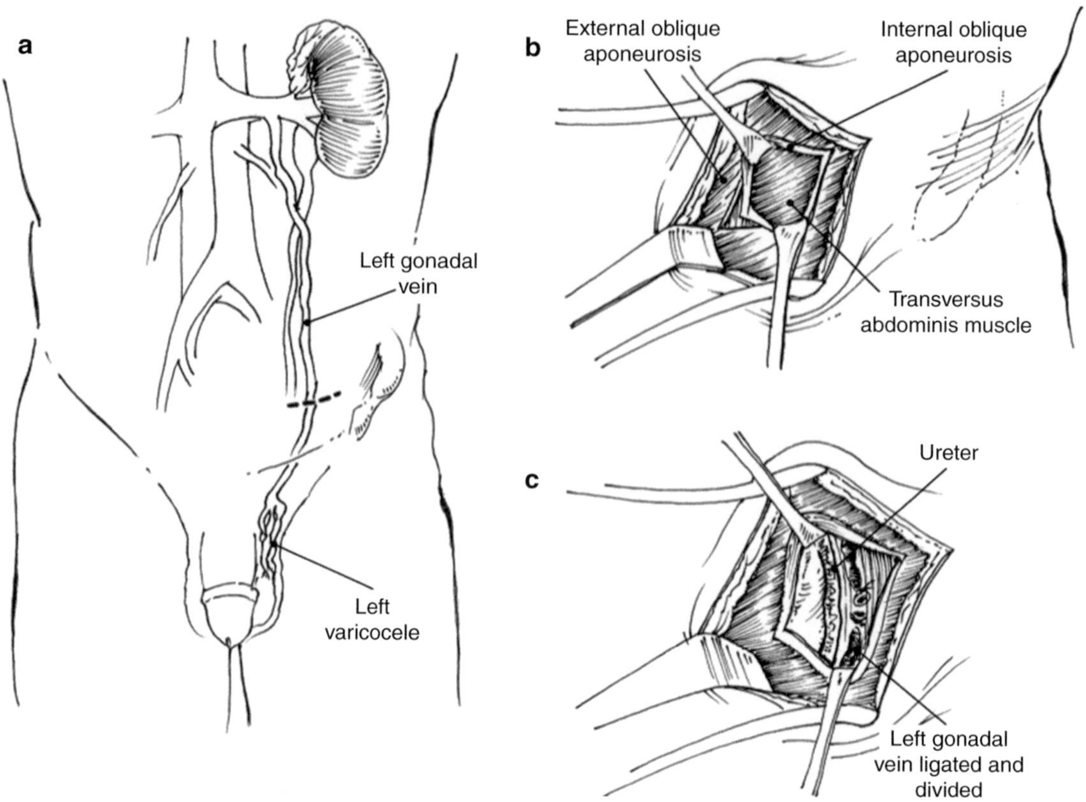

Fig. 23.4 Palomo technique. Scheme showing the level of spermatic veins ligation (**a**), the surgical access through the different anatomical structures (**b**), and location of spermatic veins at the retroperitoneum (**c**)

23.2.2 Laparoscopic Surgery

Although the more frequently used surgical techniques to repair varicocele are those of open surgery, the laparoscopic approach is possible too. The spermatic cord is located opening a small window of retroperitoneum through a transperitoneal approach. Spermatic vessels (artery and spermatic veins), vas deferens, and lymphatic vessels are identified. This identification maneuver is eased by the vision that laparoscopic optics provide. Subsequently, clips are placed in the spermatic veins, and they are cut with scissors. However, there are some detractors [13] who believe that the laparoscopic technique turns a retroperitoneal technique into a transabdominal one and makes a quick procedure to be a slower and more morbid one (by the number of incisions, optical, and working channel). Among the advantages of the laparoscopic procedure, we can mention that magnification through laparoscopic optics enables to preserve the lymphatic vessels and the gonadal artery, nothing that cannot equally be achieved by the subinguinal open microsurgery. Finally, some authors [13] believe that profitability in terms of cost-effectiveness is lower in the laparoscopic technique than in open surgery.

Nowadays, with the simplification of the laparoscopic technique to a single port, the complications associated with multiple laparoscopic ports can be avoided, achieving the same clinical efficacy than with conventional laparoscopy and open surgery [14].

Most pediatric urologists in the USA prefer the laparoscopic approach (54 %) in part because of its high success rate but also because it facilitates the preservation of lymphatics, which in turn keeps the incidence of postoperative hydroceles low [15–18]. While saving the artery can be accomplished laparoscopically, it is associated

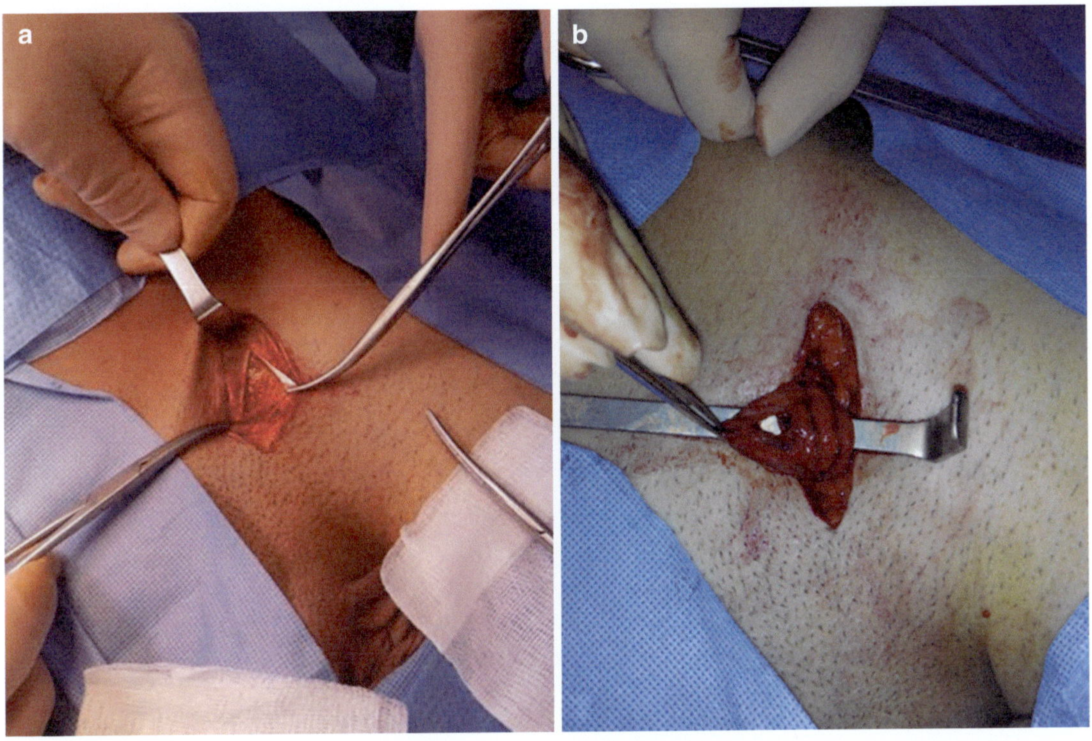

Fig. 23.5 Small right inguinal incision to perform the varicocelectomy. Note the opening of the oblique muscle aponeurosis (**a**). Exposure of pre-ligation spermatic cord elements and section of the spermatic veins (**b**) spermatic cord

with a higher recurrence rate [17–19]. However, Zampieri et al. [19] found that saving the artery led to better postoperative semen parameters than when the artery was ligated.

23.2.3 Retrograde and Antegrade Embolization or Sclerotherapy of the Spermatic Veins

Radiological techniques of occlusion or sclerotherapy have been used successfully in the treatment of varicocele. They consist of the occlusion of the internal spermatic vein by a balloon, a coil, or sclerosing substances, easy preservation of blood and lymphatic vessels that eliminate the risk of testicular atrophy, and postsurgical hydrocele. However, either by occlusion or sclerotherapy, these procedures present similar rates of recurrence than through retroperitoneal open or laparoscopic surgery.

Retrograde Endovascular Embolization The first description of the spermatic vein embolization was performed by Iaccarino et al. in 1980 [20]. Embolization to occlude the spermatic vein has varying levels depending on the anatomy of the vein itself. Embolization can be performed using coils, balloons, or gelfoam as occluding agents. It is an invasive and complex imaging technique, which can require between 1 and 3 h to be performed. Note that this technique fails to be performed in 15 % of cases. Reported technical problems with embolization include difficulty in cannulated tributaries of testicular veins and the high number of parallel collateral veins, perforation of the vein with [21].

Techniques of percutaneous transluminal approach, either femoral or jugular, represent a good alternative, with success rates of 95 % immediate and 89–95 % long term [22–25] (Figs. 23.6 and 23.7). In older adolescents that collaborate, they can be performed under local anesthesia,

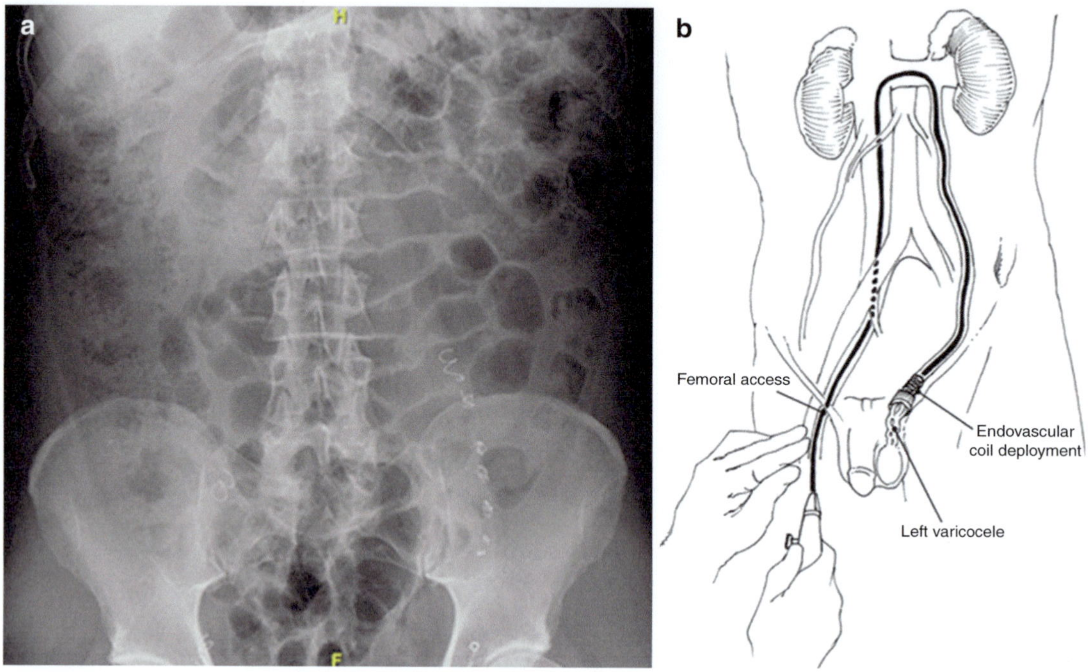

Fig. 23.6 Transfemoral approach for varicocele embolization. X-ray figure showing the coils used for retrograde transfemoral embolization (**a**). Scheme of transfemoral approach for varicocele embolization (**b**)

with return to school life almost immediately. From the technical point of view, they present some difficulties that require good equipment and experience and to assume the anatomical variability that can be found [26].

Antegrade Scrotal Sclerotherapy This surgical technique was first described by Tauber and Johnson in 1993 [27], and its results were published in 1994 [23]. It consists of the isolation of a vein in the pampiniform plexus through a scrotal incision and to inject a sclerosing agent such as ethoxysclerol into the lumen. Data reported by several authors [28, 29] confirm a high percentage of success with a very low percentage of complication, as persistent/recurrent varicocele was documented in only 5 % of the cases. A recent meta-analysis shows that anterograde scrotal sclerotherapy and microsurgical repair are superior to other techniques (open, retroperitoneal surgery, laparoscopic approach) in terms of hydrocele formation [30]. The lower risk of hydrocele formation for anterograde scrotal sclerotherapy in comparison with the open surgical approach was previously highlighted in a randomized prospective study [31].

23.3 Results of Surgical Techniques

To obtain conclusions on pregnancy rates based on the type of repair, the information must be deduced from the adult population. CAYAN et al. [32] analyzed 36 studies to define which technique affords the highest pregnancy rate after varicocele repair. They concluded that microsurgical varicocelectomy is associated with higher spontaneous pregnancy rates and less postoperative recurrence compared to other varicocelectomy techniques and radiological embolization in infertile men.

Diegidio et al. [33] reviewed pooled data from more than 5000 patients in 33 studies. Overall pregnancy rate was 38 % and the highest rate for the subinguinal (45 %) or inguinal (42 %) microsurgical technique compared to the Palomo pro-

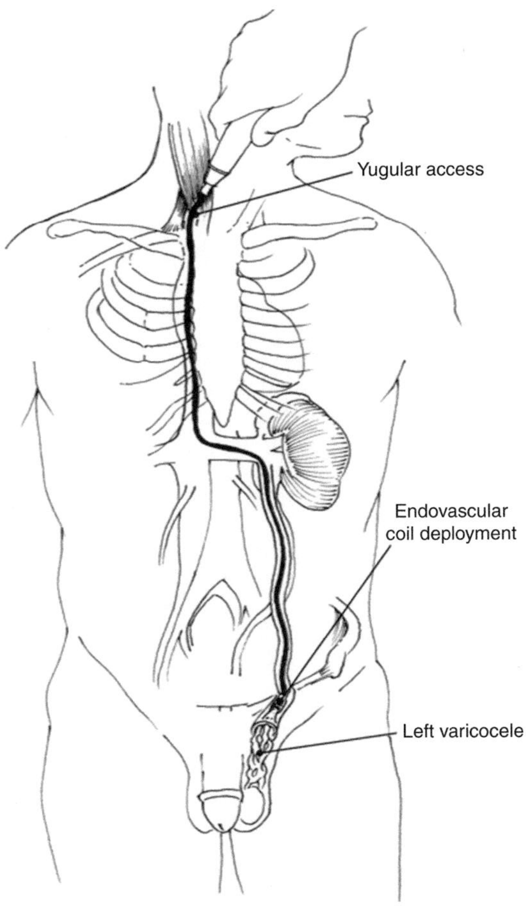

Fig. 23.7 Scheme of transjugular approach for varicocele embolization

cedure (34 %), radiological embolization (32 %), conventional inguinal repair (31 %), and laparoscopic technique (28 %).

A meta-analysis including two randomized controlled trials and three observational studies evaluated pregnancy rates after varicocelectomy among men with grade I to III varicoceles and at least one abnormal semen parameter [34]. The authors concluded that varicocele repair has beneficial effects on fertility (OR 2.87). Kim et al. performed a similar meta-analysis and found significant fixed effects (pooled OR of 4.15) [35].

The hormone response to varicocele repair has been evaluated by several authors. Fisch et al. examined the response to GnRH stimulation in boys before and after unilateral varicocele repair and associated testicular atrophy [36]. The FSH response to GnRH stimulation increased following surgery, but they noted that the GnRH stimulation test could not be used to determine which adolescent would benefit from surgical repair.

Kolon considers that the abnormal semen parameters are the most reasonable measurements that are potentially predictive of future fertility [37]. All boys with varicoceles should undergo yearly assessment of the testicular size (preferably with an orchidometer for cost savings), or every other year if the total testicular volume is normal, until the patient reaches Tanner V maturity. The patient can then be offered semen analysis and perhaps androgen hormone levels, testing pituitary, Sertoli cell, and Leydig cell function (LH, FSH, testosterone, anti-Müllerian hormone, inhibin B). A semen analysis discussion with the patient and his family should consider all individual ethical and religious concerns. If the total testicular volume is low, semen parameters are low, androgen laboratory results are abnormal, or the patient is symptomatic (uncommon), varicocele correction should be discussed.

As in adults, abnormal serial semen analyses with or without testicular hypotrophy are an indication for varicocele repair. If observation remains to be the treatment, follow-up with an adult urologist should be encouraged until paternity is achieved. It seems that all patients with varicocele should be followed until adulthood if we wish to determine during adolescence the best parameters that predict adult fertility. Only then we will really know whether we are making a difference in the overall testicular health of these patients [37].

References

1. Male Infertility Best Practice Policy Committee of the American Urological Association and Practice Committee of the American Society for Reproductive Medicine: Report on varicocele and infertility. Fertil Steril Suppl. 2004;82:S142.
2. Jungwirth A, Giwercman A, Tournaye H, Diemer T, Kopa Z, Dohle G, Krausz C. European Association of Urology Working Group on Male Infertility. European Association of Urology Guidelines on Male Infertility: the 2012 update. Eur Urol. 2012;62:324–32.
3. Palomo A. Radical cure of varicocele with a new technique: preliminary report. J Urol. 1949;61:604–7.

4. Goldstein M. Varicocelectomy: subinguinal approach surgery of male infertility, vol. 178. New York: Saunders; 1995.
5. Fretz PC, Sandlow JL. Varicocele: current concepts in pathophysiology, diagnosis, and treatment. Urol Clin North Am. 2002;29:921–37.
6. Pascual D, Rodriguez Vela L, Gonzalvo A, García Jalón A, Mallén E, Rioja LA. Treatment of varicocele by microsurgical techniques. Arch Esp Urol. 2004;57: 929–39.
7. Ivanissevich O, Gregorini H. A new operation for the cure of varicocele. Semana Med. 1918;25:575.
8. Ivanissevich O. Left varicocele due to reflux; experience with 4,470 operative cases in forty-two years. J Int Coll Surg. 1960; 34:742–755.
9. Marmar JL, De Benedictis DJ, Praiss D. The management of varicoceles by micro-dissection of spermatic cord at the external inguinal ring. Fertil Steril. 1985;43:583–8.
10. Marmar JL, Kim Y. Subinguinal microsurgical varicocelectomy: a technical critique and statistical analysis of semen and pregnancy data. J Urol. 1994;152:1127–32.
11. Cayan S, Kadioglu TC, Tefekli A, Kadioglu A, Tellaloglu S. Comparison of results and complications of high ligation surgery and microsurgical high inguinal varicocelectomy in the treatment of varicocele. Urology. 2000;55:750–4.
12. Goldstein M, Gilbert BR, Dicker AP, Dwosh J, Gnecco C. Microsurgical inguinal varicocelectomy of the testis: an artery and lymphatic sparing technique. J Urol. 1992;148:1808–11.
13. De la Peña E, Caffaratti J, Garat JM. Varicocele treatment in adolescents. Arch Esp Urol. 2004;57:995–1002.
14. Chen Q, Zhong L, S W, S S, G J, Sun J. Laparoscopic varicocelectomy with single incision in children. Laparosc Urol. 2015;12:1–4.
15. Kocvara R, Dvoracek J, Sedlacek J, Díte Z, Novák K. Lymphatic sparing laparoscopic varicocelectomy: a microsurgical repair. J Urol. 2005;173:1751–4.
16. Glassberg KI, Poon SA, Gjertson CK, De Castro GJ, Misseri R. Laparoscopic lymphatic sparing varicocelectomy in adolescents. J Urol. 2008;180:326–30.
17. Glassberg KI, Badalato GM, Fast A, et al. Laparoscopic varicocelectomy: a single surgeon's experience with over 500 cases. Pediatric Urology Fall Congress. Las Vegas, 20–22 Sept 2013.
18. Harel M, Herbst KW, Nelson E. Practice patterns in surgical approach for adolescent varicocelectomy. Springerplus. 2015;4:772.
19. Zampieri N, Zuin V, Corroppolo M, Chironi C, Cervellione RM, Camoglio FS. Varicocele and adolescents: semen quality after 2 different laparoscopic procedures. J Androl. 2007;28:727–33.
20. Iaccarino V. A nonsurgical treatment of varicocele: trans-catheter sclerotherapy of gonadal veins. Ann Radiol. 1980;23:369–70.
21. Wheatley J, Bergman W, Greeb B, Walther MM. Transvenous occlusion of clinical and subclinical varicocele. Urology. 1991;37:362–5.
22. Kaufman SL, Kadir S, Barth KH. Mechanisms of recurrent varicocele after balloon occlusion or surgical ligation of the internal spermatic vein. Radiology. 1983;147:435–40.
23. Tauber R, Johnsen N. Antegrade scrotal sclerotherapy for the treatment of varicocele: technique and late results. J Urol. 1994;151:386–90.
24. Ferguson JM, Gillespie IN, Chalmers N, Elton RA, Hargreave TB. Percutaneous varicocele embolization in the treatment of infertility. Br J Radiol. 1995;68:700–3.
25. Cornud F, Belin X, Amar E, Delafontaine D, Hélénon O, Moreau JF. Varicocele: strategies in diagnosis and treatment. Eur Radiol. 1999;9:536–45.
26. Aguilar Rivilla E, de la Peña ZE, Gallego Beuter J, Mendez JV, Santos E, Delgado JA, Blazquez J. Dificultades en el tratamiento del varicocele sintomático mediante embolizaciónpercutánea: la vena renal circumaortica. Arch Esp Urol. 2002;55:497–500.
27. Tauber R, Johnsen N. Antegrade scrotal sclerotherapy for treatment of testicular varicocele. Technique and late results. Urologe A. 1993;32:320–6.
28. Mottriea M, Matani Y, Baert J, Voges GE, Hohenfellner R. Antegrade scrotal sclerotherapy for the treatment of varicocele in childhood and adolescence. Br J Urol. 1995;76:21–4.
29. Crestani A, Giannarini G, Calandriello M, Rossanese M, Mancini M, Novara G, Ficarra V. Anterograde scrotal sclerotherapy of internal spermatic veins for varicocele treatment: technique, complications and results. Asian J Urol. 2016;18:292.5.
30. Wang J, Xia SL, Liu ZH, Tao L, Ge JF, Xu CM, Qiu JX. Inguinal and subinguinal micro-varicocelectomy, the optimal surgical management of varicocele: a meta-analysis. Asian J Androl. 2015;17:74–80.
31. Fayez A, El Shantaly KM, Abbas M, Hauser S, Müller SC, Fathy A. Comparison of inguinal approach, scrotal sclerotherapy and subinguinal anterograde sclerotherapy in varicocele treatment: a randomized prospective study. Urol Int. 2010;85:200–3.
32. Cayan S, Shavakhabov S, Kadioglu A. Treatment palpable varicocele in infertile men: a meta-analysis to define the best technique. J Androl. 2009;30: 33–40.
33. Diegidio P, Jhaveri JK, Ghannam S, Pinkhasov R, Shabsigh R, Fisch H. Review of current varicocelectomy techniques and their outcomes. BJU Int. 2011;108:1157–72.
34. Marmar JL, Agarwal A, Prabakaran S, Agarwal R, Short RA, Benoff S, Thomas Jr AJ. Reassessing the value of varicocelectomy as a treatment for male subfertility with a new meta-analysis. Fertil Steril. 2007;88:639–48.
35. Kim KH, Lee JY, Kang DH, Lee H, Seo JT, Cho KS. Impact of surgical varicocele repair on pregnancy rate in subfertile men with clinical varicocele and impaired semen quality: a meta-analysis of randomized clinical trials. Korean J Urol. 2013;54:703–9.
36. Fisch H, Hyun G, Hensle TW. Testicular growth and gonadotropin response associated with varicocele repair in adolescent males. BJU Int. 2003;91:75–8.
37. Kolon TF. Evaluation and management of the adolescent varicocele. J Urol. 2015;194:1194–201.

24 Testicular Involvement in Noninfectious Vasculitis

Manuel Nistal, Pilar González-Peramato, and
Álvaro Serrano

24.1 Polyarteritis Nodosa (PAN)

Polyarteritis nodosa is a multisystem form of necrotizing vasculitis that affects the medium- and small-size muscular arteries of the kidney, liver, heart, adrenal glands, gastrointestinal tract, joints, spleen, lungs, and central nervous system. The annual incidence is estimated at 0.7/100,000, and males between the fourth and sixth decades of life are preferably affected.

In PAN both the testis and the epididymis are affected [1]. In autopsy series its frequency is estimated, between 60 and 86 %. Only 2–18 % of cases are symptomatic [2]. In exceptional cases epididymal and/or testicular involvement is the first manifestation of the disease. In these cases the clinical symptoms may be orchitis, epididymitis, testicular torsion, or tumor [3, 4].

The definitive diagnosis is histological. The testis or epididymis usually shows arterial lesions at different evolutionary moments (fibrinoid necrosis, inflammatory reaction, thrombosis, or aneurysm) even in the same organ. The parenchyma shows areas of infarction, more or less extensive at first and tubular sclerosis with interstitial fibrosis later.

The etiology of PAN is unknown. Most cases are idiopathic. There are patients that associate PAN with autoimmune diseases (rheumatoid arthritis, lupus erythematosus), infectious diseases (hepatitis B and C, HIV), or tumor. In three patients with PAN testicular involvement, neoplasia (prostate adenocarcinoma, acute myelogenous leukemia, and hairy-cell leukemia and hepatocellular carcinoma) was associated. Contrary to microscopic polyangiitis, Wegener's disease, and Churg-Strauss syndrome, antineutrophil cytoplasmic antibodies (ANCA) are not present in classic PAN.

Isolated Arteritis of the Testis and Epididymis With the same testicular symptoms, necrotizing arteritis affecting only the testis and/or epididymis (isolated arteritis of the testis and epididymis) has been reported [5] (Fig. 24.1). In some cases involvement of either both the testes or epididymis, usually metachronous, occurs. In rare cases, testicular involvement may be recurrent [6]. Isolated arteritis of the testis and epididymis is occasionally associated with both nonseminoma [7] and seminomatous (own observation) germ cell tumors (Fig. 24.2).

The etiology of localized arteritis is unknown although the possibility has been seriously considered that isolated arteritis represents a local hypersensitivity reaction of type III. This isolated arteritis has also been described in other organs such as the appendix, gallbladder, pancreas, breast, uterus, cervix uteri, synovium, kidney, skeletal muscles, and seminal vesicle. Anyway, in the presence of histological evidence of necrotizing arteritis affecting the testis or the epididymis, clinical, hematological, and biochemical studies have to be performed as they are necessary to exclude a PAN-type systemic disease.

M. Nistal et al., *Clues in the Diagnosis of Non-tumoral Testicular Pathology*,
DOI 10.1007/978-3-319-49364-0_24

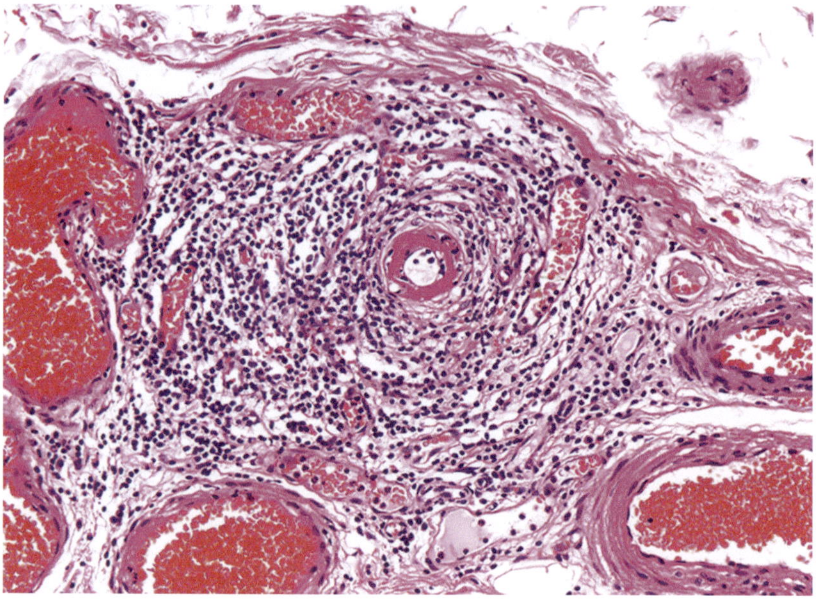

Fig. 24.1 PAN-type isolated epididymal arteritis. Small arterioles with fibrinoid necrosis are surrounded dense by lymphocyte infiltration

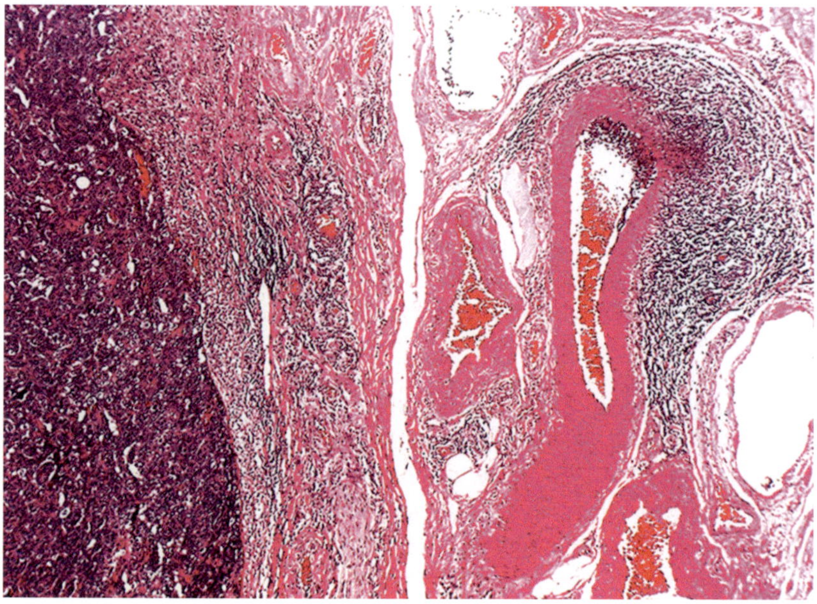

Fig. 24.2 PAN-type arteritis of the epididymis associated with a testicular germ cell tumor (embryonal carcinoma). The vascular lesion is focal and segmental

The prognosis of isolated necrotizing arteritis is excellent even without a steroid treatment [8, 9].

24.2 Henoch-Schönlein Purpura

It is a disease of unknown etiology characterized by leukocytoclastic vasculitis that mainly affects the skin, gastrointestinal tract, joints, and kidneys. It is more common in males, and the highest incidence (20 cases per 100,000) occurs between 4 and 6 years [10]. The incidence of involvement of the scrotum and its contents is between 2.4 and 38 % [11]. It may be unilateral or bilateral. The major clinical symptoms are pain and scrotal swelling, which are usually preceded 1 week before by purpuric lesions on the skin of both legs [12, 13].

The histology of lesions in the testis and epididymis is similar to that of the skin. It is a leukocytoclastic vasculitis (involvement of small vessels with endothelial swelling, red cell extravasation, and infiltration by polynuclear neutrophils with plenty of cariorrhesis).

In those cases in which scrotal pain is the first manifestation of the disease the differential diagnosis can be made with all situations that present with an acute scrotum and testicular torsion, torsion of the appendix testis and epididymis, epididymitis, orchitis, hernia, hydrocele, trauma, testicular tumor, and idiopathic scrotal edema [14]. An isotopic study with Tc99 and/or ecodoppler dismisses the most serious testicular lesion of ischemia by torsion [15, 16].

24.3 Wegener's Granulomatosis

Wegener's granulomatosis is a multisystemic disease associated with cytosplasmic antineutrophil antibody (ANCA). It presents with glomerulonephritis, necrotizing granulomatous inflammation of the medium- and small-caliber vessels of the upper and lower respiratory tract, and high ANCA levels. It is diagnosed between 45 and 60 years of age, and its prevalence is estimated at 22–157 cases per million [17]. Involvement of the urogenital tract is rare (less than 1 % of patients). Involvement of the testis occurs between 12.5 and 36 % of patients with urogenital tract involvement [18]. Clinically it mimics orchitis. The epididymis is affected in 10 % of patients with clinical epididymitis [19] and isolated epididymal lesion [20] or associated with the testicular lesion [21] that may be the only site of the disease. The arteries show fibrinoid necrosis with intense neutrophil infiltration, epithelioid cells, and multinucleated giant cells [22] (Fig. 24.3). The result is multiple testicular infarcts.

Granulomatous Vasculitis Associated with Germ Cell Tumor The presence of granulomas in the testicle is usually associated with an infection (mycobacteria, fungi), an autoimmune disease (idiopathic granulomatous orchitis), or germ cell tumors as seminoma. Granulomatous vasculitis involving both peritumoral arteries and contralateral testis has been observed in the biopsies of two patients with classic seminoma in our department, in the absence of clinical or laboratory symptoms of Wegener's granulomatosis. The infiltrate was circumferential, affected the media and adventitia of the small arteries of the epididymis and

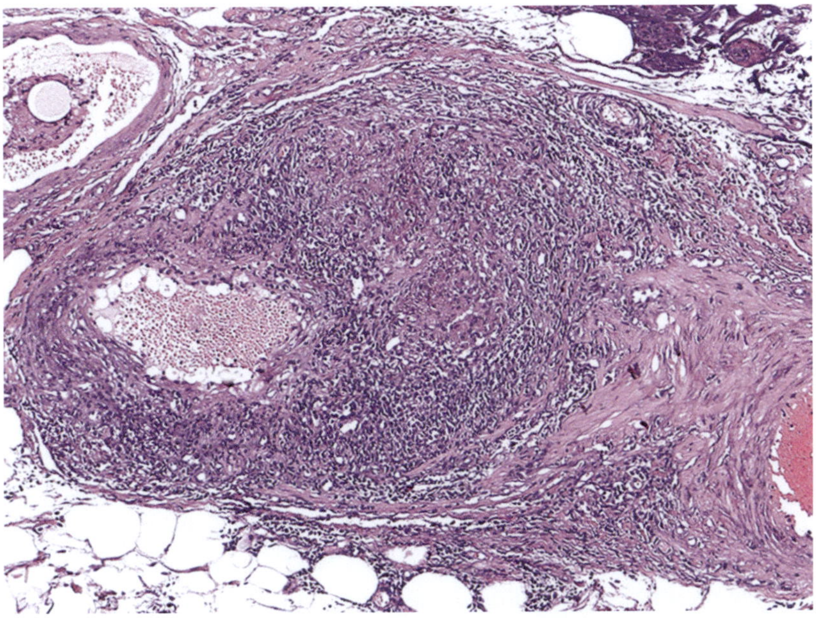

Fig. 24.3 Granulomatous arteritis in a vessel of the spermatic cord. Eccentric vascular lesion associated with an infiltrate composed of lymphoid cells, macrophages and giant cells

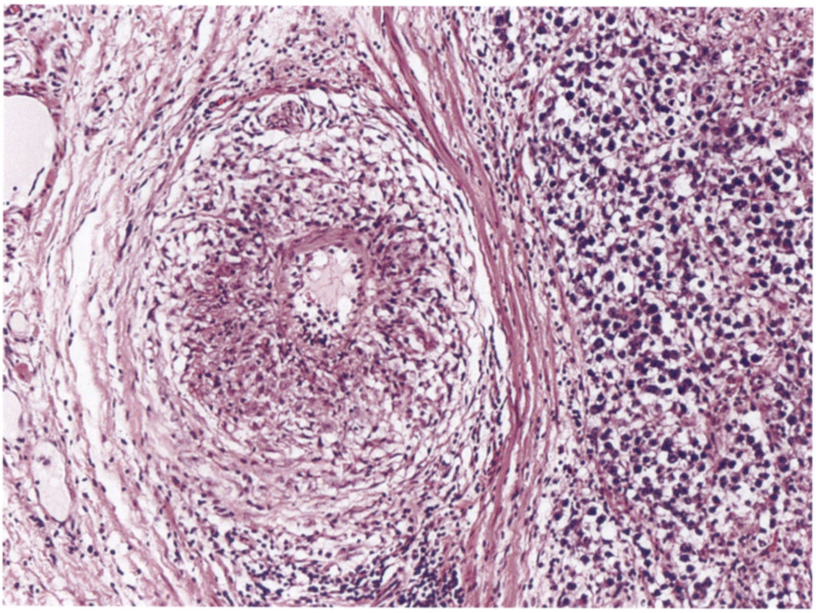

Fig. 24.4 Granulomatous arteritis with circumferential involvement of a vessel associated with seminoma. The inflammatory infiltrate locates in the media and extends to the adventitia

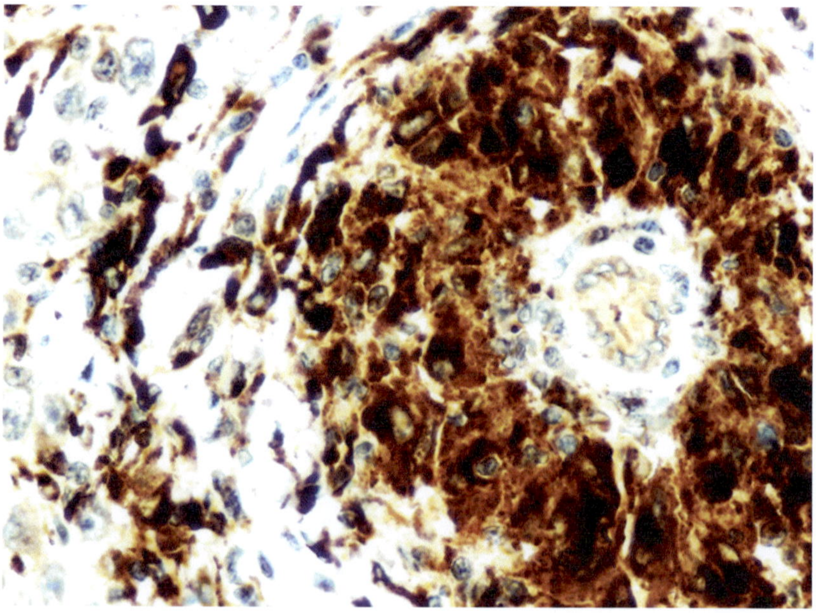

Fig. 24.5 Granulomatous arteritis associated seminoma, same case of the previous figure. The inflammatory infiltrate is rich in CD68 positive cells

the intratesticular arteries. The infiltrate was characterized by the presence of abundant epithelioid and multinucleate giant cells associated with a small number of lymphocytes that thickened the vascular wall and stenosed the vessel lumen (Figs. 24.4 and 24.5). In the contralateral testis, the most important findings of the biopsy were spermatogenesis was poor, no GCNIS, and the presence of vasculitis. In some vessels it consisted only in a dense infiltration of T lymphocytes in concentric rings. In the most advanced lesions, there were associated epithelioid cells destroying the vessel wall [23] (Fig. 24.6). As both cases were seminomas, and these often show significant sarcoid reaction, it is possible that these vasculites were the result of a reaction to circulating antigens released by tumor cells.

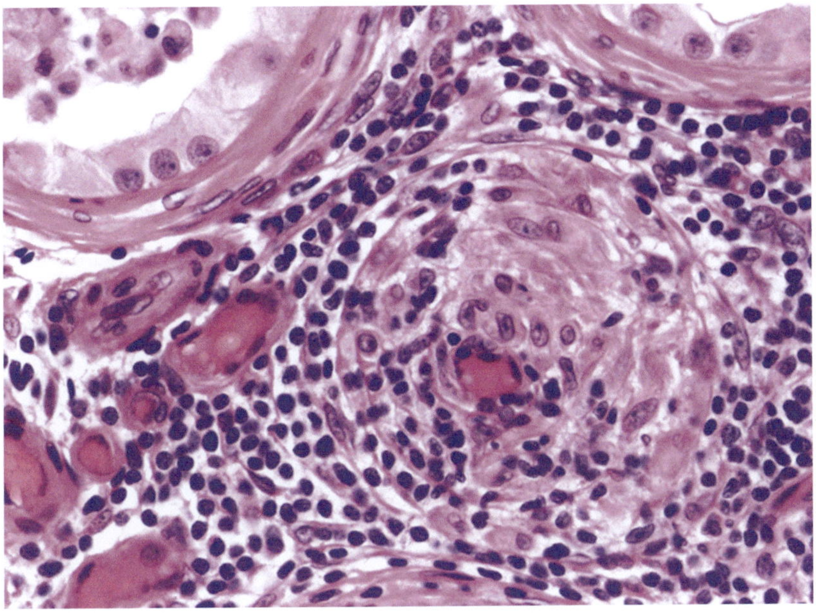

Fig. 24.6 Granulomatous arteritis in the contralateral testicular biopsy of a patient with seminoma. Dense infiltrate composed of lymphoid and epithelioid cells is shown in the wall of a small arteriole. The seminiferous tubules have no GCNIS

24.4 Giant Cell Arteritis

Granulomatous vasculitis similar to that affecting the temporal artery has been observed in other locations (heart, renal arteries, gallbladder artery and veins of the lower extremities). The spermatic cord, testis, and epididymis vessels [24] may be affected in the context of a widespread disease. The clinical symptom is a testicular mass that simulates a malignant tumor [25]. Lesions are formed by a granulomatous reaction with preferably giant cells in the intima of the vessels centered in the internal elastic that appears fragmented [26].

Another granulomatous vasculitis with a histological pattern similar to the temporal artery arteritis is Takayasu's disease. In a 7-year-old patient, testicular involvement developed in the course of the disease [27].

24.5 Thromboangiitis Obliterans (TAO)

Thromboangiitis obliterans is a rare disease that affects Asians more often than Westerners. It affects middle-aged and heavy-smoking men. The initial symptom is usually intermittent claudication as popliteal arteries and their branches usually are affected. The disease is progressive and leads to gangrene of the extremities. In some patients it also affects the coronary, cerebral, and mesenteric arteries. Thromboangiitis obliterans of the spermatic vessels can present either as part of a pattern of systemic involvement [28, 29] as an isolated manifestation of the disease [30–32] or simulating a tumor of the spermatic cord [33]. Lesions are recognized macroscopically as nodular indurations along the spermatic cord.

Histologically, affectation of both arteries and veins is observed. The injury is typically segmental. Lesions vary with disease duration. In the initial lesions, a thrombus with polymorphonuclear microabscesses and multinucleated giant cells is observed. Infiltrates extend to all layers. The internal elastic lamina remains. In the intermediate stage, there is a progressive organization of the thrombus; infiltrates are predominantly mononuclear, with occasional epithelioid cells with or without Langhans' cells. In the latter case, the thrombus is recanalized, and fibrosis of the vascular wall without loss of elastic laminae occurs. Fibrosis extends and encases veins and nerves. The adipose tissue of the spermatic cord and paratesticular structures is also affected, and often an ischemic paniculitis can be observed at the same time than steatonecrosis areas, lipogranulomas, and esteatofibrosis (Fig. 24.7).

Macroscopic differential diagnosis arises in some cases with tumors of paratesticular structures. Histologically, it has to do with PAN, arteriosclerosis obliterans (ASO), and thromboembolism. Regarding PAN, in the TAO there is no destruction of the vascular wall, aneurysms are not formed, and the internal elastic of the arteries is unaffected. The differential diagnosis between chronic lesions of TAO and ASO can be difficult. The presence of onion-like-shaped recanalizing vessels in the occluded arteries, adventitial fibrosis without medial fibrosis, swelling of the endothelium of the vasa vasorum, and edema beneath the external elastic lamina are considered to be characteristic of the TAO [34]. Thromboembolism and TAO can

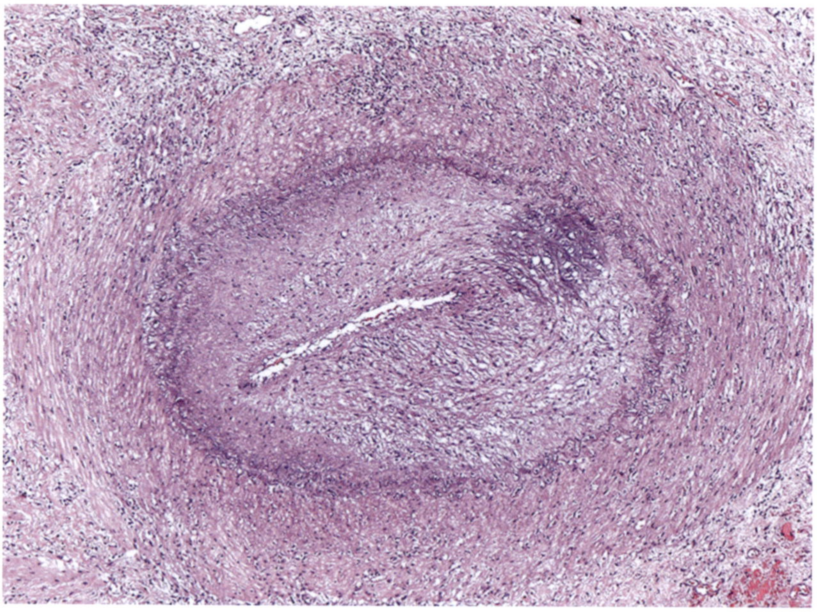

Fig. 24.7 Thromboangiitis obliterans in a vessel of the spermatic cord. Lesions affect the media and the adventitia and extend to nearby tissues as it is observed in evolved lesions

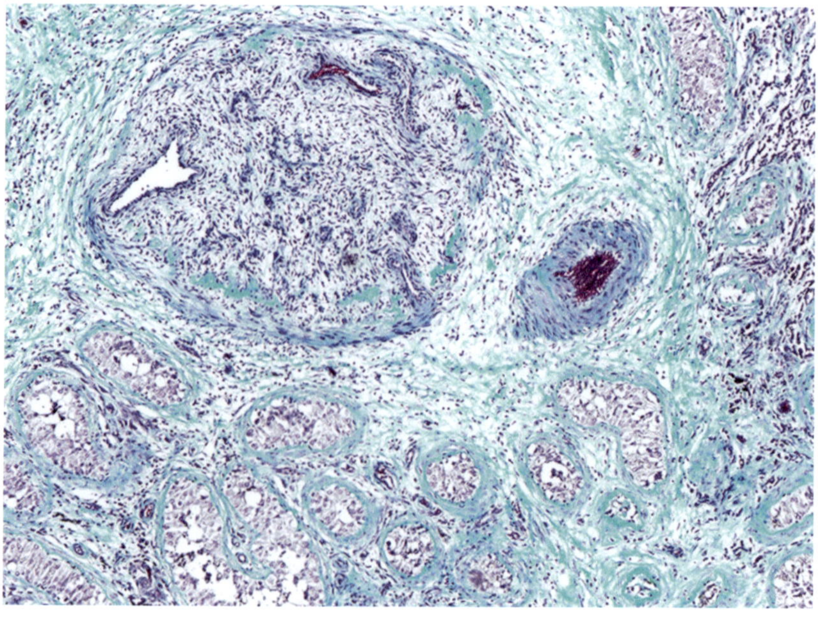

Fig. 24.8 Thromboembolism in an intraparenchymal testicular artery. Lesions preferably consist of recanalization of the thrombus. The testicular parenchyma shows an important atrophy of the seminiferous tubules

share intimal inflammation and intact media, but in thromboembolism inflammatory infiltrates are not important outside the intima, and most of the time, there is no involvement of veins and nerves (Fig. 24.8).

24.6 Kogan's Disease

Kogan's disease is an autoimmune multisystem disease that predominantly appears in children and young adults. Initially described as an association of eye (interstitial keratitis) and auditory (sensorineural deafness and vestibular dysfunction) disease, it may occur with other types of eye disease and systemic vasculitis [35, 36]. In 5 % of patients with Kogan's disease, unilateral testicular swelling can be observed [37, 38].

24.7 Behçet's Disease

It is a systemic vasculitis whose clinical manifestations are recurrent aphthous oral and genital ulcers, relapsing uveitis and skin lesions (folliculitis, erythema nodosum-like lesions), and positive pathergy test. Other frequent pathologies present are arthritis, thrombophlebitis, and various neurological syndromes. It has a higher prevalence in countries along the ancient silk route extending from Japan to the Mediterranean and Middle Eastern countries; such prevalence is considerably lower in Northern European and North American countries, which may reflect a genetic predisposition as well as environmental triggering factors [39]. There is a strong association between Behçet's disease and human leukocyte antigen (HLA) type B 51 and HLA-12. Many patients with Behcet's disease are B5101 allele carriers, so this could be a marker that predisposes to the disease [40].

Epididymal and testicular involvement simulates orchitis or epididymis-orchitis, and its variability is related to the geographic area and the age of patients. The incidence is 2 % in France, 6 % in Turkey, 12 % in Greece, 31 % Iraq, and 44 % in Russia [41]. The incidence of orchiepididymitis is higher in adult patients (11.3 %) than in young people (7.7 %). The duration of the testicular symptoms is 1–2 weeks, and it is believed to be secondary to vasculitis. One complication, as in other vasculites, is testicular infarction [42]. Very often patients with Behcet's disease develop AA-type amyloidosis, which determines a poor prognosis [43].

24.8 Vasculitis Associated with Other Processes

In dermatomyositis [44] and relapsing polychondritis [45], isolated cases of vasculitis with testicular involvement have been observed. Treatment with the antibiotic minocycline induces a variety of autoimmune pathologies, among them vasculitis. Testicular vasculitis fulfilling the histological criteria of PAN has been described in patients with rheumatoid arthritis [46, 47] and rosacea [48] treated with minocycline.

References

1. Azar N, Guillevin L, Huong Du LT, Herreman G, Meyrier A, Godeau P. Symptomatic urogenital manifestations of polyarteritis nodosa and Churg-Strauss angiitis: analysis of 8 of 165 patients. J Urol. 1989; 142:136–8.
2. Shurbaji MS, Epstein JI. Testicular vasculitis: implications for systemic disease. Hum Pathol. 1988;19: 186–9.
3. Teichman JM, Mattrey RF, Demby AM, Schmidt JD. Polyarteritis nodosa presenting as acute orchitis: a case report and review of the literature. J Urol. 1993;149:1139–40.
4. Eilber KS, Freedland SJ, Rajfer J. Polyarteritis nodosa presenting as hematuria and a testicular mass. J Urol. 2001;166:624.
5. Maričić A, Stifter S, Valenčić M, Dorđević G, Markić D, Spanjol J, Sotošek S, Fučkar Z. Primary testicular necrotizing vasculitis clinically presented as neoplasm of the testicle: a case report. World J Surg Oncol. 2011;9:63.
6. Tanuma Y, Oda T, Yokoo A, Ito S, Takeuchi K. Recurrent polyarteritis nodosa limited to the testis. J Urol. 2003;170:1953.
7. Fleischmann A, Studer UE. Isolated polyarteritis nodosa of the male reproductive system associated with a germ cell tumor of the testis: a case report. Cardiovasc Pathol. 2007;16:354–6.

8. Fraenkel-Rubin M, Ergas D, Sthoeger ZM. Limited polyarteritis nodosa of the male and female reproductive systems: diagnostic and therapeutic approach. Ann Rheum Dis. 2002;61:362–4.
9. Hernández-Rodríguez J, Tan CD, Koening CL, Khasnis A, Rodríguez ER, Hoffman GS. Testicular vasculitis: findings differentiating isolated disease from systemic disease in 72 patients. Medicine (Baltimore). 2012; 91:75-85.
10. Søreide K. Surgical management of nonrenal genitourinary manifestations in children with Henoch-Schönlein purpura. J Pediatr Surg. 2005;40:1243–7.
11. Chamberlain RS, Greenberg LW. Scrotal involvement in Henoch-Schönlein purpura: a case report and review of the literature. Pediatr Emerg Care. 1992; 8:213–5.
12. Ha TS, Lee JS. Scrotal involvement in childhood Henoch-Schönlein purpura. Acta Paediatr. 2007;96: 552–5.
13. Sakanoue M, Higashi Y, Kawai K, Sugita S, Kanekura T. Henoch-Schönlein purpura with epididymitis in an adult. J Dermatol. 2011;38:620–2.
14. Verim L, Cebeci F, Erdem MR, Somay A. Henoch-Schönlein purpura without systemic involvement beginning with acute scrotum and mimicking torsion of testis. Arch Ital Urol Androl. 2013;85:50–2.
15. Huang LH, Yeung CY, Shyur SD, Lee HC, Huang FY, Wang NL. Diagnosis of Henoch-Schönlein purpura by sonography and radionuclear scanning in a child presenting with bilateral acute scrotum. J Microbiol Immunol Infect. 2004;37:192–5.
16. Güneş M, Kaya C, Koca O, Keles MO, Karaman MI. Acute scrotum in Henoch-Schönlein purpura: fact or fiction? Turk J Pediatr. 2012;54:194–7.
17. Alba MA, Moreno-Palacios J, Beça S, Cid MC. Urologic and male genital manifestations of granulomatosis with polyangiitis. Autoimmun Rev. 2015;14:897–902.
18. Dufour JF, Le Gallou T, JF C, Aumaître O, Pinède L, Aslangul E, Pagnoux C, Marie I, Puéchal X, Decaux O, Dubois A, Agard C, Mahr A, Comoz F, Boutemy J, Broussolle C, Guillevin L, Sève P, Bienvenu B, French Center-East Internists Group, French Vasculitis Study Group. Urogenital manifestations in Wegener granulomatosis: a study of 11 cases and review of the literature. Medicine (Baltimore). 2012;91:67–74.
19. Miller DC, Koss MN. Wegener granulomatosis presenting as epididymitis. Urology. 2009;73:1225–6.
20. Al-Arfaj A. Limited Wegener's granulomatosis of the epididymis. Int J Urol. 2001;8:333–5.
21. Lee SS, Tang SH, Sun GH, Yu CP, Jin JS, Chang SY. Limited Wegener's granulomatosis of the epididymis and testis. Asian J Androl. 2006;8:737–9.
22. Agraharkar M, Gokhale S, Gupta R. Wegener's granulomatosis diagnosed by testicular biopsy. Int Urol Nephrol. 2002–2003; 34:559–64.
23. Nistal M, González-Peramato MP. Chap 15. Vascular testis pathology. In: Jezek D, editor. Atlas on the human testis. London: Springer; 2013. p. 243–51.
24. Arnillas E, de la Fuente J, Núñez M, Domínguez F. Giant cell arteritis with epididymal involvement. Med Clin (Barc). 2009;132:485.
25. Sundaram S, Smith DH. Giant cell arteritis mimicking a testicular tumour. Rheumatol Int. 2001;20:215–6.
26. Zerbino DD. Giant-cell vasculitis (arteritis and phlebitis). Arkh Patol. 1981;43:42–7.
27. Brunette MG, Bonny Y, Spigelblatt L, Barrette G. Long-term immunosuppressive treatment of a child with Takayasu's arteritis and high IgE immunoglobulins. Pediatr Nephrol. 1996;10:67–9.
28. Mathé CP. Thrombo-angiitis obliterans (Buerger's disease) of the spermatic arteries: report of a case. J Urol. 1940;44:768–70.
29. Cope E. Thrombo-angitis obliterans of the spermatic cord. S Afr Med J. 1968;42:872–3.
30. Lee McGregor A, Simson FW. Thrombo-angiitis obliterans: with special reference to a case involving the spermatic vessels. Br J Surg. 1929;16:539–41.
31. Nesbit RM, Hodgon NB. Thrombo-angiitis obliterans of the spermatic cord. J Urol. 1960;83:445–7.
32. Abercrombie GF. Thrombo-angiitis obliterans of the spermatic cord. Br J Surg. 1965;52:632–3.
33. Kuwahara M, Matsushita K, Nakamura K, Yoshinaga H, Aki M, Fujisaki N, Furihata M, Ohtsuki Y. Thromboangiitis obliterans of the spermatic cord: a case report. Hinyokika Kiyo. 1993;39:369–72.
34. Kurata A, Franke FE, Machinami R, Schulz A. Thromboangiitis obliterans: classic and new morphological features. Virchows Arch. 2000;436:59–67.
35. Olfat M, Al-Mayouf SM. Cogan's syndrome in childhood. Rheumatol Int. 2001;20:246–9.
36. García Callejo FJ, Platero Zamarreno A, Sebastian Gil E, Orts Alborch MH, Marco AJ. Atypical Cogan syndrome. Clinical and laboratory spectrum. Report of 2 cases. Acta Otorrinolaringol Esp. 2002;53:191–8.
37. Leff IL. Cogan's syndrome. NY State J Med. 1967;67: 2249–57.
38. Vollertsen RS, McDonald TJ, Younge BR, Banks PM, Stanson AW, Ilstrup DM. Cogan's syndrome: 18 cases and a review of the literature. Mayo Clin Proc. 1986;61:344–61.
39. Verity DH, Marr JE, Ohno S, Wallace GR, Stanford MR. Behcet's disease, the Silk Road and HLA-B51: historical and geographical perspectives. Tissue Antigens. 1999;54:213–20.
40. Koumantaki Y, Stavropoulos C, Spyropoulou M, Messini H, Papademetropoulos M, Giziaki E, Marcomichelakis N, Palimeris G, Kaklamanis P, Kaklamani E. HLA-B*5101 in Greek patients with Behçet's disease. Hum Immunol. 1998;59:250–5.
41. Kaklamani VG, Vaiopoulos G, Markomichelakis N, Kaklamanis P. Recurrent epididymo-orchitis in patients with Behçet's disease. J Urol. 2000;163:487–9.
42. Al-Ani Z, Suut S, Huasen B. Serial ultrasonography assessments of a testicular infarction mimicking testicular tumor in a Behcet disease patient. Urol Case Rep. 2014;2:45–7.
43. Akpolat T, Akpolat I, Kandemir B. Behcet's disease and AA-type amyloidosis. Am J Nephrol. 2000;20:68–70.

44. Jalleh RP, Swift RI, Sundaresan M, Toma A, Wood CB. Necrotising testicular vasculitis associated with dermatomyositis. Br J Urol. 1990;66:660.
45. Pannek J, Haupt G. Orchitis due to vasculitis in autoimmune diseases. Scand J Rheumatol. 1997;26:151–4.
46. Souza AW, Rosa DP, Buosi AL, Oliveira AC, Natour J. Testicular vasculitis: a rare manifestation of rheumatoid arthritis. Rev Bras Reumatol. 2013;53:365–7.
47. Lenert P, Icardi M, Dahmoush L. ANA (+) ANCA (+) systemic vasculitis associated with the use of minocycline: case-based review. Clin Rheumatol. 2013;32:1099–106.
48. Lyon TD, Ferroni MC, Casella DP, D'Agostino LA, Jackman SV. Segmental testicular infarction due to minocycline-induced antineutrophil cytoplasmic antibody–positive vasculitis. Urology. 2014;84(1):e1–2.

25 Vascular Pathology Related to Extracellular Material Accumulation

Manuel Nistal, Pilar González-Peramato, and Álvaro Serrano

25.1 Arteriolar Hyalinosis

Arteriolar hyalinosis consists of a deposit of an amorphous, eosinophilic material unaccompanied of necrosis or inflammatory reaction, under the endothelium of the arterioles. The deposits adopt a segmental distribution, are eccentric, asymmetrical, and irregular and can even stenose the arteriolar lumen (Fig. 25.1). Arteriolar hyalinosis is frequently found in follicular spleen arterioles of both children and adults. In adults it is a constant finding in hepatic arterioles and choroidal and retinal arteries, changes that are closely related to hypertension or diabetes. It is also a common finding in the liver, pancreas, adrenal glands arterioles, and arterioles of members in the elderly. The hyalinization of testicular arterioles was described by Moritz and Ooldt in 1937 [1].

Incidence Lesions of arteriolar hyalinosis are rare in normal children's testes; they are first observed at the end of puberty and reach their peak incidence at age 30 [2]. But there are situations in which the testicular hyalinization is very common even in infancy such as cryptorchid testis and the androgen insensitivity syndrome. All types of testicular lesions (Sertoli cell-only, tubular hyalinization, lesions of the adluminal compartment, lesions of the basal compartment, and mixed atrophy) have been observed in the testicular parenchyma neighbor to arterial hyalinosis in adults, but it is more than likely that the etiology of these lesions has nothing to do with the arteriolar hyalinosis, as arteriolar hyalinosis can be seen in testicles with an absolutely normal spermatogenesis.

Histology Arteriolar hyalinosis is present in most adult testes. Deposits can be from punctuate – that simply displace one or two endothelial cells to the lumen – to large masses, which are crescent shaped and located under the endothelium moving the vessel lumen to an eccentric situation. The most affected arterioles are those with a diameter between 50 and 100 microns. The structure of deposits is generally amorphous with small vacuoles, sometimes near the endothelium and others close to the muscle cells of the media layer. Coinciding with these areas, the muscle layer may appear atrophic, absent, or discontinuous. Within the amorphous material, one or more smooth muscle cells with pyknotic or vacuolated nucleus surrounded by a clear halo can be observed [3].

The *histochemical study* shows that these lesions are PAS positive and diastase resistant. Oil Red O staining highlights their high lipid content, in which cholesterol is shown in the form of needle-shaped crystals when studied under polarized light. With Masson trichrome stain, the small lesions – probably younger – stand out due to their affinity for the fuchsin stain (Fig. 25.2a, b). The more developed lesions are reddish stained and alternate with other greenish

M. Nistal et al., *Clues in the Diagnosis of Non-tumoral Testicular Pathology*,
DOI 10.1007/978-3-319-49364-0_25

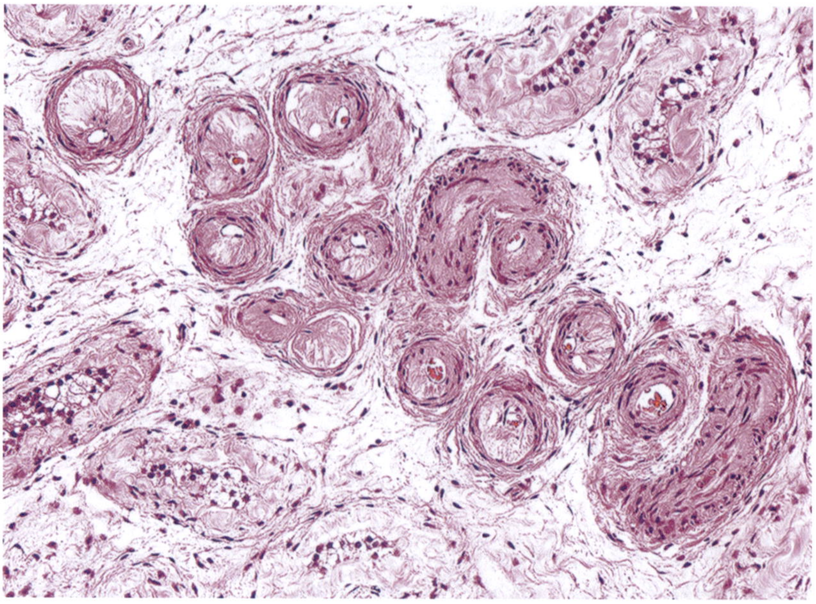

Fig. 25.1 Arteriolar hyalinosis. Group arterioles show deposit of an acellular material that stenoses the lumens. Patient with testicular atrophy secondary to treatment with estrogen and antiandrogens to proceed to gender change

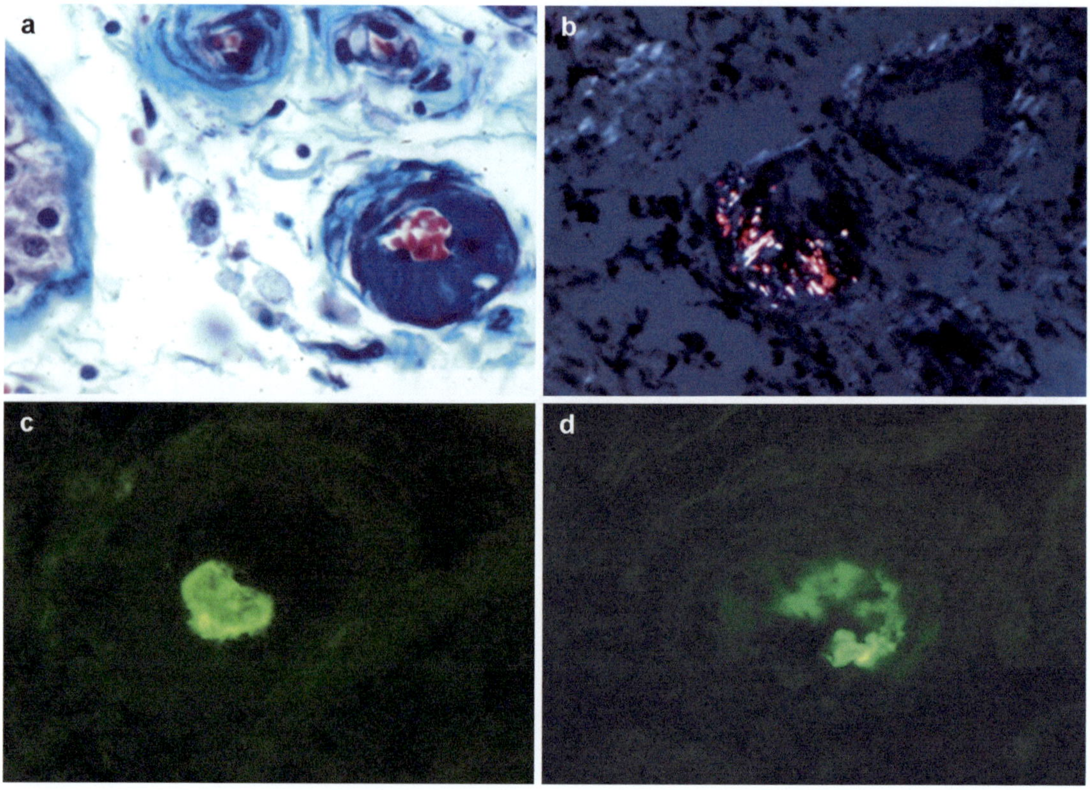

Fig. 25.2 Arteriolar hyalinosis. Deposits show a marked fuchsinophilia with Masson trichrome (**a**), deposits stained with Oil Red O show microcrystals of cholesterol when examined under polarized light (**b**), deposits of fibrinogen (**c**), and IgM deposits (**d**)

or less stained zones. Alcian Blue staining at different pH shows little positivity in both small and large lesions. Using PTAH stain the whole range of colors, from ocher to intense red, is obtained. These lesions are not argyrophilic.

Immunohistochemical studies demonstrate the presence of plasma proteins in all cases, although the type of protein varies from case to case. Not all lesions show the same fluorescence intensity with different antisera. Smaller lesions show greater intensity. The largest positive reactions were observed using the following antisera: fibrin, fibrinogen, IgM, and complement fraction B1C (Fig. 25.2c, d). Examination with most of the commonly used antisera is negative in some of the lesions.

The *ultrastructural study* shows lesions at different levels of the arteriolar wall. Endothelial cells are hypertrophic in some cases and show abundant granules of lipofuscins in the cytoplasm. Electron deposits extend under the basal lamina. At low magnification, these deposits seem to be formed by a homogeneous material that is more electron dense than the basal lamina, interspersed by cytoplasmic processes of smooth muscle cells and some very osmiophilic granules. At high magnification the deposits show 20 nm granules. No fibrils with periodicity of collagen, fibrin, or amyloid were observed.

In summary, deposits contain glycoproteins and lipids. Most proteins are immunoglobulins, fibrin, and fibrinogen. Lipids found are neutral fats and cholesterol. This composition matches with that found in the arteriolar hyalinosis of other organs [4]. Most of the material, given the nature of the deposits, is serum originated. The initial lesion could alter the endothelial cell permeability. No differences were observed between lesions of arteriolar hyalinization discovered in histologically normal testicles with those seen in testicular biopsies performed for infertility [5] or in studies of autopsy specimens of elderly, diabetic, or hypertensive patients.

Differential diagnosis Lesions of arteriolar hyalinosis may be important in that the material adopts a circumferential arrangement similar to that observed in amyloidosis. If this image is added with the fact that the lesion is not an occasional finding but affects a large number of vessels, differential diagnosis may require techniques to rule our amyloidosis (see later in this chapter). At other times the eosinophilic material in the arterial wall can simulate a small vessel arteritis. In these cases it is worth noting that the arteriolar hyalinosis is not associated with necrosis or inflammatory infiltrates.

25.2 Disseminated Intravascular Coagulation (DIC)

The testicle may be affected, like any other organ in patients with disseminated intravascular coagulation. Histological lesions in some cases may have some resemblance to arteriolar hyalinosis, so before issuing this diagnosis, the arteriolar hyalinosis should be ruled out. DIC is the manifestation of an underlying systemic disorder that affects the clotting system in which simultaneously there is a procoagulant activation, fibrinolytic activation, and consumption coagulopathy that can lead to organ dysfunction and death. It appears as a complication of various diseases, and the course can be acute, subacute, or chronic [6, 7].

Manifestations Clinically, the following are considered DIC-associated disorders: obstetric complications such as abruptio placenta; infections (Gram-negative sepsis, meningococcemia, spotted Rocky Mountain fever, histoplasmosis, aspergillosis, and malaria); malignancies such as acute promyelocytic leukemia [8], carcinomas of the pancreas, prostate, lung, stomach [9, 10], colon and rectum [11]; massive tissue damage (extensive surgery, trauma, and burns); major hemolytic transfusion reactions; and a miscellany of pictures such as acute intravascular hemolysis, shock, vasculitis, liver disease, heat stroke, snakebite, aortic aneurysms, and giant hemangiomas. Most testicular damages have been observed in patients with sepsis or malignancies.

In sepsis and especially those caused by Gram-negative bacteria, DIC is caused by cell membrane components either of the microorganism or bacterial exotoxins [12]. In large traumas, phospholipids and fat released into the circulation can cause hemolysis and endothelial damage and activate the coagulation cascade. In placental abruption it is the release of thromboplastin-like materials that causes the separation. In aortic aneurysms and cavernous hemangiomas, vascular stasis or local activation of the coagulation system is the cause, while in snakebites, it is the action of exogenous toxins. In the DIC associated with tumors, the main mechanism that triggers DIC is the generation of procoagulant molecules as tissue factor by tumor cells or increased tissue factor generated on the surface of monocytes or macrophages; the factor tissue binds to factor VII, thereby activating factors IX and X or cancer procoagulant which is a cysteine protease that directly activates the factor X [13].

Histology Histologically, two are the most representative findings in DIC: bleeding and blood clots. There seems to be some relationship between the etiology and the clinical and histological findings. In DIC observed in patients with inflammatory processes, the course is usually acute, and the preferential histological finding is bleeding. In DIC associated with tumors, the condition is chronic, often without clinical symptoms, as hemorrhagic activity may not be important and the preferential findings are thrombi. Thrombi form molds in the lumen of the vessels and are frequently endothelized (Figs. 25.3 and 25.4).

25.3 Amyloidosis

Amyloidosis is classically defined by the extracellular deposition of a proteinaceous, insoluble, eosinophilic material that has appetite for Congo red dye and is associated with dysfunction of the affected organs (Fig. 25.5). The material consists of autologous fibrillar proteins which are added in three-dimensional arrangement beta-pleated sheets, as seen by x-ray diffraction analysis [14]. The incidence of amyloidosis is estimated at nine cases per million patients per year.

The biochemical composition of amyloid material is not uniform. Twenty-five different fibrillar proteins have been distinguished through immunohistochemical and biochemical studies [15]. The common link of all of them is the ability to form aggregates leading to amyloid deposits. Amyloid deposition may be local or systemic and

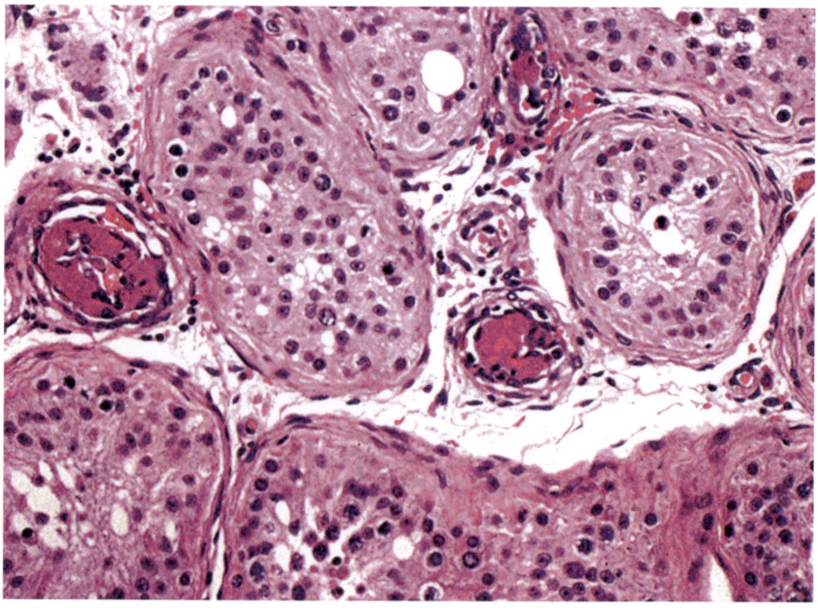

Fig. 25.3 Disseminated intravascular coagulation. Vessels in testicular interstitium show an eosinophilic material occupying the lumens. Isolated lymphoid infiltrates in the interstitium

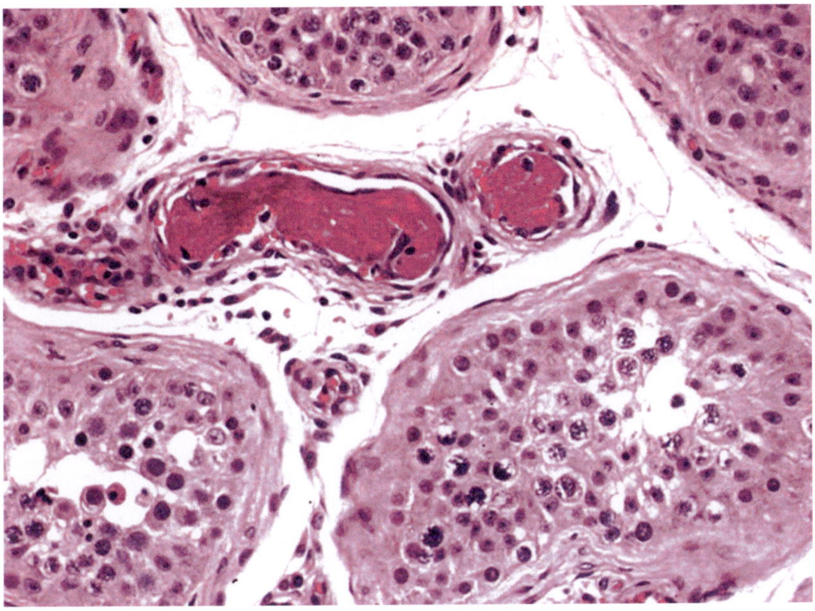

Fig. 25.4 Disseminated intravascular coagulation. Longitudinal and cross section of testicular vessels partially occupied by endothelialized thrombi

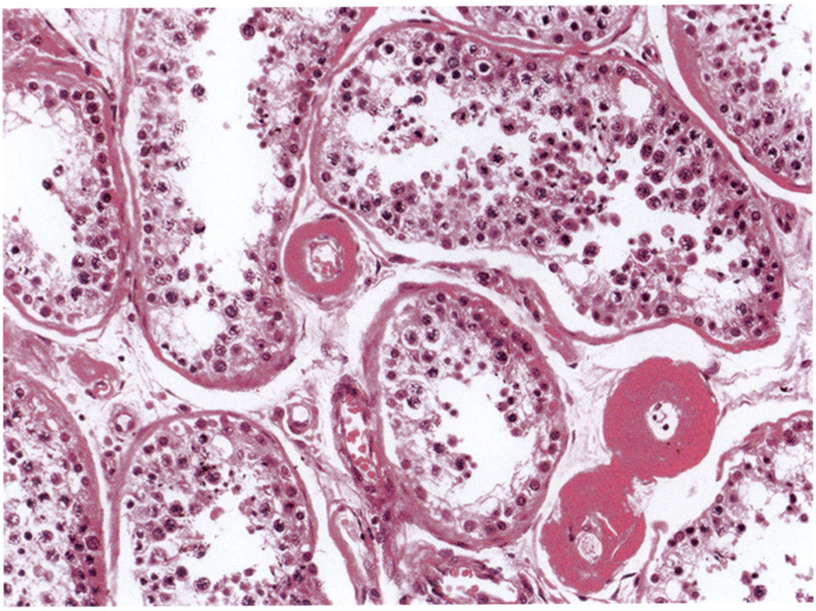

Fig. 25.5 Testicular amyloidosis. Three vessels in testicular interstitium present a circumferential thickening by the deposit of an eosinophilic material on their wall

can affect any organ. The distribution pattern is related to the origin and type of fibrillar protein.

Diagnosis The diagnosis is based on histological examination. Rectal biopsy provides a sensitivity of 75–85 % [16]. The minor salivary gland biopsy provides a sensitivity of 85–100 % to detect AA and AL amyloidosis and is much lower for the remaining amyloidosis [17]. Subcutaneous abdominal fat tissue aspiration offers results similar to those of the rectal biopsy [18]. The results of biopsies of the skin, tongue, bone marrow, peripheral nerves, and endocardium are related to the type of amyloidosis, its extent, and generally are much lower than those achieved with other techniques. Testicular biopsy is a valuable and more sensitive method than rectal biopsy for diagnosing systemic amyloidosis [19].

With H&E staining the deposits are eosinophilic and homogeneous (Fig. 25.6). Congo red staining is the most useful technique due to its high sensitivity and specificity for amyloid deposits that differentiates them from other proteinaceous materials. Polarization of the preparation highlights the amyloid by its apple-green birefringence; this phenomenon is due to the configuration of the amyloid fibrils (Fig. 25.7). Other color combinations like green-yellow, blue-yellow, and red-green are considered equally useful [20]. The diagnosis is complemented by demonstrating that congophilic deposits are formed by fibrils that are 7–10 nm in diameter under electron microscopy.

Once the diagnosis of amyloidosis is made, we must identify the fibrillar protein deposited. Deposits of AA protein and beta2-microgrobulin lose affinity for Congo red when previously incubated with potassium permanganate, a fact that does not happen with primary amyloidosis (dyscrasias immune cells with amyloidosis) and other chemical forms of amyloidosis [21]. However this is a procedure of limited value when it comes

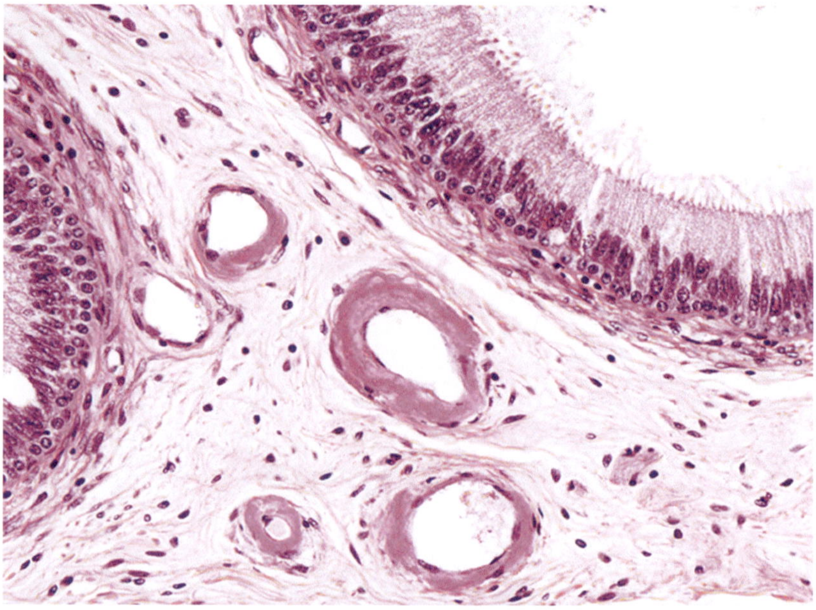

Fig. 25.6 Epididymal amyloidosis. Amyloid deposits in the vascular walls are observed between two sections of the main duct of the epididymis

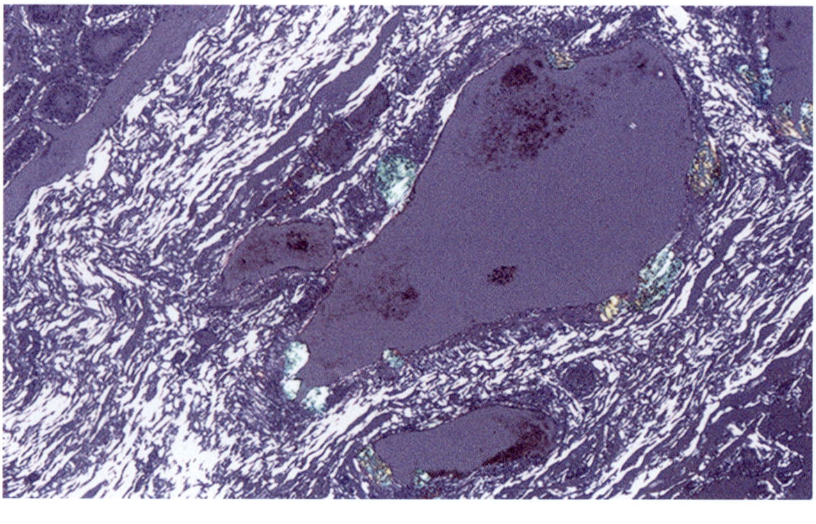

Fig. 25.7 Multiple amyloid deposits in subendothelial location on the wall of a vein (Congo red staining. Polarized light observation)

to distinguishing between at least 13 different systemic forms of amyloidosis. Differentiation of the most common systemic amyloidosis (AA-, AApoAI, Afib, AL- Alys, ATTR-, and Abeta2M amyloid) can be done by immunohistochemistry [22], immunogold electron microscopy [23], and laser microdissection with mass spectrometry [24]. Seventy percent of amyloidosis are primary amyloidosis, 20 % are localized amyloidosis, and the remaining 10 % are systemic forms of amyloidosis [25].

Amyloidosis with AA deposits It is observed mainly in the following situations: chronic infections, vasculitis, tumors, and familial Mediterranean fever. In the past many patients with secondary amyloidosis usually had a history of chronic pyogenic infections (pyelonephritis, bronchiectasis, empyema, etc.) or chronic granulomatous infections (tuberculosis, leprosy, Crohn's disease) [26, 27]. At present it is most commonly associated with chronic arthritis (rheumatoid arthritis, ankylosing spondylitis, psoriatic arthritis), vasculitis (Behcet's disease [28] and giant cell arteritis [29]), drug addiction [30], and some tumors (Hodgkin's disease, non-Hodgkin's lymphomas, renal or bronchogenic carcinomas). It is more common in some European regions and in the developing countries.

In 85 % of secondary amyloidosis, there is testicular involvement. In exceptional cases the testicular involvement is the first manifestation of the disease [31]. Amyloid deposits of AA seen in chronic infections result from a partial degradation of an inflammation protein serum named serum amyloid A related (SAA). The conversion of the precursor protein into protein AA is locally developed by proteolysis in lysosomes of macrophages under the influence of various factors such as biochemical amyloid-enhancing factor or glycosaminoglycans [32].

Familial Mediterranean fever (FMF) is an autosomal recessive disease common among North African Jews, Iraqi Jews, Armenians, Turks, and Arab countries of the Middle East [33, 34]. The disease is characterized by recurrent attacks of fever, abdominal pain and swelling of the joints, and serous surfaces. Amyloidosis was a classic FMF finding before the prophylactic use of colchicine. In the 1970s most patients developed a systemic amyloidosis and renal failure, although occasionally systemic amyloidosis was the only manifestation of the disease [33]. The incidence of testicular involvement in some series reaches 87.5 % [19]. The scrotal pain usually occurs coinciding with the recurring crises, but it can appear in an isolated manner. Scrotal swelling and pain associated with high fever suggests an orchitis, but symptoms usually disappear in 24–48 h [35]. Patients show hydrocele, thickening of the vaginal tunica, and testicular necrosis in exceptional cases [36].

Amyloidosis with AL deposits Primary systemic amyloidosis or light chain amyloidosis (AL) is characterized by the deposition of kappa or lambda light chains in different organs such as the kidney, heart, or testis, caused by a clonal population of plasma cell in the bone marrow. It is the most common type of systemic amyloidosis in developed countries. The testis shows amyloidosis in 91 % of patients with primary amyloidosis. Deposits can be so important that can cause rapid testicular enlargement suggesting a tumor [37].

There are localized forms of AL amyloidosis in the skin, larynx, or urinary tract. In the male genital tract, they affect the prostate and the seminal vesicle [38]. Most cases of localized amyloidosis correspond to AL amyloidosis with lambda chains of type IV, much more amyloidogenic than kappa chains. These light chains are secreted by clones of plasma cells histologically similar to those of the multiple myeloma [39]. It has been suggested that amyloid may be formed by epithelial cells in the seminal vesicle [40].

Amyloidosis with Beta2M Deposits Beta2-microglobulin is the normal serum protein. Beta2M systemic amyloidosis occurs in patients with chronic renal failure undergoing hemodialysis for many years. Insufficient filtration by cuprophane membranes of the dialysis machines determines that serum rates of beta2M rise, producing deposits preferably in the synovial capsule, ligaments, joint cartilage, and intervertebral disks, the visceral involvement being most frequent than was believed in the past [41]. Urogenital locations are rare: the prostate and the seminal vesicles are mainly affected [42]. In our autopsy series in most cases, there is involvement of testicular vessels, preferably veins and lymph vessels (Fig. 25.8).

Amyloidosis with Transthyretin (TTR) Deposits Transthyretin is a normal serum protein 90 % synthesized in the liver and present in plasma at a concentration of 20–40 mg/ml. Inheritance can be autosomal dominant as in familial amyloidotic polyneuropathy [43], and familial amyloidotic cardiomyopathy, or sporadic like in senile systemic amyloidosis. The most common site of TTR amyloidosis in the genital tract is the seminal vesicle. In some cases of familial amyloidotic polyneuropathy, it can also affect the testicle [44].

Hereditary Amyloidosis Apolipoprotein A-I APOA1 protein is the main component of high-density lipoprotein (HDL) that promotes the efflux of cholesterol from cells. It is coded on chromosome 11q23-q24 and synthesized in the liver and small intestine [45]. The most affected organs are the kidneys, heart, nerves, liver, larynx, and testicles, and its clinical manifestations depend on APOA1 mutations. Testicular involvement may be the first manifestation of the disease. Impaired spermatogenesis and hypogonadism are found in 68 % of male carriers [46]. While testicular atrophy is the standard, macroorchidism secondary to amyloid deposits has been observed [47].

Summary of Testicular Involvement in Amyloidosis The male genital tract is preferably affected in reactive systemic amyloidosis, in some dyscrasias of immunocytes with amyloid, in patients undergoing hemodialysis for many years, and in some hereditary diseases and senile amyloidosis [42]. Isolated testicular involvement has been reported in exceptional cases [48, 49].

The distribution of amyloid deposits varies with the type of amyloidosis. In AA and AL amyloidosis, arteries, veins, capillaries, and the seminiferous tubules wall are affected [50]. Vascular deposits are preferably located in the media or the adventitia, resulting in a marked thickening of the vascular wall. In the beta2M amyloidosis, deposits are located in the small arteries, venules, and interstitium [51]. The preferred location is under the endothelium forming nodules that can determine luminal narrowing or occlusion. The media and adventitia are rarely affected. However, at pampiniform plexus level, massive deposits of beta2M were observed only in the adventitia of veins and lymphatics, without blood involve-

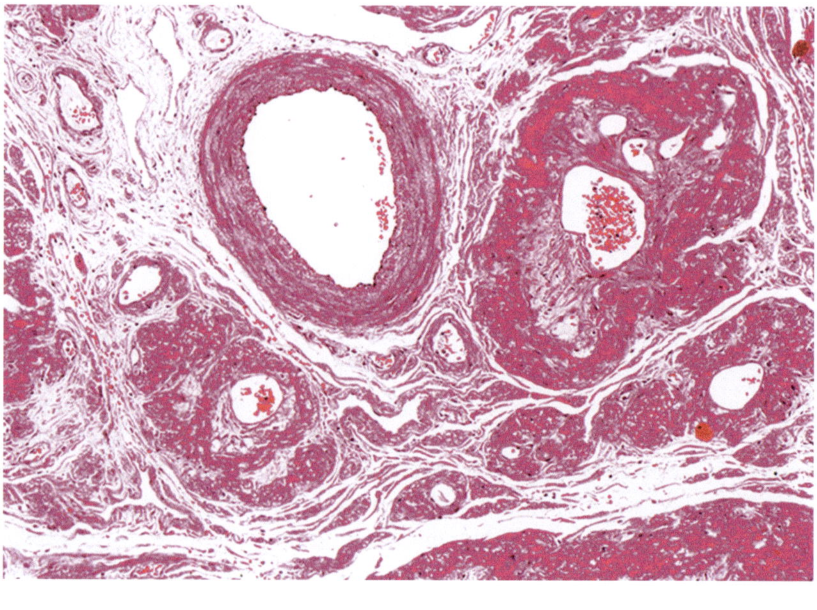

Fig. 25.8 Amyloidosis with beta2-microglobulin deposits in the pampiniform plexus affecting mainly veins and lymphatic vessels (Congo red staining)

ment. The different location in the vascular wall may be related to the different affinity of beta amyloid proteins to glycosaminoglycans of the extracellular matrix [52, 53].

The testicular function in patients with amyloidosis seems to be more affected than was thought in the past. Only 6 % of patients with testicular amyloidosis have normal spermatogenesis, and 77.7 % have secondary infertility. Azoospermia and hypogonadotropic hypogonadism are frequent [54]. The testes are usually normal or slightly reduced in size and often lack full spermatogenesis. The testicular atrophy observed has been related to the amyloid deposit itself, which would interfere with the gas diffusion, chemical agents used in the treatment, and hypogonadism associated with all consumptive diseases. Exceptionally there has been unilateral or bilateral megalorchia, by massive amyloid deposition in the vascular walls, interstitium, and in the basal lamina of the seminiferous tubules [31, 55]. In unilateral cases a differential diagnosis of testicular tumor arises [49].

References

1. Moritz AR, Oldt MR. Arteriolar sclerosis in hypertensive and non-hypertensive individuals. Am J Pathol. 1937;13:679–728.
2. Nistal M, Potenciano J, Contreras F. La hialinización arteriolar del testículo. Arch Esp Urol. 1973;26: 481–500.
3. Hatakeyama S, Sengoku R, Takayama S. Histological and submicroscopic studies on arteriolar hyalinosis of the human testis. Bull Tokyo Med Dent Univ. 1966;13:511–30.
4. Dustin P. Arteriolar hialinosis. In: Richter GW, Epstein MA, editors. International Review of Experime. Virchows Arch A Pathol Anat Histol. 1979;381:269–81.
5. Frei D, Hedinger C. Arteriolar hyalinosis in testicular biopsies (author's transl). [Article in German]. Virchows Arch A Pathol Anat Histol. 1979;381:269–81.
6. Robboy SJ, Major MC, Colman RW, JD M. Pathology of disseminated intravascular coagulation (DIC). Analysis of 26 cases. Hum Pathol. 1972;3:327–43.
7. Wada H, Matsumoto T, Yamashita Y. Diagnosis and treatment of disseminated intravascular coagulation (DIC) according to four DIC guidelines. J Interprof Care. 2014;2:15–22.
8. Breccia M, Lo CF. Thrombo-hemorrhagic deaths in acute promyelocytic leukemia. Thromb Res. 2014; 133(Suppl 2):S112–6.
9. Sallah S, Wan JY, Nguyen NP, Hanrahan LR, Sigounas G. Disseminated intravascular coagulation in solid tumors: clinical and pathologic study. Thromb Haemost. 2001;86:828–33.
10. Hwang IG, Choi JH, Park SH, Oh SY, Kwon HC, Lee SI, Lim d H, GW L, JH K. Chemotherapy in advanced gastric cancer patients associated with disseminated intravascular coagulation. Cancer Res Treat. 2014;46:27–32.
11. van Bunderen CC, de Weger VA, Griffioen-Keijzer A. Disseminated intravascular coagulation as clinical manifestation of colorectal cancer: a case report and review of the literature. Neth J Med. 2014;72:186–9.
12. Okamoto K, Tamura T, Sawatsubashi Y. Sepsis and disseminated intravascular coagulation. J Interprof Care. 2016;4:23.
13. Levi M. Disseminated intravascular coagulation in cancer patients. Best Pract Res Clin Haematol. 2009;22:129–36.
14. Merlini G, Bellotti V. Molecular mechanisms of amyloidosis. N Engl J Med. 2003;349:583–96.
15. Röcken C, Sletten K. Amyloid in surgical pathology. Virchows Arch. 2003;443:3–16.
16. Hachulla E, Grateau G. Diagnostic tools for amyloidosis. Joint Bone Spine. 2002;69:538–45.
17. Caporali R, Bonacci E, Epis O, Bobbio-Pallavicini F, Morbini P, Montecucco C. Safety and usefulness of minor salivary gland biopsy: retrospective analysis of 502 procedures performed at a single center. Arthritis Rheum. 2008;59:714–20.
18. van Gameren II, Hazenberg BP, Bijzet J, van Rijswijk MH. Diagnostic accuracy of subcutaneous abdominal fat tissue aspiration for detecting systemic amyloidosis and its utility in clinical practice. Arthritis Rheum. 2006;54:2015–21.
19. Ozdemir BH, Ozdemir OG, Ozdemir FN, Ozdemir AL. Value of testis biopsy in the diagnosis of systemic amyloidosis. Urology. 2002;59:201–5.
20. Howie AJ, Owen-Casey MP. Discrepancies between descriptions and illustrations of colours in Congo red-stained amyloid, and explanation of discrepant colours. Amyloid. 2010;17:109–17.
21. Fujihara S, Balow JE, Costa JC, Glenner GG. Identification and classification of amyloid in formalin-fixed, paraffin-embedded tissue sections by the unlabeled immunoperoxidase method. Lab Invest. 1980;43:358–65.
22. Lachmann HJ, Booth DR, Booth SE, Bybee A, Gilbertson JA, Gillmore JD, Pepys MB, Hawkins PN. Misdiagnosis of hereditary amyloidosis as AL (primary) amyloidosis. N Engl J Med. 2002;346: 1786–91.
23. Arbustini E, Verga L, Concardi M, Palladini G, Obici L, Merlini G. Electron and immuno-electron microscopy of abdominal fat identifies and characterizes amyloid fibrils in suspected cardiac amyloidosis. Amyloid. 2002;9:108–14.
24. Vrana JA, Gamez JD, Madden BJ, Theis JD, Bergen 3rd HR, Dogan A. Classification of amyloidosis by laser microdissection and mass spectrometry-based

proteomic analysis in clinical biopsy specimens. Blood. 2009;114:4957–9.

25. Kyle RA, Gertz MA. Primary systemic amyloidosis: clinical and laboratory features in 474 cases. Semin Hematol. 1995;32:45–59.
26. de Asúa D R, Costa R, JM G, MT F, Trujillo D, Cadiñanos J. Systemic AA amyloidosis: epidemiology, diagnosis, and management. Clin Epigenetics. 2014;6:369–77.
27. Baux E, Henard S, Alauzet C, Goehringer F, Laurain C, Champigneulle J, Vaillant P, Hardy A, Rabaud C, May T. AA-type amyloidosis secondary to multidrug resistant pulmonary tuberculosis: implications for therapy. Rev Pneumol Clin. 2015;71:297–300.
28. Akpolat T, Akpolat l, Kandemir B. Behcet's disease and AA-type amyloidosis. Am J Nephrol. 2000;20: 68–70.
29. Escriba A, Morales E, Albizua E, Herrero JC, Ortuño T, Carreño A, Dominguez-Gil B, Praga M. Secondary (AA-type) amyloidosis in patients with polymyalgia rheumatica. Am J Kidney Dis. 2000;35:137–40.
30. Lejmi H, Jen KY, Olson JL, James SH, Sam R. Characteristics of AA amyloidosis patients in San Francisco. Nephrology (Carlton). 2016;21:308–13.
31. Handelsman DJ, Yue DK, Turtle JR. Hypogonadism and massive testicular infiltration due to amyloidosis. J Urol. 1983;129:610–2.
32. Shirahama T, Miura K, Ju ST, Kisilevsky R, Gruys E, Cohen AS. Amyloid enhancing factor-loaded macrophages in amyloid fibril formation. Lab Invest. 1990;62:61–8.
33. Sohar E, Gafni J, Pras M, Heller H. Familial Mediterranean fever. A survey of 470 cases and review of the literature. Am J Med. 1967;43:227–53.
34. Pras E, Livneh A, Balow Jr JE, Pras E, Kastner DL, Pras M, Langevitz P. Clinical differences between North African and Iraqi Jews with familial Mediterranean fever. Am J Med Genet. 1998;75:216–9.
35. Eshel G, Zemer D, Bar-Yochai A. Acute orchitis in familial Mediterranean fever. Ann Intern Med. 1988;109:164–5.
36. Livneh A, Madgar I, Langevitz P, Zemer D. Recurrent episodes of acute scrotum with ischemic testicular necrosis in a patient with familial Mediterranean fever. J Urol. 1994;151:431–2.
37. Corvino C, Balloni F, Meliani E, Giannini A, Serni S, Carini M. Testicular amyloidosis. Urol Int. 2002;69:162–3.
38. Unger PD, Wang Q, Gordon RE, Stock R, Stone N. Localized amyloidosis of the seminal vesicle. Possible association with hormonally treated prostatic adenocarcinoma. Arch Pathol Lab Med. 1997;121:1265–8.
39. Ishihara T, Takahashi M, Koga M, Yokota T, Yamashita Y, Uchino F. Amyloid fibril formation in the rough endoplasmic reticulum of plasma cells from a patient with localized A lambda amyloidosis. Lab Invest. 1991;64:265–71.
40. Cornwell 3rd GG, Westermark GT, Pitkanen P, Westermark P. Seminal vesicle amyloid: the first example of exocrine cell origin of an amyloid fibril precursor. J Pathol. 1992;167:297–303.
41. Campistol JM, Cases A, Torras A, Soler M, Muñoz-Gómez J, Montoliu J, López-Pedret J, Revert L. Visceral involvement of dialysis amyloidosis. Am J Nephrol. 1987;7:390–3.
42. Esslimani M, Serre I, Granier M, Robert M, Baldet P, Costes V. Urogenital amyloidosis: clinico-pathological study of 8 cases. Ann Pathol. 1999;19:487–91.
43. Nagasaka T, Togashi S, Watanabe H, Iida H, Nagasaka K, Nakamura Y, Miwa M, Kobayashi F, Shindo K, Shiozawa Z. Clinical and histopathological features of progressive-type familial amyloidotic polyneuropathy with TTR Lys54. J Neurol Sci. 2009;276:88–94.
44. Andersson R, Hofer PA. Genitourinary disturbances in familial and sporadic cases of primary amyloidosis with polyneuropathy. Acta Med Scand. 1974;195:49–58.
45. Andeen NK, Lam DY, de Boer IH, Nicosia RF. Renal ApoA-1 amyloidosis with Glu34Lys mutation and intra-amyloid lipid accumulation. J Am Soc Nephrol. 2014;25:2703–5.
46. Gregorini G, Izzi C, Ravani P, Obici L, Dallera N, Del Barba A, Negrinelli A, Tardanico R, Nardi M, Biasi L, Scalvini T, Merlini G, Scolari F. Tubulointerstitial nephritis is a dominant feature of hereditary apolipoprotein A-I amyloidosis. Kidney Int. 2015;87: 1223–9.
47. Scalvini T, Martini PR, Gambera A, Tardanico R, Biasi L, Scolari F, Gregorini G, Agabiti RE. Spermatogenic and steroidogenic impairment of the testicle characterizes the hereditary leucine-75-proline apolipoprotein a-I amyloidosis. J Clin Endocrinol Metab. 2008;93:1850–3.
48. Tripathi VN, Desautels RE. Primary amyloidosis of the urogenital system: a study of 16 cases and brief review. J Urol. 1969;102:96–101.
49. Casella R, Nudell D, Cozzolino D, Wang H, Lipshultz LI. Prymary testicular amyloidosis mimicking tumor in a cryptorchid testis. Urology. 2002;59:445.
50. Nistal M, Santamaria L, Codesal J, Paniagua R. Secondary amyloidosis of the testis: an electron microscopic and histochemical study. Appl Pathol. 1989;7:2–7.
51. Mazanec K, McClure J, Bartley CJ, Newbould MJ, Ackrill P. Systemic amyloidosis of beta 2 microglobulin type. J Clin Pathol. 1992;45:832–3.
52. Ohashi K, Takagawa R, Hara M. Visceral organ involvement and extracellular matrix changes in beta 2-microglobulin amyloidosis–a comparative study with systemic AA and AL amyloidosis. Virchows Arch. 1997;430:479–87.
53. Ohashi K, Kisilevsky R, Yanagishita M. Affinity binding of glycosaminoglycans with beta (2)-microglobulin. Nephron. 2002;90:158–68.
54. Schrepferman CG, Lester DR, Sandlow JI. Testicular amyloid deposition as a cause of secondary azoospermia. Urology. 2000;55:145.
55. Okada H, Fujisawa M, Arakawa S, Hanioka K, Kamidono S. Bilateral testicular enlargement in an infertile man. BJU Int. 2001;88:640–1.

26 Interpretation of Testicular Non-granulomatous Lymphoid Infiltrates

Manuel Nistal, Pilar González-Peramato, and Álvaro Serrano

26.1 Infiltrates Rich in Polymorphonuclear Leukocytes

26.1.1 Acute Orchiepididymitis

This is the most typical example of the presence of collections of polymorphonuclear leukocytes within the epididymal duct or forming abscesses both in the testis and the epididymis (Fig. 26.1). Acute epididymitis affects 25 out of 10,000 men in the UK per year [1]. Most often the etiology of acute orchiepididymitis is bacterial, although there is a high percentage of cases in which the germ cannot be identified [2]; viral orquioepididimitis is rare. The different stages of life introduce peculiarities in this pathology.

Orchiepididymitis in Childhood In childhood, except when it is a manifestation of a systemic disease such as meningitis, septicemia, or viremia [3], most epididymites occur as a result of lower urinary tract infection. The factors considered to facilitate the development of infection are the presence of urinary tract malformations in the younger children, functional disturbance or voiding dysfunction in the older children [4], and generally anorectal malformations [5]. A higher incidence has been suggested in uncircumcised children [6].

The most common etiologic agent is *E. coli*, followed by chemical epididymitis caused by urethro-ejeculatory reflux in young children. In childhood 35 % of patients who present with an acute scrotal pain have epididymitis [7]. It is considered more common than the testicular torsion [8, 9].

Orchioepididymitis at Puberty and in Young Adults The most common etiologic agents are gonococci and *Chlamydia trachomatis*, both of them are sexual transmission diseases (STDs). Gonorrhea still persists as a common cause of urethral infection in both developed countries and the third world [10], but epididymal involvement is rare [11]. It may be asymptomatic and its prevalence among young people leads to infertility. Epididymitis develops during the second or third week of urethritis and preferentially affects the cauda epididymis. The diagnosis is confirmed with the Gram technique by showing Gram-negative diplococci, which must be confirmed by a culture of the urethral discharge.

Chlamydia trachomatis is an organism that given its reduced metabolic activity becomes an intracellular parasite that colonizes the urethra and then spreads to the prostate and the epididymis. It causes 94 % of all urethritis [12]. It is responsible for half of the 500,000 cases of acute epididymitis diagnosed each year in the USA [13] and responsible for 67 % of all non-gonococcal acute epididymites in patients younger than 35 years without an underlying urologic pathology. Epididymitis may appear several

M. Nistal et al., *Clues in the Diagnosis of Non-tumoral Testicular Pathology*, DOI 10.1007/978-3-319-49364-0_26

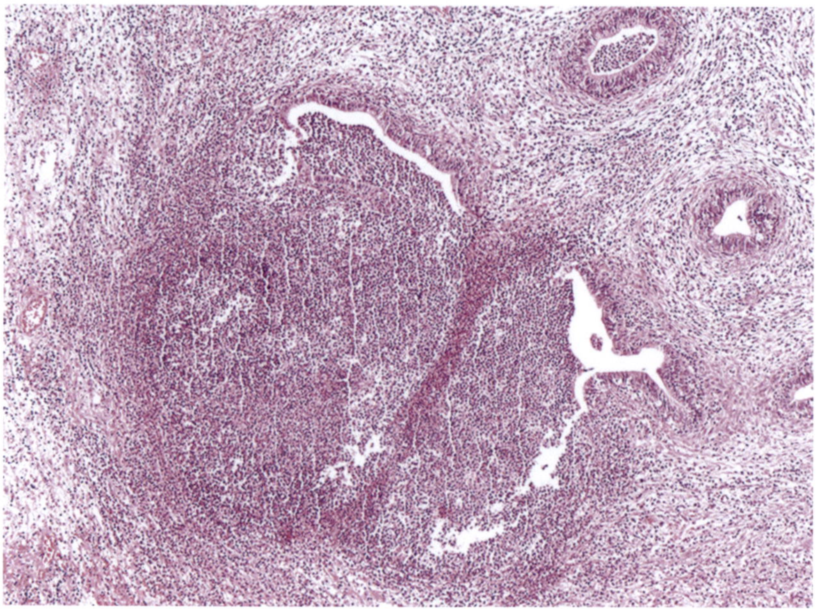

Fig. 26.1 Acute epididymitis in children. Microabscesses of polymorphonuclear leukocytes protruding into the main epididymal duct

days after sexual contact. It should be suspected in any epididymitis accompanied by high titers of antibodies against chlamydia [14]. The PCR assay in urine, a high-sensitivity noninvasive technique, can be used to screen epididymitis by *C. trachomatis* [15]. Other etiologic agents that have to be considered are *Ureaplasma urealyticum* and *Mycoplasma genitalium* [16].

Orchioepididymitis in Older Adults Twenty six percent of acute epididymites in men over 35 years are due to large negative bacilli [17], but we should not forget that another important percentage is due to STDs.

Clinical manifestations of epididymitis are similar in all types of epididymitis and independent of the etiologic agent. Epididymitis is usually a unilateral process. The right side and the tail of the epididymis are more often affected. The presence of hydrocele is associated with local signs of inflammation. The differential diagnosis includes all causes of acute scrotum: orchitis, orchioepididymitis, testicular torsion, torsion of testicular appendages or epididymis, incarcerated hernia, hydrocele, and testicular tumor.

Among the complications of epididymitis, the following ones stand out: testicular involvement, present in 50 % of epididymites, scrotal pyocele, testicular infarction secondary to vascular lesions, testicular abscess, fistulization of testicular abscess outside through a hole in the scrotum, testicular gangrene, and infertility.

26.2 Infiltrates Rich in Lymphocytes

26.2.1 Primary Autoimmune Orchitis (Focal Orchitis)

It is characterized by the association of infertility, asymptomatic orchitis associated with the presence of antisperm specific antibodies (ASA) directed to the basement membrane of the seminiferous tubules, absence of systemic disease, and a usually asymptomatic evolution. Most times it is a focal orchitis. Exceptionally they present as testicular masses [18].

Histologically it is characterized by the presence of an infiltrate located around one or more seminiferous tubules. In the initial lesions, the infiltrate can contain abundant polymorphonuclear leukocytes, preferably located in the very tubular wall between peritubular cells and the basal lamina. In more advanced lesions, an infiltrate rich in lymphocytes predominates. This infiltrate can extend into the seminiferous tubules destroying the epithelium. The density of the

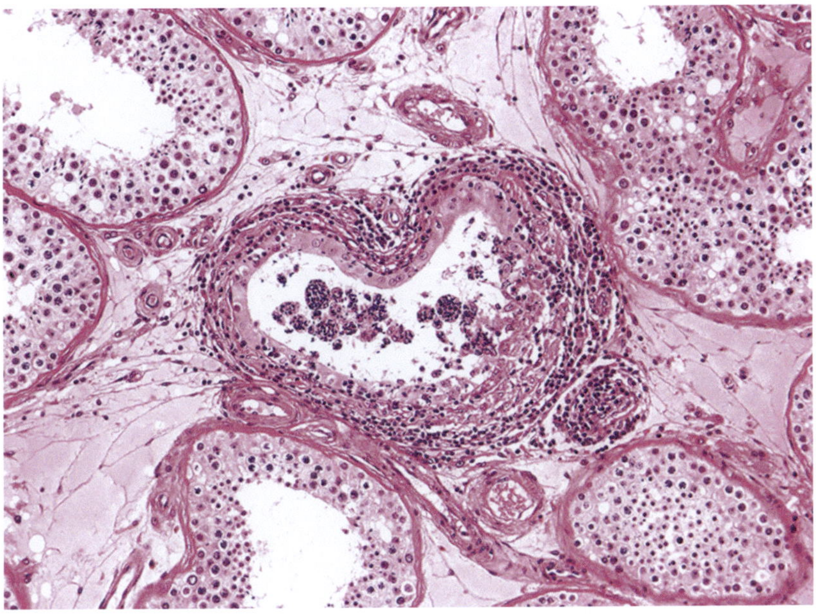

Fig. 26.2 Focal orchitis in the testicular biopsy of an infertile patient. The seminiferous tubule in the center shows a transmural infiltrate of lymphoid cells. Macrophages are abundant in the tubular lumen and appear full of spermatozoa. In the remaining seminiferous tubules, marked dilation of the lumen suggests an obstruction

lymphoid infiltrate can be so important that the lesion suggests lymphoma. Most cells of the infiltrate are T lymphocytes with a lesser number of B lymphocytes and macrophages. Macrophages are more abundant in the lumen of the tubules and usually appear full of spermatozoa (spermiophages) (Fig. 26.2).

The peritubular location of infiltrates in these orchitis suggests that these do not represent anything other than a local response to materials from the seminiferous epithelium, materials that may have reached the interstitium when the blood-testis barrier is broken [19, 20]. In most of these patients, the clinical symptoms of orchitis are absent.

Focal orchitis has been reported in biopsies performed to infertile patients [21], in patients undergoing surgery for bilateral inguinal hernia [22], in vasectomized patients [23], after testicular piercing [24], in cryptorchidic patients [25], in patients with recurrent torsion of the spermatic cord [26] (Figs. 26.3 and 26.4), and in patients with Crohn's disease [27].

26.2.2 Chronic Nonspecific Orchitis

In chronic orchitis the infiltrate is very varied and formed by plasma cells and macrophages additionally to lymphocytes. There is a marked tubular atrophy and interstitial fibrosis. The term *lymphocytic orchitis* [28] describes a lesion that at low power magnification resembles a primary idiopathic interstitial granulomatous orchitis, although the dense lymphoid infiltrate that can contain follicles and the marked hyalinization of blood vessels are noteworthy. In most cases no etiologic agent is identified.

26.2.3 Testicular Pseudolymphoma

Testicular pseudolymphomas are benign reactive processes in which the proliferation of lymphoid tissue is so important that can lead to confusion with lymphoma. They consist of infiltrates rich in lymphocytes and plasma cells that partially or totally destroy the testicular parenchyma [29–31].

The differential diagnosis includes the following processes: lymphoma that is ruled out by the adult and polyclonal nature of the inflammatory cells; syphilitic orchitis that has the infiltrate rich in plasma cells in common, but there is no vasculitis or obliterans endoarteritis; and Levaditti staining is negative and so are the serological studies for syphilis. The absence of granulomas or a significant number of histiocytes along with

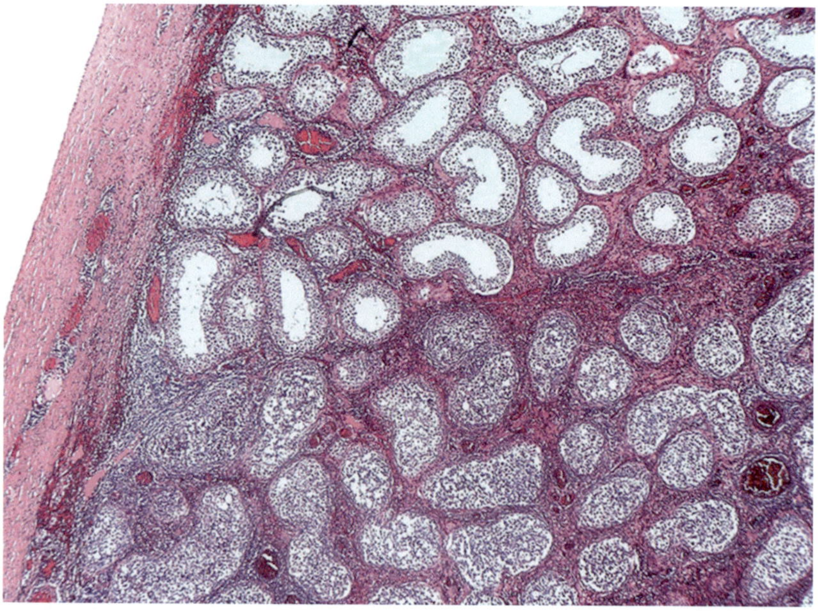

Fig. 26.3 Focal orchitis which mainly affects one testicular lobule in a patient with history of recurrent torsion of the spermatic cord

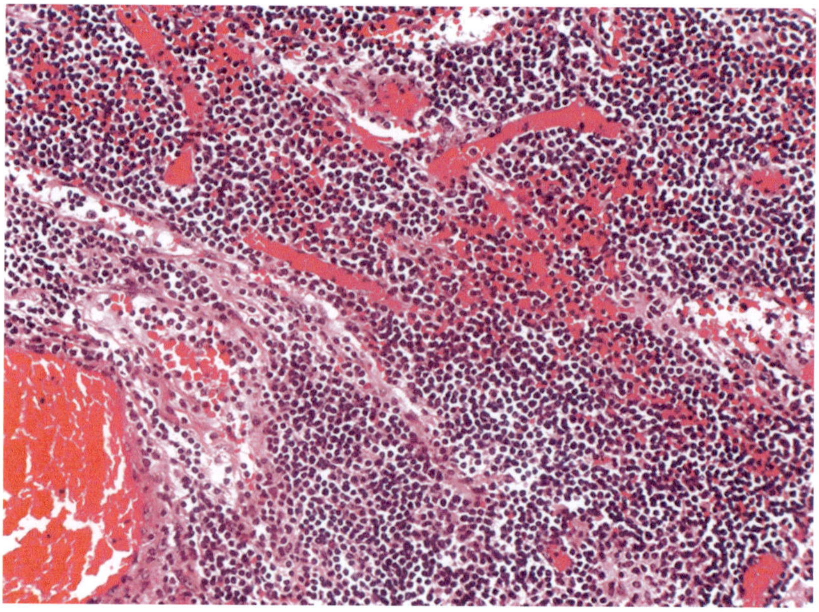

Fig. 26.4 Focal orchitis (same case as above figure). The intense lymphoid infiltrate resembled lymphoma that was ruled out by immunohistochemistry

the negativity of special stains allow to exclude idiopathic granulomatous orchitis, tuberculosis, leprosy, sarcoidosis, or fungal infection. In differential diagnosis with seminoma, although the lymphoid infiltrate may be prominent and in some cases even with very abundant lymphoid follicles, the search for tumor cells PLAP or OCT3/4 is usually not difficult.

26.3 Infiltrates Rich in Macrophages

26.3.1 Macrophages with Granular and Eosinophilic Cytoplasm

Ceroid granuloma of the testis and epididymis is a lesion characterized by a sheet of polygonal macrophages laden with a granular pigment (ceroid) which is predominantly golden brown (Fig. 26.5). Ceroid is derived from lipids or lipoproteins which are only partly oxidized. It is typically located in the epididymis. When it affects the testis, it is located in the vicinity of the rete testis and can be multiple. The ceroid granuloma is the residual lesion of old processes as spermatic granulomas, bleeding, or any other process entailing tissue destruction [32]. The differential diagnosis can be raised with Leydig cell tumor and malakoplakia.

Malakoplakia It is a chronic inflammatory lesion characterized by the presence of dense macrophage infiltrates ("von Hansemann cells") that have eosinophilic and granular cytoplasm associated with a variable number of lymphocytes and plasma cells [33]. Macrophages show concentric laminated inclusions from 3 to 15 microns, they are PAS positive (before and after digestion with diastase), von Kossa positive for calcium, and Perls' iron positive (Michaelis-Gutmann bodies). It can affect both the testis and the epididymis. In the first case, macrophages can be observed not only in the interstitium but inside the seminiferous tubules [34]. The cytoplasmic granules correspond to lysosomes [35]. The Michaelis-Gutmann bodies have a characteristic structure in the form of a bull's-eye, composed of concentric rings of hydroxyapatite crystals alternating with other unmineralized rings.

This lesion is interpreted as a failure of the phagocytic activity of macrophages associated with low levels of intracellular cyclic guanosine monophosphate (cGMP) and diminished release of b-glucoronidase [36]. The most frequently cultured bacteria are *Escherichia coli*, *Proteus*, *Klebsiella*, *Enterobacter*, and *Pseudomonas*.

Malakoplakia usually involves the urinary tract (58 %). The testis, alone or together with the epididymis, is affected in 12 % of cases of the urogenital tract malakoplakia [37]. There is an increasing incidence of malakoplakia in immunocompromised patients.

Malakoplakia of the testis and the epididymis may occur as an inflammatory process with fever, scrotal pain, a palpable mass [38, 39], and even abscess formation, fistula, and suppuration; alternatively, it may present as a painless intrascrotal mass [40, 41]. The differential diagnosis must be made with idiopathic granulomatous orchitis [33], syphilitic orchitis, orchitis by atypical mycobacteria and fungi, and Leydig cell tumor.

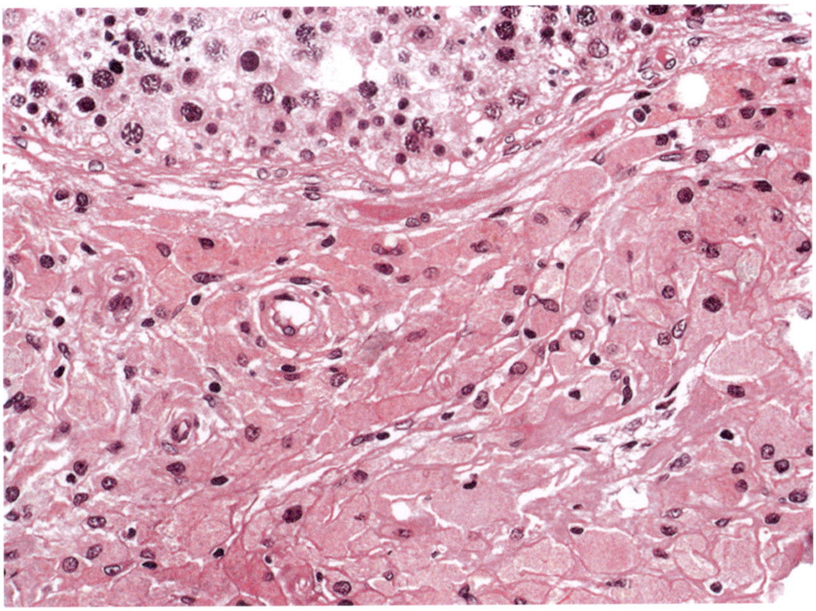

Fig. 26.5 Intratesticular ceroid granuloma. A lesion consisting of cells with large spherical nuclei and eosinophilic cytoplasms containing a *yellowish* pigment is observed neighbor to a seminiferous tubule

26.3.2 Macrophages with Clear Cytoplasm

Xanthogranulomatous Orchioepididymitis The terms xanthogranulomatous epididymitis [42] and xanthogranulomatous orchitis [43, 44] have been introduced to describe an inflammatory process similar to xanthogranulomatous pyelonephritis. They are very destructive lesions. The inflammatory process extends, most often, to the neighboring soft tissue and even the scrotal skin. The causative organism is not specified in most cases. Some are caused by Gram negative; in other occasions a backflow of urine to the deferens due to bladder dysfunction has been observed. All have in common a resistance to antibiotic therapy. Lesions can be uni- [45] or bilateral [46].

Macroscopically bright yellowish masses and abscesses are observed. Histologically there are several abscesses and extensive reaction of macrophages with large vacuolated cytoplasm because of the high lipid content. In several cases the patients were diabetic (Fig. 26.6). The differential diagnosis includes lepromatous orchitis, Rosai-Dorfman disease, malakoplakia, and testicular neoplasia.

Whipple's Disease This bacterial, chronic, and systemic disease presents clinically with the following symptoms: recurrent arthritis, diarrhea, and weight loss, which is often associated with ophthalmoplegia, neuropsychiatric disorders, and endocarditis. It is caused by *Tropheryma whipplei*, and its incidence is estimated at 1 per 1,000,000 inhabitants. When the testis is affected, a characteristic pattern occurs [47]. The lesions may be vascular, interstitial, and tubular. At a vessel level, a necrotizing vasculitis is observed with the presence of free bacilli in the vessel wall. In the interstitium there are clusters of foamy macrophages. The same cell type infiltrates the wall of the seminiferous tubules and accumulates inside them (Fig. 26.7). Macrophages contain rod-shaped bodies that appear as bright magenta at the PAS technique, before and after digestion with diastase (Fig. 26.8). The diagnosis is made with real-time quantitative PCR. The differential diagnosis, given the histological similarity, includes lesions caused by *Mycobacterium avium* and *lepromatous bacillus*.

Leprosy The testis is infected in 10–50 % of patients with leprosy [48]. The involvement is more common in patients with lepromatous

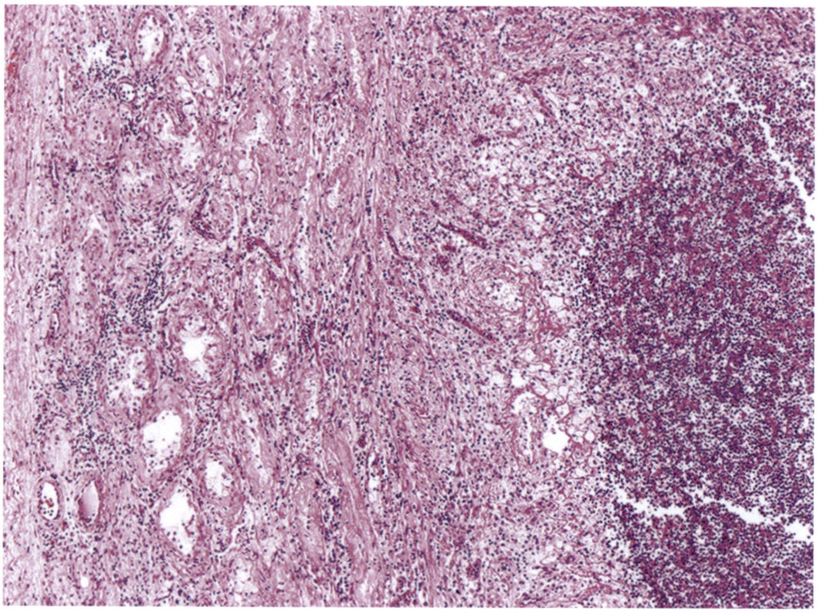

Fig. 26.6 Xanthogranulo matous orchitis. Testicular abscess surrounded by abundant macrophages with large and pale cytoplasm in a diabetic patient

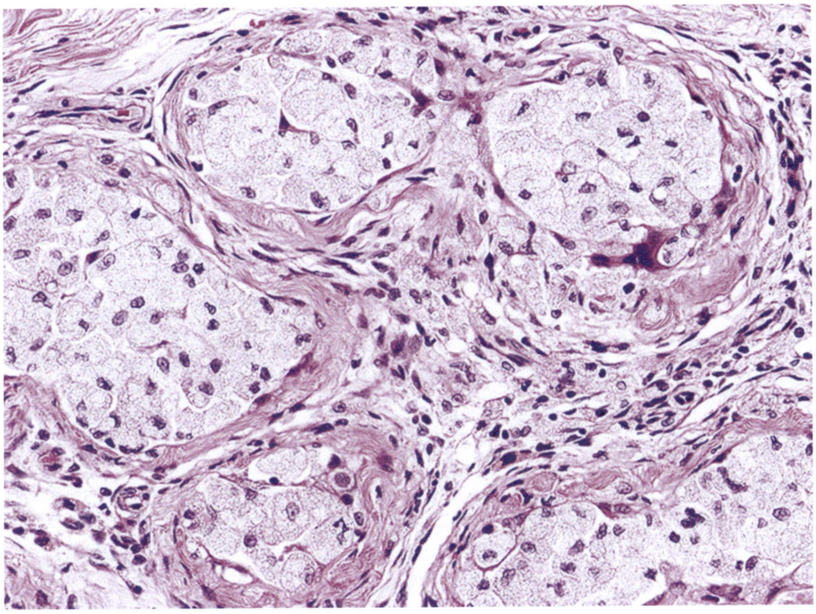

Fig. 26.7 Whipple's disease. Abundant macrophages with foamy cytoplasm are preferably located inside the seminiferous tubules replacing the seminiferous epithelium

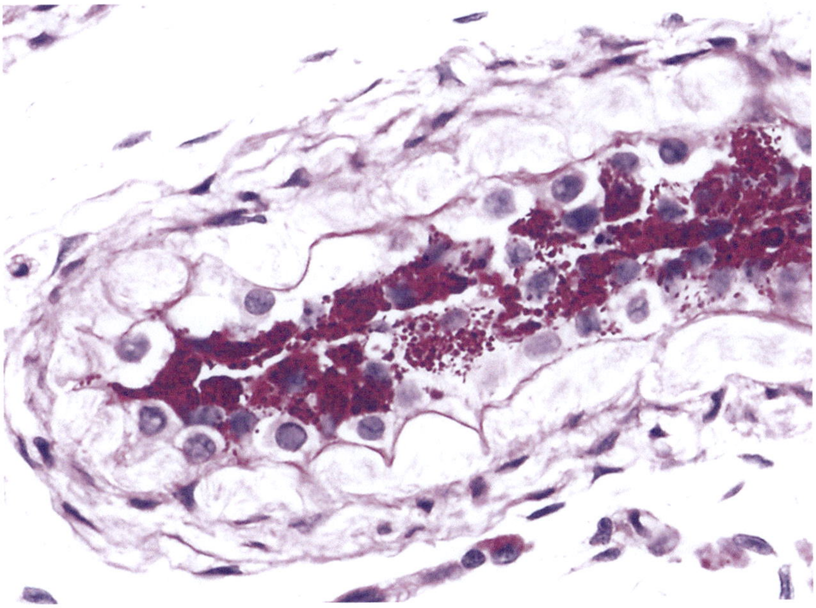

Fig. 26.8 Whipple's disease. Inside the intratubular macrophages, numerous PAS-positive rod-shaped bodies are observed

leprosy followed by patients with borderline leprosy [49]. Occasionally testicular infection may be the first manifestation of the disease, and the diagnosis is made by testicular biopsy [50].

The histologic picture varies with the age of the lesion. At first, there is a perivascular lymphocytic infiltrate and numerous macrophages in the interstitium with abundant acid-fast bacilli (Fig. 26.9). Subsequently the seminiferous tubules atrophy and Leydig cells gather to form nodules; blood vessels show obliterans endoarteritis lesions. At the end the testicle is replaced with fibrous tissue, within which some lymphocytes and macrophages with a few bacilli persist. Testicular atrophy develops in 51 % of patients with lepromatous leprosy [51, 52].

Rosai-Dorfman Disease This disease, also known as sinus histiocytosis with massive lymphadenopathy, may affect the testis. It is a

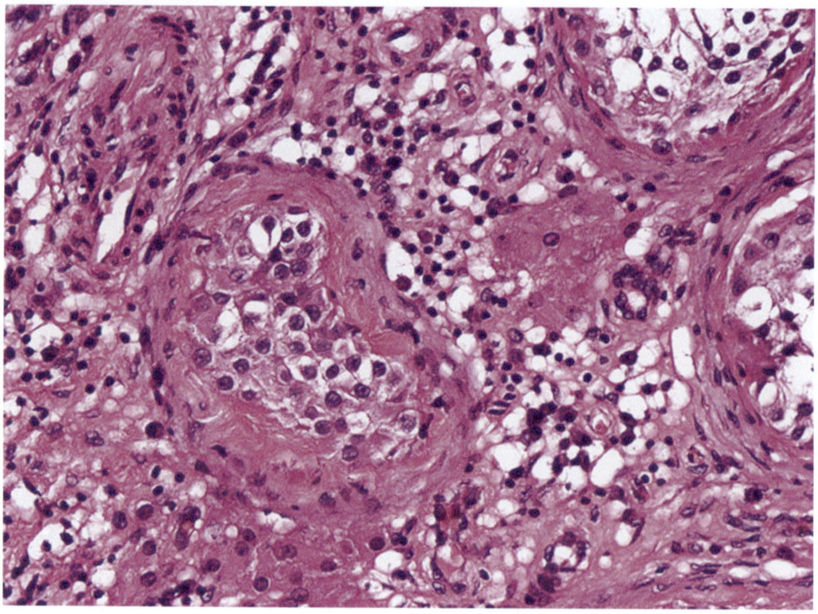

Fig. 26.9 The testis of a patient with lepromatous leprosy. Numerous macrophages in the interstitium with pale and vacuolated cytoplasm. Note the seminiferous tubules marked atrophy

disorder characterized by the abnormal proliferation of S100-positive histiocytes with phagocytosis of lymphocytes (emperipolesis). The lesions may be unilateral or bilateral. Some cases are associated with hematopoietic systemic diseases [53].

Erdheim-Chester Disease This is a non-Langerhans cell histiocytosis of unknown etiology. It is characterized by the presence of infiltrates of lipid-laden foamy hystiocytes which mainly affects the long bones of the lower extremities, the central nervous system, lung, heart, liver, spleen, retroperitoneum, testis, skin, and orbit. Patients develop hypogonadotropic hypogonadism with atrophy both of the seminiferous tubules and the Leydig cells.

Histologically there is an interstitial and intratubular infiltrate of macrophages with foamy cytoplasm. These cells show spherical nuclei without the typical configuration of Langerhans cells. These cells are CD68 positive and negative for CD1a and S100. The data considered important for clinical diagnosis are association with endocrine abnormalities, respiratory, and/or heart failure together with the radiological findings [54, 55].

Histiocytosis Secondary to Hydroxyethyl Starch Plasma Expander (HES) In more than two thirds of the autopsies of adult patients, an increase in the number of macrophages in the testicular interstitium can be seen. The causes are not known in most cases. One situation in which there is a large number of macrophages in the interstitium occurs in patients treated with HES. Macrophages are noted for their large size and multivacuolated cytoplasm, suggesting thesaurosis (Fig. 26.10). Studies to demonstrate mucopolysaccharides, starch, lipid, glycogen, and identifiable foreign body material with polarized light are negative. Ultrastructural studies show only empty vacuoles in the cytoplasm.

The commercial HES contains a heterogeneous group of molecules ranging from <10 to >1000 kDa. Their metabolism operates by hydrolysis. Most patients had no clinical symptoms derived from the HES treatment, except for the presence of pruritus and persistent erythema [56].

26.4 Infiltrates Rich in Plasma Cells

Plasma cells are an important component of the inflammatory infiltrates of chronic epididymitis and orchitis. There are three situations in which

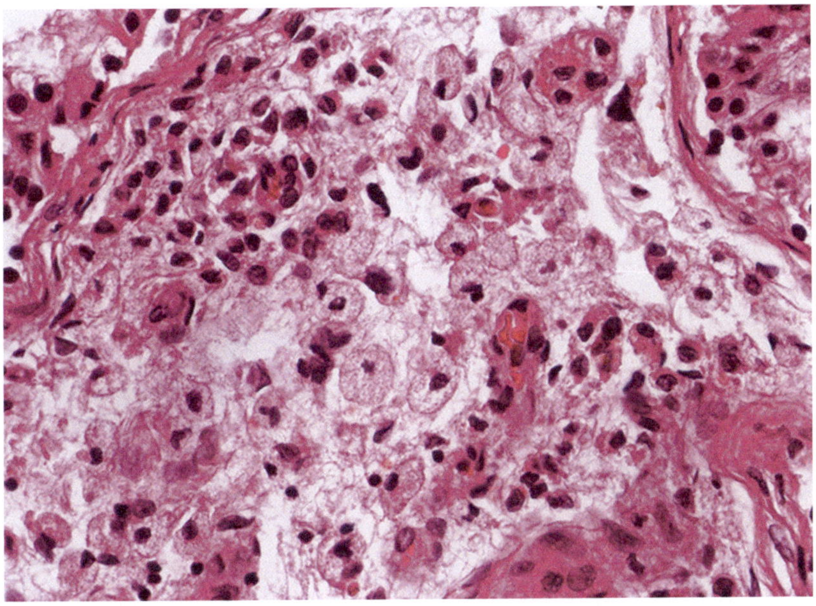

Fig. 26.10 Histiocytosis secondary to hydroxyethyl starch plasma expander. Abundant macrophages with pale and multivacuolated cytoplasm are observed in the interstitium

these infiltrates acquire specificity, and these are syphilitic interstitial orchitis, orchitis with IgG4-positive plasmacellular infiltrates, and a lesion known as plasma cell granuloma of the testicle.

Patients with interstitial syphilitic orchitis have at first a painless increase of the testicular size that can simulate a testicular tumor [57]. When cut, the testes have gray translucent areas that contrast with the yellowish color of the healthy preserved tubules. The inflammatory infiltrates, rich in plasma cells, initially are more numerous in the mediastinum testis and interlobular septa and then extend around the seminiferous tubules. The seminiferous tubules lose the seminiferous epithelium, and the tubular wall thickens until it disappears. The arteries usually show obliterans endoarteritis. Small gumma can be observed. Eventually the inflammation recedes and is replaced by fibrosis. The epididymis is usually unaffected.

IgG4-positive orchitis with testicular lesion plasmacellular infiltrates is a manifestation of IgG4-related disease [58]. The plasma cell granuloma of the testis is a reactive process of unknown etiology, with predominantly adult polyclonal plasma cells, which differentiates it from testicular plasmacytoma [59, 60].

26.5 Mast Cells and Infertility

Mast cells are present in the testis in approximately one per tubular section, and they are preferably located in the interstitium [61]. There is a significant increase in mast cells in some subfertile and infertile patients, especially carriers of Sertoli cell-only syndromes and mixed atrophy [62]. In mixed atrophy mast cell number increases amount to five per tubular section in Sertoli cell-only tubules. Mast cells are preferentially located in a peritubular situation, and since they are the main source of tryptase, a powerful fibrotic agent, they could be responsible for significant changes in the wall of the tubules and impaired spermatogenesis [63].

References

1. Nicholson A, Rait G, Murray-Thomas T, Hughes G, Mercer CH, Cassell J. Management of epididymo-orchitis in primary care: results from a large UK primary care database. Br J Gen Pract. 2010;60:e407–22.
2. Lau P, Anderson PA, Giacomantonio JM, Schwarz RD. Acute epididymitis in boys: are antibiotics indicated? Br J Urol. 1997;79:797–800.
3. Waldman LS, Kosloske AM, Parsons DW. Acute epididymoorchitis as the presenting manifestation of Hemophilus influenzae septicemia. J Pediatr. 1977;90:87–9.

4. Merlini E, Rotundi F, Seymandi PL, Canning DA. Acute epididymitis and urinary tract anomalies in children. Scand J Urol Nephrol. 1998;32:273–5.
5. VanderBrink BA, Sivan B, Levitt MA, Peña A, Sheldon CA, Alam S. Epididymitis in patients with anorectal malformations: a cause for urologic concern. Int Braz J Urol. 2014;40:676–82.
6. Bennett RT, Gill B, Kogan SJ. Epididymitis in children: the circumcision factor? J Urol. 1998;160:1842–4.
7. Lewis AG, Bukowski TP, Jarvis PD, Wacksman J, Sheldon CA. Evaluation of acute scrotum in the emergency department. J Pediatr Surg. 1995;30:277–81.
8. Bukowski TP, Lewis AG, Reeves D, Wacksman J, Sheldon CA. Epididymitis in older boys: dysfunctional voiding as an etiology. J Urol. 1995;154: 762–5.
9. Haecker FM, Hauri-Hohl A, von Schweinitz D. Acute epididymitis in children: a 4-year retrospective study. Orquioepididimitis en la pubertad y en el adulto joven. Eur J Pediatr Surg. 2005;15:180–6.
10. Taylor SN. Epididymitis. Clin Infect Dis. 2015;61(Suppl 8):S770–3.
11. Trojian TH, Lishnak TS, Heiman D. Epididymitis and orchitis: an overview. Am Fam Physician. 2009;79:583–7.
12. Pastorini E, Pastorini P, Chevallier D, Amiel J, Toubol J. Role of Chlamydia trachomatis in male urethritis. Analysis of 2,000 cases of male urethritis. J Urol (Paris). 1988;94:153–7.
13. National Institute of Health. NIAID study group on sexually transmitted diseases. 1980. Status report. Sumaries and panel recommendations. Washington, DC: Govermment Printing Office. 1981. p. 215–64.
14. Furuya R, Takahashi S, Furuya S, Kunishima Y, Takeyama K, Tsukamoto T. Is seminal vesiculitis a discrete disease entity? Clinical and microbiological study of seminal vesiculitis in patients with acute epididymitis. J Urol. 2004;171:1550–3.
15. Yamamoto M, Hibi H, Katsuno S, Miyake K. Clinical evaluation of a new polymerase chain reaction assay for detection of Chlamydia trachomatis in young patients with acute epididymitis. Hinyokika Kiyo. 1995;41:455–9.
16. Pilatz A, Hossain H, Kaiser R, Mankertz A, Schüttler CG, Domann E, Schuppe HC, Chakraborty T, Weidner W, Wagenlehner F. Acute epididymitis revisited: impact of molecular diagnostics on etiology and contemporary guideline recommendations. Eur Urol. 2015;68:428–35.
17. Berger RE, Alexander ER, Harnisch JP, Paulsen CA, Monda GD, Ansell J, Holmes KK. Etiology, manifestations and therapy of acute epididymitis: prospective study of 50 cases. J Urol. 1979;121:750–4.
18. Karam JA, Baker LA. Focal orchitis presenting as bilateral testicular masses. J Pediatr Urol. 2007;3: 337–9.
19. Suominen J, Söderström KO. Lymphocyte infiltration in human testicular biopsies. Int J Androl. 1982; 5:461–6.
20. Lehmann D, Emmons LR. Immunological phenomena observed in the testis and their possible role in infertility. Am J Reprod Immunol. 1989;19:43–52.
21. Schuppe HC, Pilatz A, Hossain H, Meinhardt A, Bergmann M, Haidl G, Weidner W. Orchitis and male infertility. Urologe A. 2010;49:629–35.
22. Suominen JJ. Sympathetic auto-immune orchitis. Andrologia. 1995;27:213–6.
23. Hendry WF, Levison DA, Parkinson MC, Parslow JM, Royle MG. Testicular obstruction: clinicopathological studies. Ann R Coll Surg Engl. 1990;72:396–407.
24. Lehmann J, Jancke C, Retz M, Loch T, Küppers F, Stöckle M, Weichert-Jacobsen K. A hypoechoic Lesion found on testicular ultrasound after testicular piercing. J Urol. 2000;164:1651.
25. Nistal M, Riestra ML, Paniagua R. Focal orchitis in undescended testes: discussion of pathogenetic mechanisms of tubular atrophy. Arch Pathol Lab Med. 2002;126:64–9.
26. Nistal M, Paniagua R, González-Peramato P. Nonneoplastic diseases of the testis. In: Bostwick DG, Cheng L, editors. Urologic Surgical Pathology. 3rd ed. Philadelphia: Elsevier Saunders Editorial; 2014.
27. Piton N, Roquet ML, Sibert L, Sabourin JC. Focal non granulomatous orchitis in a patient with Crohn's disease. Diagn Pathol. 2015;10:39.
28. Agarwal V, Li JK, Bard R. Lymphocytic orchitis: a case report. Hum Pathol. 1990;21:1080–2.
29. Gowing NFC. Malignant lymphoma of the testis. In: Pugh RCB, editor. Pathology of the testis. Oxford/ London/Edimburg/Melbourne: Blackwell; 1976. p. 334–55.
30. Jass JR, Farrell MA, Ellis H. Pseudolymphoma of the testis. Br J Urol. 1984;56:102–3.
31. Algaba F, Santaularia JM, Garat JM, Cubells J. Testicular pseudolymphoma. Eur Urol. 1986;12:362–3.
32. Nistal M, Mate A, Paniagua R. Granulomatous epididymal lesion of possible ischemic origin. Am J Surg Pathol. 1997;21:951–6.
33. McClure J. Malakoplakia of the testis and its relationship to granulomatous orchitis. J Clin Pathol. 1980;33:670–8.
34. Stevens SA. Malakoplakia of the testis. Br J Urol. 1995;75:111–2.
35. Nistal M, Echandia EL, Paniagua R. Septate junctions between digestive vacuoles in human malacoplakia. Tissue Cell. 1978;10:137–42.
36. Zurier RB, Weissmann G, Hoffstein S, Kammerman S, Tai HH. Mechanisms of lysosomal enzyme release from human leukocytes. II. Effects of cAMP and cGMP, autonomic agonists, and agents which affect microtubule function. J Clin Invest. 1974;53:297–309.
37. Kusuma V, Niveditha SR, Krishnamurthy, Ramdev K. Epididymo-testicular malacoplakia–a case report. Indian J Pathol Microbiol. 2006;49:413–5.
38. Dieckmann KP, Henke RP, Zimmer-Krolzig G. Malacoplakia of the epididymis. Report of a case and review of the literature. Urol Int. 1995;55:222–5.

39. Morgan TA, Rabban JT, Filly RA. Testicular malakoplakia: a rare sonographic mimic of malignancy. J Clin Ultrasound. 2015;43:199–202.
40. Stanton MJ, Maxted W. Malacoplakia: a study of the literature and current concepts of pathogenesis, diagnosis and treatment. J Urol. 1981;125:139–46.
41. Kang YJ, Kim SW, Lee KS, Kim KH. Malacoplakia of the epididymis. Korean J Urol. 2013;54:274–6.
42. Wiener LB, Riehl PA, Baum N. Xanthogranulomatous epididymitis: a case report. J Urol. 1987;138:621–2.
43. Hajri M, Amna MB, Derouich A, Ayed M, Zermani F, Jilani SB. Xanthogranulomatous orchitis. Report of 7 cases. Ann Urol (Paris). 2001;35:237–9.
44. Nistal M, Gonzalez-Peramato P, Serrano A, Regadera J. Xanthogranulomatous funiculitis and orchiepididymitis: report of 2 cases with immunohistochemical study and literature review. Arch Pathol Lab Med. 2004;128:911–4.
45. Ezer SS, Oguzkurt P, Temiz A, Bal N, Hicsonmez A. Xanthogranulomatous orchiepididymitis: a very uncommon cause of scrotal mass in childhood. Urology. 2013;82:228–30.
46. Val-Bernal JF, Argueta L, Fernández-Flórez A, Correas MA, Val D, Garijo MF, López-Rasines G. Bilateral xanthogranulomatous orchitis in a tetraplegic patient. Pathol Res Pract. 2012;208:62–4.
47. Dearment MC, Woodward TA, Menke DM, Brazis PW, Bancroft LW, Persellin ST. Whipple's disease with destructive arthritis, abdominal lymphadenopathy, and central nervous system involvement. J Rheumatol. 2003;30:1347–50.
48. Saporta L, Yuksel A. Androgenic status in patients with lepromatous leprosy. Br J Urol. 1994;74:221–4.
49. Nigam P, Mukhija RD, Kapoor KK, Kumar A, Sarkari NB, Gupta AK, Mishra SD. Male gonads in leprosy–a clinico-pathological study. Indian J Lepr. 1988;60: 77–83.
50. Akhtar M, Ali MA, Mackey DM. Lepromatous leprosy presenting as orchitis. Am J Clin Pathol. 1980;73: 712–5.
51. Ishikawa S, Mizushima M, Furuta M, Ishikawa A, Kawamura K. Leydig cell hyperplasia and the maintenance of bone volume: bone histomorphometry and testicular histopathology in 29 male leprosy autopsy cases. Int J Lepr Other Mycobact Dis. 2000;68:258–66.
52. Richens J. Genital manifestations of tropical diseases. Sex Transm Infect. 2004;80:12–7.
53. Wang CC, Al-Hussain TO, Serrano-Olmo J, Epstein JI. Rosai-Dorfman disease of the genito-urinary tract: analysis of six cases from the testis and kidney. Histopathology. 2014;65:908–16.
54. Sheu SY, Wenzel RR, Kersting C, Merten R, Otterbach F, Schmid KW. Erdheim-Chester disease: case report with multisystemic manifestations including testes, thyroid, and lymph nodes, and a review of literature. J Clin Pathol. 2004;57:1225–8.
55. Haroche J, Abla O. Uncommon histiocytic disorders: Rosai-Dorfman, juvenile xanthogranuloma, and Erdheim-Chester disease. Hematology Am Soc Hematol Educ Program. 2015;2015:571–8.
56. Cox NH, Popple AW. Persistent erythema and pruritus, with a confluent histiocytic skin infiltrate, following the use of a hydroxyethylstarch plasma expander. Br J Dermatol. 1996;134:353–7.
57. Nakano Y, Chokyu H, Inaba Y, Harada M, Gotoh A, Maeda S. Syphilitic orchitis: a case report. Hinyokika Kiyo. 1999;45:289–91.
58. Maillette de Buy Wenniger LJ, Doorenspleet ME, Klarenbeek PL, Verheij J, Baas F, Elferink RP, Tak PP, de Vries N, Beuers U. Immunoglobulin G4+ clones identified by next-generation sequencing dominate the B cell receptor repertoire in immunoglobulin G4 associated cholangitis. Hepatology. 2013;57:2390–8.
59. Aksoy PK, Ozdemir BH, Aygün C, Agildere M. Plasma cell granuloma of the testis: unusual localization. J Urol. 2001;166:1000.
60. Anghel G, Petti N, Remotti D, Ruscio C, Blandino F, Majolino I. Testicular plasmacytoma: report of a case and review of the literature. Am J Hematol. 2002;71: 98–104.
61. Nistal M, Santamaría L, Paniagua R. Mast cells in the human testis and epididymis from birth to adulthood. Acta Anat (Basel). 1984;119:155–60.
62. Meineke V, Frungieri MB, Jessberger B, Vogt H, Mayerhofer A. Human testicular mast cells contain tryptase: increased mast cell number and altered distribution in the testes of infertile men. Fertil Steril. 2000;74:239–44.
63. Welter H, Köhn FM, Mayerhofer A. Mast cells in human testicular biopsies from patients with mixed atrophy: increased numbers, heterogeneity, and expression of cyclooxygenase 2 and prostaglandin D2 synthase. Fertil Steril. 2011;96:309–13.

27 Histological Basis for the Interpretation of Granulomatous Orchitis

Manuel Nistal, Pilar González-Peramato, and Álvaro Serrano

27.1 Granulomatous Orchitis Destroying Testicular Architecture

27.1.1 Granulomatous Orchitis with Necrotizing Granulomas

Tuberculosis is an infectious disease caused by the bacillus *Mycobacterium tuberculosis*. In recent decades, its incidence has increased due on the one hand to its association with the pandemic of human immunodeficiency virus (HIV) and on the other hand to exposure of the population to immigration of people coming from areas where it is endemic. It is estimated to affect a third of the world population [1]. Genitourinary tuberculosis is the second of extrapulmonary sites. In 28 % of patients, the location is only genital. The organs of the male genital tract most affected by decreasing order of frequency are the epididymis, prostate, seminal vesicle, and testicle. Eighty-five percent of tuberculous epididymitis are secondary to renal tuberculosis [2]. Tuberculous orchitis is observed in 3 % of patients with genital tuberculosis usually secondary to tuberculosis of the epididymis. Isolated cases of tuberculous epididymo-orchitis with no other tuberculous foci elsewhere in the body are rare [3]. The cases in which it affects only the testis are exceptional [4]. The age of patients with tuberculous orchiepididymitis has risen: 72 % are older than 35 years and 18 % are over 65. The cases in childhood are rare.

Most of the time its *clinical symptoms* are very unspecific. Tuberculous epididymitis should be suspected in the presence of a patient with scrotal pain, few constitutional symptoms, and lack of response to conventional antibiotic or presence of a perineal sinus treatment [5]. In some cases, the sign is acute epididymitis [6], or an important increase in size of the testis and epididymis, suggesting a testicular tumor [7]. There is bilateral involvement in up to 70 % of cases depending on the duration of symptoms [8]. Diagnosis is confirmed by isolation of *M. tuberculosis* from urine or seminal fluid. In many cases the histological study of material obtained by fine needle aspiration or of the surgical specimen is required.

Histology Lesions are preferentially located in the tail of the epididymis (Fig. 27.1). The epididymis is enlarged associated with vas deferens thickening. The characteristic lesion of tuberculous granuloma consists of an eosinophilic area of granular material with nuclear debris (caseous necrosis) surrounded by epithelioid cells, Langhans' cells, peripherally by lymphocytes, and more externally a fibroblast layer (Fig. 27.2). Adjacent granulomas may coalesce causing large areas of tissue destruction. In a high percentage of cases, the presence of bacilli is disclosed by the Ziehl-Neelsen technique if care is taken to fix the material in formaldehyde. Bacilli are preferentially located in

M. Nistal et al., *Clues in the Diagnosis of Non-tumoral Testicular Pathology*,
DOI 10.1007/978-3-319-49364-0_27

younger granulomas, in the periphery of cheesy necrosis, and on the wall. In immunocompromised patients, the granulomas are composed of epithelioid cells and some lymphocytes, giant cells being rare. The number of acid-fast bacilli which in histological preparations are detected in these patients is very high.

BCG-induced tuberculous epididymo-orchitis, named "BCGitis," is rare. It results from the use of *Mycobacterium bovis* in intravesical instillations in patients with superficial bladder carcinoma [9]. Histologically it is similar to classical tuberculosis.

Syphilis There are two forms of syphilitic orchitis: congenital and acquired. In congenital orchitis both testes are enlarged at the time of birth. The histological picture is similar to interstitial

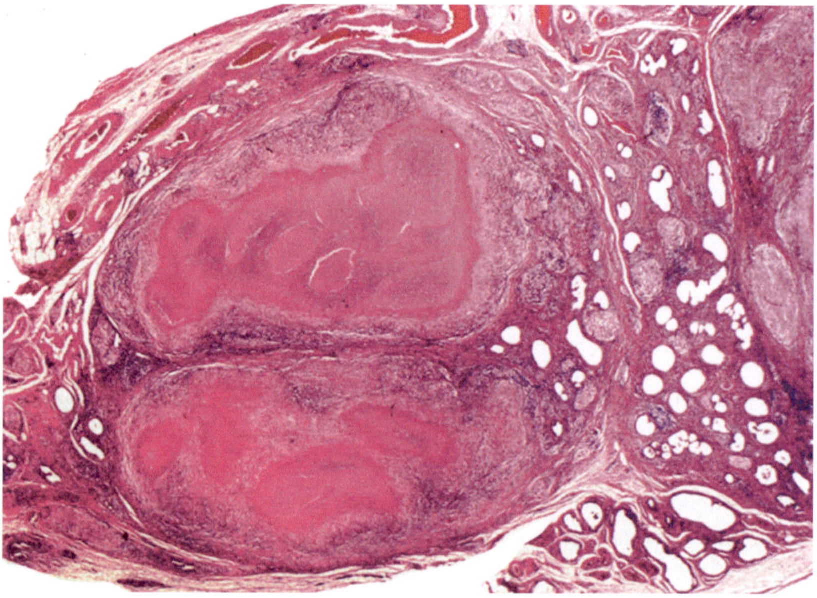

Fig. 27.1 Tuberculous epididymitis. Nodular lesion located in the tail of the epididymis. Larger nodules show central necrosis

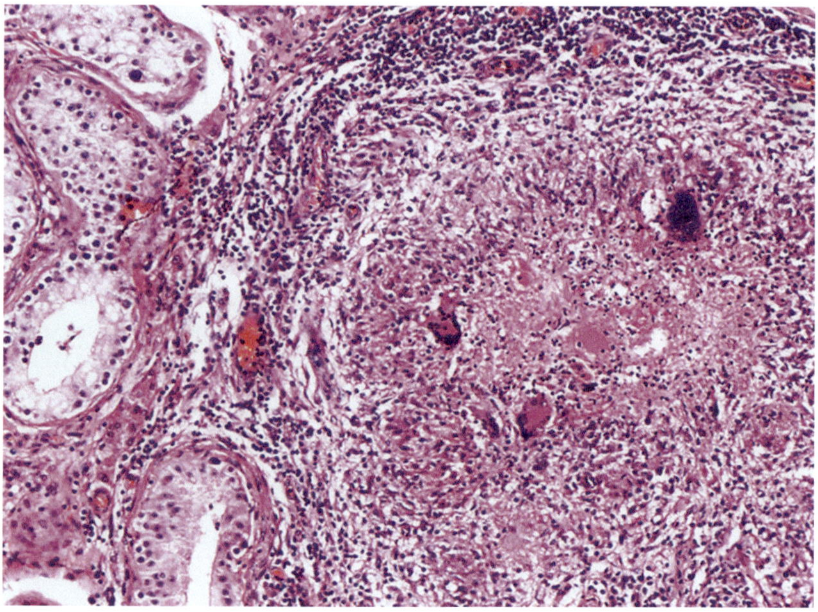

Fig. 27.2 Testicular tuberculosis. Granuloma consists of a central area of caseous necrosis surrounded by epithelioid cells, Langhans' giant cells, peripherally by lymphocytes, and more externally a fibroblast layer. Many epithelioid cells and lymphocytes extend among the neighbor seminiferous tubules

orchitis appearing in acquired syphilis. If the diagnosis is delayed until puberty, the testis undergoes atrophy and fibrosis [10]. Acquired adult orchitis is a complication of the tertiary period and shows two histological patterns, that of an interstitial inflammation (see Chap. 26) or the gummatous type [11].

Syphilitic gumma are characterized by the presence of one or more areas of necrosis, which are well defined and yellowish gray and destroy the testicular parenchyma. Their size can be so large that they form a testicular mass clinically simulating a testicular tumor. The gummatous orchitis rarely is bilateral. Histologically, the gumma shows central coagulative necrosis reminiscent of caseum, but the difference is that the silhouettes of the seminiferous tubules and other components of necrotic testicular parenchyma can be recognized. Surrounding this area there is an infiltration of lymphocytes, plasma cells, and some giant cells and more externally a myofibroblastic reaction. In HIV patients gummatous necrosis is not observed [12]. Obliterative endarteritis is a very common finding in all these lesions. To detect *Treponema pallidum* in biopsy material, some techniques can be used such as the Warthin-Starry silver stain or Levaditi, immunofluorescence, immunohistochemical, and PCR techniques in paraffin-embedded material [13].

Fungal orchiepididymitis is rare. The most common is the one caused by *Blastomyces dermatitidis*, *Coccidioides immitis*, *Histoplasma capsulatum*, and *Cryptococcus* [14]. Isolated cases of abscessified epididymitis by *Candida albicans* and *Torulopsis glabrata* have been reported, and testicular affectation by *Aspergillus fumigatus*, *Paracoccidioides brasiliensis*, *Exophiala jeanselmei, and Sporothrix schenckii* is known. All of them share the characteristic of being destructive lesions with necrosis or abscesses and granulomas similar to those of tuberculosis.

Blastomycosis Most cases are caused by *Blastomyces dermatitidis*. Blastomycosis is endemic in the valleys of the Mississippi, Missouri, and Ohio rivers. Unlike other inflammatory processes, blastomycosis can affect patients without immune defects.

The lung affectation is the most common manifestation. The genitourinary apparatus is affected in up to 20 % of systemic infections [15]. In decreasing order of frequency, prostate, epididymis, testes, and seminal vesicles are involved. The affected organs have small abscesses, which provide a cheesy appearance at the section. Histologically, inside the inflammatory cells or in the cytoplasm of giant cell of granulomas, there are fungi 8–15 microns in diameter with a double refraction contour, positive for PAS and silver methenamine [16].

Coccidioidomycosis It is an endemic disease in the semiarid regions of Western USA, Mexico, Central America, and South America. It is caused by *Coccidioides immitis*. Extrapulmonary sites are rare (1 %). It may present as a localized disease in the epididymis [17] after the general symptoms have ceased. Epididymal lesions can fistulize outside. Granulomas produced by *Coccidioides immitis* are similar to those of tuberculosis. The diagnosis is made with the PAS technique, whereupon spheres of 30–60 microns in diameter containing numerous endospores can be observed [18].

Histoplasmosis Histoplasma capsulatum has a worldwide distribution. Infection is more prevalent in the valleys of the Mississippi and Ohio rivers. In 90 % of cases, it manifests by a mild respiratory condition that may be asymptomatic. In the remaining cases, its severity is greater, and the germ is able to bring about a disseminated infection with serious complications in various organs and even death [19]. In the pre-AIDS era, testicular affectation appeared in 6 % of autopsies of patients with disseminated histoplasmosis. Epididymitis by *Histoplasma* may be the only manifestation of the disease [20]. The affected organs often show areas of necrosis or abscesses reminiscent of a sperm granuloma where it is easy to identify the fungus. The latter measures two to five microns in diameter and becomes more apparent with silver techniques [21]. In some cases it has also been diagnosed by culturing *Histoplasma capsulatum* taken from semen [22].

Cryptococcosis Genital involvement is the manifestation of a disseminated infection whose initial focus is usually the lung. It is a well-known complication after steroid therapy, orchitis being described as the only manifestation of cryptococcosis [23]. *Cryptococcus* is identified by its characteristic mucicarmine cover.

27.1.2 Granulomatous Orchitis with Non-necrotizing Granulomas

Brucellosis is a multisystem infectious disease. It is endemic in the Mediterranean countries, the Middle East, Central and South America, and India, where it causes great losses of domestic animals [24, 25]. The disease spreads by ingestion of products such as non-pasteurized milk or cheese or through skin wounds.

Epididymo-orchitis is its most common genitourinary complication, affecting more frequently young males [26, 27]. Genitourinary involvement occurs between 2 and 20 % of systemic brucellosis in endemic areas. In 2 to 14 % of cases, epididymitis which may be bilateral develops. The percentage of patients who develop orchitis is very low, but it has to be suspected when there is an increase in testicular size in a patient with undulant fever, malaise, chills, sweating, arthralgia, weight loss, and headache [28]. In other cases these symptoms are not as alarming and can be confused with a testicular tumor.

The histological picture is that of a granulomatous orchitis with a lympho-histiocytic infiltrate and occasional noncaseating granulomas in the interstitium. The seminiferous tubules are infiltrated by inflammatory cells and eventually undergo atrophy. The diagnosis is made through the clinical and laboratory findings: blood culture or high *Brucella* agglutination titers or in a faster way with real-time polymerase chain reaction assay in urine samples [29]. Improper diagnosis can lead to serious complications, which in some series reach 39 % of cases, such as testicular abscess, testicular infarction or atrophy, suppurative necrosis, and infertility [30].

Sarcoidosis is a granulomatous systemic disease, which mainly affects the skin, lymph nodes, lung, liver, and uvea. The etiology is unknown but has been linked to immune dysregulation in genetically predisposed individuals after exposure to infectious agents or environmental antigen. It is more prevalent in black people (20: 1), affecting individuals from 20 to 40 years [31]. It is estimated to affect 1: 10,000 in USA with about 22,500 cases annually. The genitourinary tract is affected only in 0.5 % of the clinically diagnosed cases, in 5 % of the postmortem studies [32]. In descending order of frequency epididymis, the testis and prostate are affected. Around 70 cases have been reported in English literature. Only 75 % have epididymal affectation and up to 50 % of the testis is affected [33]. The cases of isolated testicular involvement are exceptional [34].

Most often it manifests clinically as epididymitis (with bilateral involvement in one third of the cases), and it is almost asymptomatic with nodular increase of the epididymis; other cases present as orchiepididymitis and some as a tumor.

The histological picture is characteristic and consists of non-necrotizing granulomas composed of epithelioid cells, Langhans' cells, and foreign body giant cells peripherally surrounded by fibroblasts. Typical granulomas do not have a ring of lymphocytes (Fig. 27.3). The giant cells may contain asteroid bodies, Schaumann bodies, or cytoplasmic birefringent crystals.

Before issuing a diagnosis of sarcoidosis, a long list of processes should be ruled out that includes all granulomatous orchitis both bacterial and those produced by fungi and parasites, as well as granulomatous angiitis, spermatic granuloma, and some germ cell tumors. Tuberculosis differs by the presence of caseating granulomas that tend to coalesce. In spermatic granuloma spermatozoa can be recognized for many years inside the giant cells. In idiopathic granulomatous orchitis, the granulomas are preferably intratubular, while in sarcoidosis they are interstitial. In seminomas the sarcoid reaction can be very important, and even sarcoidosis and seminoma

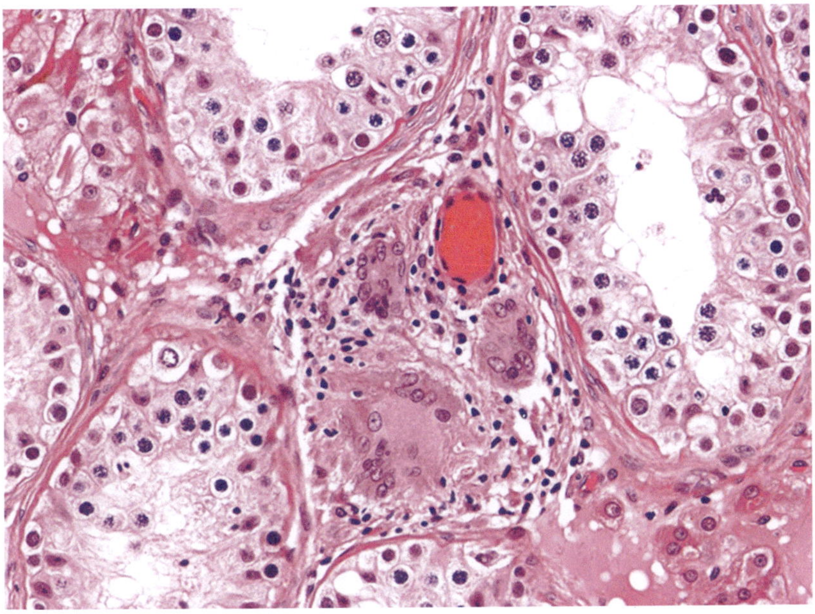

Fig. 27.3 Sarcoidosis. Granuloma consists of several giant cells and few lymphocytes. The surrounding seminiferous tubules still show spermatogenesis

can be associated [35]. Immunohistochemical markers for seminoma cells (Oct3/4, PLAP) facilitate the diagnosis.

27.1.3 Granulomatous Orchitis by Foreign Bodies

Orchiepididymitis by Parasites Parasitic infections are rare even in the areas where parasites are endemic. The agents most frequently affecting the genital tract are filarial worms and schistosomes. Lesions are basically characterized by the presence of a chronic inflammatory infiltrate with abundant eosinophils and foreign body giant cells related to parasite eggs or rests of dead worms.

Filariasis Filariasis is caused by *Wuchereria bancrofti*, a nematode that lives in the tropical and subtropical regions of Africa, South America, Caribbean islands, Southeastern Asia, and the Pacific islands, where it is a major public health issue [36].

Mosquitoes transmit larvae that develop in the human host. Adult worms migrate to the lymphatic vessels of the inguinal region causing funiculitis and orchiepididymitis [37]. The vascular endothelium proliferates; the lymphatic vessel's lumen occludes, and an infiltrate rich in eosinophils develops around the worm. The lymphatic stasis determines varicose lymphatic vessels and elephantiasis [38]. The lesions may become fibrous or calcify. The lesions may be recognized as hard nodules in the epididymis or along the spermatic cord. Testicular lesions are secondary to vascular lesions caused by the worm [39].

Schistosomiasis Schistosomiasis is endemic in Africa, the Middle East, India, China, and Latin America. It is estimated that 8 % of the world population is infected [40].

Involvement of the genitourinary tract is usually caused by *S. haematobium*. Prostatic and seminal vesicle involvement leads to calcifications, easily observed by transrectal ultrasonography. Worms can move to the epididymis or spermatic cord via the spermatic or deferential vein but usually do not enter the testes [41].

The most important lesion is a funiculitis [42], which can be granulomatous (reaction to eggs) or arteritic [43]. The lesions consist of an infiltration of inflammatory cells in the spermatic arteries without thrombosis or eggs. They present clinically as a testicular infarction and polypoid endophlebitis [44] (Fig. 27.4). The lesion consists of subendothelial granulomas and sclerosis of veins distal to the segment containing dead worms. Testicular massive involvement by *Schistosoma*, clinically simulating a testicular tumor, has also been observed [45].

Other parasites that cause testicular lesions are *Angiostrongylus costaricensis*, *Dirofilaria repens*, *Enterobius vermicularis*, *Echinococcosis*, and spargana. Testicular involvement has also been reported in visceral leishmaniasis; trypanosomiasis, both African and American; amebiasis; acanthamebiasis; malaria; and toxoplasmosis (Fig. 27.5).

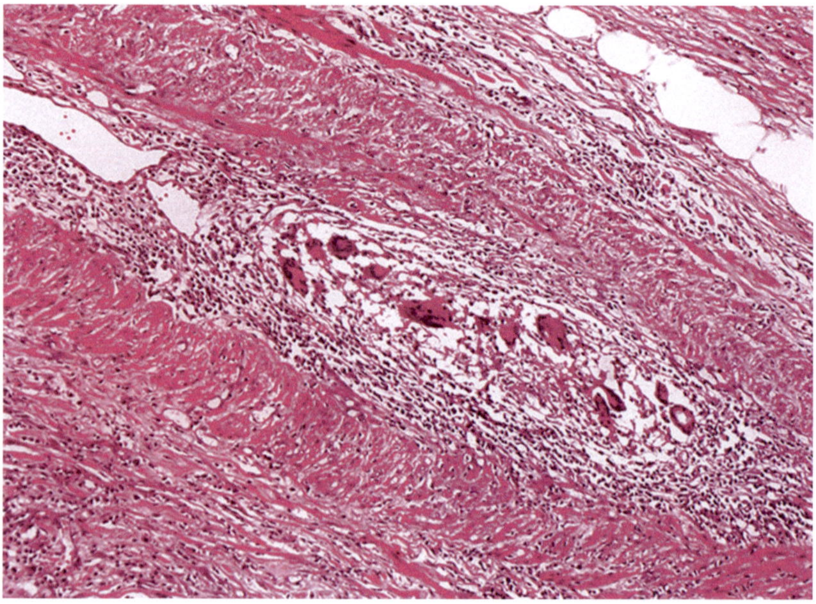

Fig. 27.4 Granulomatous endophlebitis in a vessel of the spermatic cord in a patient with schistosomiasis. Numerous giant cells in the intima are observed

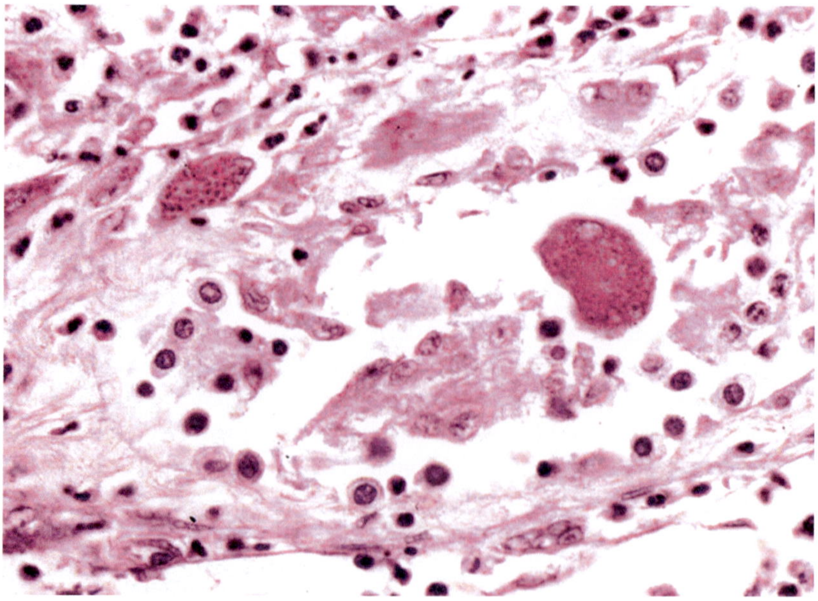

Fig. 27.5 Orchitis in toxoplasmosis. Oblique section of a seminiferous tubule in which some germ cells can be recognized. Two giant cells, one inside the tubule, another in its wall with numerous parasites, stand out

27.2 Granulomatous Orchitis Preserving Testicular Architecture

27.2.1 Idiopathic Granulomatous Orchitis (IGO)

This is a chronic inflammatory granulomatous lesion of senior persons (fifth–sixth decade, average 59.2 years) [46], which simulates a tumor [47]. Clinically it can present in different ways: with acute testicular pain, testicular pain associated with recurrent increased testicular size, or more frequently with an asymptomatic increase of the testicular size suggesting a tumor. Although it is generally a unilateral process, it can affect both testes. The right testis is affected with a slightly higher frequency (55 %) than the left one [48]. Its etiology is unknown, the following assumptions having been considered: traumatic, infectious, ischemic, and immunological.

The testicle is enlarged; the cut surface is nodular with areas of necrosis or infarction. Histologically two forms are distinguished, one predominantly tubular and the other one interstitial. In some cases the damage is focal and diffuse in others [49].

The primary tubular granulomatous orchitis is characterized by lesions that are centered on the seminiferous tubule. Germ cells degenerate; Sertoli cells show a vacuolated cytoplasm and vesicular nucleus. The tubular wall adopts a structure in concentric rings as it is infiltrated by lymphocytes, plasma cells, and histiocytes. Multinucleated giant cells appear in the old tubular lumen and also sometimes in the interstitium [50] (Fig. 27.6). Vascular thrombosis and arteritis are common findings. Spermatozoa have never been observed in the interstitium.

In the primary interstitial granulomatous orchitis, the interstitial infiltrate predominates for long over the seminiferous epithelium lesion. The infiltrate characteristics are similar to those of the tubular granulomatous orchitis. Finally, in both cases, and without observing any phagocytosis of spermatozoa, tubular atrophy and interstitial fibrosis occur (Fig. 27.7).

The histological pattern of these two forms of IGO has been linked to two classic models of experimental allergic orchitis [51]. The primary tubular granulomatous orchitis reproduces the orchitis transmitted by injection of serum of affected animals, while primary interstitial orchitis reminds the orchitis caused by the transference of sensitized T lymphocytes.

The IGO diagnosis requires ruling out bacterial granulomatous orchitis, orchitis by spiro-

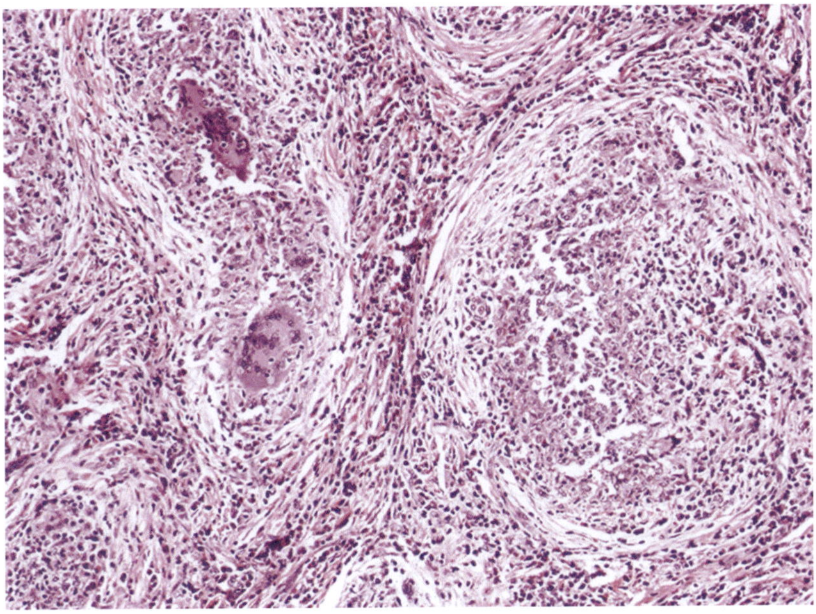

Fig. 27.6 Idiopathic granulomatous orchitis. Two seminiferous tubules show marked wall thickening and large clusters of inflammatory cells in the lumen. The seminiferous epithelium is not recognized. Two giant multinucleated cells are inside a tubule

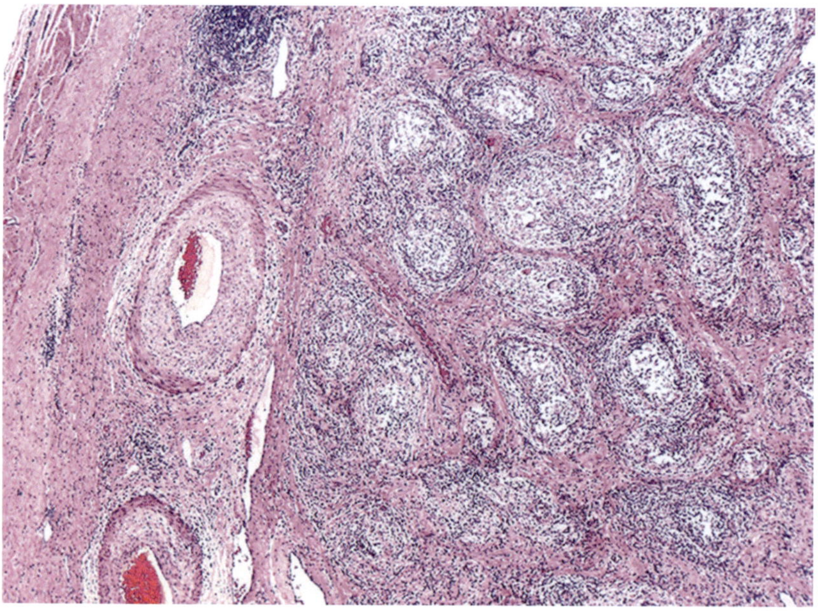

Fig. 27.7 Idiopathic granulomatous orchitis in a 65-year-old patient. The tunica albuginea is thickened. Vascular lesions of arteriosclerosis are severe. The testicular parenchyma has an abundant infiltrate both tubular and interstitial

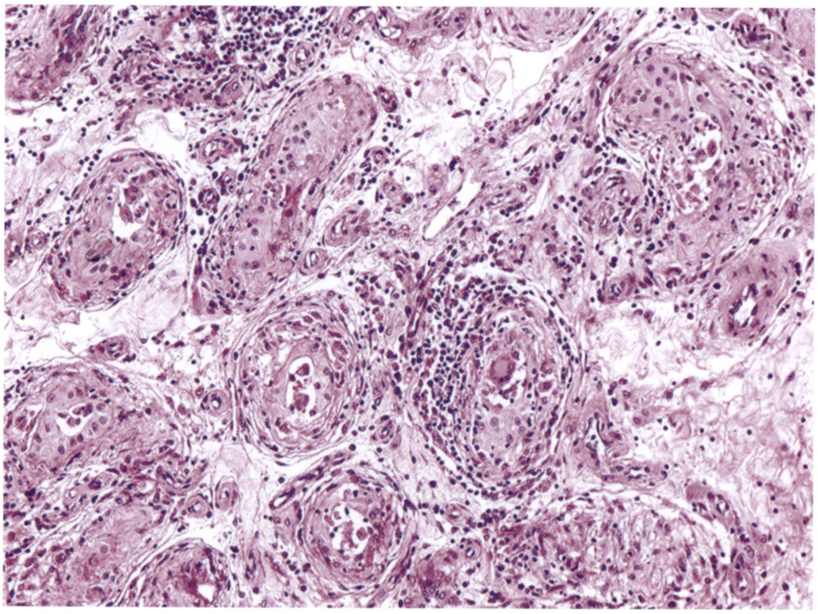

Fig. 27.8 Peritubular granulomatous orchitis associated with germ cell tumor. Lesions are centered on seminiferous tubules. Tubules are atrophic and of small caliber and show lymphocytes and giant cells both in the wall and inside the tubule

chetes, fungi, and parasites as well as testicular tumors such as seminomas and lymphomas.

27.2.2 Peritumoral Granulomatous Orchitis. Granulomatous Tubulitis

This is an infrequent lesion that develops in the testicular parenchyma surrounding certain germ cell tumors, especially seminoma. Granulomatous tubulitis is characterized by the presence of a granulomatous reaction that develops in the tubular wall. The lesions begin with lymphocytic infiltrates that are located among myoid cells and the basal lamina. These infiltrates soon contain a large number of epithelioid cells. At the end, in the same area, granulomas with multinucleated giant cells develop. Co-incidentally with the seminiferous epithelium atrophy, the Sertoli cells

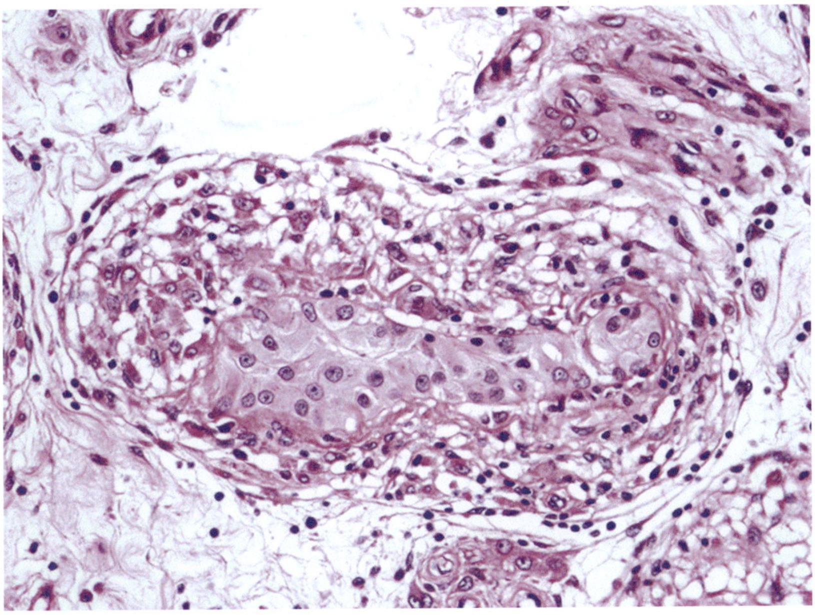

Fig. 27.9 Peritubular granulomatous orchitis associated with germ cell tumor. The inflammatory infiltrate is located in the tubular wall among myoid cells. It is composed of epithelioid cells and lymphocytes

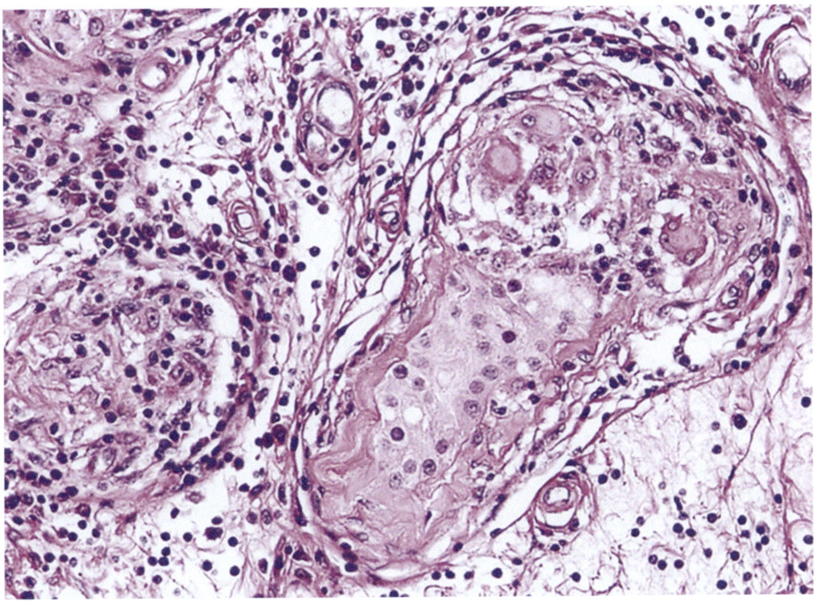

Fig. 27.10 Peritubular granulomatous orchitis associated with germ cell tumor. Granulomatous reaction with giant cells is developing in the thickness of the tubular wall. The seminiferous epithelium show secondary atrophy

undergo oncocytic changes and disappear as the granulomatous infiltrate goes through the tubular epithelium and reaches the lumen. Everything suggests that it is a reaction to the tubular wall materials (Figs. 27.8, 27.9, and 27.10).

This granulomatous tubulitis differs from both the sarcoid reaction associated with seminomas and the idiopathic granulomatous orchitis of the tubular type. The sarcoid reaction in the seminoma can be important enough to make the diagnosis of seminoma difficult, but it has no preference for the seminiferous tubules. In the idiopathic granulomatous orchitis of the tubular type, the granulomatous lesion develops concentrically affecting all tubular structures. The giant cells appear in the central part of the tubules and not only in the thickness of the peritubular myoid cells.

References

1. Furlow B. Tuberculosis: a review and update. Radiol Technol. 2010;82:33–52.
2. Kapoor R, Ansari MS, Mandhani A, Gulia A. Clinical presentation and diagnostic approach in cases of genitourinary tuberculosis. Indian J Urol. 2008;24:401–5.
3. Shenoy VP, Viswanath S, D'Souza A, Bairy I, Thomas J. Isolated tuberculous epididymo-orchitis: an unusual presentation of tuberculosis. J Infect Dev Ctries. 2012;6:92–4.
4. Lamichaney R, Das D, Sherpa M. Koch's disease presenting as an isolated testicular mass – an unusual occurance. J Clin Diagn Res. 2014;8:FD13–5.
5. Kim SH, Pollack HM, Cho KS, Pollack MS, Han MC. Tuberculous epididymitis and epididymo-orchitis: sonographic findings. J Urol. 1993;150:81–4.
6. Kinnear N, Hoh I, Campillo P, Bolt J. Tuberculous epididymo-orchitis masquerading as acute scrotum. BMJ Case Rep. 2016. pii: bcr2015214060.
7. Badmos KB. Tuberculous epididymo-orchitis mimicking a testicular tumour: a case report. Afr Health Sci. 2012;12:395–7.
8. Petersen L, Mommsen S, Pallisgaard G. Male genitourinary tuberculosis. Report of 12 cases and review of the literature. Scand J Urol Nephrol. 1993;27:425–8.
9. Harada H, Seki M, Shinojima H, Miura M, Hirano T, Togashi M. Epididymo-orchitis caused by intravesically instillated bacillus Calmette-Guérin: genetically proven using a multiplex polymerase chain reaction method. Int J Urol. 2006;13:183–5.
10. Oppenheimer EH, Hardy JB. Congenital syphilis in the newborn infant: clinical and pathological observations in recent cases. Johns Hopkins Med J. 1971;129:63–82.
11. Mackenzie H, Mahmalji W, Raza A. The gumma and the gonad: syphilitic orchitis, a rare presentation of testicular swelling. Int J STD AIDS. 2011;22:531–3.
12. Chu CY, Chen WY, Yeh SD, Yeh HM, Fang CL. Syphilitic orchitis mimicking a testicular tumor in a clinically occult HIV-infected young man: a case report with emphasis on a challenging pathological diagnosis. Diagn Pathol. 2016;11:4.
13. Nakano Y, Chokyu H, Inaba Y, Harada M, Gotoh A, Maeda S. Syphilitic orchitis: a case report. Hinyokika Kiyo. 1999;45:289–91.
14. Orr WA, Mulholland SG, Walzak Jr MP. Genitourinary tract involvement with systemic mycosis. J Urol. 1972;107:1047–50.
15. Lam WL, Dashefsky SM, Levi CS, MacLennan GT, Quinonez G. US case of the day. Right epididymo-orchitis due to disseminated Blastomyces dermatitidis. Radiographics. 1994;14:931–3.
16. Seo R, Oyasu R, Schaeffer A. Blastomycosis of the epididymis and prostate. Urology. 1997;50:980–2.
17. Sohail MR, Andrews PE, Blair JE. Coccidioidomycosis of the male genital tract. J Urol. 2005;173:1978–82.
18. Dykes TM, Stone AB, Canby-Hagino ED. Coccidioidomycosis of the epididymis and testis. AJR Am J Roentgenol. 2005;184:552–3.
19. Tichindelean C, East JW, Sarria JC. Disseminated histoplasmosis presenting as granulomatous epididymo-orchitis. Am J Med Sci. 2009;338:238–40.
20. Kauffman CA, Slama TG, Wheat LJ. Histoplasma capsulatum epididymitis. J Urol. 1981;125:434–5.
21. Schuster TG, Hollenbeck BK, Kauffman CA, Chensue SW, Wei JT. Testicular histoplasmosis. J Urol. 2000;164:1652.
22. Randhawa HS, Chaturvedi S, Khan ZU, Chaturvedi VP, Jain SK, Jain RC, Bazaz-Malik G. Epididymal histoplasmosis diagnosed by isolation of Histoplasma capsulatum from semen. Mycopathologia. 1995;131:173–7.
23. James CL, Lomax-Smith JD. Cryptococcal epididymo-orchitis complicating steroid therapy for relapsing polychondritis. Pathology. 1991;23:256–8.
24. Fallatah SM, Oduloju AJ, Al-Dusari SN, Fakunle YM. Human brucellosis in Northern Saudi Arabia. Saudi Med J. 2005;26:1562–6.
25. Yetkin MA, Erdinc FS, Bulut C, Tulek N. Epididymoorchitis due to brucellosis in central Anatolia. Turkey Urol Int. 2005;75:235–8.
26. Savasci U, Zor M, Karakas A, Aydin E, Kocaaslan R, Oren NC, Coskun O, Turhan V, Gul HC, Cicek AF, Aydur E, Eyigun CP. Brucellar epididymo-orchitis: a retrospective multicenter study of 28 cases and review of the literature. Travel Med Infect Dis. 2014;12(6 Pt A):667–72.
27. Bosilkovski M, Kamiloski V, Miskova S, Balalovski D, Kotevska V, Petrovski M. Testicular infection in brucellosis: Report of 34 cases. J Microbiol Immunol Infect. 2016. pii: S1684–1182(16)30004–4.
28. González Sánchez FJ, Encinas Gaspar MB, Napal Lecumberri S, Rajab R. Brucellar orchiepididymitis with abscess. Arch Esp Urol. 1997;50:289–92.
29. Queipo-Ortuño MI, Colmenero JD, Muñoz N, Baeza G, Clavijo E, Morata P. Rapid diagnosis of Brucella epididymo-orchitis by real-time polymerase chain reaction assay in urine samples. J Urol. 2006;176:2290–3.
30. Memish ZA, Venkatesh S. Brucellar epididymo-orchitis in Saudi Arabia: a retrospective study of 26 cases and review of the literature. BJU Int. 2001;88:72–6.
31. Naseem S, Lindley R, Mufti GR. Testicular sarcoid. Urol Int. 2001;67:100–1.
32. Turk CO, Schacht M, Ross L. Diagnosis and management of testicular sarcoidosis. J Urol. 1986;135:380–1.
33. Kodama K, Hasegawa T, Egawa M, Tomosugi N, Mukai A, Namiki M. Bilateral epididymal sarcoidosis presenting without radiographic evidence of intrathoracic lesion: Review of sarcoidosis involving the male reproductive tract. Int J Urol. 2004;11:345–8.
34. Wong JA, Grantmyre J. Sarcoid of the testis. Can J Urol. 2006;13:3201–3.
35. Droz JP, Ruffie P, Piot G, Ghosn M, Caillaud JM, Elias D, Perrin JL, Levasseur P. Sarcoidosis and testicular germ cell tumor. Case report. Scand J Urol Nephrol. 1990;24:171–3.
36. WHO. Fourth report of the WHO Expert Committee on filariasis. Wld Hlth Org Techn Rep Ser No. 702. 1984, p. 112.

37. Arora VK, Bhatia A. Adult filarial worm in fine needle aspirate of an epididymal nodule. Acta Cytol. 1989;33:421.
38. Tripathi FM, Sinha JK, Bhattacharya V. Elephantine scrotum and pseudoscrotum in endemic filariasis. Lymphology. 1990;23:198–9.
39. Pacella M, Corbu C, Naselli A, Quilici P, Carmignani G. Acute scrotum secondary to filarial infection: a case report. Int Urol Nephrol. 2002;34:385–6.
40. Webbe G. The six diseases of WHO. Schistosomiasis: some advances. Br Med J (Clin Res Ed). 1981;283: 1104–6.
41. Alves LS, Assis BP, Rezende MM. Schistosomal epididymitis. Int Braz J Urol. 2004;30:413–5.
42. Makar N. Urological aspects of bilharziasis in Egypt. SOP Pres: Cairo; 1955. p. 1–208.
43. Steinberger RM, Lindsay KG, Alassandri R, Wise GJ. Infarction of testicle and *Schistosoma mansoni*. Urology. 1975;5:567–9.
44. Elbadawi A, Khuri FJ, Cockett AT. Polypoid granulomatous and sclerosing endophlebitis of spermatic cord: new pathologic type of schistosomal funiculitis. Urology. 1979;13:309–14.
45. Soans B, Abel C. Ultrasound appearance of schistosomiasis of the testis. Australas Radiol. 1999;43:385–7.
46. Wegner HE, Loy V, Dieckmann KP. Granulomatous orchitis–an analysis of clinical presentation, pathological anatomic features and possible etiologic factors. Eur Urol. 1994;26:56–60.
47. Martínez-Rodríguez M, Navarro Fos S, Soriano Sarrió P, Alcalá-Santaella Casanova C, Ramos Soler D, Llombart Bosch A. Idiopathic granulomatous orchitis: pathologic study of one case. Arch Esp Urol. 2006;59:725–7.
48. Pekindil G, Hüseyin Atakan I, Kaya E, Bilgi S, Inci O. Bilateral synchronous granulomatous orchitis: gray-scale and colour Doppler sonographic findings. Eur J Radiol. 1999;31:201–3.
49. Roy S, Hooda S, Parwani AV. Idiopathic granulomatous orchitis. Pathol Res Pract. 2011;207:275–8.
50. Grüneberg H. Über drei ungewöhnliche Fälle von chronischer Orchitis unter dem klinischen Bilde eines Hodentumors. Frankf Z Pathol. 1926;33:217–27.
51. Sato K, Hirokawa K, Hatakeyama S. Experimental allergic orchitis in mice. Histopathological and Immunological studies. Virchows Arch A Pathol Anat Histol. 1981;392:147–58.

28 Rete Testis Dysgenesis as a Marker of Undescended Testis

Manuel Nistal, Pilar González-Peramato, and Álvaro Serrano

28.1 Normal Rete Testis

The rete testis is an elongated, slightly curved comma-shaped structure. The thickened end is located in the upper pole of the testis. The rete testis connects the seminiferous tubules with the ductuli efferentes [1].

The rete testis is a network of interconnected channels and flattened cavities which are empty normal under conditions. According to its topography, three parts are distinguished: septal, mediastinal, and extratesticular.

Septal Rete

The septal rete is composed of the tubuli recti which are short tubular structures that connect the seminiferous tubules to the mediastinal rete. The cranial tubuli recti end perpendicular to the mediastinal rete testis, while those in the caudal testicular region end in progressively more obtuse angles. Tubuli recti are trumpet shaped with a widened area in continuity with the seminiferous tubules called transition segment [2]. The diameter of the tubular zone is less than 25 microns. Tubuli recti are lined with cuboidal epithelial cells. Transition segments are lined with columnar cells similar to Sertoli anchored obliquely and with the apical pole directed toward the testicular mediastinum. Some tubuli recti are very short or even can be missing; in this case the seminiferous tubules connect directly into the mediastinal rete. There are approximately 1400 holes in the septal rete for drainage of secretions from the seminiferous tubules [3].

Mediastinal Rete

The mediastinal rete is lodged at the testicular mediastinum, a structure composed of dense fibrous connective tissue rich in collagen and elastic fibers. It comprises flattened and largely interconnected cavities that run parallel to the testicular surface. The lining of these cavities is an epithelium with two types of cells, squamous and columnar cells. Squamous cells are the most abundant; the columnar cells form small islets preferably located in the angled ends of the cavities (Fig. 28.1).

Both types of cells have a deep fold in the nucleus, isolated microvilli, a single cilium at the apical pole, and junctions in the lateral surfaces. In the cytoplasm there are some mitochondria, rough reticulum, and Golgi complex. Both cell types express immunostaining for vimentin and keratin. The epithelium lies on a basement membrane, surrounded by some myofibroblasts.

The cavities of the rete testis are crossed obliquely by the chordae of the rete testis (Fig. 28.1). They are structures formed by parallel filiform bundles of collagen fibers with occasional fibroblasts. The chordae are covered by the epithelium of the rete. Capillaries can be observed in the thicker ones [4].

M. Nistal et al., *Clues in the Diagnosis of Non-tumoral Testicular Pathology*,
DOI 10.1007/978-3-319-49364-0_28

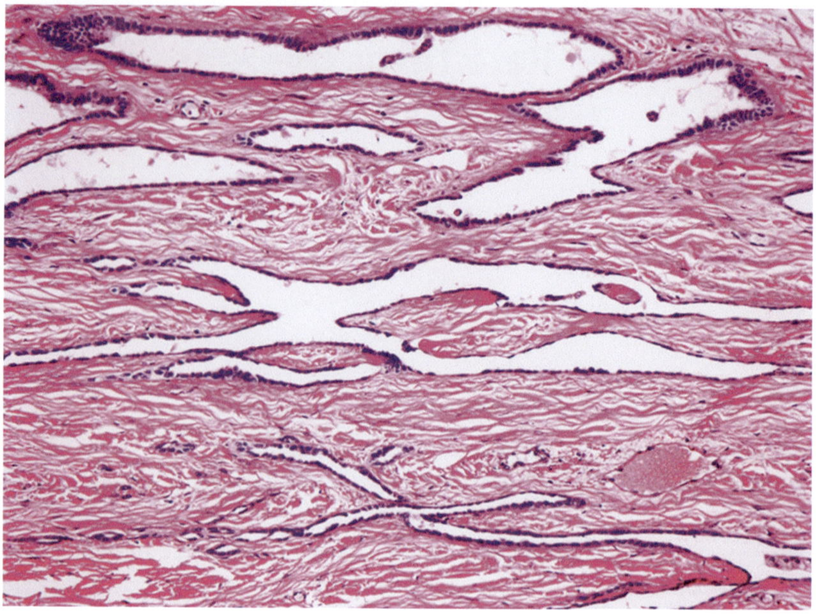

Fig. 28.1 Normal adult rete testis. Flattened mediastinal rete cavities lined by squamous epithelium. Some cavities are crossed by the chordate of the rete testis

Extratesticular Rete

The extratesticular rete connects the mediastinal rete with the efferent ductules. It starts coinciding with lacks of continuity present in the testicular albuginea for the passage of the spermatic pathway. It comprises cavities showing a certain degree of dilatation. The epithelium is similar to the mediastinal rete testis.

In addition to constituting the first part of the spermatic pathway, the rete testis contributes to homogenize testicular secretions and is involved in the secretion of various electrolytes [5] and in defective sperm phagocytosis [6].

28.2 Rete Testis Dysgenesis

28.2.1 Definition

Dysgenesis of the rete testis is a nonneoplastic lesion characterized by an inadequate maturation of the rete testis with persistence of infantile or pubertal histological characteristics in adults, associated with proliferation of its components.

The expression of dysgenesis of the rete testis is a wide spectrum of images ranging from poor development of the cavities to hyperplasia [7]. All of them have in common the changes in the epithelial lining which becomes cuboidal or columnar instead of the characteristic flattened epithelium with areas of cuboidal cells.

This disorder involves the three segments of the rete testis known as septal, mediastinal, and extratesticular. The involvement of the septal rete is constant. At this level, a marked twisting of tubuli recti can be observed, and it is expressed in the histological sections as cords and tubular or glandular proliferations. The transitional segments do not end abruptly at the start of the seminiferous tubules but do it in an irregular fashion. In this way, a variable length of the seminiferous tubules is lined with both epithelial and Sertoli cells. This double cell types is easily detected by immunohistochemistry as, unlike Sertoli cells, the epithelial cells of the rete express AE1/AE3 cytokeratin.

28.2.2 Histological Patterns of Dysgenesis of the Rete Testis

Three histological patterns of dysgenesis of the rete testis can be distinguished depending on the degree of development of the mediastinal and extratesticular rete testis, referred to as diffuse hypoplasia, cystic hypoplasia, and adenomatous hyperplasia (Table 28.1).

Diffuse Hypoplasia

Testes with diffuse hypoplasia show an infantile pattern of the rete testis. It consists of winding cords of cuboidal cells. The lumina of the cavities are absent in the mediastinal rete and very scant in the extratesticular rete. The connective tissue of the mediastinum does not show the characteristic high grade of collagenization of adult testis. On the contrary, it is frequently loose and abundant (Figs. 28.2 and 28.3).

Cystic Hypoplasia

Testes with cystic hypoplasia of the rete testis share some features with diffuse hypoplasia, such as poor development and extension of the rete and abundance of ductal or pseudoglandular structures, but they differ in the microcystic dilatation undergone by the cavities (Fig. 28.4). The microcystic dilatation can reach up to 500 microns. This disorder is present in 50 % of undescended testes.

Difficulties in drainage of the testicular fluid of seminiferous tubules could be the cause of the cystic transformation of hypoplastic rete testis. Multiple epididymal anomalies have been reported in cryptorchidic patients [8]. Even in the absence of significant anomalies, hypoplasia of the efferent ductules and immaturity of the muscular wall of the principal epididymal duct can be microscopically observed [9]. However,

Table 28.1 Clues in the differential diagnosis of dysgenesis of the rete testis

	Diffuse hypoplasia	Cystic hypoplasia	Adenomatous hyperplasia
Pattern	Infantile	Infantile	
Architecture	Cords	Ducts	Solid
		Pseudoglands	Glandular
			Papillary
			Cribriform
Lumen of cavities	Absent RM	Dilated microcysts	Variable
	Scant RE		Spermatozoa
Lining cells	Cuboidal	Flattened/cuboidal	Cuboidal/columnar

RM rete mediastinal, *RE* rete extratesticular

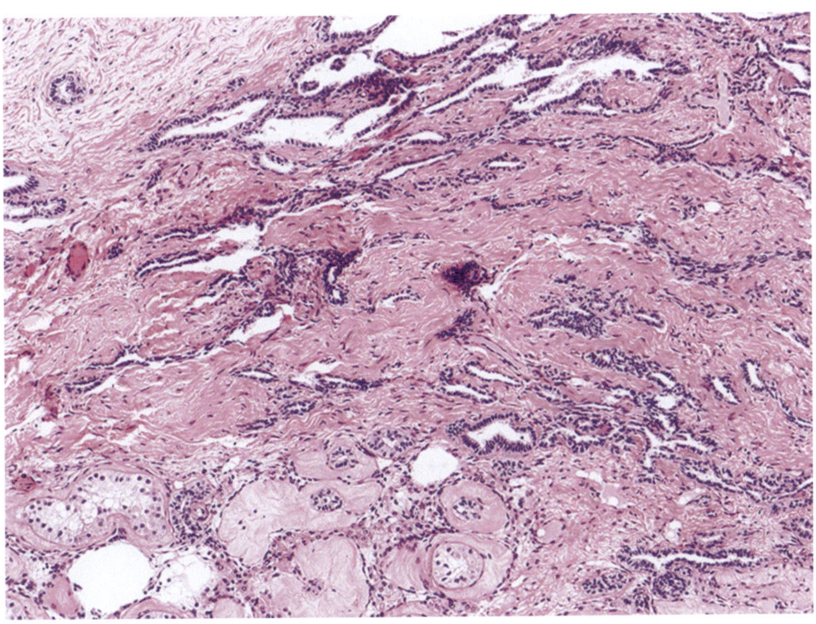

Fig. 28.2 Diffuse hypoplasia of the rete testis. Undescended testicle of an adult showing atrophy of the seminiferous tubules. The rete testis cavities are small and appear well separated from each other by an apparent increased mediastinum testis tissue

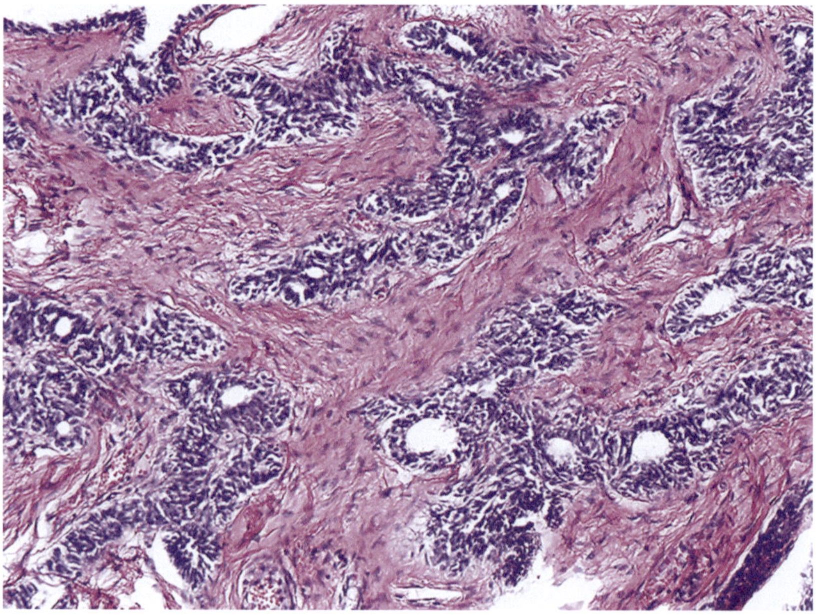

Fig. 28.3 Diffuse hypoplasia of the rete testis in a 27-year-old cryptorchid patient. Most of the rete testis consists of epithelial cords or small ducts lined by cuboidal epithelium

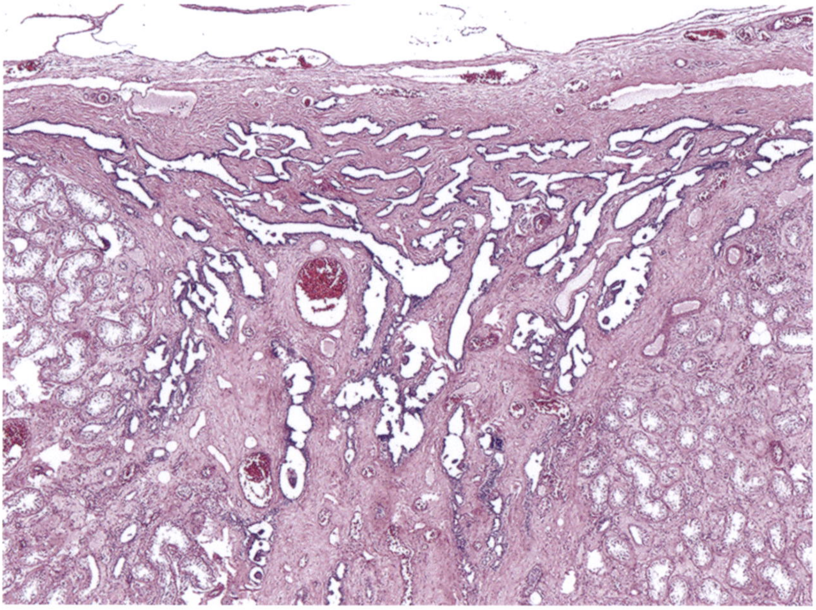

Fig. 28.4 Cystic hypoplasia of the rete testis. The two most characteristic findings are the small size of the cavities and ectasia. All cavities are lined by a cuboidal epithelium

this does not seem to be the single reason of microcystic dilatation, as testes with cystic hypoplasia of the rete testis frequently show seminiferous tubules lined with dysgenetic Sertoli cells which are unable to produce testicular fluid after puberty. Moreover, the possibility of a limited capacity of fluid production by cells of the rete testis and a retrograde repletion of epididymal fluid cannot be ruled out. The last possibility is improbable because these epididymides are frequently hypoplastic and the ectasia should produce atrophy and flattening of the epithelium that is not present in this dysgenesis of the rete testes.

Adenomatous Hyperplasia Testes with adenomatous hyperplasia of the rete testis show a solid/glandular, papillary, or cribriform epithelial proliferation that preferentially involves mediastinal rete similar to the adenomatous hyperplasia reported by Nistal in 1988 [10]. The epithelium is cuboidal or columnar; the cells have ovoid nuclei with a deep nuclear fold and peripheral nucleoli, are devoid of atypia, and do not show mitosis (Figs. 28.5, 28.6, and 28.7). In some cases spermatozoa can be observed inside the cavities, suggesting that this epithelial proliferation is connected with the seminiferous tubules.

28.2.3 Relationship Between Dysgenesis of the Rete Testis and Other Primary Anomalies of the Undescended Testis

The dysgenetic nature of these rete testes is in accordance with other anomalies frequently observed in undescended testis and in the extra-testicular ductal system.

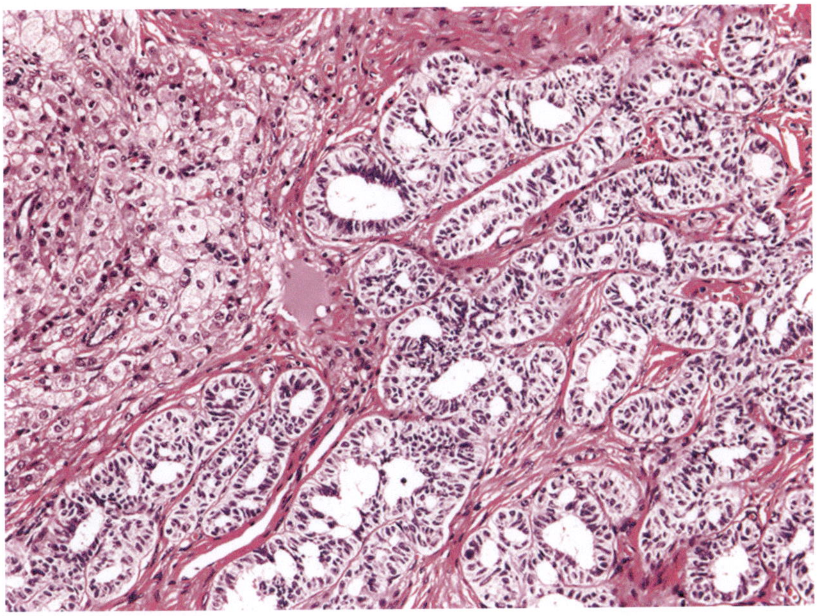

Fig. 28.5 Adenomatous hyperplasia of the rete testis with glandular pattern. The normal arrangement of the rete testis in flattened cavities has been replaced by glandular structures lined by columnar epithelium

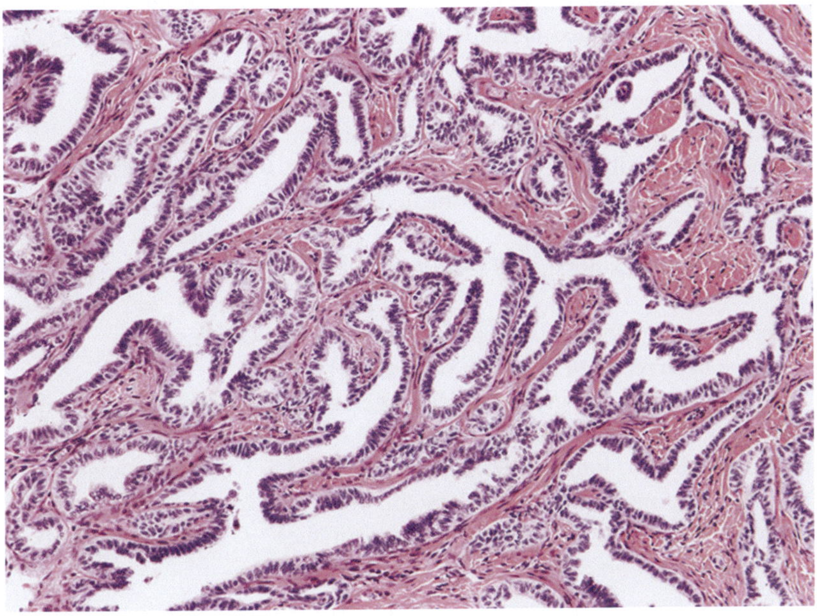

Fig. 28.6 Adenomatous hyperplasia of the rete testis with papillary pattern. Numerous papillary projections lined by cuboidal epithelium protrude inside the cavities of the rete testis

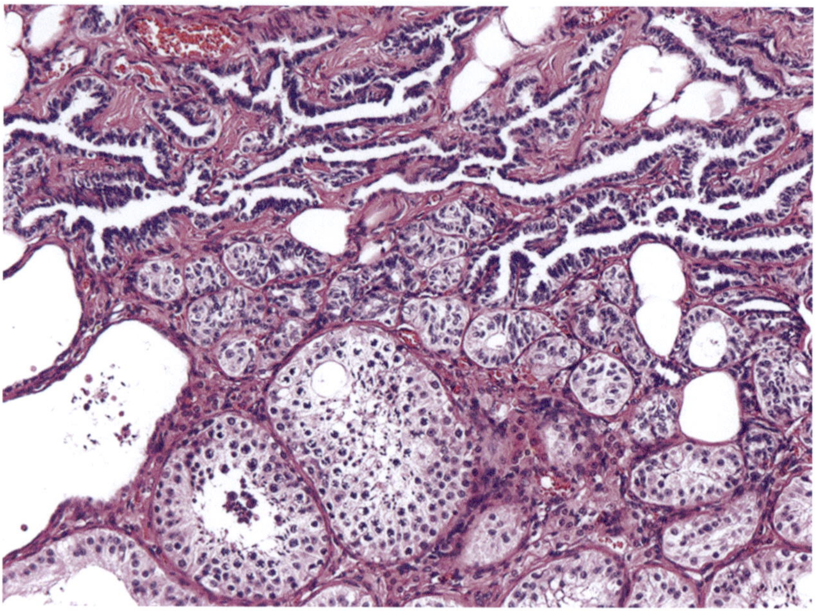

Fig. 28.7 Adenomatous hyperplasia of the rete testis with glandular and papillary patterns. Seminiferous tubules with spermatogenesis side by side with others showing cystic transformation

In a 40-case series [11], the lesions observed in the seminiferous tubules were Sertoli cell-only syndrome (57.5 %), diffuse tubular hyalinization (20 %), mixed tubular atrophy (7.5 %), maturation arrest at spermatogonia level (10 %), and adluminal compartment pathology (5 %).

When studying in more detail the different components of the seminiferous tubules and the interstitium, the following anomalies have been observed:

- Dysgenetic Sertoli cells [11]
- Poorly differentiated peritubular myoid cells [12]
- Scarce elastic fibers [13, 14]
- Low quantity of collagen IV and laminin in the tubular wall [15]
- Morphological anomalies in Leydig cells [16, 17]
- Low immunoexpression of testosterone [18]

In human cryptorchidism, epididymal anomalies have been reported in 36–79 % of cases [19–21]. Some of them are grossly evident such as an elongated loop-like epididymis, separation of the testis, angulation, long mesocardium, or atresia [20, 22]. The most frequent lesions are efferent ductules hypoplasia, delayed maturation of the epithelium, and poor development of the muscular layers of the principal duct of the epididymis [9, 23]. In about one third of cases, the epididymis show marked luminal dilation with or without association with atresia of the epididymis [8].

Everything indicates that both derivatives of the anastomosis of the testicular cords in the mesonephros area – primordium of the rete testis – and the mesonephros would undergo an injury early during development. This abnormality, although present at birth, in most cases would not be fully developed until adulthood, perhaps influenced by hormonal changes associated with puberty.

28.2.4 Differential Diagnosis

Dysgenesis of the rete testis with a microcystic pattern, and especially the adenomatous pattern, has to be distinguished mainly from three entities:

1. Secondary pseudohyperplasia of the rete testis associated with atrophic testes usually through an inflammatory or ischemic mechanism
2. Adenocarcinoma of the rete testis
3. Metastatic adenocarcinoma

In the pseudohyperplasia, the lesions are focal, microscopic, and more often located in the septal rete. The mediastinal rete show minimal alterations. This lesion is associated with a pronounced atrophy of the seminiferous tubules, which in turn may even cause tubular sclerosis.

Benign tumors of the rete testis such as adenomas in their solid and papillary variants, as well as cystadenomas, are unique and focal lesions [24], while hyperplasia of the rete testis is a diffuse lesion.

Adenocarcinoma of the rete testis is a tumor with abundant mitosis infiltrating adjacent structures [25]. Prostate carcinoma metastases are ruled out as they preserve the rete testis architecture. Prostatic acid phosphatase and PSA immunostaining are also useful for the differential diagnosis.

28.2.5 Situations in Which Dysgenesis of the Rete Testis Can Be Observed

Most cases of rete testis dysgenesis have been reported in undescended testes removed in adults. Careful study of the rete testis in the testicles with germ cell tumors shows that even in cases in which a pagetoid pattern of infiltration of GCNIS is not seen, lesions resembling those of the dysgenesis of the rete testis with a microcystic or an adenomatous or a papillary pattern are frequently observed. This fact does not seem to be fortuitous and could be another finding to be added to the injuries presented by the testes of patients with testicular dysgenesis syndrome [26] (see Chap. 13).

References

1. Ilio KY, Hess RE. Structure and function of the ductuliefferentes: a review. Microsc Res Tech. 1994;29: 432–67.
2. Osman DI, Ploën L. The mammalian tubuli recti: ultrastructural study. Anat Rec. 1978;192:1–17.
3. Roosen-Runge EC, Holstein AF. The human rete testis. Cell Tissue Res. 1978;189:409–33.
4. Bustos-Obregon E, Holstein AF. The rete testis in man: ultrastructural aspects. Cell Tissue Res. 1976;175:1–15.
5. Waites GMH, Gladwell RT. Physiological significancy of fluid secretion in the testis and blood-testis barrier. Physiol Rev. 1982;62:624–69.
6. Holstein AF. Spermatophagy in the seminiferous tubules and excurrent ducts of the testis in Rhesus monkey and in man. Andrologia. 1978;10:331–52.
7. Nistal M, Jiménez-Heffernan JA. Rete testis dysgenesis. A characteristic lesion of undescended testes. Arch Pathol Lab Med. 1997;121:1259–64.
8. Mollaeian M, Mehrabi V, Elahi B. Significance of epididymal and ductal anomalies associated with undescended testis: study in 652 cases. Urology. 1994;43:857–60.
9. DePalma L, Carter D, Weiss RM. Epididymal and vas deferens immaturity in cryptorchidism. J Urol. 1988;140:1194–6.
10. Nistal M, Paniagua R. Adenomatous hyperplasia of the rete testis. J Pathol. 1988;154:343–6.
11. Nistal M, Paniagua R, Abaurrea MA, Santamaría L. Hyperplasia and the immature appearance of Sertoli cells in primary testicular disorders. Hum Pathol. 1982;13:3–12.
12. Hadziselimović F. Cryptorchidism. Ultrastructure of normal and cryptorchid testis development. Adv Anat Embryol Cell Biol. 1977;53:3–7.
13. Gotoh M, Miyake K, Mitsuya H. Elastic fibers in tunica propria of undescended and contralateral scrotal testes from cryptorchid patients. Urology. 1987;30:359–63.
14. Paniagua R, Martinez-Onsurbe P, Santamaria L, Saez FJ, Amat P, Nistal M. Quantitative and ultrastructural alterations in the lamina propria and Sertoli cells in human cryptorchid testes. Int J Androl. 1990;13:470–87.
15. Santamaria L, Martinez-Onsurbe P, Paniagua R, Nistal M. Laminin, type IV collagen, and fibronectin in normal and cryptorchid human testes.An immunohistochemical study. Int J Androl. 1990;13:135–46.
16. Nistal M, Paniagua R, Abaurrea MA. Multivacuolated leydig cells in human adult cryptorchid testes. Andrologia. 1981;13:436–9.
17. Paniagua R, Nistal M, Bravo MP. Leydig cell types in primary testicular disorders. Hum Pathol. 1984;15: 181–90.
18. Regadera J, Codesal J, Paniagua R, Gonzalez-Peramato P, Nistal M. Immunohistochemical and quantitative study of interstitial and intratubular Leydig cells in normal men, cryptorchidism, and Klinefelter's syndrome. J Pathol. 1991;164:299–306.
19. Mininberg DT, Schlossberg S. The role of the epididymis in testicular descent. J Urol. 1983;129:1207–8.
20. Koff WJ, Scaletscky R. Malformations of the epididymis in undescended testis. J Urol. 1990;143:340–3.
21. Elder JS. Epididymal anomalies associated with hydrocele/hernia and cryptorchidism: implications regarding testicular descent. J Urol. 1992;148:624–6.
22. Scorer CG, Farrington GH, editors. Congenital deformities of the testis and epididymis. London: Bütterworths; 1971. p. 136–46.

23. De Miguel MP, Mariño JM, Gonzalez-Peramato P, Nistal M, Regadera J. Epididymal growth and differentiation are altered in human cryptorchidism. J Androl. 2001;22:212–25.
24. Badoual C, Cohen C, Michenet P, Maître F, Delavierre D, Vieillefond A. Adenoma of the rete testis. Ann Pathol. 1999;19:80–1.
25. Nochomovitz LE, Orenstein JM. Adenocarcinoma of the rete testis. Case report, ultrastructural observations, and clinicopathologic correlates. Am J Surg Pathol. 1984;8:625–34.
26. Nistal M, Gonzalez-Peramato P, Regadera J, Serrano A, Tarin V, De Miguel MP. Primary testicular lesions are associated with testicular germ cell tumors of adult men. Am J Surg Pathol. 2006;30:1260–8.

29 Congenital Cystic Pathology of the Rete Testis

Manuel Nistal, Pilar González-Peramato, and Álvaro Serrano

29.1 Cysts of the Rete Testis

Three types of cysts, malformative in nature, can be observed in the testis [1]: rete testis cysts, simple testicular cysts, and tunica albuginea cysts. The first two are intraparenchymal and unrelated to the tunica albuginea. Cysts of the tunica albuginea originate in its thickness but can grow to the testicular parenchyma or outward.

Macroscopically, what rete testis cysts have in common with simple cysts is the fact that both can be unilateral or multicameral and can be located some distance from the rete testis (Fig. 29.1). Histologically, what identifies them is the epithelial lining as it is similar to the rete testis epithelium, with two cell types, flat and columnar. Immunohistochemically the cells, such as the epithelium of the rete testis, express cytokeratin and vimentin. Chronic inflammation, fibrosis, or teratomatous elements should not be observed on the cyst walls. Sperm are very often found inside, so these cysts are also known as intratesticular spermatoceles [2–4] (Fig. 29.2).

Most rete testis cysts, as happens with simple testicular cysts and albuginea cysts, are incidentally discovered during a routine testicular ultrasound exploration [5] or are autopsy findings. In some patients the rete testis cysts are associated with cystic transformation of the rete testis and multiple epididymal cysts. Cyst size ranges from 8 to 12 mm, although there are rete testis cysts of several cm, presenting a differential diagnosis with malignant tumors.

The differential diagnosis of rete testis cysts has to be done with the simple testicular cyst, the epidermoid cyst, and cystic teratomas (Table 29.1). The simple testicular cyst contains a clear fluid and no sperm; it is lined with flat or cubic cells that immunohistochemically express, in addition to cytokeratin, mesothelial markers such as calretinin, D2-40, HBME-1, mesothelin, and thrombomodulin [6]. Under their ultrastructure they show multiple irregular microvilli at the luminal cell surface [7]. At ultrasound the epidermoid cyst has the characteristic image of a bull's eye, and histologically it is made up of three to five layers of keratinized squamous epithelium. Cystic teratomas always have other mesodermal derivatives associated with cystic formations.

29.2 Cystic Dysplasia of the Rete Testis

29.2.1 Definition

Cystic dysplasia of the rete testis is a congenital lesion characterized by the cystic transformation of an overdeveloped rete testis that can partially or totally replace the testicular parenchyma.

It was described in 1973 by Leissring and Oppenheimer [8], who named it "cystic dysplasia of the testis" in a 4-year-old boy that also had agenesis of the right kidney.

Cystic dysplasia of the rete testis has been observed in the scrotal undescended testes, in

M. Nistal et al., *Clues in the Diagnosis of Non-tumoral Testicular Pathology*,
DOI 10.1007/978-3-319-49364-0_29

both childhood and adulthood [9–15]. It may be unilateral or bilateral [16]. About 50 cases have been reported, most of them in childhood [17]. The mean age at diagnosis is 6.1 years (range 0–63).

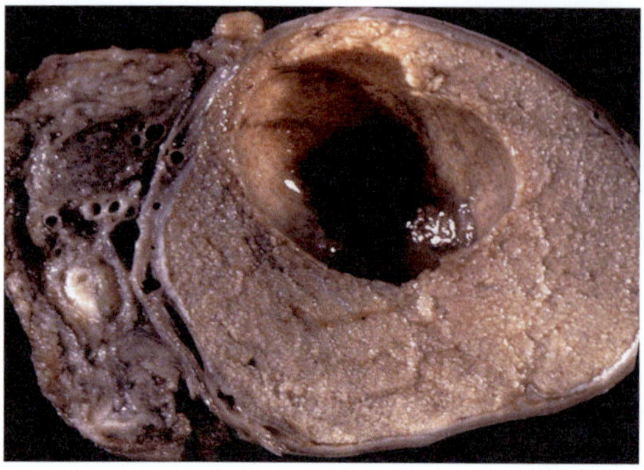

Fig. 29.1 Unicameral cyst of the rete testis with smooth and shiny surface. Autopsy finding

The diagnosis is suspected by clinical and ultrasound findings. The most common clinical symptom is the increased testicular size, while pain is very rarely seen. About 35 % of patients have abdominal cryptorchidism. Ultrasound imaging of the cystic dysplasia of the rete testis is characteristic: small cystic formations of different diameters located in the mediastinum testis and proximal parenchymal area that compress the rest of the surrounding parenchyma and small hyperechoic foci arising from the interface between the walls of the distal cysts and the surrounding parenchyma. High-resolution ultrasound is the best diagnostic approach to cystic dysplasia of the rete testis especially when genitourinary anomalies are associated [18]. The

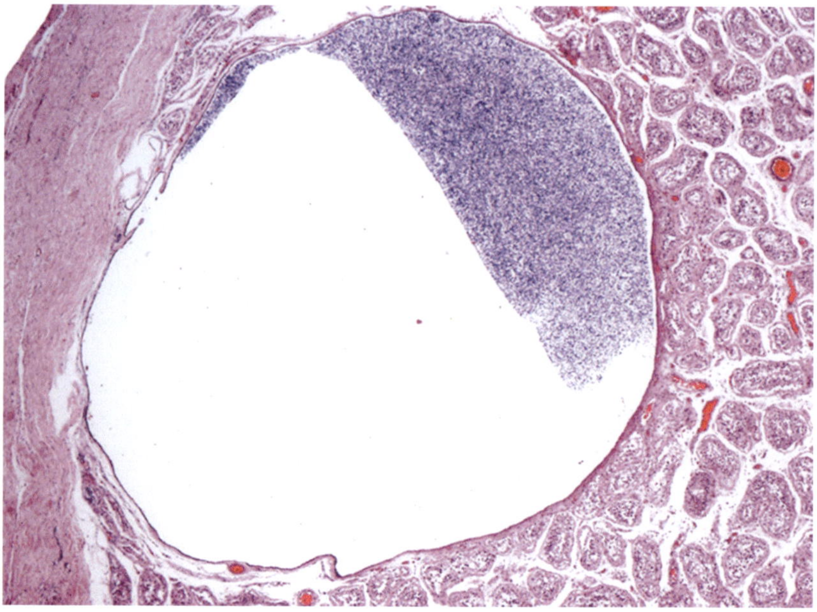

Fig. 29.2 Cyst of the rete testis with large accumulations of spermatozoa (intratesticular spermatocele)

Table 29.1 Clues in the differential diagnosis of rete testis cysts

	Rete testis cyst	Simple testicular cyst	Epidermoid cyst	Cystic teratomas
Containing	Clear fluid	Clear fluid	Keratin	Keratin, mucus
Sperm	Yes	No	No	No
Lining cells	Flat	Flat	3–5 layers of squamous epithelium	Other mesodermal derivatives
	Columnar	Cuboidal		
IHC	CK and vimentin	CK and mesothelial markers	HMW CK	CK

IHC immunohistochemistry, *CK* cytokeratin, *HMW* high molecular weight

MRI study shows cystic changes revealed by low and high signal intensities on short and long TE sequences, respectively, with no contrast uptake on postcontrast series [19].

29.2.2 Histological Features

The extent of the cystic transformation varies from case to case. It goes from lesions just beyond the testicular mediastinum to the involvement of the greatest part of the testicle; in these cases it is barely recognized as a peripheral crescent with preserved seminiferous tubules (Figs. 29.3 and 29.4). In this case the macroscopic aspect of the testis is characteristic of a sponge [20].

The size of the lesion varies from microscopic to 7 cm. Cystic expansions are uniform in size in the first situation and several cm in the other scenarios. Cystic formations are located in the septal and mediastinal rete testis; they are

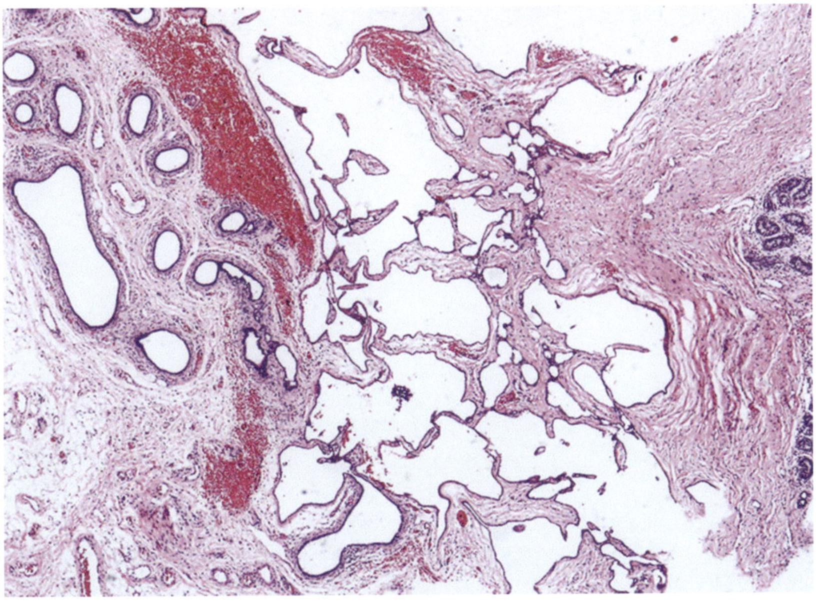

Fig. 29.3 Cystic dysplasia of the rete testis in a child. Marked dilatation of the rete testis cavities and irregular dilation of the efferent ductules are shown

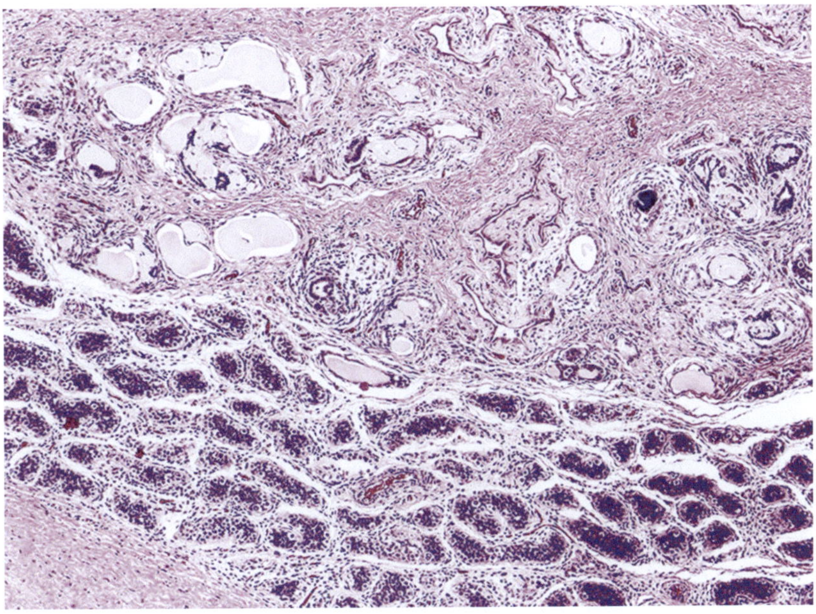

Fig. 29.4 Cystic dysplasia of the rete testis in a child. Rete testis cavities with cystic transformation have replaced the testicular parenchyma. The testicular parenchyma is recognized as a peripheral crescent

interconnected and contain eosinophilic, acellular, periodic acid-Schiff (PAS)-positive material. The covering epithelium is cuboidal or flattened and their cells are ultrastructural [21]; immunohistochemically (they express cytokeratin, vimentin and WT1) they are similar to those of the normal rete testis [22]. The connective tissue that remains between the cavities is generally poor in collagen and elastic fibers, similar to that of the testicular interstitium (Fig. 29.5). In some cases of cystic dysplasia of the rete testis, the connective tissue may be so abundant that it partially collapses the cavities. Beneath the epithelium in these areas, abundant psammoma bodies and small lymphoid infiltrates can be observed.

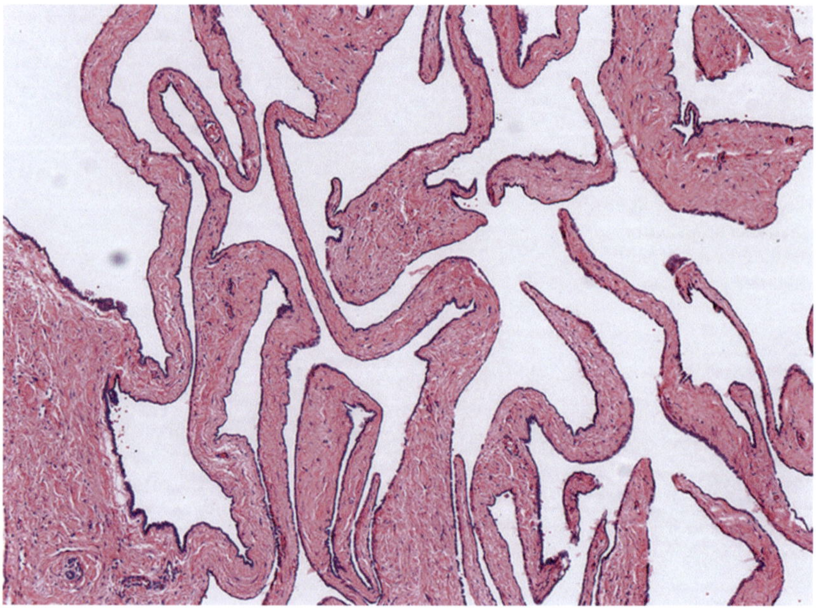

Fig. 29.5 Cystic dysplasia of the rete testis in an adult. The cavities are interconnected. Its epithelium is flat and are separated by thin connective septa

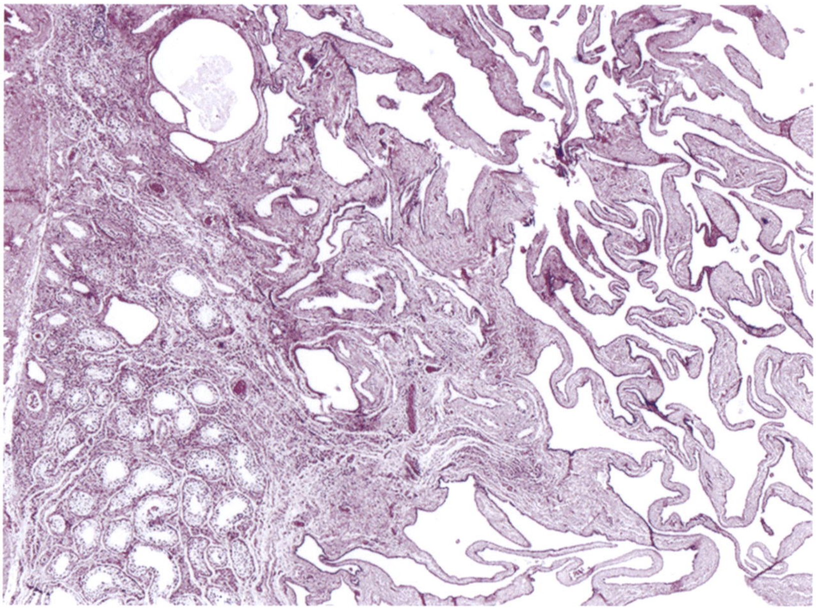

Fig. 29.6 Cystic dysplasia of the rete testis in an adult. A small group of tubules with complete spermatogenesis is located just under the tunica albuginea

The development of the residual testicular parenchyma during childhood is normal in some cases, there is a marked spermatogonia decrease in the undescended testes, and a small expansion of the proximal part of the seminiferous tubules (the opening to the rete testis) is steadily shown. In adults with cystic dysplasia of the rete testis, the testes develop the characteristic pattern of an obstructive lesion: tubular ectasia, loss of seminiferous epithelium, tubular hyalinization, and Leydig cell pseudohyperplasia (Fig. 29.6).

The epididymis shows alterations in most cases [23]. The head of the epididymis is usually small; there is a small number of efferent ductules that continue to present irregular contours, expanded lumen, and abundant loose stroma. In most cases the main epididymis duct shows lumen dilation, epithelial atrophy that is reduced to a cubic epithelium with no stereocilia, and wall thickening. This thickening is developed at the expense of connective tissue (Fig. 29.7). The vas deference may also be dilated, and exceptionally there is ipsilateral absence of the vas deferens. In other cases there is a marked hypoplasia of the epididymis.

There is a small number of cases where the overdeveloped rete testis does not show any cystic transformation. The rete testis consists of cordonal or tubular structures that may take one third of the testicular volume. This lesion, described as adenomatous hyperplasia of the rete testis, can affect the testicles of both newborn babies and children. It may be unilateral or bilateral. In the unilateral cases, it is associated with an undescended or evanescent testicle. In the bilateral cases, it is associated with bilateral renal dysplasia. The efferent ductules may show an enlarged lumen and irregular contours [24].

29.2.3 Differential Diagnosis

The differential diagnosis arises in childhood with all cystic testicular lesions that preferably affect the prepubertal testis, such as epidermoid cysts, cystic teratomas, juvenile granulose cell tumors, testicular lymphangiectasis, simple cysts of the testis, and post-torsion cystic testicular degeneration [14, 25, 26] (Table 29.2). The diagnosis is suggested by a combination of ultrasound scanning (mediastinal or preferentially near the location of the cystic lesions and ipsilateral absence of renal and urinary tract abnormalities) and normal rates of tumor markers (alphafetoprotein, lactate dehydrogenase, and beta subunit of HCG) [27, 28].

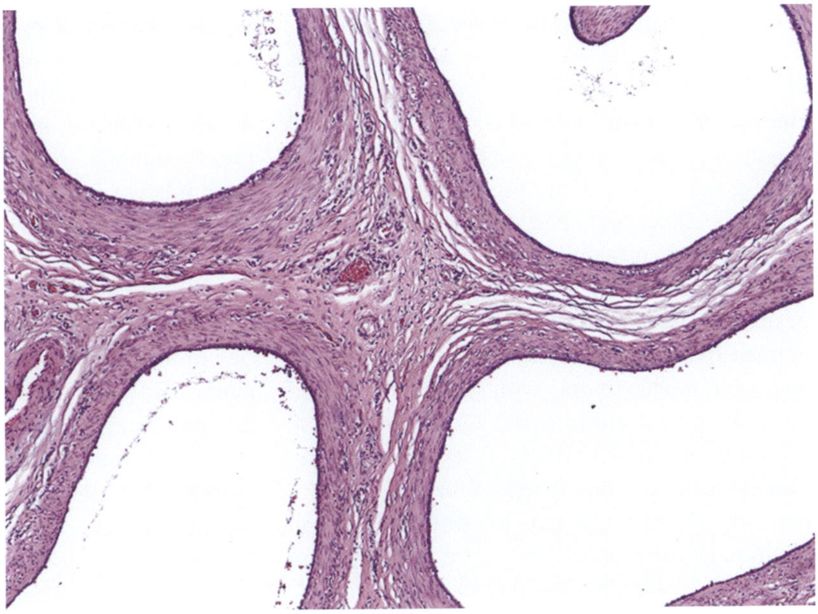

Fig. 29.7 Sections of the main duct of the epididymis show dilated lumen, epithelial atrophy, and fibrosis of the muscle layers

Table 29.2 Differential diagnosis of cystic dysplasia of the rete testis

Children	Clues
Epidermoid cyst	Ultrasound scanning
Cystic teratoma	
Juvenile granulosa cell tumor	
Testicular lymphangiectasis, simple testicular cysts	Tumor markers
Post-torsion cystic testicular degeneration	
Adults	**Clues**
Cystic transformation of RT	Middle-aged/elderly men. No UG malformation
Cystadenoma of RT	Well-defined ovoid lesion/small uniform cysts
Sertoliform cystadenoma	Solid areas beside cysts
Cystadenocarcinoma of RT	Solid areas besides cysts

RT rete testis
UG Urogenital

The differential diagnosis in adults has to be made with cystic transformation of the rete testis (ectasia of the rete testis) and rete testis tumors such as cystadenomas and cystadenocarcinomas. Ectasia of the rete testis is an acquired condition, which often affects middle-aged and elderly men, caused by an obstruction of the spermatic ducts, and not associated with malformations of the urogenital system. Tumors of the rete testis are rare. The cystadenoma is suggested in ultrasound by the image of a well-defined ovoid lesion, frequently located in the testicular mediastinum, with an extratesticular component and confirmed by the histological presence of small uniform cysts separated by thin connective septa. In sertoliform cystadenomas and adenocarcinomas of the rete testis, in addition to the presence of cystic lesions, there are always solid areas on ultrasound.

29.2.4 Associated Pathology

The major problem of patients with cystic dysplasia is, more than the lesion itself, the high degree of association with ipsilateral anomalies of the kidney or the urinary system. The most frequent of these anomalies are renal agenesis (51 %) [8, 21, 29–31], renal dysplasia (21 %), hydronephrosis (8 %), dilated or cystic epididymis (8 %), absence of ipsilateral ureteral orifice (6 %), ureteral duplication (4 %), urethral stenosis [32], ectopic ureter draining into the seminal vesicle [33], ipsilateral renal agenesis and contralateral crossed ectopia [34], and the VATER association (ipsilateral vertebra/anus/cardiac/trachea/esophagus/radius/renal anomalies) [35]. In isolated cases diagnosed both in children [19] and adults [36] renal anomalies have not been observed.

29.2.4.1 Etiopathogenesis

The etiology and pathogenesis of this lesion are unknown. However there are data to suggest that they are due to an early insult affecting the mesonephric duct development. The insult might have occurred between the fourth and eighth weeks of pregnancy. A failure might have occurred during the embryonic period in the connection between the efferent ductules (mesonephric origin) and the primordium of the rete testis, a result of the anastomosis of the testicular cords in the area of influence of the mesonephros. Under normal conditions, the rete testis cavities are devoid of lumen during childhood, and only just as puberty progresses do they become properly tunneled. In the adult it is not just a step structure for the passage of tubular fluid and spermatozoa, but it has the ability to modify fluid from the seminiferous tubules [37]. Various ions, proteins, and steroids are incorporated at this level. A primary pathology of the cells of the rete testis could lead to an abnormal function that is revealed by the production of a fluid at an inappropriate time and probably of a pathological composition. The fluid secreted from the rete testis is unable to escape, which results in cystic dilatation. Since most of the associated renal malformations, renal agenesis and renal dysplasia, can be considered as the result of a lack of induction of the metanephric blastema by the ureteral bud, which is another derivative of Wolff duct, it can be concluded that both injuries are due to a defect in the caudal and cephalic ends of this conduit [16].

A similar cystic dysplasia of the rete testis has been experimentally induced by sodium intoxication after administration of a salt-retaining hormone or deoxycorticosterone acetate in fowls [38], as well as by estradiol administration in newborn rats [39] and in deficiency of lunatic fringe mice [40].

29.2.5 Treatment

The treatment of choice of cystic dysplasia was classically orchidectomy; subsequently a testis-sparing surgery was considered [41], and currently a conservative therapy is recommended if the ultrasound diagnosis is highly suggestive of the disease and tumor markers (α-fetoprotein and hCG β-subunit) are negative [18, 42]. However, it is not yet clear whether these attempts to save the testis are effective for preserving spermatogenesis. Physical examination and ultrasound control are recommended annually. When most of the testicle is replaced by cystic formations, orchiectomy may be the best option [28]. Spontaneous regression has been reported in several cases [17, 43].

A similar cystic dysplasia involving the epididymis has been observed by our group in a large collection of perinatal specimens [44] (see Chap. 32 "Congenital Epididymis Anomalies").

References

1. Nistal M, Iñiguez L, Paniagua R. Cysts of the testicular parenchyma and tunica albuginea. Arch Pathol Lab Med. 1989;113:902–6.
2. Tejada E, Eble JN. Simple cyst of the rete testis. J Urol. 1988;139:376–7.
3. Yalowitz BR, Eble JN, Wilks DC. Spermatozoa-containing simple cysts of the rete testis. J Urol. 1989;142:1572–3.
4. Davis RS. Intratesticular spermatocele. Urology. 1998;51(5A Suppl):167–9.
5. Höbarth K, Kratzik C. High resolution ultrasonography in the diagnosis of simple intratesticular cysts. Br J Urol. 1992;70:546–9.
6. Kuwamoto S, Okuno K, Kato M, Hayashi K. Simple cysts of testis with immunohistochemical evidence of mesothelial origin. Pathol Int. 2009;59:656–9.
7. García CJ, Zúñiga S, Rosenberg H, Arce JD, Zúñiga F. Simple intratesticular cysts in children: preoperative sonographic diagnosis and histological correlation. Pediatr Radiol. 1999;29:851–5.
8. Leissring JC, Oppenheimer ROF. Cystic dysplasia of the testis: a unique congenital anomaly studied by microdissection. J Urol. 1973;110:362–3.
9. Zaragoza MR, Buckler LB, Parikh MJ. Cystic dysplasia of the testis: an unusual cause of a pediatric scrotal mass. Urology. 1996;47:244–7.
10. Poddevin F, Courrèges P, Lecoutre D, Bayart M. Ectasiekystique du rete testis: à proposd'un cas. J d'Urologie. 1996;102:92–4.
11. Wojcik LJ, Hansen K, Diamond DA, Koyle M, Koff SA, Coplen DE, Caldamone AA. Cystic dysplasia of the rete testis: a benign congenital lesion associated with ipsilateral urological anomalies. J Urol. 1997;158:600–4.
12. Kajo K, Matoska J, Javorka K, Machalekova K, Tomaskin R, Kliment K. Cystic dysplasia of the rete testis. Case report. APMIS. 2005;113:720–3.
13. Nanni L, Buonuomo V, Gessi M, Lauriola L, Pintus C. Cystic dysplasia of the rete testis associated to cryptorchidism: a case report. Arch Ital Urol Androl. 2005;77:199–201.
14. Mac New HG, Terry NE, Fowler CL. Cystic dysplasia of the rete testis. J Pediatr Surg. 2008;43:768–70.
15. Smith PJ, DeSouza R, Roth DR. Cystic dysplasia of the rete testis. Urology. 2008;72:230.e7–10.
16. Nistal M, Regadera J, Paniagua R. Cystic dysplasia of the testis: light and electron microscopic study of three cases. Arch Pathol Lab Med. 1984;108:579–83.
17. Jeyaratnam R, Bakalinova D. Cystic dysplasia of the rete testis: a case of spontaneous regression and review of published reports. Urology. 2010;7:687–90.
18. Toffolutti T, Gamba PG, Cecchetto G, Talenti E, Tchaprassian Z. Testicular cystic dysplasia: evaluation of 3 new cases treated without surgery. J Urol. 1999;162:2146–8.
19. Emam AT, Awad FM, Elsayed EA, Alghashi M. Cystic dysplasia of the rete testis: ultrasound and magnetic resonance imaging findings. Saudi J Kidney Dis Transpl. 2012;23:559–61.
20. Cho CS, Kosek J. Cystic dysplasia of the testis: sonographic and pathologic findings. Radiology. 1985; 156:777–8.
21. Glantz L, Hansen K, Caldamone A, Madeiros LJ. Cystic dysplasia of the testis. Hum Pathol. 1993;24:1142–5.
22. Loo CKC, Yung T. Cystic dysplasia of the testis: a report of three cases and review of the literature. Pediatr Pathol Lab Med. 1995;15:885–93.
23. Robson WL, Thomason MA, Minette LJ. Cystic dysplasia of the testis associated with multicystic dysplasia of the kidney. Urology. 1998;51:477–9.

24. Nistal M, García-Villanueva M, Sanchez J. Displasia quístuica del testículo. Anomalía en la diferenciación del parénquima testicular por probable fallo de la conexión entre los conductos de origen mesonéfrico y los cordones testiculares. Arch Esp Urol. 1976;29: 431–44.
25. Garrett JE, Cartwright PC, Snow BW, Coffin CM. Cystic testicular lesions in the pediatric population. J Urol. 2000;163:928–36.
26. Meirás FC, Fraile AG, Ruiz GD, Tomás IE, Robinot DC, Bramtot AA. Cystic dysplasia of the rete testis: case report. J Pediatr Urol. 2009;5:513–5.
27. Bonnet JP, Aigrain Y, Ferkadji L. Cystic dysplasia of the testis with ipsilateral renal agenesis. A case report and review of the literature. Eur J Pediatr Surg. 1997;7:57–9.
28. Kogan SJ. Testicular cystic dyplasia–a diagnostic and therapeutic enigma? J Urol. 1999;162:2149.
29. Fisher JE, Jewett Jr TC, Nelson SJ, Jockin H. Ectasia of the rete testis with ipsilateral renal agenesis. J Urol. 1982;128:1040–3.
30. Wegmann W, Illi O, Kummer-Vago M. Zystische Hodendysplasie mit ipsilataler Nierenagenesie. Schweiz Med Wochenschr. 1984;114:144–8.
31. Keetch DW, Mcalister WH, Manley CB, Dehner LP. Cystic dysplasia of the testis. Sonographic features with pathological correlation. Pediatr Radiol. 1991;21:501–3.
32. Tesluk H, Blankenberg TA. Cystic dysplasia of testis. Urology. 1987;29:47–9.
33. McGee SM, Hutcheson JC, Vandersteen DR, Reinberg Y, Wolpert JJ. Cystic dysplasia of testis associated with ectopic ureter causing chronic orchalgia. Urology. 2008;73:1423.e7–8.
34. Burns JA, Cooper CS, Austin JC. Cystic dysplasia of the testis associated with ipsilateral renal agenesis and contralateral crossed ectopia. Urology. 2002;60:344.
35. Park E, Morrison S. Cystic dysplasia of the rete testis in an adolescent with VATER association. Pediatr Radiol. 2008;38:123.
36. Kang KS, Cho DY, Park MG, Yeo JK. Cystic dysplasia of the rete testis accompanying an inguinal hernia: a 63-year-old man. Korean J Urol. 2011;52:502–4.
37. Tuck RR, Setchell BP, Waites GMH, Young JA. The composition of fluid collected by micropuncture and catheterization from the seminiferous tubules and rete testis of rats. Pflugers Arch. 1970;318:225–43.
38. Siller WG, Dewar WA, Whitehead CC. Cystic dilatation of the seminiferous tubules in the fowl: a sequel of sodium intoxication. J Pathol. 1972;107:191–7.
39. Aceitero J, Llanero M, Parrado R, Peña E, Lopez-Beltran A. Neonatal exposure of male rats to estradiol benzoate causes rete testis dilation and backflow impairment of spermatogenesis. Anat Rec. 1998;252: 17–23.
40. Hahn KL, Beres B, Rowton MJ, Skinner MK, Chang Y, Rawls A, Wilson-Rawls J. A deficiency of lunatic fringe is associated with cystic dilation of the rete testis. Reproduction. 2009;137:79–93.
41. Noh PH, Cooper CS, Snyder III HM. Conservative managemet of cystic dysplasia of the testis. J Urol. 1999;162:2145.
42. Cimador M, Rosone G, Castagnetti M, Libri M, Bertozzi M, Lima M, De Grazia E. Cystic dysplasia of rete testis associated with ipsilateral renal agenesis. Case report. Minerva Pediatr. 2003;55:175–9.
43. Thomas AD, Wu HY, Canning DA, Snyder 3rd HM. Spontaneous regression of cystic dysplasia of the testis. J Urol. 2003;169:645.
44. Nistal M, González-Peramato P, Sousa G, García-Cabezas MA, Rodríguez JI, Cajaiba MM. Cystic dysplasia of the epididymis: a disorder of mesonephric differentiation associated with renal maldevelopment. Virchows Arch. 2010;456:695–702.

30 Acquired Cystic Transformation of the Rete Testis (Cystic Ectasia of the Rete Testis)

Manuel Nistal, Pilar González-Peramato, and Álvaro Serrano

30.1 Defense Mechanisms of the Testis Against Testicular Fluid Obstruction

There are a number of barriers along the spermatic ducts whose purpose is to minimize the injuries caused by a potential obstruction. These are primarily located at the head of the epididymis, the efferent ducts, and secondarily in the rete testis itself, lodged in the testicular mediastinum.

Epididymis

Among the multiple functions of the epididymis, there are those related to sperm transport, maturation, and subsequent storage in the tail; another very important function is to absorb the bulk of the testicular fluid. Testicular fluid is produced in the seminiferous tubules by the Sertoli cells when they achieve complete maturation, i.e., after puberty. Through a mechanism of active transport, water moves from the basal to the apical pole and is drained to the tubular lumen. The contractile activity of myoid peritubular cells and the tone and spontaneous contractions of the tunica albuginea are responsible for the testicular fluid to reach the rete testis and epididymis through the rete testis.

Efferent Ducts

The efferent ducts originate in the extratesticular rete testis and end in the epididymal duct. They are 10–15 conduits that as they draw away from the testicle fold over themselves in ever-widening spirals (*vasculose cones*). Then they branch and re-anastomose resulting in a network. Up to seven kinds of tubes have been described with different epithelia and eight different types of connections [1]. At the end, the ducts terminate in the epididymal duct with both termino-terminal and termino-lateral junctions [2].

They are lined with simple columnar epithelium formed by principal cells and ciliated cells and a wall with contractile cells [3].

The *principal cells* have a pale nucleus, basal, with deep folds. They have numerous microvilli on the apical pole forming a brush border and under it a well-developed endocytic apparatus consisting of coated pits, apical tubules, endosomes, multivesicular bodies, and lysosomes. The tubular fluid is internalized into lysosomes where it is subjected to the action of proteolytic enzymes [4].

The *ciliated cells* are 25–40 microns tall. The nucleus is large, spherical, and euchromatic, and it is located in the middle portion of the cytoplasm. Most organelles are located at the apical pole. These include mitochondria, distributed

M. Nistal et al., *Clues in the Diagnosis of Non-tumoral Testicular Pathology*,
DOI 10.1007/978-3-319-49364-0_30

between the basal bodies of cilia. These cells have, although in small amounts, one endocytic apparatus. While the ciliated cells are joined by a well-developed juxtaluminal complex union (occludens zonule, zonula adherens, and macula adherens), among the principal cells, of which there are different types, tight junctions (occludens zonules) dominate, so that the joints are segmental or incomplete. This gives the epithelium multiple weaknesses that may facilitate fluid movement [5].

An important role in the absorption of tubular fluid depends on the collaboration of different aquaporin water channels that allow the quick removal of the tubular fluid and the coexistence of lectin-reactive apical cytoplasmic granules and vacuoles that form part of an endophytic unit specialized in capturing materials from the lumen. This mechanism is similar to what happens in the proximal convoluted tubules of the kidney where more than 80 % of the glomerular fluid is absorbed [6].

The trophic state of the efferent ducts is mainly due to androgens that arrive by the canalicular pathway [7]. Epithelial cells have estrogen receptors. ESR1 has a crucial role in the regulation of testicular fluid reabsorption [8].

Other mechanisms that prevent retrograde flow are in the testicular mediastinum and involve both the rete testis and the stroma where they are located. Two structures are involved in the rete testis, the chordae rete and the initial segment of the tubuli recti (septal rete). The chordae rete is anchored obliquely to the side walls of the cavities of the mediastinal rete and prevents the loosening of same. The initial segment of the tubuli recti is funnel shaped with its widest part coupled to the seminiferous tubules. It is just at this level that there is a coating of cylindrical cells, modified Sertoli cells, whose major axis is inclined toward the rete testis acting as a valve that prevents the fluid from rete testis from reversing into the seminiferous tubules [9]. The connective tissue of the testicular mediastinum is a dense connective tissue with fibroblasts, myoid cells, and abundant collagenous and elastic fibers that prevent the expansion of the structures that traverse it.

30.2 Concept of Acquired Cystic Transformation of the Rete Testis (ACTRT)

30.2.1 Definition

Acquired cystic transformation of the rete testis is defined by the presence of cystic dilations in the testicular mediastinum containing sperm, associated with partial or complete epididymal obstruction.

This lesion is also known as "cystic ectasia of the rete testis" and "tubular ectasia of the rete testis." It was discovered on ultrasound in 1992 by Weingarten, who named it "tubular ectasia within the mediastinum testis" [10]. The lesion was observed in 11 patients, and, although there was no histological evidence, the author advanced its benign nature. Histological studies are rare [11]. The lesion size varies from 10 to 43 mm.

It is a benign condition usually found in patients older than 50 years. The mean age of patients is 62 years [12]. The incidence of ACTRT is higher than previously thought. It is observed in 2.6 % [13] to 4.3 % [14] of ultrasound studies in adults. According to histological studies in adult autopsies, the incidence is 11.9 % [15]. Most often it is an incidental finding on scrotal sonograms with a variety of presentations. The most frequent presentation is scrotal swelling and enlargement with physical findings consistent with testicular tumor, suspected hydrocele, epididymal cysts or spermatoceles, epididymitis, traumatic injuries, and infertility. It is bilateral in one third of cases. Its presentation may be asymmetrical [14].

30.2.2 Diagnosis

The diagnosis is made by ultrasonography, when an ovoidal tight cluster of small and anechoic cystic lesions located in the mediastinum testis is observed. No solid component is visible between the cystic spaces [16–18]. Its sonographic appearance varies according to the size of the lesion. In mild cases a tiny branching pattern of the rete testis is seen, making it difficult in some cases to differentiate it from the normal sonographic appearance of the rete testis [19]. At the opposite pole, cysts of more than 1 cm in diameter surrounding the central area of cystic transformation can be observed. In over half of the cases, there are epididymal cysts [20] and occasionally rete testis cysts. The advantage of MRI is that the test can be done with application of contrast agents (gadolinium), and the organ can be examined in several signal qualities. First used in 1993 [21], it may be useful in some cases, but its high cost and the fact of being a time-consuming operation make it unnecessary in most cases [22]. Testicular biopsy or orchiectomy seems unnecessary in most cases.

30.2.3 Differential Diagnosis of the Cystic Transformation of the Rete Testis

In general, the ultrasound image is diagnostic; however it would be considered in the differential diagnosis of the following conditions: cystic dysplasia of the rete testis, intratesticular varicocele, cystadenomas and cystadenocarcinomas of the rete testis, rete testis dilatation associated with testicular tumors, and simple testicular cyst.

- *Cystic dysplasia of the rete testis* is a malformative condition characteristic of childhood that entails the cystic transformation of an overdeveloped rete testis that shows a similarity with acquired cystic transformation of the rete testis on the ultrasound [23]. This lesion is most often associated with lack of kidney or urinary tract disease. Its etiology appears to be an abnormal development of the proximal and distal ends of the Wolff duct. Some cases reported in adults actually correspond to acquired cystic changes of the rete testis.
- The *intratesticular varicocele* is always associated with extratesticular varicocele. The ultrasound image may resemble the ectasia of the rete testis, but the diagnosis of varicocele is confirmed by showing a vascular flow in the cystic formations on Doppler studies [24–26].
- The *rete testis cystadenoma* has a characteristic ultrasound image. It is a well-circumscribed lesion located in the mediastinum testis with an often extratesticular component that can be associated with ectasia of the rete testis. Cysts are of small size with a delicate septation. There is absence of solid component [27].
- The *cystadenoma sertoliform*, the *papillary cystadenoma*, and the *adenofibroma* are rare tumors. All of them are located in the mediastinum testis and show ultrasound findings similar to cystic transformation of the rete testis; the differential diagnosis is based on the search of the solid areas that most of them show [28].
- The *adenocarcinomas of the rete testis* are rare tumors; most often they result in a palpable stony mass. When associated with cysts, these cysts are larger, and there are associated solid areas on ultrasound [29].
- *Dilations associated with testicular tumors.* Approximately, 10 % of all testicular tumors contain a teratoma component. In these cases the symptoms are mainly a clear increase of the testicular size and a palpable tumor. On ultrasound solid areas are always observed together with cystic formations. The location of the cysts is usually eccentrical [30]. Germ cell tumors appear at an earlier age and are rarely bilateral.

30.3 Histological Types of Cystic Transformation of the Rete Testis

This entity is well described in the radiologic literature; however, its mention in the urologic literature is scant and even rarer in histological studies. The ACTRT can occur in three ways [11].

30.3.1 Simple Cystic Transformation of the Rete Testis

It is the most common lesion. Cystic transformation of the rete testis occurs while preserving the normal characteristics of the epithelium. It is a diffuse and symmetric alteration that causes a harmonic expansion (Figs. 30.1 and 30.2). Its origin is secondary to an obstructive process that causes obliteration of the efferent ducts, either in binding testis-epididymis, in epididymal itself, or in the initial portion of the vas deferens. This obstruction is explained by the following mechanisms:

- *Ischemic*. In patients with arteriosclerosis, the upper epididymal artery, a small collateral branch of the testicular artery, is frequently injured making most of the caput of the epididymis ischemic [31]. The atrophy of the efferent ducts determines not only a loss of the absorptive capacity of their cells but obstruction of testicular fluid, which accumulates in the rete testis.

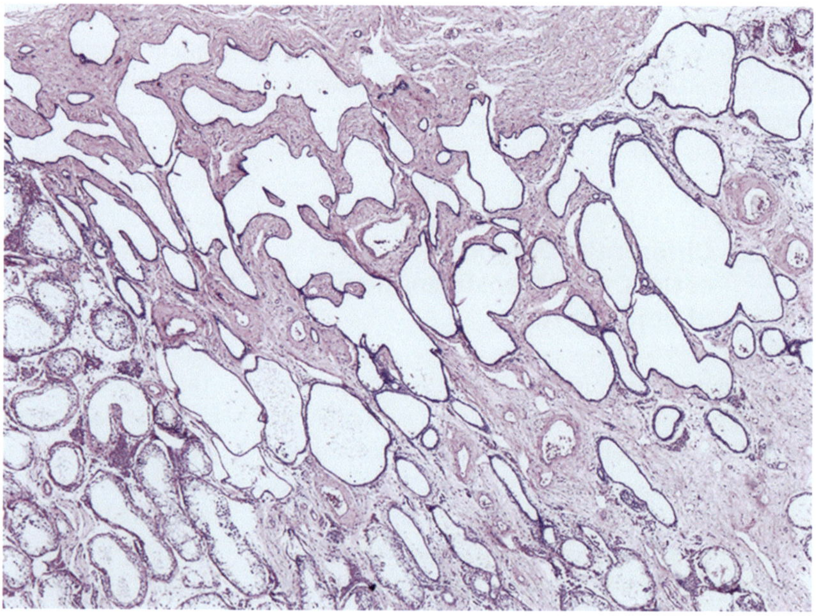

Fig. 30.1 Simple cystic transformation of the rete testis. Testicular mediastinum is widened with displacement of the seminiferous tubules

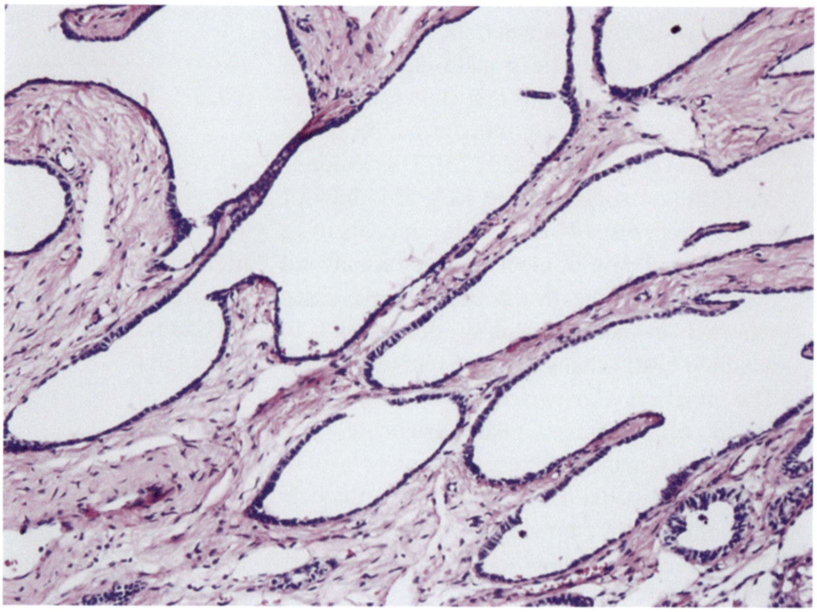

Fig. 30.2 Simple cystic transformation of the rete testis. The epithelium of the rete testis retains the two types of epithelial cells, predominantly squamous cells

- *Mechanic*. Epididymal obstruction occurs in the following situations:
  - By extrinsic compression, as occurs in patients with cysts [32] and tumors of the epididymis and the spermatic cord, in long-term hematocele cases, and in some varicoceles. In the varicocele ectasia of the rete testis may occur either at an extratesticular level with compression of efferent ducts by varicose veins or at an intratesticular level with compression and distortion of the rete testis by centripetal veins. This dilation of the rete testis is never as intense as in the previously mentioned etiologies, and it is always asymmetric [33].
  - By interruption of epididymal flow, similarly to patients who have undergone epididymectomy [34].
- *Inflammatory*. It occurs only when the head of the epididymis is injured either directly (by inflammation) or indirectly (by a residual obstruction).
- *Malformation*. Malformations that more frequently cause cystic transformation of the rete testis are the epididymis-testicular dissociation and partial or total initial segment epididymis or vas agenesis. Among the causes of these malformations, there is cystic fibrosis [35].
- *Iatrogenic*. Vasectomy by itself only causes ectasia of the main duct of the epididymis and the efferent ducts, with little impact on the testicle. As the expression of a greater absorptive activity, the cells of the efferent ducts develop granular changes in their cytoplasm (Panet-like changes). In some patients these passages rupture, inducing the development of multiple small sperm granulomas. In these cases, where there is a clear destruction of the epididymis, cystic transformation of the rete testis happens. ACTRTs described in a patient who consulted for chronic testicular pain after epididymal cyst removal [36] or epididymectomies [34] have been reported.

30.3.2 Cystic Transformation of the Rete Testis with Epithelial Changes

Cystic transformation of the rete testis with epithelial changes is a common finding in the study of autopsy pathology and not uncommon in the study of surgical specimens [11]. Two lesions are combined, cubic or cylindrical metaplasia of the rete testis and cystic transformation of same (Figs. 30.3, 30.4, and 30.5). Both lesions can

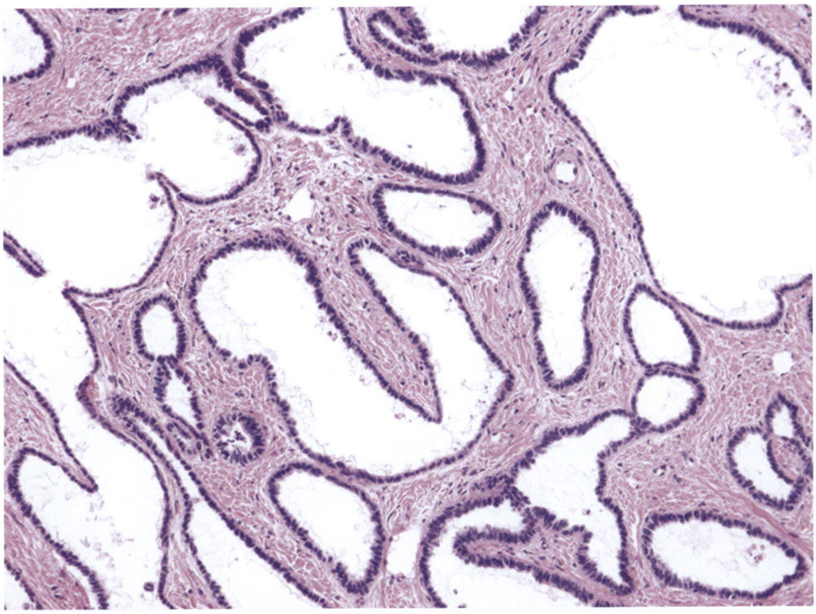

Fig. 30.3 Cystic transformation of the rete testis with epithelial changes. Pronounced dilatation of the rete testis cavities lined by an epithelium of uniform height

obey to the same causating mechanism, or a match may occur when several mechanisms are combined. It is observed in patients with chronic liver failure, hormonally active testicular tumors, and some orchitis. The most plausible mechanisms are:

- *Hormonal*. Experimental data are in favor of the hormonal theory. Varying degrees of hyperplasia of the rete testis have been observed in mice exposed prenatally to diethylstilbestrol [37, 38]; when diethylstilbestrol was administered in the neonatal period, cystic transformation of the rete testis was seen [39] and also obstructive azoospermia [40].

In chronic liver failure, epithelial changes of the rete testis could be secondary to increased estrogen, whereas cystic transformation could be due to atrophy of the caput epididymis by hypoandrogenism that usually accompanies these patients [41]. The efferent ducts are very

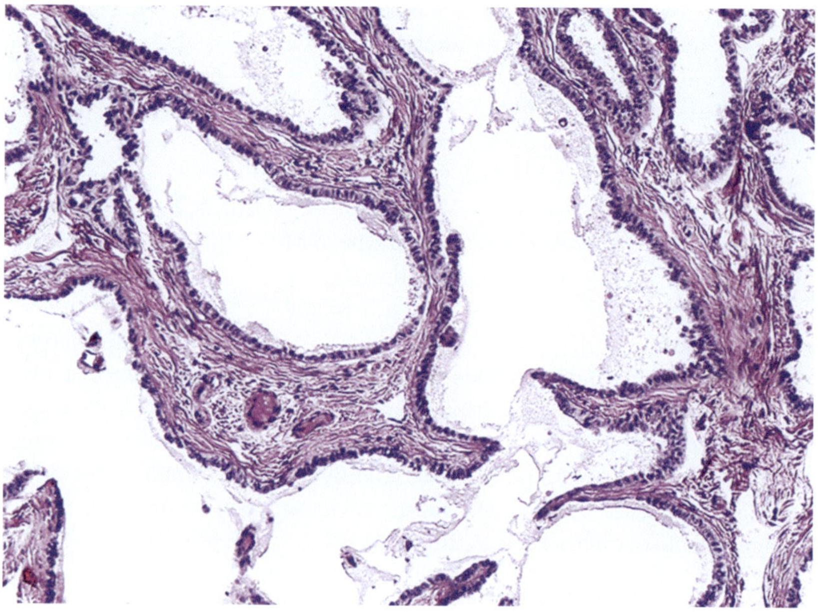

Fig. 30.4 Cystic transformation of the rete testis with epithelial changes. The cavities contain a slightly eosinophilic fluid. The lining of the cavities consists of cuboidal and columnar cells

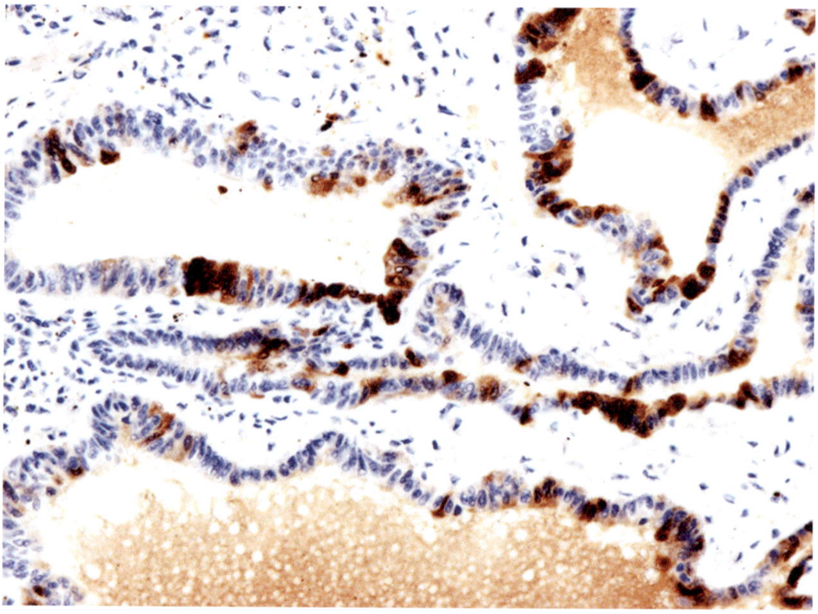

Fig. 30.5 Cystic transformation of the rete testis with epithelial changes. Groups of cubic and cylindrical cells express calretinin

sensitive to androgen deprivation structures. Neither can it be ruled out that in some of the elderly ACTRT patients, ischemia secondary to atherosclerosis emphasizes their cystic lesions.

In estrogen-producing or HCG testicular tumors, epithelial metaplasia of rete testis could also have a hormonal mechanism. Cystic transformation in these cases, in the absence of atrophy or epididymal sperm pathway obstruction, could be explained by a hyperproduction of fluid by the testicles with tumor, beyond the capacity of reabsorption of the efferent ducts.

- *Inflammatory*. In some chronic orchitis with extension to the mediastinum testis and testicular tumors with abundant lymphoid reaction, cystic transformation of the rete testis is observed that is generally irregular and asymmetrical. Epithelial changes have a reactive character. Not infrequently, inside the partially cystic cavities, an inflammatory exudate being reabsorbed is observed.

30.3.3 Cystic Transformation of the Rete Testis with Crystalline Deposits

This is also named "cystic transformation of the rete testis secondary to renal failure" [15]. It is a bilateral lesion of the adult testis characterized by the association of three facts: metaplasia of the epithelium of the rete testis, urate and oxalate crystal deposits, and cystic transformation of the rete testis (Fig. 30.6). It is a pathognomonic lesion of patients with chronic renal failure on dialysis.

The crystalline deposits begin to be seen under the epithelium and usually do not trigger an inflammatory reaction or the appearance of giant cells (Fig. 30.7). When they acquire certain size, they protrude into the cavities of the rete testis, dragging part of the epithelium as they penetrate. Then they reach the efferent ducts and even occlude them. At this level, they are often surrounded by foreign body giant cells. Crystalline deposits can also be found initially beneath the efferent ducts epithelium, but not in the main duct of the epididymis. The large amount of deposits in this secondary oxalosis, sometimes associated with sperm granulomas, may mimic a testicular tumor [42].

The CTRT developed in these patients is related sometimes to obstruction of the efferent ducts with these and other materials and on other occasions to atrophy of the efferent ducts by ischemia secondary to arteriosclerosis or hypertension that is frequent in these patients.

This lesion is somewhat similar to the cystic kidney lesions described in these same patients [43], and this is not surprising since the embryological origin of the mesonephric tubules and its derivatives at the level of the testis (rete testis and

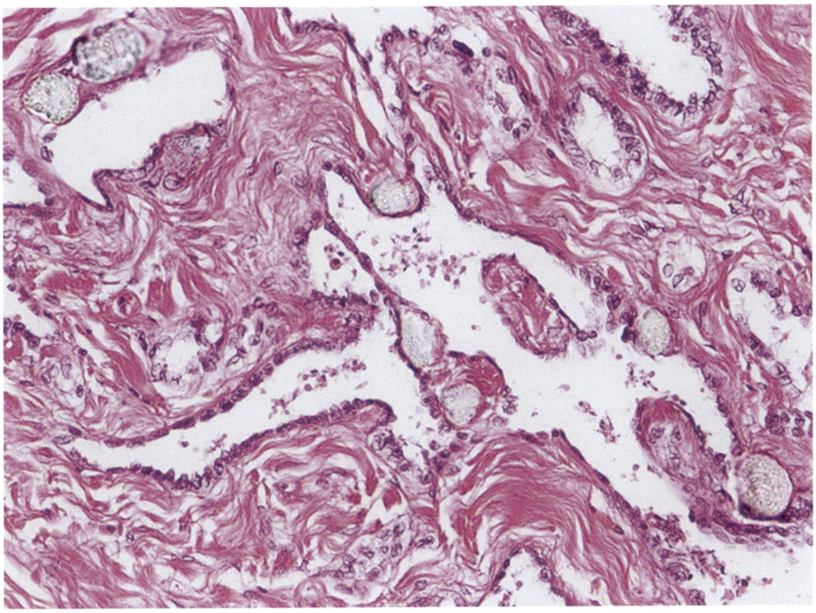

Fig. 30.6 Rete testis shows mildly dilated cavities and refractile subepithelial crystalline deposits

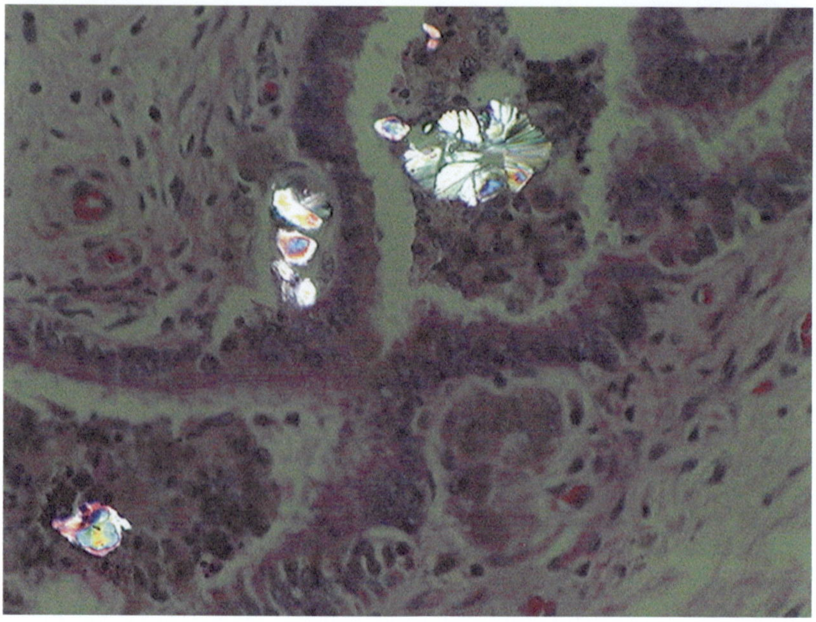

Fig. 30.7 Subepithelial oxalate's deposits in the rete testis. Polarized light observation

efferent ducts) are related to the embryological origin of the kidney.

Cystic transformation of the rete testis with crystalline deposits needs some time to develop – the earliest lesions were observed 30 months after dialysis start, but they may occur earlier. The lesion is not observed in patients who were transplanted.

References

1. Yeung CH, Cooper TG, Bergmann M, Schulze H. Organization of tubules in the human caput epididymidis and the ultrastructure of their epithelia. Am J Anat. 1991;191:261–79.
2. Jonté G, Holstein AF. On the morphology of the transitional zones from the rete testis into the ductuli efferentes and from the ductulie fferentes into the ductus epididymidis. Investigations on the human testis and epididymis. Andrologia. 1987;19:398–412.
3. Saitoh K, Terada T, Hatakeyama S. A morphological study of the efferent ducts of the human epididymis. Int J Androl. 1990;13:369–76.
4. Hermo L, Morales C. Endocytosis in nonciliated epithelial cells of the ductuliefferentes in the rat. Am J Anat. 1984;171:59–74.
5. Ilio KY, Hess RA. Structure and function of the ductuliefferentes: a review. Microsc Res Tech. 1994;29: 432–67.
6. Arrighi S, Ventriglia G, Aralla M, Zizza S, Di Summa A, Desantis S. Absorptive activities of the efferent ducts evaluated by the immunolocalization of aquaporin water channels and lectin histochemistry in adult cats. Histol Histopathol. 2010;25:433–44.
7. Pelliniemi LJ, Dym M, Gunsalus GL, Musto NA, Bardin CW, Fawcett DW. Immunocytochemical localization of androgen-binding protein in the male rat reproductive tract. Endocrinology. 1981;108: 925–31.
8. Pereira MF, Fernandes SA, Nascimento AR, Siu ER, Hess RA, Oliveira CA, Porto CS, Lazari MF. Effects of the oestrogen receptor antagonist Fulvestrant on expression of genes that affect organization of the epididymal epithelium. Andrology. 2014;2:559–71.
9. Osman DI. On the ultrastructure of modified Sertoli cells in the terminal segment of seminiferous tubules in the boar. J Anat. 1978;127:603–13.
10. Weingarten BJ, Kellman GM, Middleton WD, Gross ML. Tubular ectasia within the mediastinum testis. J Ultrasound Med. 1992;11:349–53.
11. Nistal M, Mate A, Paniagua R. Cystic transformation of the rete testis. Am J Surg Pathol. 1996;20:1231–9.
12. Brown DL, Benson CB, Doherty FJ, Doubilet PM, DiSalvo DN, Van Alstyne GA, Vickers MA, Loughlin KR. Cystic testicular mass caused by dilated rete testis: sonographic findings in 31 cases. AJR Am J Roentgenol. 1992;158:1257–9.
13. Gooding GA, Leonhardt W, Stein R. Testicular cysts: US findings. Radiology. 1987;163:537–8.
14. Rouvière O, Bouvier R, Pangaud C, Jeune C, Dawahra M, Lyonnet D. Tubular ectasia of the rete testis: a potential pitfall in scrotal imaging. Eur Radiol. 1999;9:1862–8.

15. Nistal M, Santamaría L, Paniagua R. Acquired cystic transformationof the rete testis secondary to renal failure. Hum Pathol. 1989;20:1065–70.
16. Colangelo SM, Fried K, Hyacinthe LM, Fracchia JA. Tubular ectasia of the rete testis: an ultrasound diagnosis. Urology. 1995;45:532–4.
17. Ortega Herrera R, Medina Benítez A, López Milena G. Tubular ectasia of the rete testis: ultrasonography findings in 19 patients. Arch Esp Urol. 2000;53:455–9. [in Spanish].
18. Pascual Mateo C, Fernández González I, LujánGalán M, Rodríguez García N, Espinales Castro G, Berenguer Sánchez A. Cystic ectasia of the rete testis. Arch Esp Urol. 2006;59:55–8. [in Spanish].
19. Thomas RD, Dewbury KC. Ultrasound appearances of the rete testis. Clin Radiol. 1993;47:121–4.
20. Pavlica P, Ramini R, Barozzi L. Tubular ectasia of the rete testis. The echographic aspects. Radiol Med. 1994;87:493–7.
21. Tartar VM, Trambert MA, Balsara ZN, Mattrey RF. Tubular ectasia of the testicle: sonographic and MR imaging appearance. AJR Am J Roentgenol. 1993;160:539–42.
22. Meyer DR, Huppe T, Lock U, et al. Pronounced cystic transformation of the rete testis: MRI appearance. Invest Radiol. 1999;34:600–3.
23. Eberli D, Gretener H, Dommann-Scherrer C, Pestalozzi D, Fehr JL. Cystic dysplasia of the testis: a very rare paediatric tumor of the testis. Urol Int. 2002;69:1–6.
24. Weiss AJ, Kellman GM, Middleton WD, Kirkemo A. Intratesticular varicocele: sonographic findings in two patients. AJR Am J Roentgenol. 1992;158:1061–3.
25. Stewart VR, Sidhu PS. The testis: the unusual, the rare and the bizarre. Clin Radiol. 2007;62:289–302.
26. Hansen N, Sanchez R, Ivancic V. Unusual combination of bilateral testicular microlithiasis and tubular ectasia of the rete testis with left intra- and extratesticular varicocele in a 17-year-old boy. J Clin Ultrasound. 2012;40:314–8.
27. Gabriel H, Marko J, Nikolaidis P. Cystadenoma of the rete testis: sonographic appearance. AJR Am J Roentgenol. 2007;189:W67–9.
28. Sahnan K, Manjunath A, Vaughan-Shaw PG, Mitsopoulos G. An unexpected finding of a rare intrascrotal lesion: the sertoliform cystadenoma of the rete testis. BMJ Case Rep. 2013. pii: bcr2012008439.
29. Stein JP, Freeman JA, Esrig D, Chandrasoma PT, Skinner DG. Papillary adenocarcinoma of the rete testis: a case report and review of the literature. Urology. 1994;44:588–94.
30. Hamm B, Fobbe F, Loy V. Testicular cysts: differentiation with US and clinical findings. Radiology. 1988;168:19–23.
31. Regadera J, Nistal M, Paniagua R. Testis, epididymis, and spermatic cord in elderly men. Correlation of angiographic and histologic studies with systemic arteriosclerosis. Arch Pathol Lab Med. 1985;109:663–7.
32. Jimenez-López M, Ramírez-Garrido F, López-González Garrido JD, Mantas-Avila JA, Nogueras-Ocaña M, Jimenez-Verdejo A, Fernández-Mena J. Dilatation of the rete testis: ultrasoundstudy. Eur Radiol. 1999;9:1327–9.
33. Nistal M, Paniagua R, Regadera J, Santamaria L. Obstruction of the tubuli recti and ductuliefferentes by dilated veins in the testes of men with varicocele and its possible role in causing atrophy of the seminiferous tubules. Int J Androl. 1984;7:309–23.
34. Tchetgen MB, Wolf Jr JS. Postsurgical changes in the testis: a diagnostic dilemma. Urology. 1998;51:333–4.
35. Wilschanski M, Corey M, Durie P, et al. The diversity of reproductive tract abnormalities in males with cystic fibrosis. JAMA. 1996;276:607–8.
36. Mayfield M, Edwards P, Dundas S. An unusual case of testicular pain. Br J Urol. 1996;77:471–2.
37. Newbold RR, Bullock BC, McLachlan JA. Lesions of the rete testis in mice exposed prenatally to diethylstilbestrol. Cancer Res. 1985;45:5145–50.
38. Bullock BC, Newbold RR, McLachlan JA. Lesions of testis and epididymis associated with prenatal diethylstilbestrol exposure. Environ Health Perspect. 1988;77:29–31.
39. Aceitero J, Llanero M, Parrado R, Peña E, Lopez-Beltran A. Neonatal exposure of male rats to estradiol benzoate causes rete testis dilation and backflow impairment of spermatogenesis. Anat Rec. 1998;252:17–33.
40. Naito M, Hirai S, Terayama H, Qu N, Hayashi S, Hatayama N, Kawamura H, Nakano T, Itoh M. Neonatal estrogen treatment with β-estradiol 17-cypionate induces in post-pubertal mice inflammation in the ductuliefferentes, epididymis, and vas deferens, but not in the testis, provoking obstructive azoospermia. Med Mol Morphol. 2014;47:21–30.
41. Karagiannis A, Harsoulis F. Gonadal dysfunction in systemic diseases. J Clin Endocrinol Metab. 1988; 67:639–43.
42. Coyne J, al-Nakib L, Goldsmith D, O'Flynn K. Secondary oxalosis and sperm granuloma of the epididymis. J Clin Pathol. 1994;47:470–1.
43. Concolino G, Lubrano C, Ombres M, et al. Acquired cystic kidney disease: the hormonal hypothesis. Urology. 1993;41:170–5.

31 Acquired Pathology of the Rete Testis

Manuel Nistal, Pilar González-Peramato, and Álvaro Serrano

31.1 Reactive Hyperplasia

Reactive hyperplasia is an unspecific way of rete testis reaction. It consists of a proliferation of epithelial cells in the cavities of the rete testis. The proliferation may take a solid or a cribriform pattern (Fig. 31.1). The cells in the solid pattern are polyhedral and have an ovoid nucleus and an eosinophilic cytoplasm. Isolated mitosis can be seen. In the cribriform form, a lattice pattern is observed in the cavities of the rete testis; it is cubic on the periphery and spindle shaped in the central part (Fig. 31.2). Both forms of proliferation can be associated with the presence of granulation tissue filling some cavities or showing intracavitary polypoid growth.

Reactive hyperplasia can be observed virtually in all non-tumor and tumor processes of the testis, as in the adult testicular torsion, orchitis, epidermoid cysts, stromal tumors, germ cell tumors, and even primary lymphomas.

The differential diagnosis includes three situations: intratesticular adenomatoid tumor, adenocarcinoma of the rete testis, and intracavitary extension of a germ cell tumor. The clearly intraductal arrangement of the proliferation and its multicentrality distinguish reactive hyperplasia from adenomatoid tumor. The absence of an infiltrative component is an important criterium to differentiate adenocarcinoma of the rete testis. Intracavitary proliferation could remind an infiltration by an embryonic carcinoma. The absence of a pagetoid pattern of infiltration by germ cell neoplasia in situ, and of testicular tumor in the neighboring parenchyma, enables to distinguish them. A negative CD30 immunostaining rules out embryonic carcinoma. The cells of the reactive hyperplasia express immunostaining for AE1/AE3cytokeratin (Fig. 31.3).

31.2 Hyperplasia with Hyaline Globules

This is a reactive lesion characterized by the presence of accumulations of hyaline eosinophilic globules in the epithelial cells of the rete testis (Fig. 31.4). The architecture of the rete testis is hardly affected [1].

In most cases the epithelium is hyperplastic and may sometimes adopt a cribriform or microcystic pattern. The cells show spherical nuclei without folds with a prominent nucleolus, and they lack atypia and mitosis.

Hyaline globules measure from less than 1 micron to over 10 microns, and they move to the nucleus and bulge the plasma membrane. Cells having multiple hyaline bodies usually have hyperchromatic nuclei with irregular contours.

In the lumen of the rete testis, an eosinophilic material and sometimes tumor cells can be observed.

M. Nistal et al., *Clues in the Diagnosis of Non-tumoral Testicular Pathology*, DOI 10.1007/978-3-319-49364-0_31

This lesion is associated with both tumors and inflammation adjacent to the mediastinum testis. It is observed in 75 % of mixed testicular germ cell tumors, in 47 % of seminomas, and 20 % of non-germ cell testicular tumors, tumors of the epididymis that infiltrate the testicle (adenomatoid tumor) [2]. This lesion does not appear to be induced by a neoplastic invasion of the rete testis. The globules could correspond to intracytoplasmic accumulation of proteins extracted by the epithelial cells from the rete testis fluid.

Knowledge of this lesion is useful as a similar image can be produced by infiltration of the rete testis by the endodermal sinus tumor. The positive staining of hyaline globules of this tumor for alphafetoprotein and the presence of atypia are very useful criteria to difference this tumor from hyperplasia of the rete testis with hyaline globules.

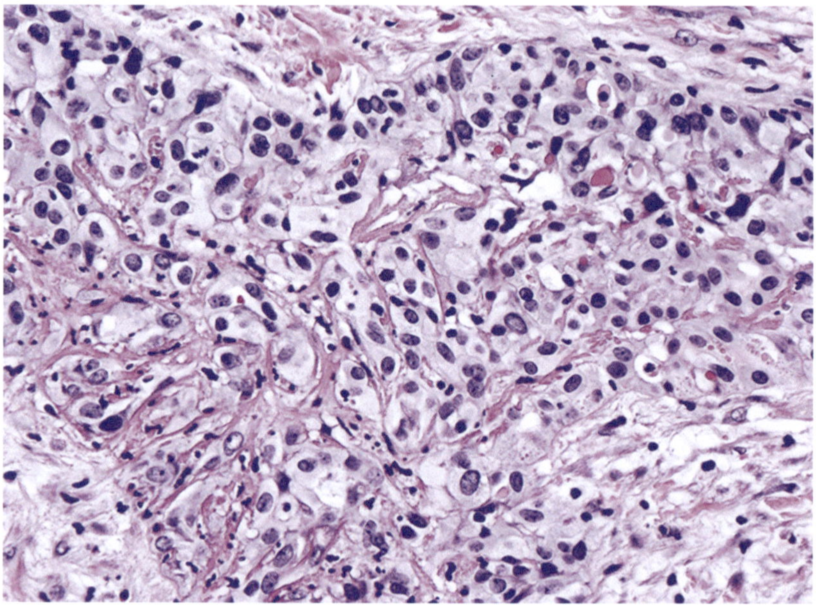

Fig. 31.1 Reactive hyperplasia of the rete testis. Pseudotumoral proliferation of epithelial cells of the rete testis taking a solid pattern

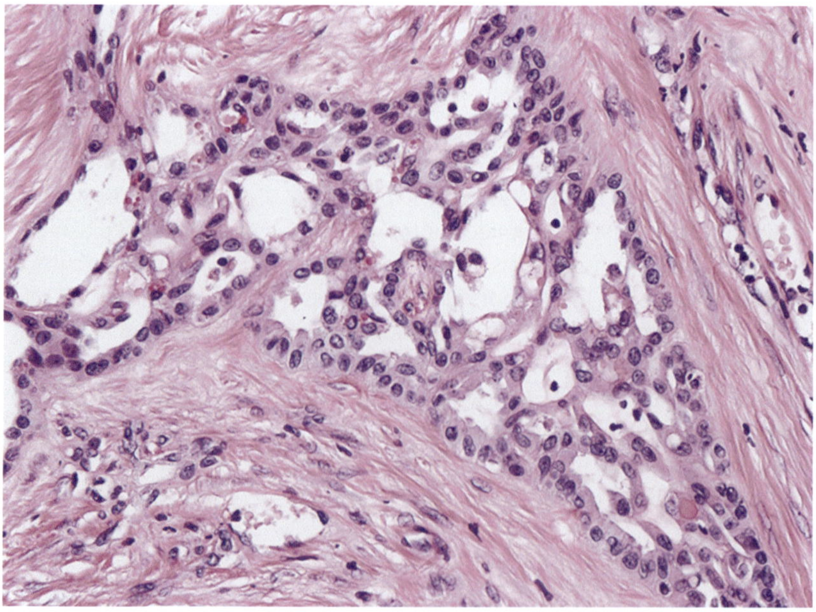

Fig. 31.2 Reactive hyperplasia of the rete testis. The epithelium of the rete testis adopts a cribriform pattern

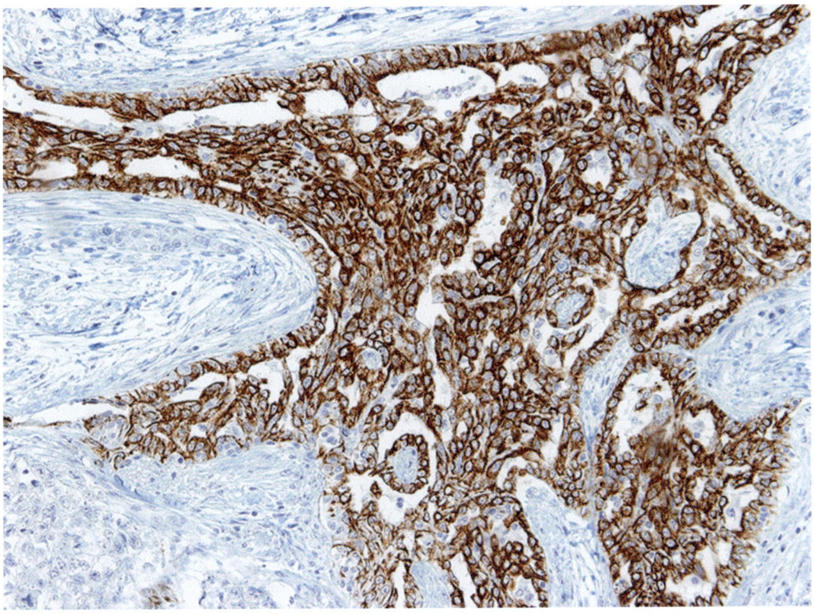

Fig. 31.3 Reactive hyperplasia of the rete testis. The cells of the intracavitary proliferation express immunostaining for AE1/AE3cytokeratin

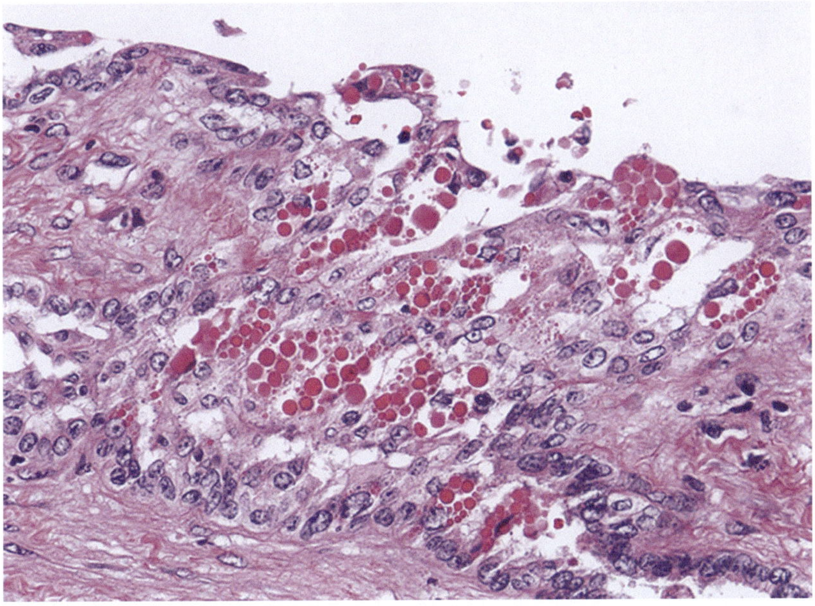

Fig. 31.4 Hyperplasia with hyaline globules. The distribution of hyaline globules varies widely in epithelial cells of the intracavitary proliferation

31.3 Adenomatous Hyperplasia of the Rete Testis

The term "adenomatous hyperplasia of rete testis" (AHRT) was used by M. Nistal et al. in 1976 [3] for the first time in an article about the cystic dysplasia of the testis in childhood to refer to an overdeveloped rete testis that took much of the testicular parenchyma and with which renal malformations were associated (see Chap. 29). In the adult, adenomatous hyperplasia of the rete testis is a lesion characterized by diffuse proliferation of the tubular structures or papillary derived rete testis. It is preferentially located in the septal and mediastinal rete testis [4] (Fig. 31.5).

The epithelium of the rete testis sometimes forms nodular unencapsulated growths, and other adopts a diffuse pattern. The size of the nodules can be sufficiently large to make us think of a tumor. The cells are cubic or cylindrical with a deeply folded ovoid nucleus and a peripheral nucleolus, there is lack of atypia, and they do not show mitosis. There is continuity between the hyperplastic epithelium and the epithelium of a normal rete testis. The ultrastructure and immunophenotype of this epithelium is similar to that of the normal rete testis (Fig. 31.6). In some cases sperm are observed inside the cavities, suggesting that this proliferation is connected to the seminiferous tubules. Most of the testes show some degree of atrophy of the seminiferous tubules.

On a color Doppler echo, it is described as a well-circumscribed and hypoechogenic solid mass located in the upper pole of the testis with a great perilesional vascularization pattern [5].

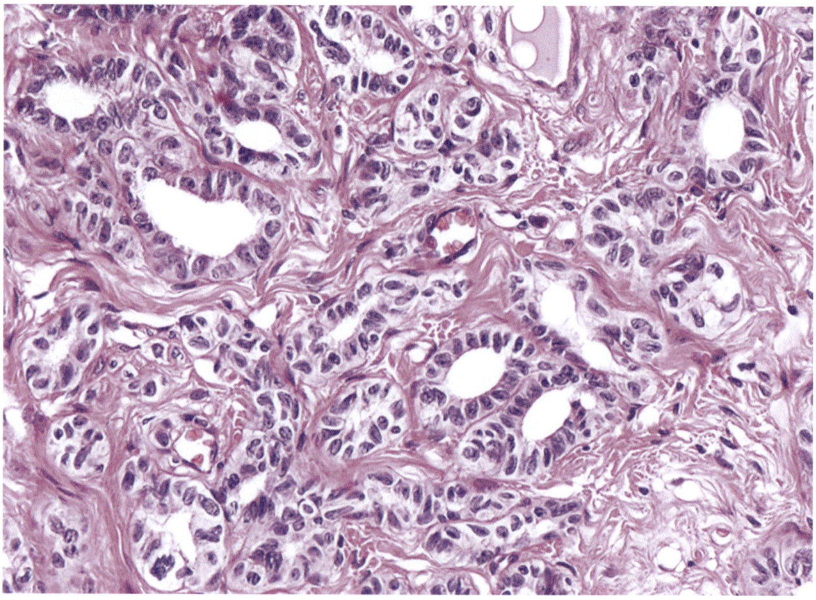

Fig. 31.5 Adenomatous hyperplasia of the rete testis. Mediastinal rete testis has lost his organization in flat cavities arranged parallel to the surface; instead there is a cordonal and pseudoglandular proliferation. The epithelial lining of the cavities is cubic and lacks atypia

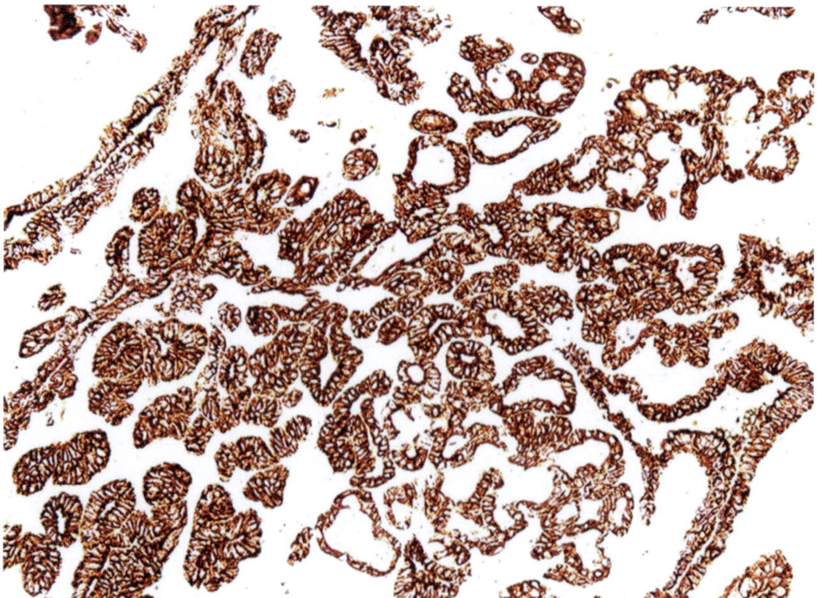

Fig. 31.6 Adenomatous hyperplasia of the rete testis. The cells in cordonal structures and glandular formations express cytokeratins (immunostaining for AE1/AE3)

Adenomatous hyperplasia is usually an incidental finding in the study of the testes at autopsy [6], in undescended testicles [7, 8] or in testicles with germ cell tumors.

The etiology of adenomatous hyperplasia in cases where it is an incidental finding of the autopsy is unknown, but it has been linked to hormonal changes or the action of chemical agents [9–11]. Adenomatous hyperplasia, which is observed in many undescended testis and testicular tumors, is probably a primary anomaly and is part of the testicular dysgenesis syndrome [12].

A problem emerges in connection with the testicular dysgenesis syndrome at whose base an androgen/estrogen imbalance lies – to consider to what extent the adenomatous hyperplasia may be a precursor lesion of adenocarcinoma of the rete testis. Although experimentally in male mice the rete testis develops various degrees of epithelial hyperplasia, proliferation, and papillary adenocarcinoma after exposure to diethylstilbestrol [13], there is no record of any human case of adenocarcinoma of the rete testis attributed to exposure to diethylstilbestrol. In the reported cases of coexistence of the two lesions, the patients had no history of exposure to estrogen [14, 15].

Adenomatous hyperplasia must be distinguished from the rete testis pseudohyperplasia shown in atrophic testes, from primary tumors of the testis and from metastatic adenocarcinomas. For a differential diagnosis, see Chap. 28.

31.4 Lithiasis of the Rete Testis

The presence of calcifications in the rete testis is uncommon. They can adopt two different patterns. Sometimes calcifications are amorphous, very variable in size, and arranged within the cavities, and they are observed in the lesion described later as calcifying nodular intracavitary polypoid proliferation. At other times they are small concentric laminated formations that take the shape of microliths (Fig. 31.7). The microliths can be seen in the rete testis in different processes, malformation, tumors, and elderly men, and in these cases their meaning is completely different.

The malformation that is often accompanied by microliths is cystic dysplasia of the rete testis. Calcifications isolated or forming clusters are arranged in the periphery of the cystic lesions in relation to the residual testicular parenchyma. Both are located under the epithelium of the rete testis and inside it in relation to the eosinophilic material of its lumen.

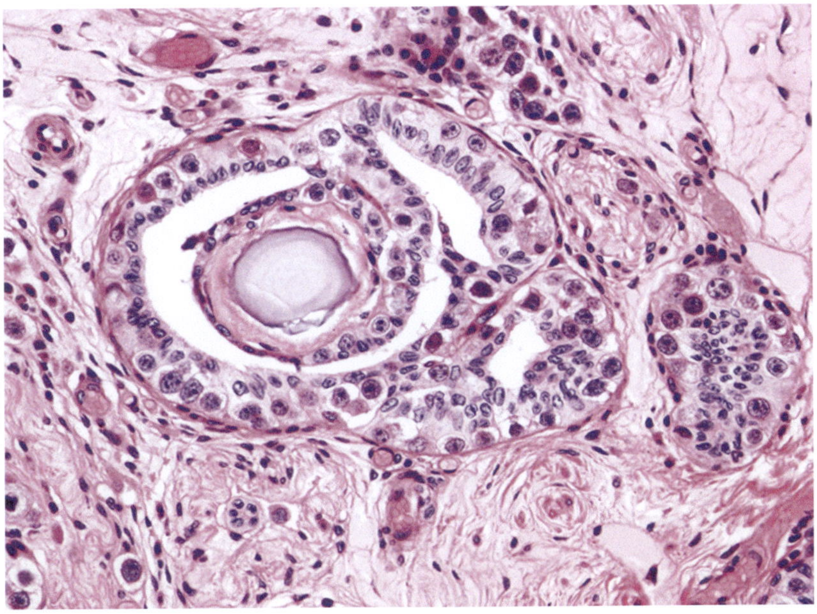

Fig. 31.7 Microlithiasis, a chordae associated with pagetoid infiltration of rete testis by GCNIS

Calcifications associated with testicular tumors are located subepithelially; they are also characteristic of microliths and are generally associated with testicular microlithiasis, so they can be considered as part of the histological lesions of the testicular dysgenesis syndrome.

In elderly patients, coinciding with testicular atrophy of ischemic etiology, in which the rete adopts a cordonal appearance, a large number of microliths can be seen in the fibrous stroma beneath the epithelium. In these cases it is common to observe microlithiasis in the epididymis and vas deferens [16].

31.5 Intracavitary Nodular Polypoid Calcifying Proliferations

These are bilateral lesions characterized by the presence of pedunculated or sessile masses inside the cavities of the rete testis. They are formed of a loose connective tissue in the implantation base, coated with a fibrin-like cap material. The surface is covered by the epithelium of the rete testis. They are not associated with inflammation and may appear partially or completely calcified. They are observed in adult patients with poor peripheral perfusion (arteriosclerosis, hypertension, gastrointestinal or brain hemorrhage, myocardial infarction). The lesions can be observed either isolated or associated with other acquired processes of the rete testis.

Selective localization in both walls of the cavities of the rete testis and chordae may be related to the poor vascularization of these structures, which only reach the terminal branches of the centripetal testicular arteries. The pathogenic mechanism could be the following: anoxia, necrosis, fibrin deposits, conjunctiva proliferation, and dystrophic calcification (Fig. 31.8). Differently from the growth toward the mediastinum testis, the intracavitary growth may depend on the lower hydrostatic pressure inside the cavities of the rete testis and the very rigid structure of the mediastinum testis [17].

31.6 Atrophy of the Rete Testis

Atrophy of the rete testis presents with a marked decrease of the space taken by their cavities. The epithelium lining can be flat or cubic. The septal rete testis may adopt a pseudoglandular pattern as a result of the tubuli recti shortening. This pseudohyperplasia has been misdiagnosed as

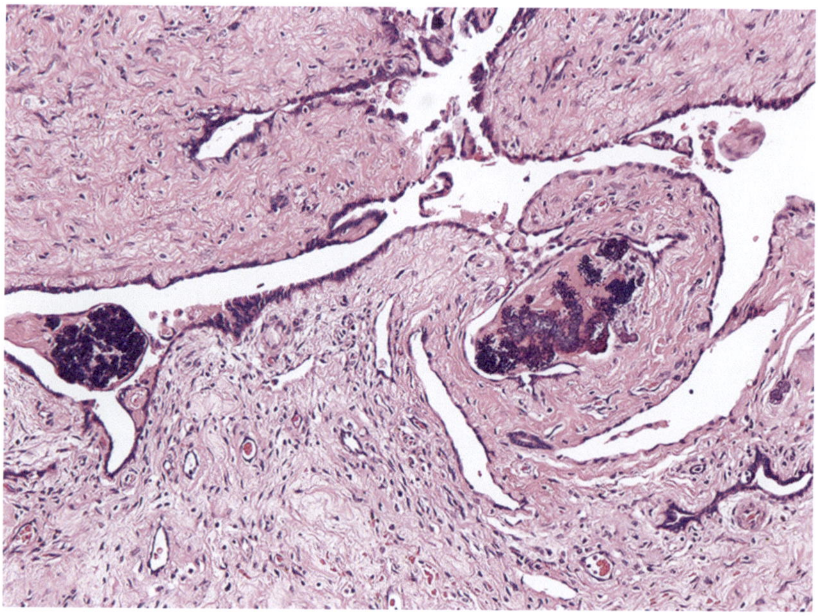

Fig. 31.8 Intracavitary nodular polypoid proliferation associated with dystrophic calcification of nodular formations

adenomatous hyperplasia. It represents only the result of the collapse of the rete after the atrophy of seminiferous tubules. The epithelial changes can associate focal proliferation myofibroblasts arranged in bundles between the cavities of the atrophic rete.

This is typical of patients with a lesion of the hypothalamic-pituitary-testicular axis, and it is caused by hypogonadotropic hypogonadism. It is also observed in patients with arteriosclerosis. In this case it is usually associated with mediastinal fibrosis and hyalinization and subepithelial microliths.

References

1. Ulbright TM, Gersell DJ. Rete testis hyperplasia with hyaline globule formation. A lesion simulating yolk sac tumor. Am J Surg Pathol. 1991;15:66–74.
2. Skinnider BF, Young RH. Infarcted adenomatoidtumor: a report of five cases of a facet of a benign neoplasm that may cause diagnostic difficulty. Am J Surg Pathol. 2004;28:77–83.
3. Nistal M, García-Villanueva M, Sanchez J. Displasia quística del testículo: anomalía en la diferenciación del parénquima testicular por probable fallo de la conexión entre los conductos de origen mesonéfrico y los cordones testiculares. (Abstrac in English). Arch Esp Urol. 1976;29:431–44.
4. Nistal M, Paniagua R. Adenomatous hyperplasia of the rete testis. J Pathol. 1988;154:343–6.
5. Martino G, Pasta V, Ciardi A, Palmieri A, Marinaccio L, Malavenda MS, Monti M. Rete testis adenomatous hyperplasia: our experience. Ann Ital Chir. 2013;6:84 (ePub) pii:S2239253X13019877.
6. Nistal M, Castillo MC, Regadera J, García-Cabezas MA. Adenomatous hyperplasia of the rete testis. A review and report of new cases. Histol Histopathol. 2003;18:741–52.
7. Uguz A, Gönlüşen G, Ergin M, Tunali N. Adenomatous hyperplasia of the rete testis: report of two cases. Int Urol Nephrol. 2002;34:87–9.
8. Ozgur T, Akin MM, Gokce H, Davarci M. Adenomatous hyperplasia of the rete testis: not a true hyperplasia, just proliferation! Contemp Oncol (Pozn). 2013;17:466–7.
9. Channer JL, MacIver AG. Glandular changes in the rete testis: metastatic tumour or adenomatous hyperplasia? J Pathol. 1989;157:81–2.
10. Srigley JR, Hartwick RW. Tumors and cysts of the paratesticular region. Pathol Annu. 1990;25(Pt 2):51–108.
11. Hartwick RW, Ro JY, Srigley JR, Ordoñez NG, Ayala AG. Adenomatous hyperplasia of the rete testis. A clinicopathologic study of nine cases. Am J Surg Pathol. 1991;15:350–7.
12. Nistal M, Gonzalez-Peramato P, Regadera J, Serrano A, Tarin V, De Miguel MP. Primary testicular lesions are associated with testicular germ cell tumors of adult men. Am J Surg Pathol. 2006;30:1260–8.
13. Newbold RR, Bullock BC, McLachian JA. Adenocarcinoma of the rete testis. Diethylstilbestrol-induced lesions of the mouse rete testis. Am J Pathol. 1986;125:625–8.
14. Gruber H, Ratschek M, Pummer K, Breinl E, Spuller E, Hubmer G. Adenocarcinoma of the rete testis: report of a case with surgical history of adenomatous hyperplasia of the rete testis. J Urol. 1997;158:1525–6.
15. Lin XY, Yu JH, Xu HT, Wang L, Fan CF, Liu Y, Wang EH. A case of adenocarcinoma of the rete testis accompanied by focal adenomatous hyperplasia. Diagn Pathol. 2013;8:105.
16. Nistal M, García-Cabezas MA, Regadera J, Castillo MC. Microlithiasis of the epididymis and the rete testis. Am J Surg Pathol. 2004;28:514–22.
17. Nistal M, Paniagua R. Nodular proliferation of calcifying connective tissue in the rete testis: a study of three cases. Hum Pathol. 1989;20:1231–9.

32 Congenital Cystic Pathology of the Epididymis

Manuel Nistal, Pilar González-Peramato, and Álvaro Serrano

32.1 Cysts

The cysts are the most common pathology of the epididymis. In principle, they could be considered to represent a banal pathology, and this is true in most cases. But we should not forget that they may be the only expression, at a testicular level, of genetic alterations responsible for serious chronic diseases.

The incidence of epididymal cysts in pediatric patients who have undergone a scrotal ultrasound varies from 5 % [1] to 15 % of children presenting with scrotal pain or mass [2]. The group next to puberty or at puberty is the one with the highest incidence [3]. The rates are even higher in patients who have been exposed in utero to diethylstilbestrol (20 %) [4] or with cystic fibrosis [5], hepatorenal polycystic disease [6], or von Hippel-Lindau disease [7–9]. The incidence increases with age.

32.1.1 Histological Types

From the pathological point of view, cysts can be classified in five types: simple cysts, spermatoceles, epidermoid cyst, nonpapillary cystadenomas, and papillary cystadenomas. For the epidermoid cyst, see Chap. 37 on paratesticular acquired tumor-like lesions.

Simple Cysts

Simple cysts are usually of small size, more frequently unilateral, uni- or multilocular, and approximately 1 cm in diameter. They are located in the caput epididymis (Fig. 32.1), although cysts in the corpus and the cauda have also been reported [10]. Some cysts of larger size can cause scrotal discomfort, pain, or mass although most of them are asymptomatic. Exceptionally, an acute scrotum secondary to torsion of the cyst may occur [11, 12].

Histologically, all cysts are lined with a simple epithelium that may have different characteristics according to their embryological origin: mesothelial, Müllerian or Wolffian remnants, efferent ductules, or aberrant ducts. Mesothelial cysts have a simple flattened epithelium that immunoexpresses calretinin, WT1, and D240. The Wolffian and Müllerian cysts have a columnar or pseudostratified epithelium with isolated ciliated cells. Wolffian-derived cysts can be distinguished from Müllerian-derived cysts by a lineal positive CD10 immunoexpression in the apical border of epithelial cells. Most of the cysts in boys are considered to be originated in hormonal disorders during embryonic life. It has even been suggested that cysts of the epididymis might be part of a dysgenesis syndrome [13]. The treatment should be conservative, except for symptomatic cysts, those larger than 3 cm and torsioned cysts.

M. Nistal et al., *Clues in the Diagnosis of Non-tumoral Testicular Pathology*,
DOI 10.1007/978-3-319-49364-0_32

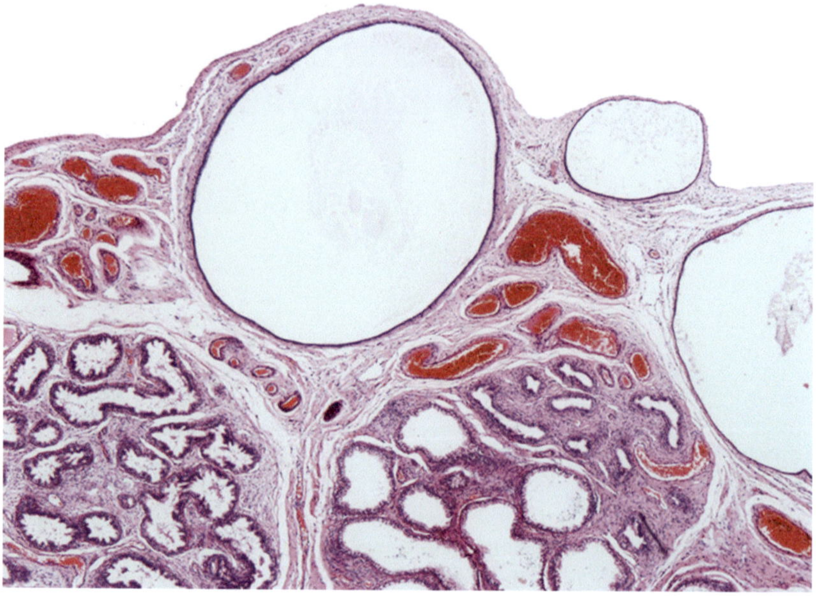

Fig. 32.1 Multiple cysts in the caput of the epididymis probably originated from embryonic remnants. Cystic formations are separated from the efferent ductules

Spermatoceles

This term refers to any type of cyst containing sperm [14]. Cysts can appear in the efferent ductules, in the aberrant ducts, or in the spermatic cord. Spermatoceles are common in the caput epididymis and originate from a lack of connection to the main duct of the epididymis of an efferent ductule. Even under normal conditions, by microdissection techniques, a blind bottom ending has been observed. In exceptional cases the lack of connection is complete, and the head of the epididymis is thickened by cystic transformation of the efferent ductules. It is probable that in childhood, some spermatoceles would have been diagnosed as simple cysts [15].

The epithelium of spermatoceles is cubic or columnar and formed by two cell types: ciliated and secretory. They contain abundant spermatozoa in histological preparations can also appear in the pericystic tissue structures due to artifact. Among the sperm there are also macrophages full of them (spermiophages) [16], immature epithelial cells, and epithelial cells detached from the rete testis (small blue cells) or from the efferent ductuli [17, 18]. Spermatoceles are not always originated in a congenital alteration, and there are spermatoceles secondary to infection, traumatism, or vasectomy. An infrequent complication of spermatocele is torsion [19] or intracystic hemorrhage [20]. Spermatoceles larger than 4 cm should be removed.

Extra care must be taken while removing epididymal cysts, whether there are spermatoceles or not, because the damage that can be caused to the efferent ductules may originate or even aggravate an obstruction of the spermatic pathway; that is why a conservative approach when the cysts do not cause discomfort has been imposed [21]. However, there are cases in which, left to their evolution, they increase in size, compress the epididymis until causing atrophy, or bring about epididymal obstruction that has to be surgically treated. There are series of patients with olizoospermia that after surgical removal of the cyst show improvement, not only in numbers but in the sperm motility too.

Cystadenomas

Nonpapillary Serous Cystadenomas Are rare cystic lesions in adults, and their content is a thick fluid without sperm. They were first reported by Pick and Galliano in 2005 [22]. The age at presentation varies from 12 to 64 years. They can be single or multiple and are preferably located in the caput epididymis. Except for one case, cystadenomas are unilateral.

The cystadenoma lining is an epithelium similar to nonpapillary serous tumors of the ovary. It is a cubic or columnar epithelium with ciliated cells, apical snouts, and vacuolated cytoplasm without papillae. They can also show lipofuscin pigment. The epithelium is positive for CK7, vimentin, EMA, estrogen receptors, progesterone receptors, CD15, Ca-125, MOC-31, and focally for CD10, and it is negative for S100, CK20, and calretinin [23].

This neoplasia is considered to originate from the testicular appendix or from some of the numerous Müllerian remnants that can be observed along the epididymis and paratesticular structures [24].

The treatment consists in the removal of the cyst. The histological study should be especially careful, as if an infiltrative growth is demonstrated, although focal, a diagnosis of cystadenocarcinoma should be made because distant metastasis can develop.

Papillary Cystadenoma This is a hamartomatous lesion of the caput epididymis consisting in papillary proliferations developed within ecstatic efferent ductules that arise from the epithelium of these ducts [25]. The first cases were reported by Brandt in 1921 [26], Lindau in1924 [27], and Sherrick in1956 [28].

Incidence: They account for 4 % of all epididymal tumors [29]. The presentation is bilateral in about 40 % of cases. The age of presentation varies from 7 to 81 years [30], although they are most frequently diagnosed during the second and the third decades of life. Approximately 60 % of papillary cystadenomas of the epididymis occur in patients with von Hippel-Lindau disease (VHL); in fact, papillary cystadenoma of the epididymis has been revealed as an initial stage of the VHL disease in several cases [31].

Usually, the clinical presentation is either as an incidental finding or in patients with von Hippel-Lindau disease (VHL). Papillary cystadenoma of the epididymis has also been reported associated with infertility in patients with severe oligozoospermia [32] or an obstructive azoospermia [33] caused by the intratubular growth of this lesion [34]. It has also been reported as found during vasectomy in a patient with a spermatic cord tumor located more than 4 cm away from the superior testicular pole [35]. Other cases have been found in necropsy. The most common sign among symptomatic patients is a painless slowly growing scrotal swelling.

VHL disease is an autosomal, dominant inherited disease with high penetrance. The prevalence is estimated at 2–3 per 100,000 persons [36], which accounts for approximately 7000 patients in the USA. A germline mutation in the VHL gene predisposes carriers to tumors in multiple organs. These tumors may include hemangioblastoma in the retina and central nervous system, renal cell carcinoma, paraganglioma, meningiomas, pheochromocytomas, endolymphatic sac tumor of the inner ear, islet cell tumor of the pancreas, adrenal cortex adenomas, and the development of cysts in different organs (liver, kidney, pancreas, adrenal gland, epididymis, and broad ligament) [37, 38].

The VHL disease gene is mapped to chromosome 3, in the locus 3p25-26 [39], and it is a suppressor gene that encodes a 213-amino acid sequence. The VHL disease gene plays an important role in the suppression of the vascular endothelial growth factor (VEGF) [40]. About 75–80 % of patients with VHL disease have a germline mutation of the VHL gene, while somatic mutations of this gene have also been reported in sporadic cases of hemangioblastomas, clear cell renal carcinomas [41], pheochromocytoma [42], endolymphatic sac tumor, and papillary cystadenomas of the epididymis. Therefore, diagnosis of one of these tumors should prompt finding out the presence of VHL disease.

Diagnosis Ultrasonography is the easiest method to diagnose epididymal papillary cystadenoma. The ultrasound image shows a predominantly solid mass, which contains small cysts or echogenic foci located in the caput epididymis, usually associated with cystic transformation of the rete testis [43]. The lesion may be asymptomatic for months or even years.

Pathology A conservative treatment is recommended, and that is why, pathological studies of epididymal papillary cystadenomas are rare. Macroscopically, the lesion is well delimited, grayish or yellowish, with cystic or solid formations, measuring 0.5–8 cm in diameter, and located in the caput epididymis.

No histological differences have been found between the isolated forms of epididymal papillary cystadenoma and those forms associated with VHL disease. The lesion consists of cysts with papillary formations growing inside that occasionally can occupy the whole cystic lumen [44]. The cysts and the papillary formations are lined with identical epithelium derived from the efferent ductule epithelium. It comprises two cell types that recall the epithelium of the efferent ductules both under light microscopy and electronic microscopy: columnar and ciliated cells. The columnar cells show a hyperchromatic and spherical nucleus and a glycogen-rich, clear cytoplasm. The apical cytoplasm contains lipid droplets, and the luminal plasma membrane displays long microvilli and some cilia. The basal plasma membrane forms hemidesmosomes with the basal lamina. The axis of the papillae is formed by loose connective tissue that contains fenestrated capillaries [45]. The lumen of cysts and ecstatic efferent ductules contains a granular, intensely PAS-positive, proteinaceous, colloid-like material (Fig. 32.2). The stroma that surrounds the cysts can appear hyalinized and sometimes contains some psammoma bodies. Histological images similar to hemangioblastoma as well as lipogranuloma and inflammatory lymphoid infiltrates can be observed at the periphery of the lesion [46].

Some lesions are totally [47] or partially solid, and their cells show the same characteristics as those of the cystic or the papillary areas, although they can also adopt a pseudoinfiltrative growing pattern (Fig. 32.3). The cells of the papillary cystadenoma show immunoexpression for AE1/AE3, CAM5.2, CEA, HIF-alpha, VEGF, alphaSMA, and CD34. Cells are positive for cytokeratin 7 [48] and negative for cytokeratin 20. The cells are variably positive for S100, renal cell marker, and vimentin [49, 50]. One case showed positive expression for PAX2 [51] and CD10, calretinin and WT-1 having been negative in all cases [52]. The stroma next to epithelial cells shows an intense vascular neoformation with CD31 [53].

Epididymal tumorigenesis in VHL patients occurs in two sequential steps as it has been shown in detailed histologic and molecular pathologic analysis of tumor-free epididymal tissues. The first stage is characterized by the

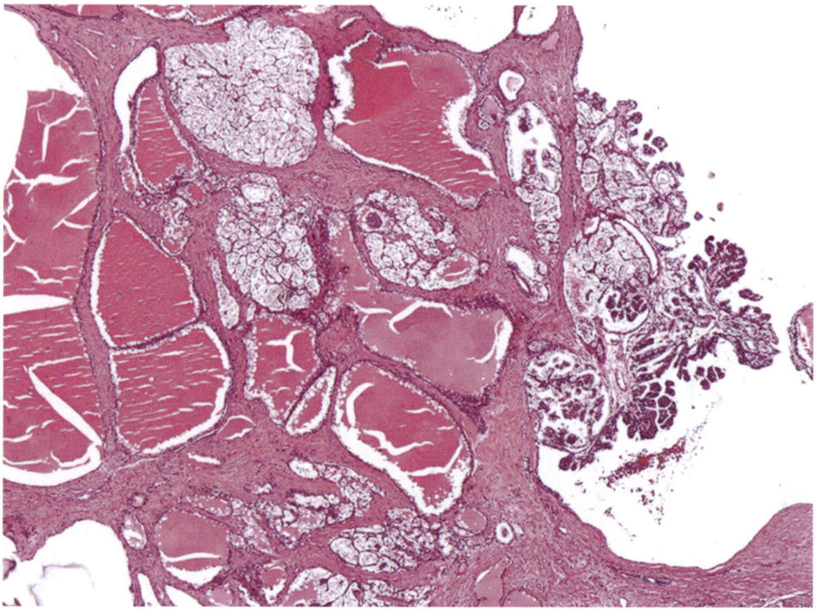

Fig. 32.2 Papillary cystadenoma of the epididymis. The head of the epididymis is markedly enlarged. The efferent ductules are dilated and show a content ranging from a granular and eosinophilic fluid to a solid or papillary epithelial proliferation

developmental arrest of VLH-deficient mesonephric cells with subsequent structural-anatomic alterations of the epididymal tissue. The second stage is characterized by slow proliferation of a subset of VHL-deficient cells with activation/upregulation of hypoxia-inducible factor (HIF) and VEGF, associated with continuous reactive fibrovascular proliferation that determines the neoplastic papillary proliferation [54].

Differential Diagnosis Mural papilloma and metastasis of either thyroid papillary carcinoma or clear cell renal carcinoma should be included in the differential diagnosis of this hamartomatous lesion (Fig. 32.4). Mural papilloma is a focal lesion, developed in a spermatocele wall (see later). Metastasis of thyroid papillary carcinoma to the epididymis is exceptional. The characteristic nuclear changes of thyroid papillary

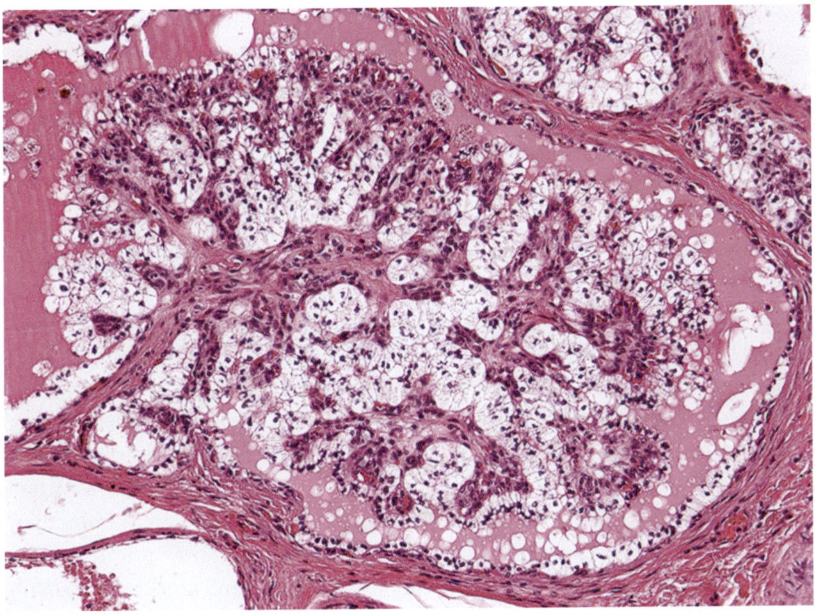

Fig. 32.3 Papillary cystadenoma of the epididymis. Dilated efferent ductule housing a papillary proliferation lined by cells of clear cytoplasm

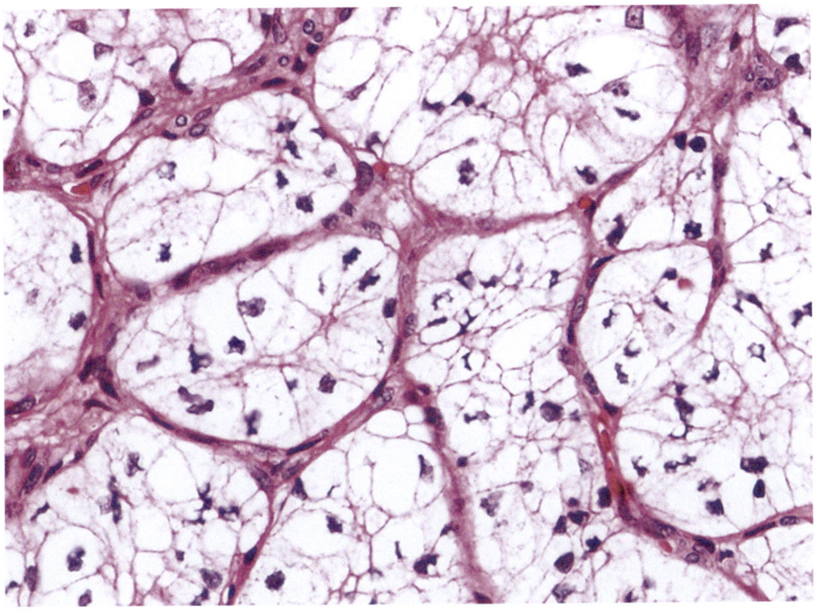

Fig. 32.4 Papillary cystadenoma of the epididymis. Proliferation of cells with large pale cytoplasms and vesicular nuclei simulating a renal tumor metastasis

carcinoma and immunoexpression for TTF1 are useful for the differential diagnosis. The possibility of epididymal metastasis of a clear cell renal cell carcinoma should always be taken into account because this tumor has been reported in association with VHL disease and can metastasize to the epididymis. The higher nuclear pleomorphism, the presence of solid areas, and the absence of granular, PAS-positive material in the papillary zones are characteristics of renal cell carcinoma. Immunohistochemically, both CK 7 and CD10 are useful as all the epididymal cystadenomas have a CK7-positive and a CD10-negative profile [55], while clear cell renal cell carcinoma has the opposite immunophenotype.

32.1.2 Peculiar Findings in Epididymal Cysts

Among the curious findings within the epididymal cysts, we have observed the following: mural papilloma, Liesegang rings, crystalloid and crenellated membranes.

Mural Papilloma The mural papilloma is a very rare lesion and only two cases have been reported [56, 57]. In both of them, the cyst wall was lined by a simple cubical epithelium together with some ciliated cells and others with hyperchromatic nuclei. Papillary neoformation had a thin base of implantation and an arborescent growth inside the cyst. Multiple papillary fronds and multilobar blebs with a core of edematous or hyalinized connective tissue were found. The papillae were lined with a columnar epithelium positive for cytokeratin 7 and negative for cytokeratin 20, with intense CD10 antigen expression observed in the epithelial papillary proliferative cells (Fig. 32.5). This immunophenotype suggests a Wolffian origin.

Liesegang Rings Is the name given to eosinophil bodies observed inside the cystic formations by RE Liesegang, a German biochemist who produced them in vitro more than a century ago [58]. They are concentric laminated bodies of variable size from 10 to 800 microns that in addition to a laminar structure usually have radial striations [59]. Liesegang rings have been observed in renal and perirenal hemorrhagic cysts and in various inflammatory and necrotic lesions in the kidney, nasal sinus, pleura, pericardium, omentum, extraovarian and ovarian endometriosis, breast, synovium conjunctiva, and eyelid.

They are formed by precipitation around a central nidus alternating cycles of subsaturation

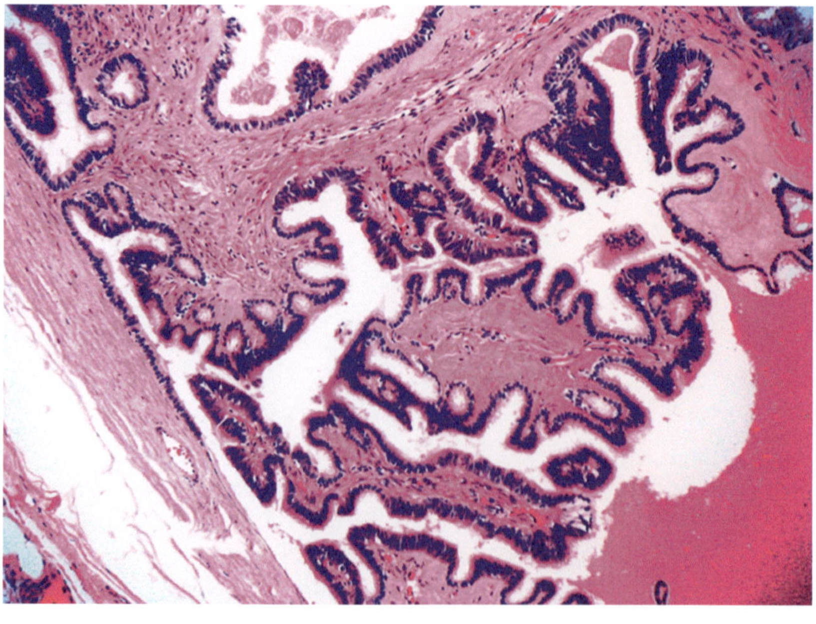

Fig. 32.5 Mural papilloma inside an epididymal cyst. Lining cells show immunostaining for CD10 and CK7

and supersaturation of an insoluble product in a colloidal system. The mechanisms by which precipitation occurs are not well known although they should include the electrical charge, pH, chemical concentration, temperature, and the presence of cellular debris [60] (Fig. 32.6). From a practical point of view, the structure of Liesegang rings reminds amylaceous bodies, Michaelis-Guttman bodies as those observed in malacoplakia, calcium deposits, hyaline globules, and even parasites like the giant kidney worm Dioctophyma renale, but none of them meets the following three characteristics: eosinophilia, concentric structure, and radial laminar striation.

Crystalloid

Eosinophilic rectangular formations of up to 20 microns in length and 4 microns in width that resemble crystals can be observed in some cysts. They are probably the result of a dystrophic process, possibly related to inflammation, although the mechanism of crystalloid formation is uncertain.

Crenellated Membranes

Some epididymal cysts in adults present many membranous formations lining the cyst, with the peculiarity of showing a bristled surface with many small protrusions of the same size and relatively regularly arranged. These membranes have histological and histochemical characteristics similar to those observed in membranes of lipomembranous fat necrosis. They are eosinophilic, PAS positive (before and after digestion with diastase), refractive, and orcein and Sudan black positive and have autofluorescence when examined under ultraviolet light (Fig. 32.7). The mechanism occurring in the absence of inflammation and necrosis suggests that the starting point may be the peeling and cell death of lining cells of the cyst and perhaps secretion materials from the lining epithelial cells accumulated for years. The transformation of these lipid-rich materials would be similar to that suggested for the lipomembranous fat necrosis [61].

32.2 Cystic Dysplasia of the Epididymis

Cystic dysplasia of the epididymis (CDE) is a malformative anomaly recently described by Nistal [62]. It is characterized by the presence of irregular, segmental cystic dilatation of the efferent ductules with aberrant forms and an

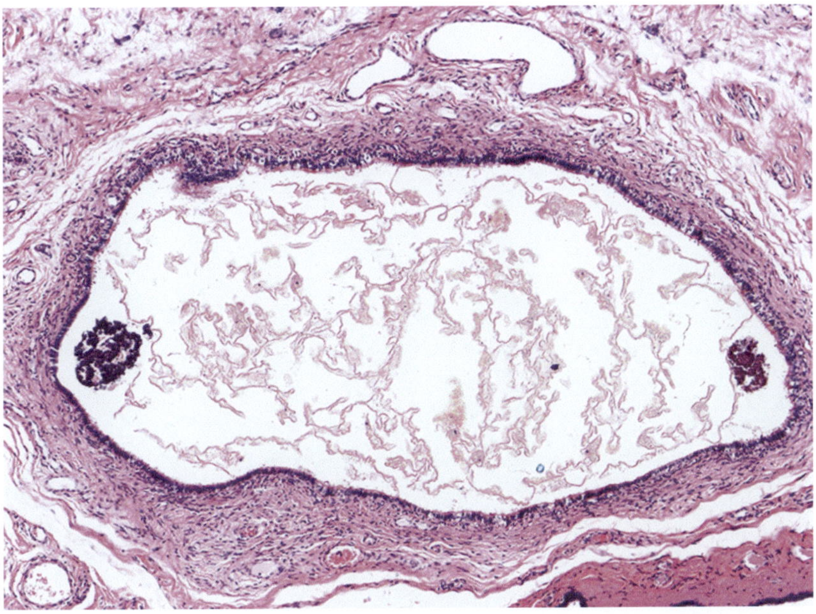

Fig. 32.6 Epididymal cyst with probable origin in embryonic remnants filled with eosinophilic membranous formations and calcified cellular debris

immature aspect associated with an important decrease in the number of sections of efferent ductules without lesions in the lining epithelium. In seven cases gross examination showed loss of the typical hemispherical shape of the epididymis head caused by the irregular cystic dilatations. The lesions may affect one segment of the epididymal duct in association with the lesions in the head of the epididymis or as an isolated lesion (Fig. 32.8).

CDE was observed in 19 fetal and neonatal autopsies of male subjects with ages ranging from 27 weeks of gestation to 10 days of life and one surgical specimen corresponding to a 4-year-old boy. The lesion was bilateral in all 13 cases in which both epididymides were available for review. Eighteen out of 20 cases presented with either renal and/or urinary tract anomalies including renal dysplasia (eight cases), renal agenesis (four cases), autosomal recessive polycystic renal disease (one

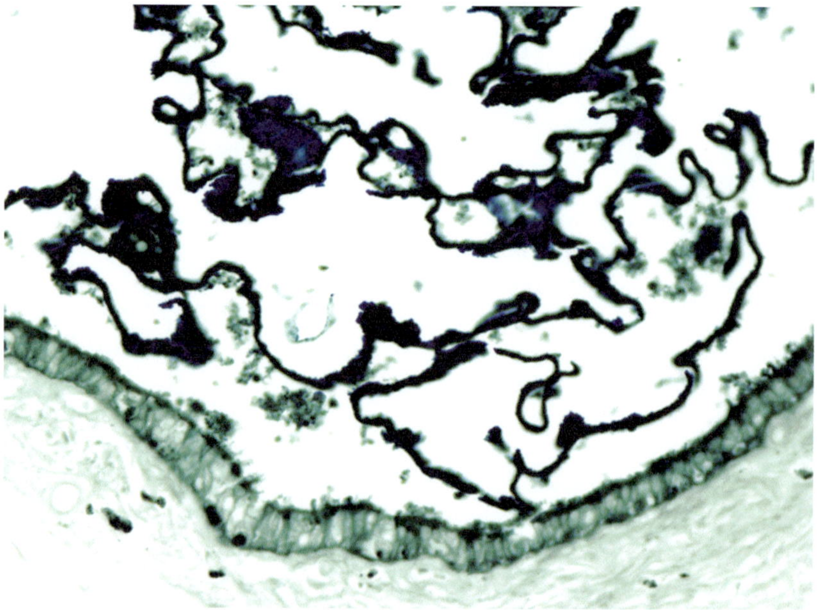

Fig. 32.7 Crenellated membranous formations are Oil Red O positive, similar to those observed in lipomembranous fat necrosis

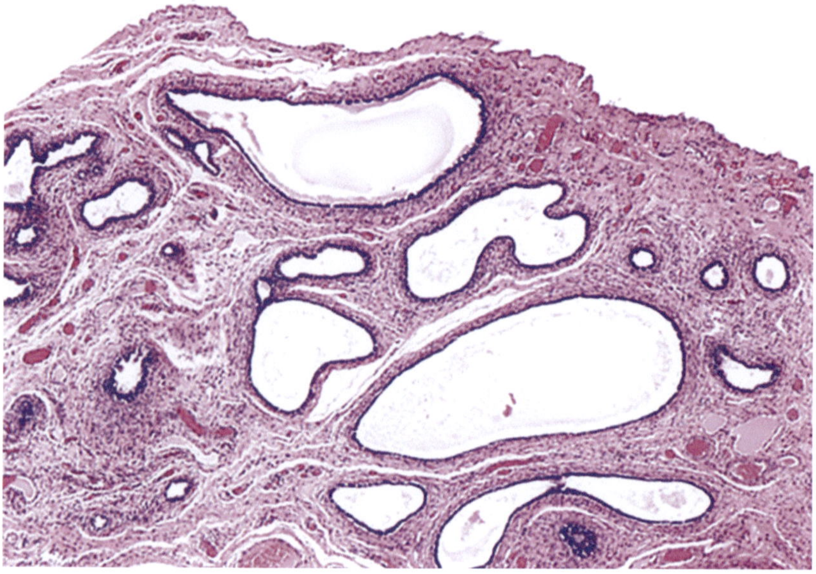

Fig. 32.8 Cystic dysplasia of the epididymis associated with dysplasia of the rete testis. The epididymis caput consists in cystic dilations of efferent ductules with irregular size and shape

case), and renal hypoplasia (one case). In eight cases the testes were cryptorchidic. One patient associated ipsilateral testicular cystic dysplasia.

Cystic dysplasia of the epididymis presents a novel congenital anomaly of the mesonephric differentiation that should be added to the spectrum of male excretory system disorders associated with renal and urinary malformations.

References

1. Finkelstein MS, Rosenberg HK, Snyder 3rd HM, Duckett JW. Ultrasound evaluation of scrotum in pediatrics. Urology. 1986;27:1–9.
2. Aragona F, Pescatori E, Talenti E, Tomà P, Malena S, Glazel GP. Painless scrotal masses in the pediatric population: prevalence and age distribution of different pathological conditions – a 10 year retrospective multicenter study. J Urol. 1996;155:1424–6.
3. Posey ZQ, Ahn HJ, Junewick J, Chen JJ, Steinhardt GF. Rate and associations of epididymal cysts on pediatric scrotal ultrasound. J Urol. 2010;184:1739–42.
4. Palmer JR, Herbst AL, Noller KL, Boggs DA, Troisi R, Titus-Ernstoff L, Hatch EE, Wise LA, Strohsnitter WC, Hoover RN. Urogenital abnormalities in men exposed to diethylstilbestrol in utero: a cohort study. Environ Health. 2009;18:8–37.
5. Blau H, Freud E, Mussaffi H, Werner M, Konen O, Rathaus V. Urogenital abnormalities in male children with cystic fibrosis. Arch Dis Child. 2002;87: 135–8.
6. Leclerc JP, Canet J, Lancret P, Chelloul N, Le Bont H, Pesnel G, Fabre A, Lajouanine P. Thoracic asphyxiating dystrophia and hepato-pancreatico-epididymo-renal polycystosis. A case. Arch Fr Pediatr. 1969;26:1160–2.
7. Gill WB, Schumacher GF, Bibbo M, Straus II FH, Schoenberg HW. Association of diethylstilbestrol exposure in utero with cryptorchidism, testicular hypoplasia and semen abnormalities. J Urol. 1979;122:36–9.
8. Whitehead ED, Leiter E. Genital abnormalities and abnormal semen analyses in male patients exposed to diethylstilbestrol in utero. J Urol. 1981;125:47–50.
9. Caballero Martínez MC, Cuesta Alcalá JA, Amat Villegas I, Gómez Dorronsoro ML, Ruiz de AzúaCiria Y, Martínez-Peñuela JM. Papillary cystadenoma of the epididymis: report of 2 new cases. Arch Esp Urol. 2003;56:297–9.
10. Ushida H, Hayashida H, Kim CJ, Park KI, Okada Y. Bilateral synchronous multilocular epididymal cysts: a case report. Nippon Hinyokika Gakkai Zasshi. 1999;90:692–5.
11. Yilmaz E, Batislam E, Bozdogan O, Basar H, Basar MM. Torsion of an epididymal cyst. Int J Urol. 2004;11:182–3.
12. Karaman A, Afşarlar CE, Arda N. Epididymal cyst: not always a benign condition. Int J Urol. 2013;20: 457–8.
13. Skakkebaek NE, Rajpert-De Meyts E, Main KM. Testicular dysgenesis syndrome: an increasingly common developmental disorder with environmental aspects. Hum Reprod. 2001;16:972–8.
14. Walsh TJ, Seeger KT, Turek PJ. Spermatoceles in adults: when does size matter? Arch Androl. 2007;53:345–8.
15. Homayoon K, Suhre CD, Steinhardt GF. Epididymal cysts in children: natural history. J Urol. 2004;171: 1274–6.
16. Castelino-Prabhu S, Ali SZ. Spermiophages in a giant spermatocele. Diagn Cytopathol. 2010;38:816–7.
17. Lane Z, Epstein JI. Small blue cells mimicking small cell carcinoma in spermatocele and hydrocele specimens: a report of 5 cases. Hum Pathol. 2010;41:88–93.
18. Marotti JD, Seigne JD, Gutmann EJ. Presence of benign germ cells in a fine needle aspirate of a spermatocele. Diagn Cytopathol. 2013;41:342–3.
19. Takimoto K, Okamoto K, Wakabayashi Y, Okada Y. Torsion of spermatocele: a rare manifestation. Urol Int. 2002;69:164–5.
20. Cozcolluela MR, Sarria L, Martinez-Berganza MT, Ripa L, Monzón F, Sanz LA, Fernandez J. Espermatocele complicado como causa de masa escrotal de aspecto sólido. Hallazgosecográficos. Actas Urol Esp. 1996;20:750–2.
21. Kliesch S. Hydrocele, spermatocele, and vasectomy: management of complications. Urologe A. 2014;53: 671–5.
22. Pich A, Galliano D. Pure (non-papillary) serous cystadenoma of the epididymis: a histologic and immunohistochemical study. Pathol Res Pract. 2005;201:65–9.
23. Fernández-Aceñero MJ, Renedo G, Fortes J, Manzarbeitia F. Nonpapillary serous cystadenoma of the epididymis: report of 2 cases of a rare entity. Urology. 2010;75:563–5.
24. Abdull Gaffar B, Al-Hasani S, El-Fayomy A. Multiple bilateral nonpapillary serous cystadenoma of the epididymis. Urology. 2013;82:e24–5.
25. Mostofi FK, Price Jr EB. Tumors and tumor-like conditions of testicular adnexal structures (epididymis, spermatic cord, capsule, and supporting structures). In: Tumors of the male genital system, Atlas of tumor pathology, fasc. 8, 2nd series. Armed Forces Institute of Pathology: Washington, DC; 1973. p. 143–75.
26. Brandt R. Zur Frage der Angiomatosisretinea. V Graefe's Arch Ophthal. 1921;106:127–30.
27. Lindau A. ZurFrage der Angiomatosis retinae undihrer Hirnkomplikationen. Acta Opthal. 1927;4: 193–6.
28. Sherrick JC. Papillary cystadenoma of the epididymis. Cancer. 1956;9:403–6.
29. Richard S, Beroud C, Joly D, Chretien Y, Benoit G. Von Hippel-Lindau disease and renal cancer: 10 years of genetic progress. GEFVHL (French-Speaking Study Group on von Hippel-Lindau disease). Prog Urol. 1998;8:330–9.

30. Wernert N, Goebels R, Prediguer L. Papillary cystadenoma of the epididymis: case report and review of the literature. Pathol Res Pract. 1986;181:260–4.
31. Lamiell JM, Salazar FG, Hsia YE. Von Hippel-Lindau disease affecting 43 members of a single kindred. Medicine (Baltimore). 1989;68:1–29.
32. Crisp JC, Roberts PF. A case of bilateral cystadenoma of the epididymis presenting as infertility. Br J Urol. 1975;47:–682.
33. De Souza Andrade J, Bambirra EA, Bicalho OJ, De Souza AF. Bilateral papillary cystadenoma of the epididymis as a component of von Hippel-Lindau's syndrome: report of a case presenting as infertility. J Urol. 1985;133:288–9.
34. Pozza D, Masci P, Amodeo S, Marchionni L. Papillary cystadenoma of the epididymis as a cause of obstructive azoospermia. Urol Int. 1994;53:222–4.
35. Geenen RWF, Bevers RFM, Gielis C, Boon TA. Papillary cystadenoma located in the spermatic cord. J Urol. 1997;158:546.
36. Béroud C, Joly D, Gallou C, Staroz F, Orfanelli MT, Junien C. Software and database for the analysis of mutations in the VHL gene. Nucleic Acids Res. 1998;26:256–8.
37. Hes FJ, Van Der Luijt RB, Lips CJ. Clinical management of Von Hippel-Lindau (VHL) disease. Neth J Med. 2001;59:225–34.
38. Künzli BM, Shrikhande SV, Büchler MW, Friess H. Pancreatic lesions in von Hippel-Lindau syndrome: report of a case. Surg Today. 2004;34:626–9.
39. Latif F, Tory K, Gnarra J, Yao M, Duh FM, Orcutt ML, Stackhouse T, Kuzmin L, Modi W, Geil L, et al. Identification of the von Hippel-Lindau disease tumor suppressor gene. Science. 1993;260:1317–20.
40. Leung SY, Chan AS, Wong MP, Yuen ST, Fan YW, Chung LP. Expression of vascular endothelial growth factor in von Hippel-Lindau syndrome-associated papillary cystadenoma of the epididymis. Hum Pathol. 1998;29:1322–4.
41. Zhuang Z, Gnarra JR, Dudley CF, Zbar B, Linehan WM, Lubensky IA. Detection of von Hippel-Lindau disease gene mutations in paraffin-embedded sporadic renal cell carcinoma specimens. Mod Pathol. 1996;9:838–42.
42. Murgia A, Martella M, Vinanzi C, Polli R, Perilongo G, Opocher G. Somatic mosaicism in von Hippel-Lindau disease. Hum Mutat. 2000;15:114.
43. Choyke PL, Glenn GM, Wagner JP, Lubenski IA, Thakore K, Zbar B, Linehan M, Walther MM. Epididymal cystadenomas in von Hippel-Lindau disease. Urology. 1997;49:926–31.
44. Chan YH, Schinella RA, Draper JW. Papillary clear cell cystadenoma of the epididymis. J Urol. 1968;100:661–5.
45. Torikata C. Papillary cystadenoma of the epididymis. An ultrastructural and immunohistochemical study. J Submicrosc Cytol Pathol. 1994;26:387–93.
46. Price Jr EB. Papillary cystadenoma of the epididymis.A clinicopathologic analysis of 20 cases. Arch Pathol. 1971;91:456–70.
47. Yang L, Xu WS, Melamed J, Zhou M, Deng FM. Solid variant of papillary cystadenoma of the epididymis. Histopathology. 2015;67:138–41.
48. Gilcrease MZ, Schmidt L, Zbar B, Truong L, Rutledge M, Wheeler TM. Somatic von Hippel-Lindau mutation in clear cell papillary cystadenoma of the epididymis. Hum Pathol. 1995;26:1341–6.
49. Calder CJ, Gregory J. Papillary cystadenoma of the epididymis: a report of two cases with an immunohistochemical study. Histopathology. 1993;23: 89–91.
50. Yaqoob N, Ahsan A, Ahmad Z, Khan AN. Clear cell papillary cystadenoma of epididymis, a mimic of metastatic renal cell carcinoma. J Pak Med Assoc. 2008;58:209–11.
51. Gokden N, Kemp SA, Gokden M. The utility of Pax-2 as an immunohistochemical marker for renal cell carcinoma in cytopathology. Diagn Cytopathol. 2008;36:473–7.
52. Odrzywolski KJ, Mukhopadhyay S. Papillary cystadenoma of the epididymis. Arch Pathol Lab Med. 2010;134:630–3.
53. Sano T, Horiguchi H. Von Hippel-Lindau disease. Microsc Res Tech. 2003;60:159–64.
54. Mehta GU, Shively SB, Duong H, Tran MG, Moncrief TJ, Smith JH, Li J, Edwards NA, Lonser RR, Zhuang Z, Merrill MJ, Raffeld M, Maxwell PH, Oldfield EH, Vortmeyer AO. Progression of epididymal maldevelopment into hamartoma-like neoplasia in VHL disease. Neoplasia. 2008;10:1146–53.
55. Mehta GU, Shively SB, Gläsker S, Bechert CJ, Zhuang Z, Raffeld M, Lonser RR, Oldfield EH, Vortmeyer AO. von Hippel-Lindau disease: epididymal cystadenoma targeted by metastatic events. Urology. 2007;69:1209.e9–12.
56. Mostofi FK, Price EB. Tumors of the male fenital system, Atlas of tumor pathology, Second Series, Fascicle 8. Washington, DC: Armed Forces Institute of Pathology; 1973. p. 165.
57. Nistal M, González-Peramato P, Serrano A, Vega-Perez M, De Miguel MP, Regadera J. Paratesticular cysts with benign epithelial proliferations of wolffian origin. Am J Clin Pathol. 2005;124:245–51.
58. Liesegang RE. Uber einige Eigenschaften von Gallerton. Nature Wochschr. 1896;11:353–62.
59. Glazier DB, Murphy DP, Cummings KB, Morrow FA. Liesegang rings. J Urol. 1997;157:940–1.
60. Raso DS, Greene WB, Finley J, Silverman JF. Morphology and pathogenesis of Liesegang rings in cyst aspirates: report of two cases wich ancillary studies. Diagn Cytopathol. 1998;19:116–9.
61. Nistal M, González-Peramato P, Paniagua R. Lipomembranous fat necrosis in three cases of testicular torsion. Histopathology. 2001;38:443–7.
62. Nistal M, González-Peramato P, Sousa G, García-Cabezas MA, Rodriguez JI, Cajaiba MM. Cystic dysplasia of the epididymis: a disorder of mesonephric differentiation associated with renal maldevelopment. Virchows Arch. 2010;456:695–702.

33 Reactive Pathology of the Epididymis

Manuel Nistal, Pilar González-Peramato, and Álvaro Serrano

33.1 Epididymal Ectasia

Epididymal ectasia results from an increase in epididymal intraluminal pressure. It can be congenital (malformation, mucoviscidosis) or acquired (vasectomy, inguinal hernia repair, epididymitis, prostatitis or extrinsic compression by a tumor mass). The most common cause is vasectomy (Fig. 33.1). In over 50 % of cases, it is associated with spermatocele, spermatic granuloma, dilated vas deferens, and ectasia of the rete testis.

Ectasia brings about histological changes in the epididymal duct itself, in the efferent ductules, in the vas deferens, and even in the rete testis. These changes are classified as early, intermediate, and late. The initial changes are the result of increased intraductal pressure secondary to the obstruction. Efferent ductules are dilated. The absorption increases, the ciliated cells disappear, and spermatoceles can be formed. Intermediate changes occur when the absorption capacity has been exceeded and an important expansion has been reached. The wall shows thickening with collagen and ground substance accumulation. The myoid cells in the efferent ductules acquire a phenotype characteristic of smooth muscle cells of distal areas of the epididymis [1]. A large number of macrophages traverse the epididymis to aid in the clearance of sperm and fluid. The latest post-vasectomy findings begin with sperm extravasations into the interstitium of the epididymis or vas deferens. The answer is twofold; on the one side, a reaction with giant foreign body cells on groups of sperm takes place leading to spermatic granulomas (Fig. 33.2), and on the other side, attempts of epithelial regeneration result in numerous ductal structures that are known as nodosa vasitis or epididymitis depending on their location [2, 3].

A late complication of ectasia of the epididymis in vasectomy patients is the post-vasectomy pain syndrome that occurs 5–7 years after vasectomy in 10 % [4] to 33 % of patients [5]. It is characterized by scrotal pain during ejaculation or sexual intercourse, or both. The potential etiologic factors considered are mechanical obstruction with perineural fibrosis and compression of the epididymis by adjacent cysts.

The ultrasound study reveals an enlarged epididymis with linear hypoechoic structures with echogenic walls giving a speckled appearance to the epididymis [6–8]. The lesion is typically avascular in color Doppler sonography, which rules out epididymitis. MRI is able to contribute another step toward the knowledge of the epididymis contents. In cases of tubular ectasia, increased epididymal T1 intensity [9] is observed.

In 12.5 % of vasectomized patients, the ultrasound examination of the epididymis shows the presence of mobile echogenicities [10]. These mobile echogenicities bear a strong resemblance to the random to-and-fro movements of countless tiny echogenic particles in a distended epididymis

M. Nistal et al., *Clues in the Diagnosis of Non-tumoral Testicular Pathology*,
DOI 10.1007/978-3-319-49364-0_33

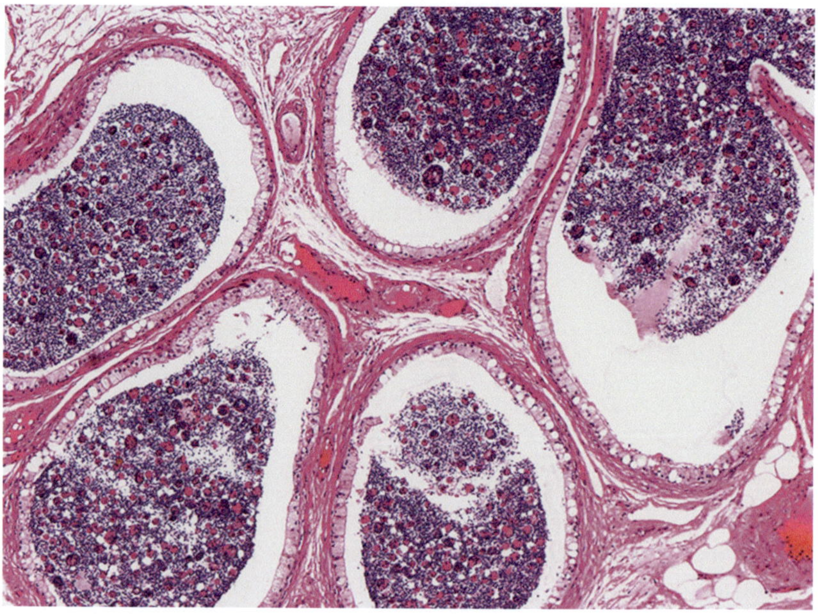

Fig. 33.1 Epididymal ectasia secondary to vasectomy. The epididymis had to be removed by severe painful discomfort (late post-vasectomy syndrome). Abundant spermatozoa free or inside spermiophages are seen inside the epididymal ducts. Most epithelial cells have a pale apical cytoplasm

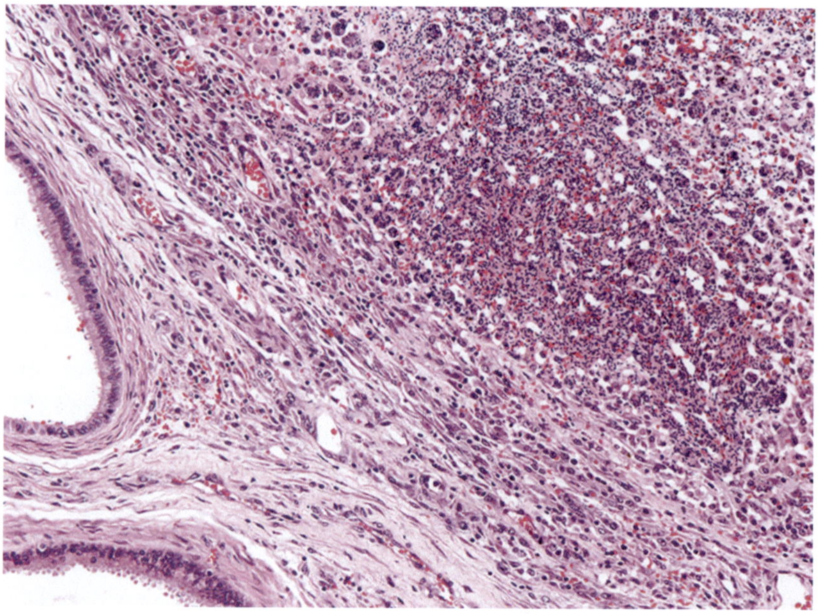

Fig. 33.2 Spermatic granuloma. Sperm extravasations into the interstitium of the epididymis trigger an inflammatory reaction with abundant macrophages and giant foreign body cells that engulf and degrade the spermatozoa

of men infected with adult *Wuchereria bancrofti*, a phenomenon described as "filarial dance" [11]. Histological studies have linked this finding to the presence of numerous macrophages with or without sperm in their cytoplasm that may reach 100 microns and are located in the lumen of the dilated epididymis [12]. Similar findings may be observed in post-inflammatory obstruction. Another finding observed in histological sections of enlarged epididymis is the presence of Liesegang rings.

33.2 Paneth-Like Metaplasia

Granular changes in epididymal cells known as Paneth cell-like metaplasia refer to the resemblance of the eosinophilic granulations of the epididymis cells with the Paneth cells of the intestinal glands. It is a typical lesion of the efferent ductules that may affect all or just some of them. The changes may appear in the two types of epithelial cells, principal and secretory cells. The cells show an increase in cytoplasmic size due to the presence of numerous eosinophilic inclusions preferably located in the supranuclear region, which are fluorescent when examined under ultraviolet light and are also intensely PAS positive (Fig. 33.3).

Although these histological findings are common with intestinal Paneth cells, there are a number of important immunohistochemical differences. Epididymal cells with granular changes are positive for alpha1-antitripsin (alpha-1 AT), alpha1-antichemotripsin (alpha-1 AChT), and CD68, which suggests a lysosomal nature of the granules. Conversely, the granules of the intestinal Paneth cells are negative for alpha-1 AChT and CD68, and so secretory vesicles of antimicrobial peptides correspond [13]. These immunohistochemical differences suggest the most appropriate term could be Paneth metaplasia-like [14].

Both benign and malignant processes have been described in the epididymis. They have been associated with obstructive processes of the spermatic ducts and have even been identified as markers of obstruction [15]. However, there are many cases in which an obstruction of the sperm pathway is not shown and could have another explanation as, e.g., a mismatch between the amount of fluid reaching the epididymis and the reabsorption capacity of the epithelial cells. This is the case of the Paneth-like changes seen in patients with testicular tumors. In these cases there are alterations in the amount of fluid produced by the testes and in its composition. Most testicular fluid production would be secondary to the intense congestion that accompanies tumors. The tumor necrosis that may be involved causes a massive release of substances for which the endocytic machinery of epithelial cells of the efferent ductules is not ready. Excessive endocytosis probably leads to an increase in secondary lysosomes in their cytoplasm.

33.3 Ischemic Granulomatous Epididymitis

The term ischemic granulomatous epididymitis refers to a lesion, preferably located at the head of the epididymis, noninfectious in nature, observed in elderly patients [16].

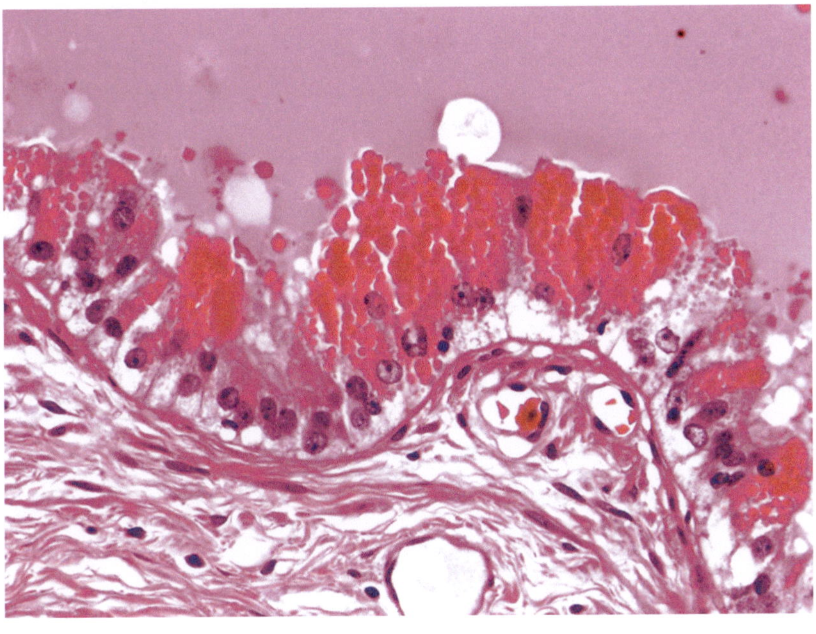

Fig. 33.3 Paneth-like metaplasia of one efferent ductule epithelium. The apical cytoplasms of all epithelial cells show numerous eosinophilic granulations

Histologically, in the initial stages of this lesion, there is necrosis affecting both the efferent ductules and the intertubular connective tissue (Fig. 33.4). As the lesion progresses, several facts occur such as sperm extravasations, the necrotic material tends to be removed into the lumen of the best preserved efferent ductules, forming polypoid masses. An infiltrate of macrophages can be observed, either engulfing the necrotic material, or being removed to the lumen, or becoming giant cells engulfing cholesterol crystals or sperm resulting in sperm microgranulomas (Fig. 33.5).

In the epididymal fibrosis final stages, an accumulation of lipofuscins in epithelial cells of the residual efferent ductules and ceroid granulo-

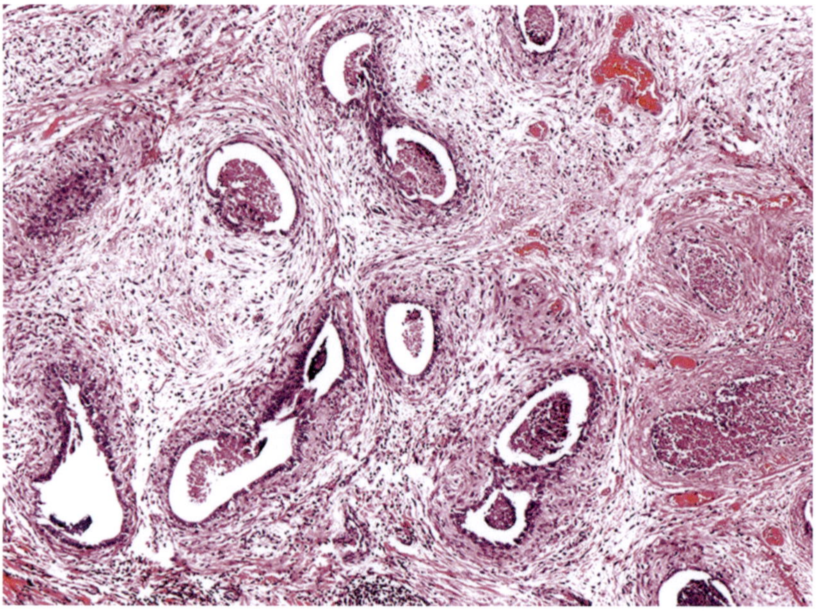

Fig. 33.4 Ischemic epididymitis. Necrosis of efferent ductules at different stages of evolution. There are ductules with necrosis of both the epithelium and the muscular wall adjacent to others with epithelial necrosis, and even some of them show signs of regeneration

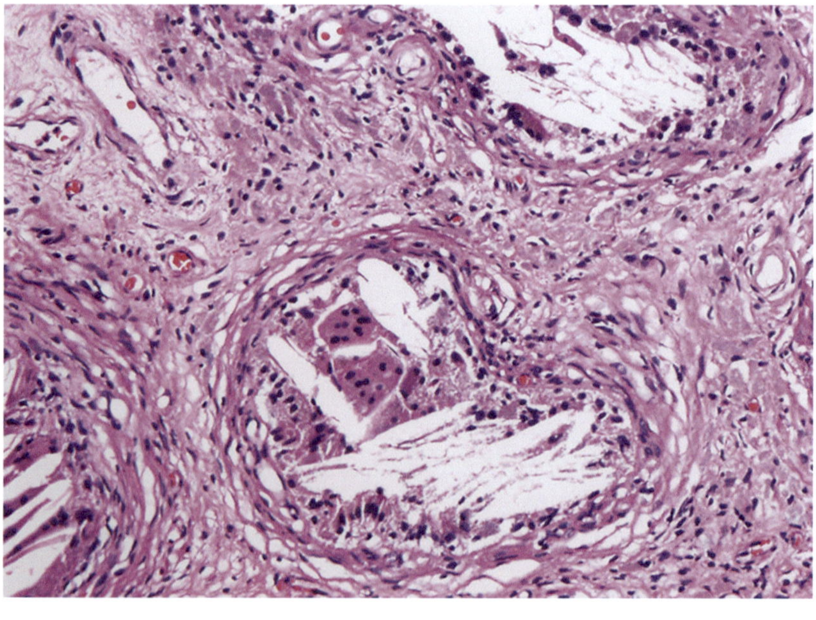

Fig. 33.5 Ischemic epididymitis. Efferent ductules full of cholesterol crystals and multinucleated giant cells. In the intertubular interstitium, only isolated lymphocytes and macrophages are recognized

mas is observed in some cases. These lesions give the epididymis an appearance of brown patches [17]. In other cases a cavitation of the epididymis or neoformation of ductal structures similar to epididymitis nodosa occurs. Although the cause is unknown, given the age of the patients and the distribution of the lesions, the hypothesis of ischemia is highly suggestive. The territory that presents the most important changes is supplied by the superior epididymal artery, a collateral branch of the testicular artery. The age of patients and the atherosclerosis observed in autopsy cases would support the hypothesis of ischemia [18]. The lesion is asymptomatic in most cases.

33.4 Epididymal Metaplasia

The main epididymal duct is constituted by a pseudostratified epithelium and one or two layers of smooth muscle cells around. The epithelium cells are of several types: basal cells, principal cells, narrow cells, clear cells, halo cells, and dendritic cells. The basal cells are attached to the basement membrane; they are small, flattened, and ovoid with a hyperchromatic nucleus. The principal cells are the most numerous; they have many stereocilia in the apical pole and frequent intranuclear eosinophilic inclusions. Their secretory and endophytic machinery is highly developed. Narrow cells make protrusion toward the lumen and reach the basement membrane through a fine cytoplasmic extension. They have numerous vesicles involved in endocytosis, and their function is to secrete H + ions into the lumen. Clear cells are cylindrical with basal nuclei, few microvilli, abundant endocytic system with multivesicular bodies, and a large number of lysosomes. The halo cells correspond to lymphocytes and macrophages that cross the epithelium. The dendritic cells form a network throughout the epididymis, and, as at other locations, they are antigen-presenting cells. Two types of metaplasia were observed in the epididymis: prostatic and squamous metaplasia.

33.4.1 Prostatic Metaplasia

The presence of prostatic tissue outside the urinary tract is rare; the cases published in English barely exceed a dozen. Most of the time, it is an incidental finding in the study of surgical specimens or in autopsy, but it can be the cause of lower gastrointestinal bleeding, constipation, urinary symptoms, and a retroperitoneal mass [19, 20].

The presence of prostatic tissue in the epididymis has previously been observed only in three cases to which we now add another one observed in our department. The first case was found at autopsy in the normal epididymis of a 30-year-old organ donor [21]. The second case was found in an orchiectomy specimen of an undescended testicle [22]. The third patient was an 11-year-old male who presented with an asymptomatic supratesticular mass in the right hemiscrotum [23]. And the fourth case (our case) was found in a cryptorchidic testicle of a 58-year-old patient (Figs. 33.6 and 33.7).

Prostatic tissue may be seen in different forms: (1) as a node separated from the epididymal duct, (2) as a mixed arrangement of prostate glands and duct sections, and (3) consisting in the presence of multiple small areas along the main duct where the main duct epithelium of the epididymis is replaced by the prostate glands.

The first two forms are considered ectopias of prostatic parenchyma and the third one a form of metaplasia. The presence of ectopic prostatic parenchyma in mesonephric derivatives perhaps may be related, following McNeal hypothesis [24], to the different sources in the different areas of the prostate, as while the peripheral zone derives from the urogenital sinus and the central zone originates from the mesonephric duct. Remnants of this duct would differentiate in the prostate tissue. The hypothesis of a metaplasia to explain prostate glands in the epithelium of the epididymal duct finds its best support in the juxtaposition of prostate glands with epithelial cells of the epididymis. The fact that both testes were cryptorchidic may not be a coincidence. We must remember that in cryptorchidism, the epididymis has alterations in cell

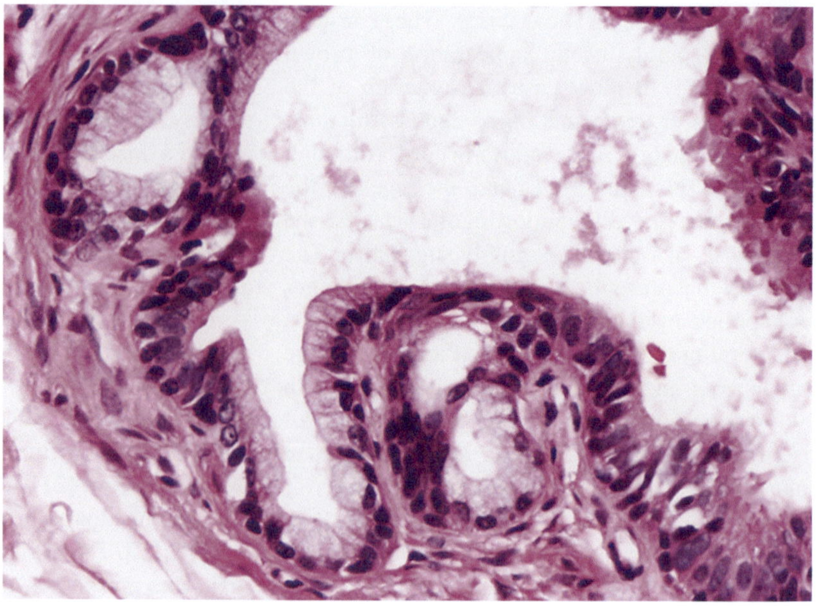

Fig. 33.6 Prostatic metaplasia. Section of the main duct of the epididymis. The pseudostratified epithelium with stereocilia has been replaced by columnar epithelium with cells of basal nuclei and pale cytoplasm

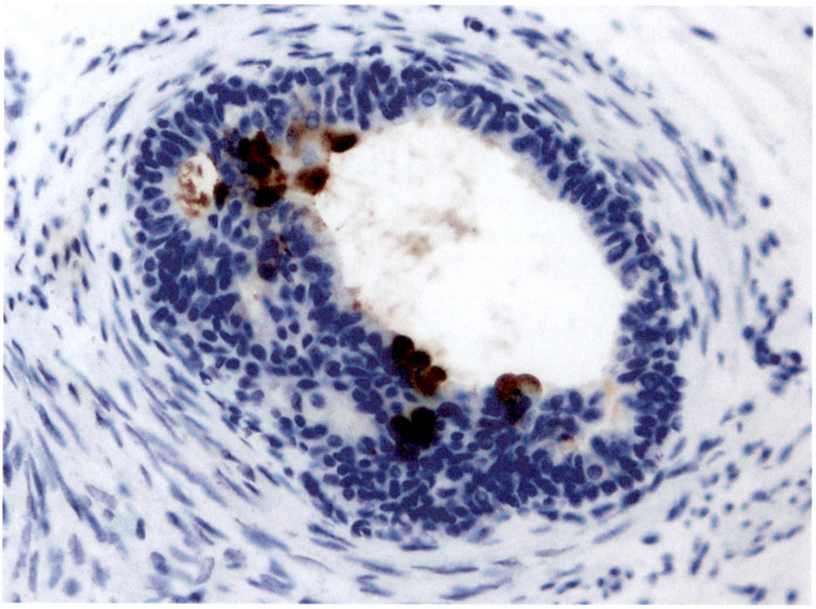

Fig. 33.7 Prostatic metaplasia. Positive immunostaining of single cells or groups cells for prostatic acid phosphatase (same case of the previous figure)

growth and differentiation, which could aid the development of metaplasia in the absence of a reactive process [25].

33.4.2 Squamous Metaplasia

This is an uncommon lesion related to the present or former presence of an inflammatory process. The part of the epididymis that most often shows squamous metaplasia is the tail. The epithelium is sometimes nonkeratinized stratified squamous, and other times it shows a thick layer of keratin. In these cases an obstruction of the lumen occurs. The masses of keratin can calcify (Fig. 33.8). The tubular wall is thickened; it shows fibrosis and inflammatory cell debris. The differential diagnosis can be raised with epidermoid cysts and carci-

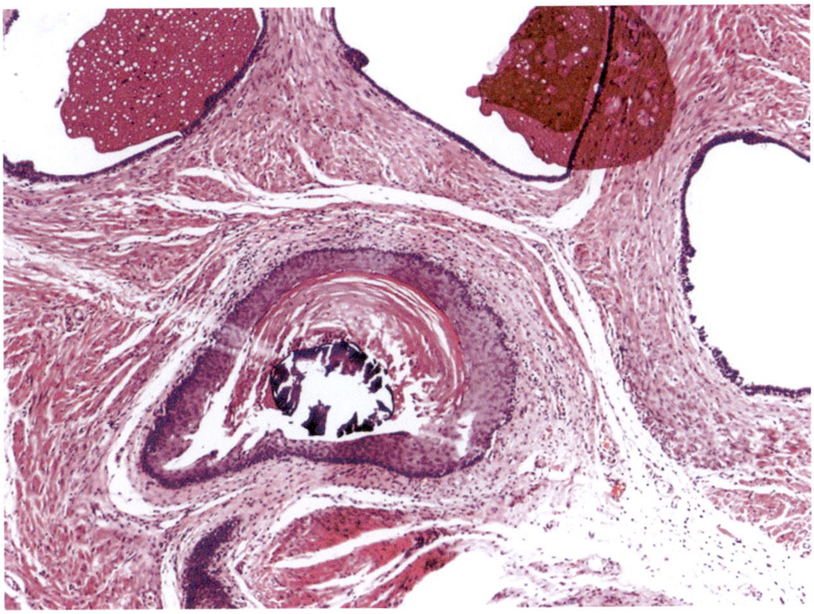

Fig. 33.8 Squamous metaplasia with dystrophic calcification of the keratin in a section of the epididymal duct

nomas of the epididymis. The presence of a muscular layer together with the multifocality of the lesion rules out the first one, and the absence of cellular atypia facilitates the exclusion of a carcinoma diagnosis [26].

References

1. Pelliccione F, Cordeschi G, Giuliani V, D'Abrizio P, Necozione S, Negri L, Mancini M, Sagone P, Francavilla F, Colpi GM, Francavilla S. The contractile wall of the caput epididymidis in men affected by congenital or postinflammatory obstructive azoospermia. J Androl. 2004;25:417–25.
2. McDonald SW. Vasectomy review: sequelae in the human epididymis and ductus deferens. Clin Anat. 1996;9:337–42.
3. Woodward PJ, Schwab CM, Sesterhenn IA. From the archives of the AFIP: extratesticular scrotal masses: radiologic-pathologic correlation. Radiographics. 2003;23:215–40.
4. Christiansen CG, Sandlow JI. Testicular pain following vasectomy: a review of postvasectomy pain syndrome. J Androl. 2003;24:293–8.
5. McMahon AJ, Buckley J, Taylor A, Lloyd SN, Deane RF, Kirk D. Chronic testicular pain following vasectomy. Br J Urol. 1992;69:188–91.
6. Ishigami K, Abu-Yousef MM, El-Zein Y. Tubular ectasia of the epididymis: a sign of postvasectomy status. J Clin Ultrasound. 2005;33:447–51.
7. Reddy NM, Gerscovich EO, Jain KA, Le-Petross HT, Brock JM. Vasectomy-related changes on sonographic examination of the scrotum. J Clin Ultrasound. 2004;32:394–8.
8. Cho SH, Min SK, Lee ST. Associations of ultrasonographic features with scrotal pain after vasectomy. Korean J Urol. 2011;52:782–6.
9. McCammack KC, Aganovic L, Hsieh TC, Guo Y, Welch CS, Gamst AC, Cassidy F. MRI of the epididymis: can the outcome of vasectomy reversal be predicted preoperatively? AJR Am J Roentgenol. 2014;203:91–8.
10. Frates MC, Benson CB, Stober SL. Mobile echogenicities on scrotal sonography: is the finding associated with vasectomy? J Ultrasound Med. 2011;30:1387–90.
11. Amaral F, Dreyer G, Figueredo-Silva J, Noroes J, Cavalcanti A, Samico SC, Santos A, Coutinho A. Live adult worms detected by ultrasonography in human Bancroftian filariasis. Am J Trop Med Hyg. 1994;50:753–7.
12. Wang Z, Yang Z, Lei YY, Zhang YD, Chen LD, Xie XY, Lu MD, Wang W. Who is doing the dance in epididymis: the principle of moblile echogenicities without filarial infection: case report. Medicine (Baltimore). 2015;94(34):e1418.
13. Bykov VL. Paneth cells: history of discovery, structural and functional characteristics and the role in the maintenance of homeostasis in the small intestine. Morfologiia. 2014;145:67–80.
14. Nistal M, Mariño-Enríquez A, De Miguel MP. Granular changes (Paneth cell-like) in epididymal epithelial cells are lysosomal in nature and are not markers of obstruction. Histopathology. 2007;50:944–7.
15. Shah VI, Ro JY, Amin MB, Mullick S, Nazeer T, Ayala AG. Histologic variations in the epididymis: findings in 167 orchiectomy specimens. Am J Surg Pathol. 1998;22:990–6.

16. Nistal M, Mate A, Paniagua R. Granulomatous epididymal lesion of possible ischemic origin. Am J Surg Pathol. 1997;21:951–6.
17. Mitchinson MJ, Sherman KP, Stainer-Smith AM. Brown patches in the epididymis. J Pathol. 1975;115:57–62.
18. Regadera J, Nistal M, Paniagua R. Testis, epididymis, and spermatic cord in elderly men. Correlation of angiographic and histologic studies with systemic arteriosclerosis. Arch Pathol Lab Med. 1985;109:663–7.
19. Fulton RS, Rouse RV, Ranheim EA. Ectopic prostate: case report of a presacral mass presenting with obstructive symptoms. Arch Pathol Lab Med. 2001;125:286–8.
20. Tekin K, Sungurtekin U, Aytekin FO, Calli N, Erdem E, Ozden A, Yalcin N. Ectopic prostatic tissue of the anal canal presenting with rectal bleeding: report of a case. Dis Colon Rectum. 2002;45:979–80.
21. Bromberg WD, Kozlowski JM, Oyasu R. Prostate-type gland in the epididymis. J Urol. 1991;145:1273–4.
22. Lee LY, Tzeng J, Grosman M, Unger PD. Prostate gland-like epithelium in the epididymis: a case report and review of the literature. Arch Pathol Lab Med. 2004;128:e60–2.
23. VanBeek CA, Peters CA, Vargas SO. Ectopic prostate tissue within the processus vaginalis: insights into prostate embryogenesis. Pediatr Dev Pathol. 2005;8:379–85.
24. McNeal JE. Prostate anatomy and BPH morphogenisis. Prog Clin Biol Res. 1984;145:27–54.
25. De Miguel MP, Mariño JM, Gonzalez-Peramato P, Nistal M, Regadera J. Epididymal growth and differentiation are altered in human cryptorchidism. J Androl. 2001;22:212–25.
26. Aydin A, Aksoy HZ, Reis A, Ozdemir F. Undifferentiated carcinoma of the epididymis. Acta Clin Croat. 2011;50:415–8.

34 Metaplasias of the Testicular Tunica Vaginalis

Manuel Nistal, Pilar González-Peramato, and Álvaro Serrano

34.1 Histological Types of Metaplasia

Five types of metaplasia have been observed: urothelial metaplasia, Müllerian metaplasia, mucinous metaplasia, squamous metaplasia, and gastric metaplasia.

34.1.1 Urothelial Metaplasia

Urothelial metaplasia is the most common one. It was observed in 17 % of the cases studied by Sundarasivarao [1]. A similar incidence is seen in the mesothelial lining of the female reproductive tract and particularly in the serosa of the Fallopian tube [2, 3]. It is a localized phenomenon in the serosa of the testis and epididymis close to the implantation of the epididymis (sinus, close to the base of the appendix of the epididymis or the head of the epididymis).

The size of these lesions varies from macroscopic plaques to histological findings (Fig. 34.1). The epithelium varies in height from bilayered cubic to half a dozen strata. The cells have eosinophilic cytoplasm and imprecise boundaries. The nuclei have a central fold with the aspect of coffee beans. Glove finger-like projections that penetrate the underlying connective tissue can often be seen protruding from the epithelium lining, generally in the epididymis. Some of these digitations may suffer a cystic transformation very similar to von Brunn nests in cystic cystitis (Figs. 34.2 and 34.3) or Walthard's nests of the ovarian tube [1, 4, 5]. The nature of the epithelium from which this metaplasia derives is quite controversial – while some authors consider it mesothelial, others believe it might originate in Müllerian remnants. In some cases the presence of ciliated cells would support this second possibility. It is likely that some cysts of testicular tunics as well as the Brenner tumors described in the testicles derive from this form of metaplasia with a cubic stratified epithelium [6, 7].

34.1.2 Müllerian Metaplasia

Müllerian metaplasia is a focal and multiple lesion that mainly affects the parietal layer. It consists of plaques of cylindrical cells that have replaced the mesothelium. In most cases two cell types, one of them with spherical euchromatic nuclei and the other one with elongated nuclei disposed in palisade, are distinguished. These nuclei have heterochromatin granulations and deep folds. Many of these cells are ciliated (Figs. 34.4, 34.5, and 34.6).

A lesion in the testicular tunica vaginalis was recently described as *florid cystic müllerianosis of the testis* [8]. It has a great similarity with the one reported as endosalpingiosis in the Fallopian tubes, cervix, abdominal cavity, and bladder [9]. This lesion was observed in three patients aged between 47 and 81 years. The testes were atro-

M. Nistal et al., *Clues in the Diagnosis of Non-tumoral Testicular Pathology*, DOI 10.1007/978-3-319-49364-0_34

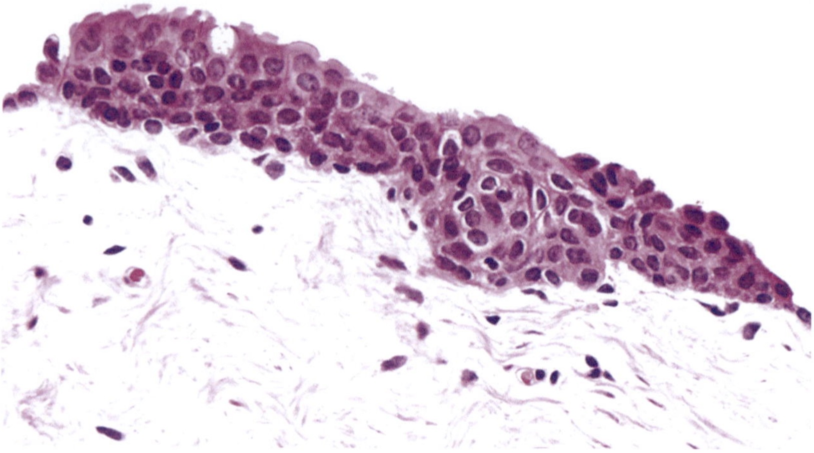

Fig. 34.1 Urothelial metaplasia of the tunica vaginalis showing in plaques. Note the characteristic appearance of the most superficial cells

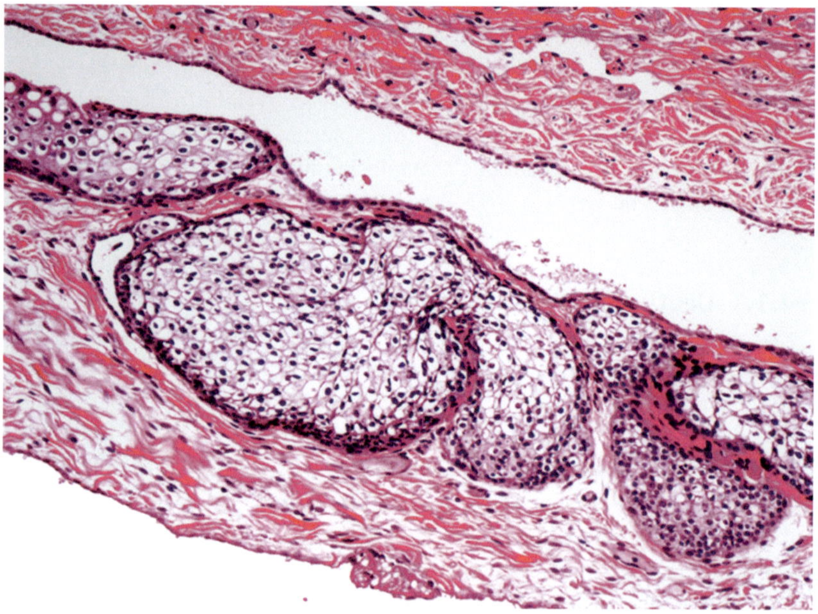

Fig. 34.2 Urothelial metaplasia of the parietal layer of the tunica vaginal. Cell proliferation takes a pseudoinfiltrative nodular pattern having a strong resemblance to von Brunn nests

phic in two of them. There was no history of varicocele, epididymitis, or testicular tumor. The mesothelium changes were associated with a Müllerian proliferation of small cysts of varying sizes, from microscopic to 5 mm. Most cysts were located in the parietal layer of the tunica vaginalis, which was markedly thickened. The contents of the cysts were a liquid whose color varied from clear to yellow. Cysts were usually unicameral and were generally arranged in two or three layers, not exceeding 5 mm in depth. Most cysts showed both ciliated and non-ciliated cells, but ciliated cells were less abundant. In some cysts, non-ciliated cells showed cytoplasmic protrusions toward the lumen, which caused an apocrine appearance. Those cysts with columnar or pseudostratified epithelium also showed "peg" cells (basal triangular cells typical of Fallopian tubes and endosalpingiosis in women) and small papillary proliferations. Neither cellular atypia nor mitoses were observed. In one case isolated lymphocytes were observed on the cyst wall.

The immunohistochemical pattern of these metaplastic cells differs in many respects from the mesothelium it derives from. Metaplastic mesothelial cells do not express markers such as calretinin or D2-40, but they still share the low-molecular-weight mesothelial cytokeratin (CK8,18,19).

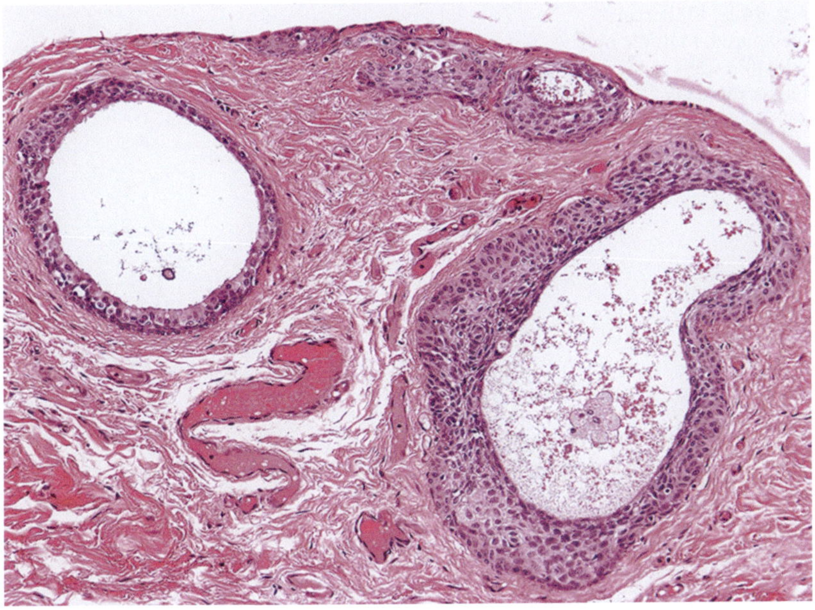

Fig. 34.3 Urothelial metaplasia with cystic transformation of von Brunn-like nests

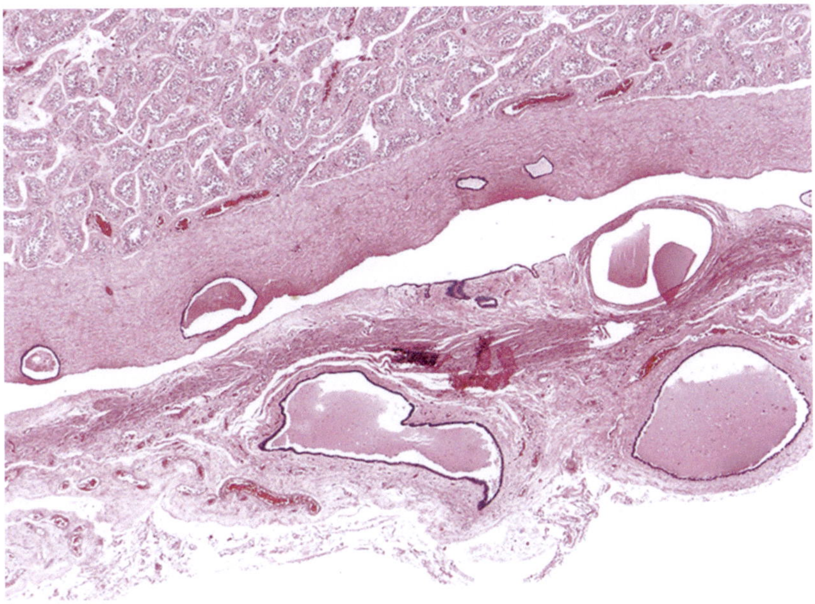

Fig. 34.4 Müllerian metaplasia of both layers of the tunica vaginalis. Several cystic formations both in the tunica albuginea testis and in the parietal layer of the tunica vaginalis are shown

Metaplastic cells have androgen and progesterone receptors but do not express estrogen receptors. The connective tissue surrounding the cyst cells is CD10 positive and has progesterone receptors.

This form of metaplasia may be responsible for many cysts of the tunica vaginalis which are not lined by mesothelium and rare cases of endometriosis [10]. It is also possible that they may undergo malignant transformation leading to cases of ovarian-like serous tumors (serous cystadenomas and cystadenocarcinomas) as described in the paratesticular structures [11, 12].

34.1.3 Mucinous Metaplasia

It is characterized by the presence of mesothelium areas that have been replaced with mucinous

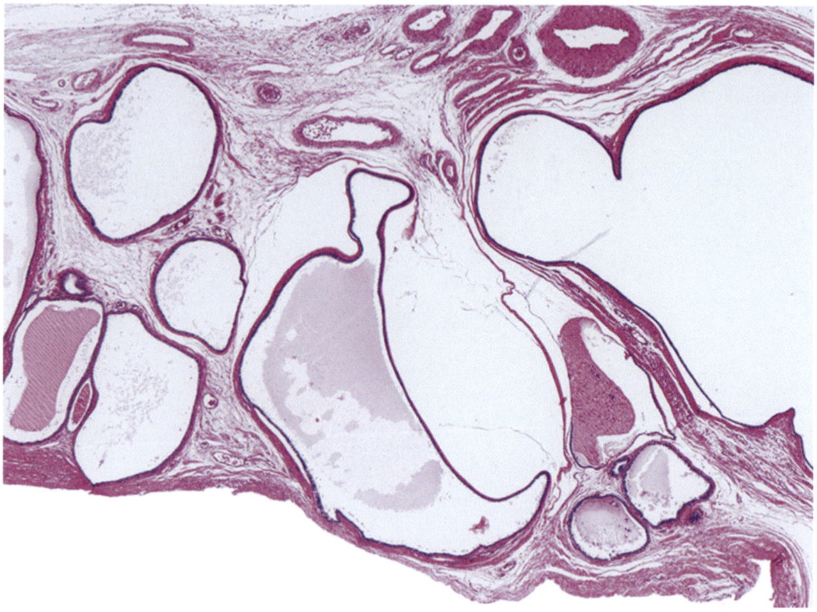

Fig. 34.5 Müllerian metaplasia. Multiple cysts with thin walls in the tunica vaginalis

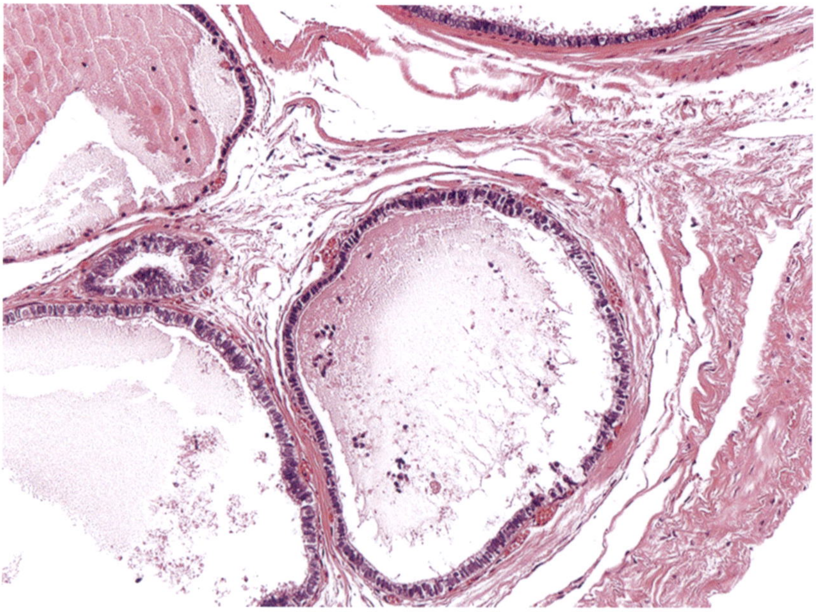

Fig. 34.6 Müllerian metaplasia. Cysts are lined by columnar epithelium and contain an eosinophilic material

columnar epithelium (Fig. 34.7). These cells have basal nuclei and pale apical cytoplasm which stains intensely with PAS. The epithelium shows no pseudostratification, and cells lack nuclear hyperchromasia or pleomorphism. The epithelium focally invaginates into the connective tissue, providing a pseudoglandular aspect. Light edema and small nonspecific lymphoid infiltrates stand out in the underlying tissue. We have observed this lesion in the wall of hydroceles that recur again and again in both childhood and adulthood. But it is unknown whether they may progress toward a tumor as happens in the mucinous metaplasia of the urothelial tract [13].

34.1.4 Squamous Metaplasia

Squamous metaplasia of the tunica vaginalis is very rare indeed. It has been described in chronic inflammatory processes [14]. Among the proposed mechanisms, reactions to mechanical

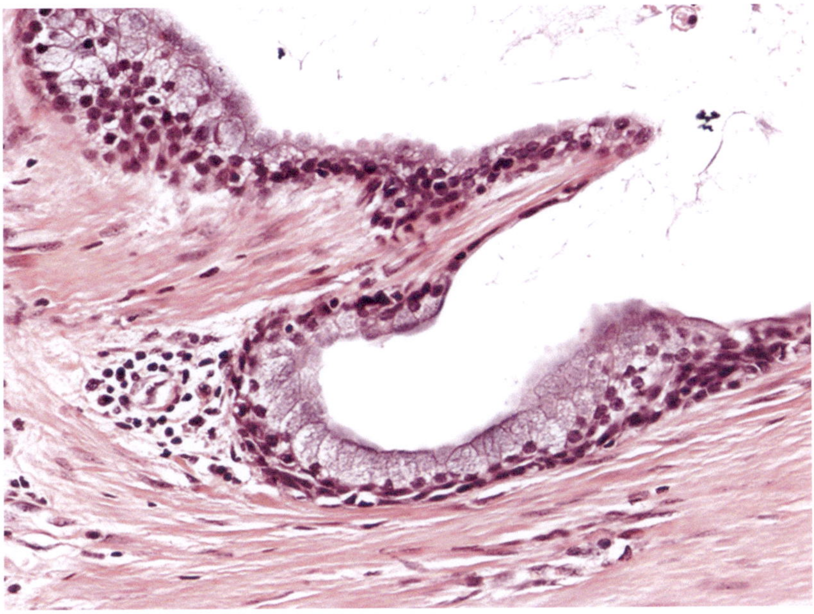

Fig. 34.7 Mucinous metaplasia in the tunica vaginalis of long-term hydrocele. The mesothelium has been replaced by an mucinous columnar epithelium

irritation, inflammation, or infection are included, similarly to the peritoneum [15–17]. In cases being studied in frozen section biopsies where the lesion is very showy, a metastatic squamous cell carcinoma should be ruled out. The absence of atypia, the good epithelial differentiation, and the tendency of the lesions to be very superficial dismiss a squamous carcinoma.

34.1.5 Gastric Metaplasia

This metaplasia has also been described with the name of gastric heterotopia. It has been observed in an adult and also in a 12-year-old child with hydrocele [18]. It may be originated from an in situ metaplasia from pluripotent cells or a true heterotopia. Gastric heterotopia has been reported throughout the gastrointestinal tract including the hepatobiliary system as well as the skin of the abdominal wall. The gastric mucosa would have to migrate to the peritoneum and then to the scrotum when the testes descend.

References

1. Sundarasivarao D. The mullerian vestiges and benign epithelial tumors of the epididymis. J Pathol. 1953;66:417–32.
2. Weir MM, Bell DA, Young RH. Transitional cell metaplasia of the uterine cervix and vagina: an underrecognized lesion that may be confused with high-grade dysplasia: a report of 59 cases. Am J Surg Pathol. 1997;21:510–7.
3. Rabban JT, Crawford B, Chen LM, Powell CB, Zaloudek CJ. Transitional cell metaplasia of fallopian tube fimbriae: a potential mimic of early tubal carcinoma in risk reduction salpingooophorectomies from women with BRCA mutations. Am J Surg Pathol. 2009;33:111–9.
4. Hartz PH. Occurrence of Walthard cell in Brenner-like epithelium in the serosa of the epididymis. Am J Clin Pathol. 1947;17:654–6.
5. Teoh TB. The structure and development of Walthard nests. J Pathol Bacteriol. 1953;66:433–9.
6. Ross L. Paratesticular Brenner-like tumor. Cancer. 1968;21:722–6.
7. Nogales Jr FF, Matilla A, Ortega I, Alvarez T. Mixed Brenner and adenomatoid tumor of the testis: an ultrastructural study and histogenetic considerations. Cancer. 1979;43:539–43.
8. Nistal M, González-Peramato P, De Miguel MP. Florid cystic mullerianosis of the testis: new pathological entity originating from a peculiar Müllerian differentiation of the testicular vaginal mesothelium. Histopathology. 2015;66:1037–41.
9. Clement PB, Young RH. Florid cystic endosalpingiosis with tumor-like manifestations: a report of four cases including the first reported cases of transmural endosalpingiosis of the uterus. Am J Surg Pathol. 1999;23:166–75.
10. Zámečník M, Hoštáková D. Endometriosis in a mesothelial cyst of tunica vaginalis of the testis. Report of a case. Cesk Patol. 2013;49:134–6.
11. Albino G, Nenna R, Inchingolo CD, Marucco EC. Hydrocele with surprise. Case report and review of literature. Arch Ital Urol Androl. 2010;82:287–90.

12. Geramizadeh B, Farzaneh MR, Pakbaz S, Zeighami S. Testicular papillary serous cystadenocarcinoma: a rare case report and review of the literature. Rare Tumors. 2011;3:e44.
13. Zhang BY, Aguilar J, Yang M, Wang P, Li B. Mucinous metaplasia in urothelial tract may be the precancerous lesion of mucinous adenocarcinoma: report of two cases and review of literature. Int J Clin Exp Med. 2014;7:285–9.
14. Kirk D, Gingell JC, Feneley RC. Infarction of the testis: a complication of epididymitis. Br J Urol. 1982;54:311–2.
15. Crome L. Squamous metaplasia of the peritoneum. J Pathol Bacteriol. 1950;62:61–8.
16. Schatz JE, Colgan TJ. Squamous metaplasia of the peritoneum. Arch Pathol Lab Med. 1991;115:397–8.
17. Mourra N, Nion I, Parc R, Flejou JF. Squamous metaplasia of the peritoneum: a potential diagnostic pitfall. Histopathology. 2004;44:621–2.
18. Khan MA, Fitzgerald RJ. Heterotopic gastric tissue in the scrotum. J Urol. 1996;155:2061.

Reactive Mesothelial Hyperplasia Versus Mesothelioma

35

Manuel Nistal, Pilar González-Peramato, and Álvaro Serrano

35.1 Histopathology: Types of Reactive Mesothelial Hyperplasia

Mesothelial hyperplasias are reactive processes that can be seen on the wall of hydroceles, hematoceles, and inguinal hernia sacs, associated with pseudotumoral processes as fibrous pseudotumor or tumors either testicular or from testicular covers. Several growth patterns have been described: solid, papillary, nodular, and pseudoinfiltrative [1].

Mesothelial cells, regardless of their growth pattern, show the same characteristics. They are large columnar or low cuboidal cells that have spherical, central, or basal nuclei. The nuclear membrane may have small folds; the nucleolus is small and has regularly dispersed chromatin. The cytoplasm is pale or eosinophilic, sometimes vacuolated, and positive with PAS (glycogen) and Alcian Blue pH2.5 (hyaluronic acid). The number of mitosis is generally low although there have been cases with a high proliferation [2]. Sometimes there are multinucleated cells with hyperchromatic nuclei and prominent nucleoli.

35.1.1 Solid and Papillary

The solid and papillary proliferations arise from the surface of the mesothelial tunic. In the first case, the mesothelial cells are arranged in compact masses, except in the most superficial layers where they tend to flake isolated or in small groups. In the second case, they are arranged in one or more layers over connective tissue papilla (Fig. 35.1). At the axis of the papillae and the underlying tissue, an inflammatory infiltrate is usually present.

35.1.1.1 Nodular

The nodular growths can be placed not only on the mesothelial surface as in the previous case, but without apparent communication with it. The architecture of these nodules is more variegated and solid, papillary and glandular patterns can coexist, and psammomas can also be shown [3] (Fig. 35.2).

35.1.2 Pseudoinfiltrative: Florid Mesothelial Hyperplasia

Pseudoinfiltrative reactive mesothelial hyperplasia is characterized by the presence of tubular formations, glandular-like solid nest, or cysts in the thickness of a thickened vaginal wall [4]. Apparently these epithelial structures are randomly arranged, but they all have in common that the infiltration stops abruptly at a shallow level (Figs. 35.3, 35.4, and 35.5). The surrounding stroma is generally fibrous, but it can show chronic inflammatory infiltrates preferably around vessels. Its layered structure represents the organization of fibrinous exudates trapping mesothelial cells.

M. Nistal et al., *Clues in the Diagnosis of Non-tumoral Testicular Pathology*,
DOI 10.1007/978-3-319-49364-0_35

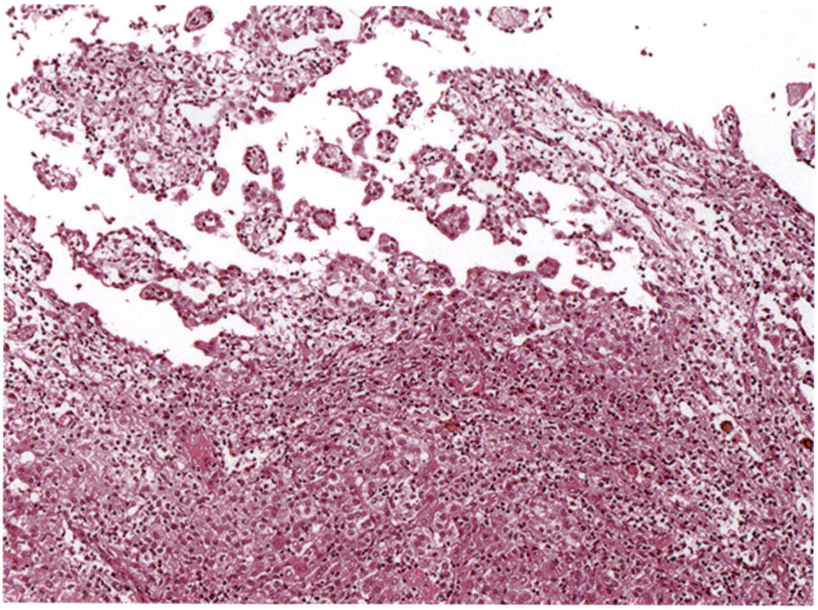

Fig. 35.1 Reactive solid and papillary mesothelial hyperplasia is observed in the wall of a hydrocele

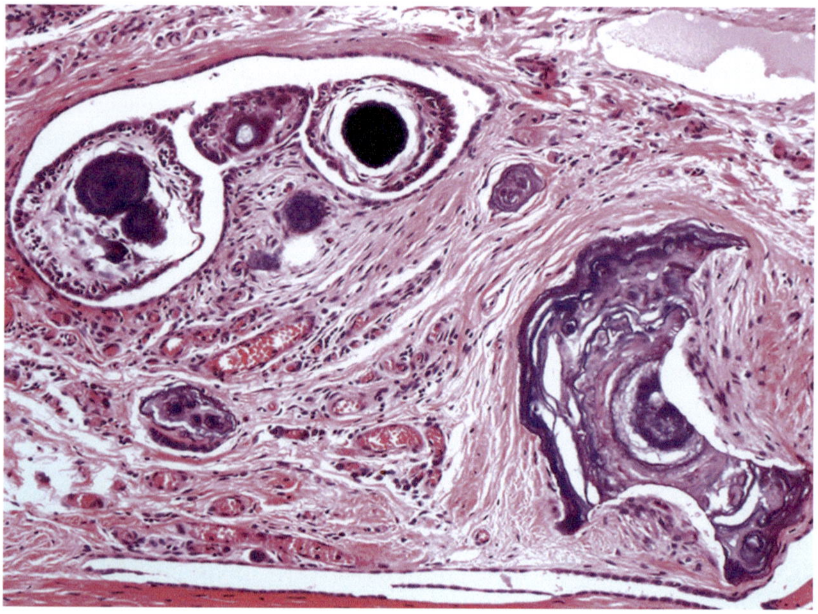

Fig. 35.2 Nodular mesothelial hyperplasia. Nodules are constituted by a fibrous stroma in which proliferations, preferably papillary with numerous psammoma bodies, protrude

35.2 Clinical Features

The mesothelial hyperplasia is an incidental finding in most cases although some are present as a tumor, and what is more worrying, they have been previously diagnosed as malignant mesotheliomas.

35.3 Differential Diagnosis

The differential diagnosis of reactive mesothelial hyperplasia should be established with mesotheliomas (well-differentiated papillary mesothelioma, malignant mesothelioma, and mesothelioma of

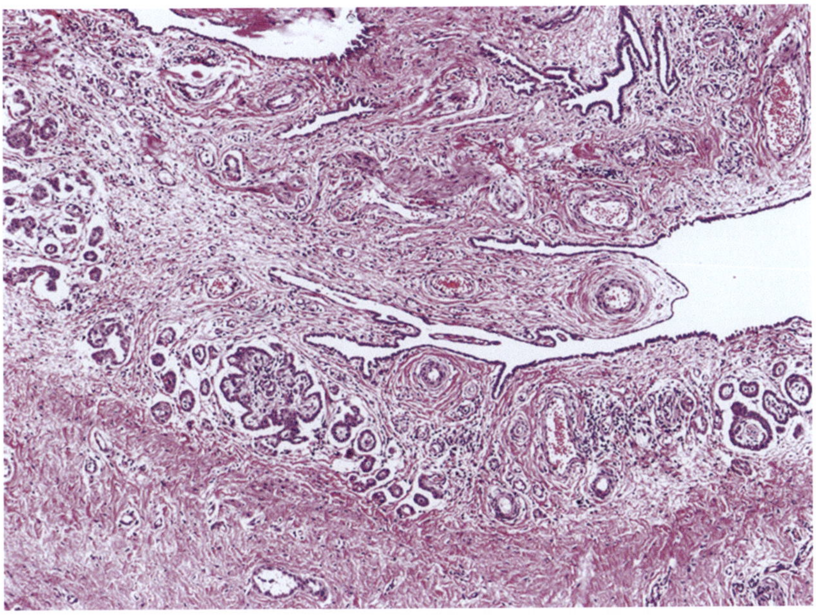

Fig. 35.3 Pseudoinfiltrative mesothelial hyperplasia. Cordonal, solid, and glandular mesothelial cell proliferations which are arranged parallel to the surface in a band. The mesothelial proliferation stops abruptly in depth without infiltrating the underlying tissue

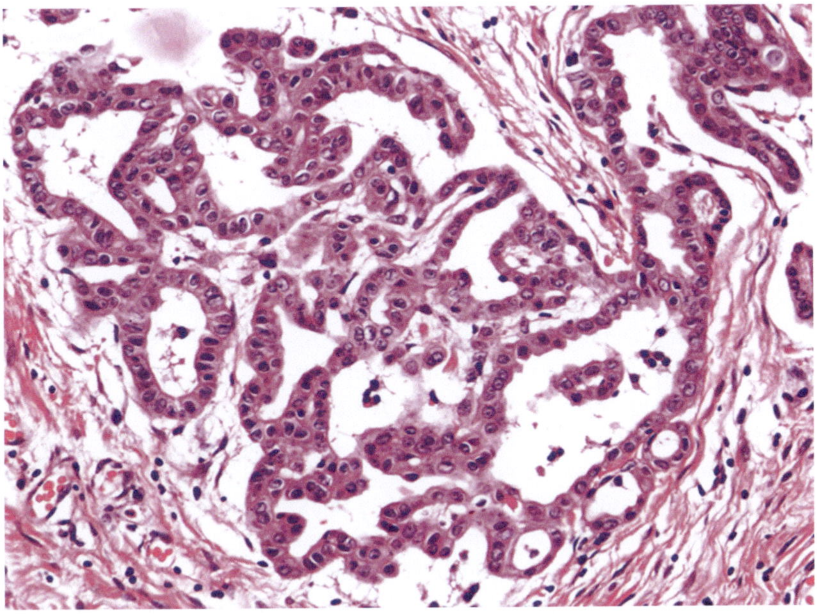

Fig. 35.4 Pseudoinfiltrative mesothelial hyperplasia. Cords and glandular structures lined by cuboidal cells of hyperchromatic nuclei and eosinophilic cytoplasm

uncertain malignant potential) [5–9] and metastatic adenocarcinoma.

35.3.1 Mesotheliomas

Well-Differentiated Papillary Mesothelioma Well-differentiated papillary mesothelioma is a low malignant potential lesion that may progress to malignant mesothelioma [10, 11]. It has a papillary structure with a treelike pattern, where the fibrous axis branches into papillary processes of varying complexity. They are lined by a single layer of bland epithelial cuboid lining cells with a mild degree of atypia with rare mitosis. Some may show more com-

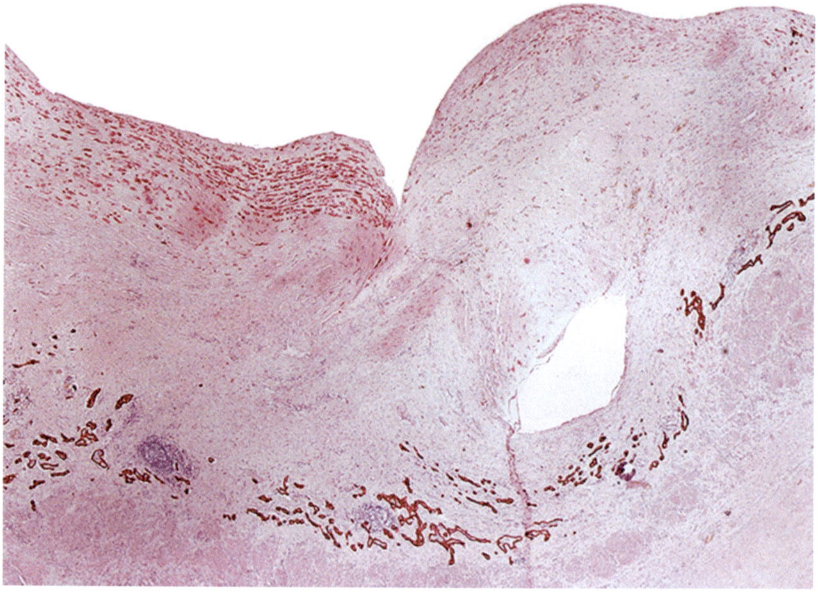

Fig. 35.5 Pseudoinfiltrative mesothelial hyperplasia. Immunostaining for cytokeratin (AE1/AE3) clearly shows the characteristic pseudoinfiltrative pattern of the mesothelial proliferation and the abrupt plane that reaches in depth

plex pathologic features as tubulopapillary areas or solid nests [12]. The absence of stromal infiltration differentiates from malignant mesothelioma. And the complexity of the papillae and cellular atypia, when they are present, is not observed in the papillary mesothelial hyperplasia.

Malignant Mesothelioma Malignant mesothelioma and above all the epithelioid variant, the most frequent variant in this location, pose a difficult differential diagnosis with florid mesothelial hyperplasia. In favor of a malignant mesothelioma, the clinical or sonographic presence of a tumor mass inside a long-standing hydrocele can be seen [13]. The mass is a thickening of the vaginal wall with one or more irregular nodules. In most cases reactive mesothelial hyperplasia is not macroscopically recognized due to its extremely small size. The age of presentation is also different as the malignant mesothelioma is most common between 55 and 75 years, while hyperplasias usually appear in younger patients.

Most of the time, the differential diagnosis of malignant mesothelioma and reactive mesothelial hyperplasia must be done only with histologic criteria (Table 35.1). There are no immunohistochemical or cell biology data to guide the diagnosis.

Table 35.1 Criteria for the differential diagnosis in favor of reactive mesothelial hyperplasia

Proliferation in a tissue with fibrosis and inflammation
Tubular and glandular proliferations parallel to the surface oriented
The absence of cellular atypia in the rest of the mesothelium lining of the vaginal cavity
Sparse epithelial proliferation
No back-to-back growth
Low tendency to branching of tubular and glandular structures
Sharp delimitation of lesion in depth
No infiltration of submesothelial layer
Cytological data: no atypia

Histologically, the presence of tubular, glandular, and papillary formations arranged back to back in a scarce stroma is characteristic of the malignant mesothelioma [14]. The infiltration of the underlying structures, parietal layer of tunica vaginalis, testis, epididymis, or spermatic cord is also characteristic [2]. Cytologically, most mesotheliomas have cells with prominent nucleoli, coarse chromatin, and frequent and atypical mitosis. Malignant mesothelioma presents necrosis and invasion of vessels [15]. Although these data are

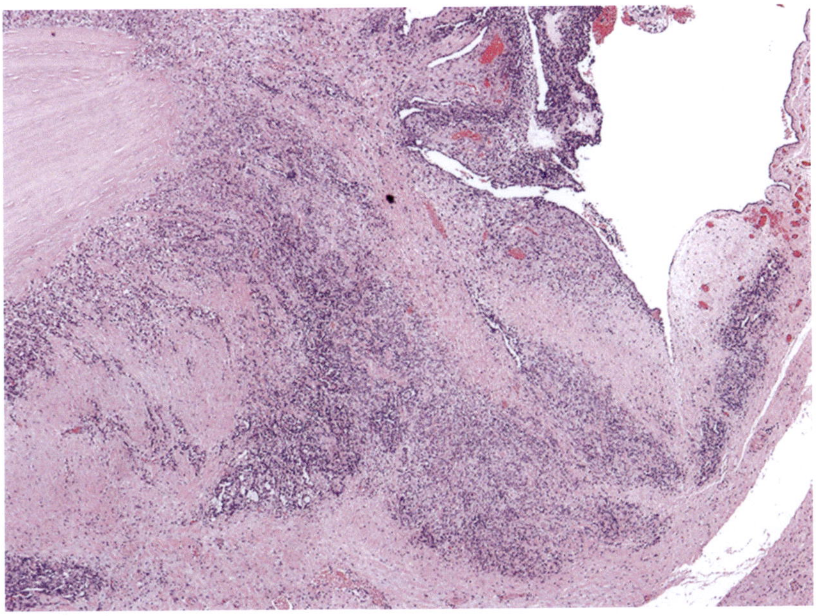

Fig. 35.6 Malignant mesothelioma. The tumor has variable thickness from one to other areas of the tunica vaginalis. Cellular areas alternate with other more fibrous

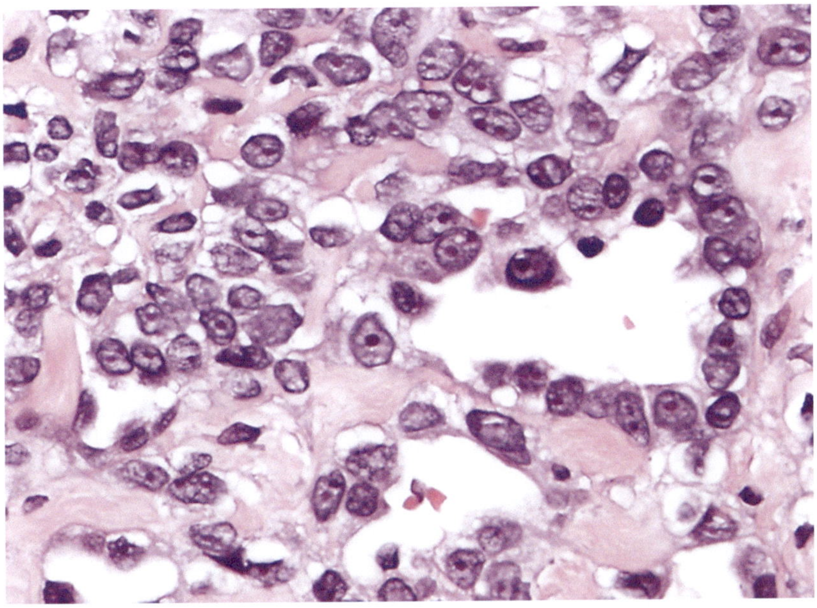

Fig. 35.7 Malignant mesothelioma. Solid and glandular cell proliferation showing spherical nucleus with a large central nucleolus

absent in reactive mesothelial hyperplasia, we must be careful as some mesotheliomas may be cytologically bland with cells with spherical nuclei and prominent nucleoli [16] (Figs. 35.6 and 35.7).

Although infiltrating the underlying tissues is a criterion of malignancy, it is necessary to bear in mind that in many hyperplasias, there are images of pseudoinvasion when mesothelial cells trapped in the thickness of underlying reactive fibrous tissue proliferate [17] (Fig. 35.8).

Immunohistochemical Data No antibody has an absolute value in the differential diagnosis. Mesothelioma cells have a strong positivity for EMA in contrast with the low or absent positive immunoexpression of mesothelial cells in reactive mesothelial hyperplasia [18]. p53 has a sensitivity of 45 % and a specificity of 100 % for diffuse malignant mesothelioma [19]. Ki-67 is higher (mean 24.6 %) in diffuse mesothelioma than in reactive mesothelial hyperpla-

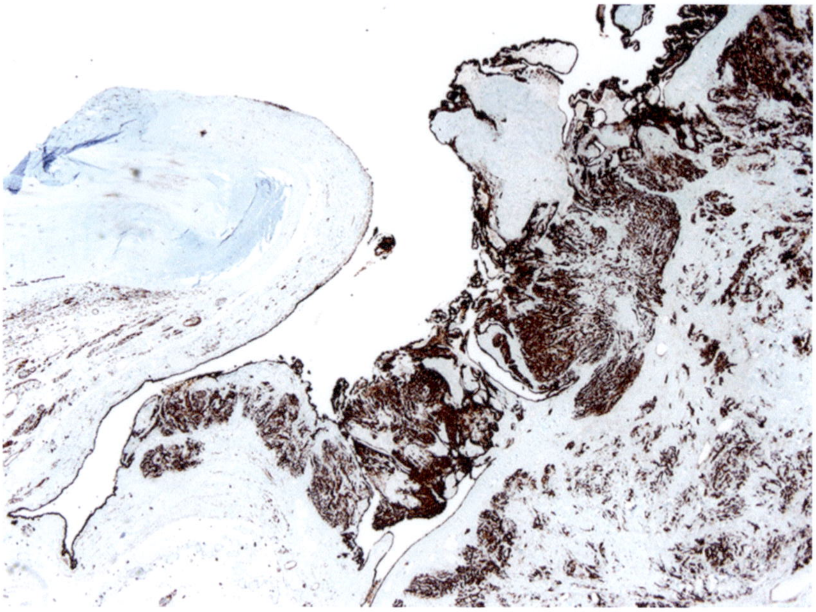

Fig. 35.8 Malignant mesothelioma. Immunostaining for AE1/AE3 cytokeratin reveals three important features: (1) the continuity of the tumor with the mesothelial lining, important for the differential diagnosis with other neoplasias, (2) the irregular thickness of the mesothelial proliferation, and (3) the infiltration of the underlying structures. These latter two details are important for the differential diagnosis with pseudoinfiltrative mesothelial hyperplasia

sia (mean 6.2 %) [20]. GLUT-1 shows high expression in diffuse malignant mesothelioma (60–100 %) compared to the low expression in reactive hyperplasia (0–27 %) [21, 22].

Upon investigating the molecular pathogenesis of malignant mesothelioma, it has been observed that homozygous deletion of the 9p21 locus is one of the most common genetic alterations as it is present using FISH between 67 and 83 % of mesotheliomas and it is not observed in any case of reactive mesothelial hyperplasia [23, 24].

35.3.2 Metastasis of Adenocarcinoma

The differential diagnosis with metastatic adenocarcinoma usually does not offer much difficulty. Metastases show a cellular atypia, high mitotic activity, stromal and vascular invasion, and areas of necrosis. The cells are positive for CEA and EMA and negative for calretinin and D2-40. Reactive mesothelial hyperplasia and metastasis of adenocarcinoma can coexist [25].

References

1. Rosai J, Dehner LP. Nodular mesothelial hyperplasia in hernia sacs: a benign reactive condition simulating a neoplastic process. Cancer. 1975;35:165–75.
2. Churg A, Colby TV, Cagle P, Corson J, Gibbs AR, Gilks B, Grimes M, Hammar S, Roggli V, Travis WD. The separation of benign and malignant mesothelial proliferations. Am J Surg Pathol. 2000;24:1183–200.
3. Nistal M, Santamaría L. Hiperplasia mesotelial en los sacos herniarios. Med Esp. 1981;80:43–6.
4. Moliniè V, Girodroux C, Seytor A. Pseudotumoral hyperplasia of the tunica vaginalis. Apropos of a case in an 18-year-old adolescent. Arch Anat Cytol Pathol. 1994;42:304–6. [Article in French].
5. Brimo F, Illei PB, Epstein JI. Mesothelioma of the tunica vaginalis: a series of eight cases with uncertain malignant potential. Mod Pathol. 2010;23:1165–72.
6. Bisceglia M, Dor DB, Carosi I, Vairo M, Pasquinelli G. Paratesticular mesothelioma. Report of a case with comprehensive review of literature. Adv Anat Pathol. 2010;17:53–70.
7. Churg A. Paratesticular mesothelial proliferations. Semin Diagn Pathol. 2003;20:272–8.
8. Tolhurst SR, Lotan T, Rapp DE, Lyon MB, Orvieto MA, Gerber GS, Sokoloff MH. Well-differentiated papillary mesothelioma occurring in the tunica vaginalis of the testis with contralateral atypical mesothelial hyperplasia. Urol Oncol. 2006;24:36–9.

9. Chekol SS, Sun CC. Malignant mesothelioma of the tunica vaginalis testis: diagnostic studies and differential diagnosis. Arch Pathol Lab Med. 2012;136:113–7.
10. Xiao SY, Rizzo P, Carbone M. Benign papillary mesothelioma of the tunica vaginalis testis. Arch Pathol Lab Med. 2000;124:143–7.
11. Fukunaga M. Well-differentiated papillary mesothelioma of the tunica vaginalis: a case report with aspirate cytologic, immunohistochemical, and ultrastructural studies. Pathol Res Pract. 2010;206:105–9.
12. Chetty R. Well differentiated (benign) papillary mesothelioma of the tunica vaginalis. J Clin Pathol. 1992;45:1029–30.
13. Akin Y, Bassorgun I, Basara I, Yucel S. Malignant mesothelioma of tunica vaginalis: an extremely rare case presenting without risk factors. Singapore Med J. 2015;56:e53–5.
14. Henderson DW, Shilkin KB, Whitaker D. Reactive mesothelial hyperplasia vs mesothelioma, including mesothelioma in situ: a brief review. Am J Clin Pathol. 1998;110:397–404.
15. Grove A, Jensen ML, Donna A. Mesotheliomas of the tunica vaginalis testis and hernial sacs. Virchows Arch A Pathol Anat Histopathol. 1989;415:283–92.
16. Lee S, Illei PB, Han JS, Epstein JI. Florid mesothelial hyperplasia of the tunica vaginalis mimicking malignant mesothelioma: a clinicopathologic study of 12 cases. Am J Surg Pathol. 2014;38:54–9.
17. McCaughey WT, Al-Jabi M. Differentiation of serosal hyperplasia and neoplasia in biopsies. Pathol Annu. 1986;21(Pt 1):271–93.
18. Di Naro N, Puliga G, Olla L, Tolu GA. Reactive pseudoglandular mesothelial hyperplasia in testis tunica vaginalis: a case report. Pathologica. 2011;103:304–6.
19. Attanoos RL, Griffin A, Gibbs AR. The use of immunohistochemistry in distinguishing reactive from neoplastic mesothelium. A novel use for desmin and comparative evaluation with epithelial membrane antigen, p53, platelet-derived growth factor-receptor, P-glycoprotein and Bcl-2. Histopathology. 2003;43: 231–8.
20. Taheri ZM, Mehrafza M, Mohammadi F, Khoddami M, Bahadori M, Masjedi MR. The diagnostic value of Ki-67 and repp86 in distinguishing between benign and malignant mesothelial proliferations. Arch Pathol Lab Med. 2008;132:694–7.
21. Kato Y, Tsuta K, Seki K, Maeshima AM, Watanabe S, Suzuki K, Asamura H, Tsuchiya R, Matsuno Y. Immunohistochemical detection of GLUT-1 can discriminate between reactive mesothelium and malignant mesothelioma. Mod Pathol. 2007;20:215–20.
22. Lagana SM, Taub RN, Borczuk AC. Utility of glucose transporter 1 in the distinction of benign and malignant thoracic and abdominal mesothelial lesions. Arch Pathol Lab Med. 2012;136:804–9.
23. Chiosea S, Krasinskas A, Cagle PT, Mitchell KA, Zander DS, Dacic S. Diagnostic importance of 9p21 homozygous deletion in malignant mesotheliomas. Mod Pathol. 2008;21:742–7.
24. Takeda M, Kasai T, Enomoto Y, Takano M, Morita K, Nakai T, Iizuka N, Maruyama H, Ohbayashi C. Comparison of genomic abnormality in malignant mesothelioma by the site of origin. J Clin Pathol. 2014;67:1038–43.
25. Wai HP, Yau TK, Sze WM, Yeung MW, Hioe F, Lee AW. Metastatic tumour of the tunica vaginalis testis from carcinoma of the stomach. Int J Clin Pract. 2000;54:685–6.

36 Paratesticular Tumor-Like Congenital Lesions

Manuel Nistal, Pilar González-Peramato, and Álvaro Serrano

36.1 Adrenal Cortex Ectopia

This is one of the more frequent incidental findings in male urological surgery. The incidence of adrenal rests in paratesticular structures in pediatric autopsies is 15 [1] and 3.8 % in patients submitted to inguinal-scrotal surgery [2]. The rate is even higher (5.1 %) in patients with undescended testicles [3]. The ectopic adrenal tissue can be located in the tunica albuginea, epididymis, testis [4], hernial sacs, and spermatic cord [5]. They are more common on the right side.

Pathology

Macroscopically, the ectopic adrenal formations are yellowish nodules measuring 1–4 mm in diameter and spherical or ovoid in shape, sometimes umbilicated, and they show a firm consistency. They can be single or multiple. Histologically, the nodules are formed only by the adrenal cortex and usually show a radial structure that is only lost in some elderly patients (Figs. 36.1, 36.2, 36.3, and 36.4). The cellular proliferation grows in a trabecular pattern. The cytoplasms vary from eosinophilic to xanthomized. Atypical nuclear features and mitosis are infrequent [6]. The ectopic nodules can develop causing a testicular enlargement that suggests a tumor in two disorders: adrenogenital syndrome and Nelson's syndrome (see Chap. 7). Particularly interesting are the nodules of intratesticular adrenal tissue. Intratesticular adrenal ectopies have been observed between the rete testis and the adjacent seminiferous tubules [7, 8].

When associated with adrenal cytomegaly, both in patients with the Wiedemann-Beckwith syndrome and with isolated adrenal cytomegaly, adrenal cortex ectopia may also show cytomegalic cells. The paratesticular adrenal ectopias are interpreted as an entrapment of cells of the adrenal cortex during the testicular descent [9]. The origin of the intratesticular nodules could be secondary to the activation of testicular steroid hilus pluripotential cells [10].

Clinical Features

Ectopies of the adrenal cortex are an incidental finding and elicit no symptoms. In certain circumstances they can be functioning and acquire a large size. These compensatory hyperplasias have been reported in patients with Addison's disease [11] and signs of hyperfunction in patients with Cushing's syndrome [12]. Tumors can reach several centimeters in size. Macroscopically, the tumors are encapsulated and show a yellowish variegated surface.

M. Nistal et al., *Clues in the Diagnosis of Non-tumoral Testicular Pathology*,
DOI 10.1007/978-3-319-49364-0_36

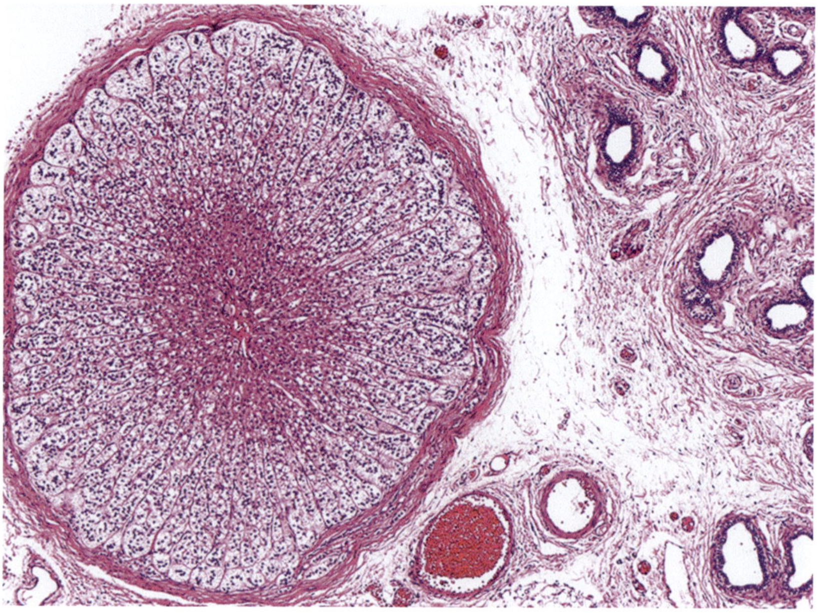

Fig. 36.1 Ectopic adrenal cortex in the epididymis. The radial arrangement of cells and the presence of a capsule are characteristic. Finding in a undescended testicle of a 2-year-old child

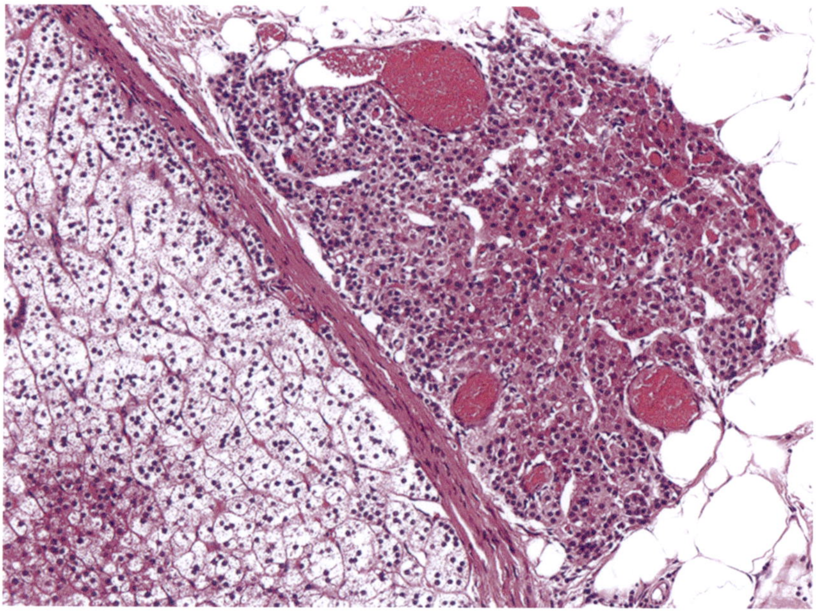

Fig. 36.2 Ectopic adrenal tissue in the spermatic cord. Cell groups located outside the capsule surrounded by fatty tissue are observed in some cases as in normal adrenal

36.2 Splenic Ectopia (Splenogonadal Fusion)

Although infrequent, it is important to keep paratesticular ectopic splenic tissue in mind as clinically it can be interpreted as a tumor. The first description of splenic-gonadal fusion was made by Boestroem in 1883 [13] and was followed by a detailed description by Pommer in 1889 [14]. It is predominant in males with a male to female ratio of 15/1. About 200 cases have been reported [15], 16.8 % of which are autopsy findings [16, 17]. The remaining cases were observed in orchiopexy or surgery for inguinal hernia repair. Other presentations are painful scrotal swelling second-

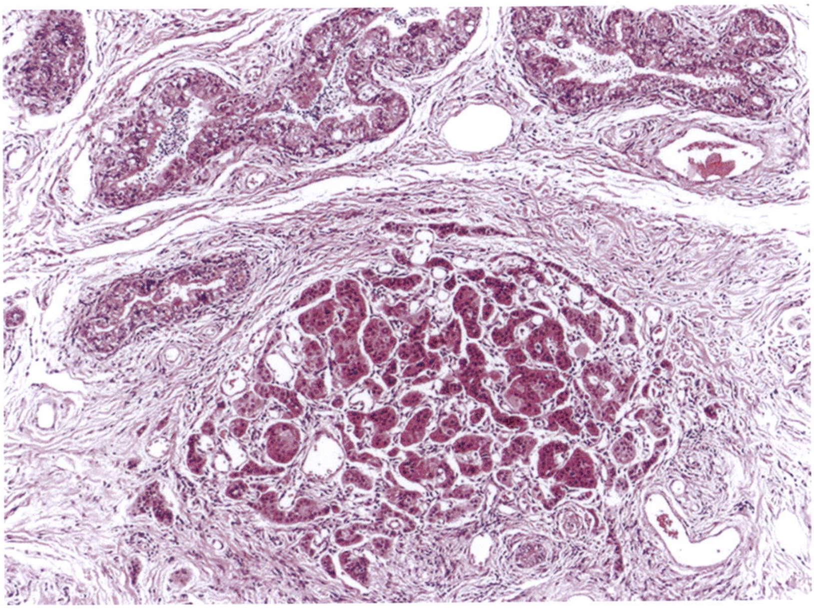

Fig. 36.3 Adrenal cortex ectopia located between the testis and epididymis in a of 72-year-old patient. The radial arrangement of the cells is lost in this poorly defined nodular formation

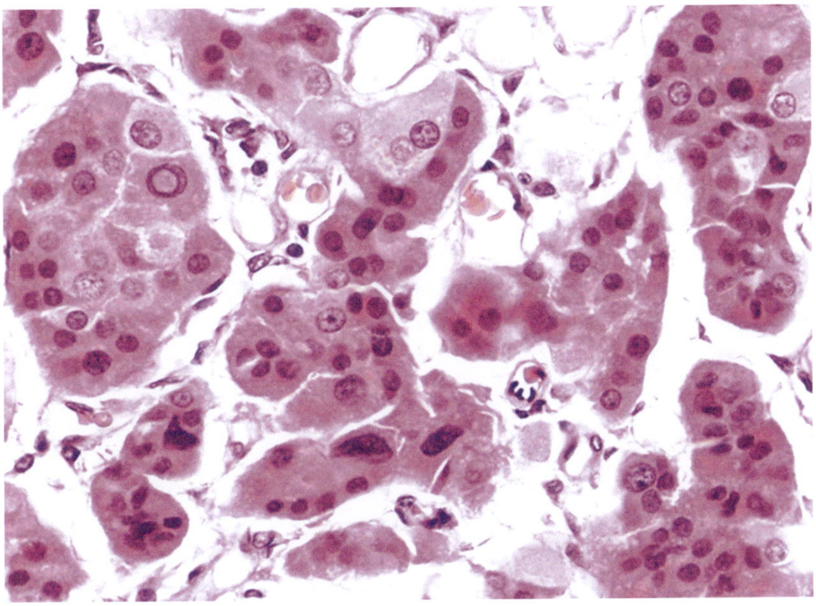

Fig. 36.4 Adrenal cortex ectopia (same case as above figure). The cellular groups are separated by abundant sinusoids

ary to malaria, mumps, traumatic rupture of ectopic splenic tissue [18], and scrotal tumor [19] associated with germ cell tumor [20], with infertility [21], or with contralateral displaced intra-abdominal testis [22]. Only a minority of cases were suspected before surgery [23]. The age of patients ranges from newborn children to 81 years [24]. More than 70 % of the reported cases were younger than 20 years, and approximately 50 % were younger than 10 years [25], although the reported ages vary from birth up to 81-year-old men. Splenogonadal fusion usually occurs on the left side (98 % of cases).

Types of Splenogonadal Fusion

They have been classified in two types: continuous and discontinuous [26]. In the continuous type, the ectopic splenic tissue is connected to the eutopic spleen by a cord that can be either splenic tissue or fibrous tissue. In the discontinuous presentation, the splenic tissue is not joined to the eutopic spleen. The continuous splenogonadal fusion is more frequent (55 %) than the discontinuous type [27].

The most frequently associated anomalies are inguinal hernia and cryptorchidism (one third of cases). In half the cases of cryptorchidism, this is bilateral [28]. In isolated cases contralateral testicular aplasia [29] or hypospadias [30] has been observed. Other anomalies associated primarily with the continuous type [31] are ectromelia, micrognathia, hypoglosia, spina bifida, craniosynostosis, cardiac malformations, anal atresia, pulmonary hypoplasia, intestinal malrotation, fissures of the liver, and bilobated spleen [32].

Continuous splenogonadal fusion (with or without extremity malformations or micrognathia) has been recognized as a syndrome (splenogonadal fusion-limb defect syndrome) [33, 34]. The discontinuous type is nearly always associated with congenital anomalies apart from some isolated cases with coexistence of cardiac defects [35]; thus it can be considered as a rare variant of accessory spleen.

Histology

The ectopic splenic tissue has a reddish appearance and is usually well delimitated by a connective tissue capsule joined to the testis, the epididymis, or the spermatic cord (Figs. 36.5 and 36.6). Only exceptionally, this tissue shows continuity with the seminiferous tubules.

Pathogenesis

The presence of splenic tissue in the testicle has an embryological base [36], and two hypotheses have been proposed to explain how such different structures became fused. The fusion should occur between the 5 and 8 weeks of gestation before testicular descent begins, when the splenic anlage is located in the dorsal mesogastrium opposite to the genital anlage. The process could be caused either by a fusion between the peritoneal surface of the spleen and the gonadal ridge or by an inflammation of the peritoneal surface over the spleen and the gonadal ridge [37]. When the descent of the testis begins, the splenic tissue attached follows the gonadal path.

Cryptorchidism and splenogonadal fusion might be the result of a lack of cranial suspensory ligament involution. This persistent ligament might be colonized by splenic cells and could hinder the testicular migration [28].

Diagnosis

Ultrasonography [33, 38] helps in the diagnosis, but this must be confirmed by Tc99m sulfur colloid imaging [39], and if there remained any doubt regarding the diagnosis during the operation, frozen sections should be considered to avoid unnecessary orchiectomies. Doppler ultrasound of the scrotum in patients with a palpable mass may show a hypervascular image on the upper pole of the testis [15]. This technique is useful in cases of high suspicion. Contrast-enhanced CT can help diagnosis, but its use is limited due to high exposure to radiation [40]. Magnetic resonance imaging has been used in isolated cases [41]. Laparoscopy is the most accurate method for diagnosing when the testis is not palpable. This exploration also allows surgical treatment and in many cases to know the intra-abdominal abnormalities that are associated [42, 43].

Treatment

The treatment of splenogonadal fusion consists in removing the splenic tissue, while the testis, epididymis, and vessels should be separated and preserved. If the location is scrotal, no surgery is required.

The trend is to reduce the high number of orchiectomies (37 %) made in the past. Removal of the cord as close to the spleen as possible is important to prevent complications such as small bowel obstruction, by entanglement with the bowel loops or colonic obstruction at the splenic flexure by compressing the colon [44]. Germ cell tumors (less than one dozen publications) associated with splenic-gonadal fusion have been linked to the presence of cryptorchidism and require appropriate treatment [45].

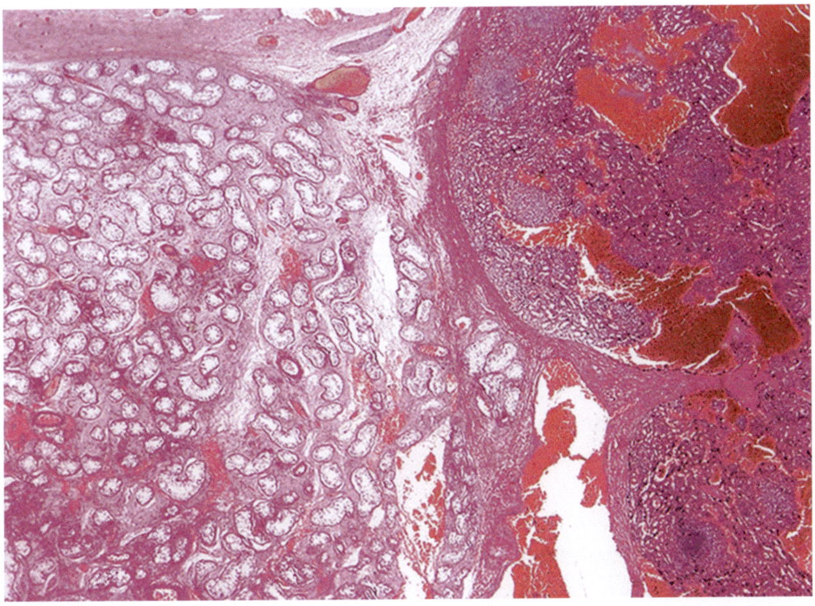

Fig. 36.5 Splenogonadal fusion in an adult undescended testicle

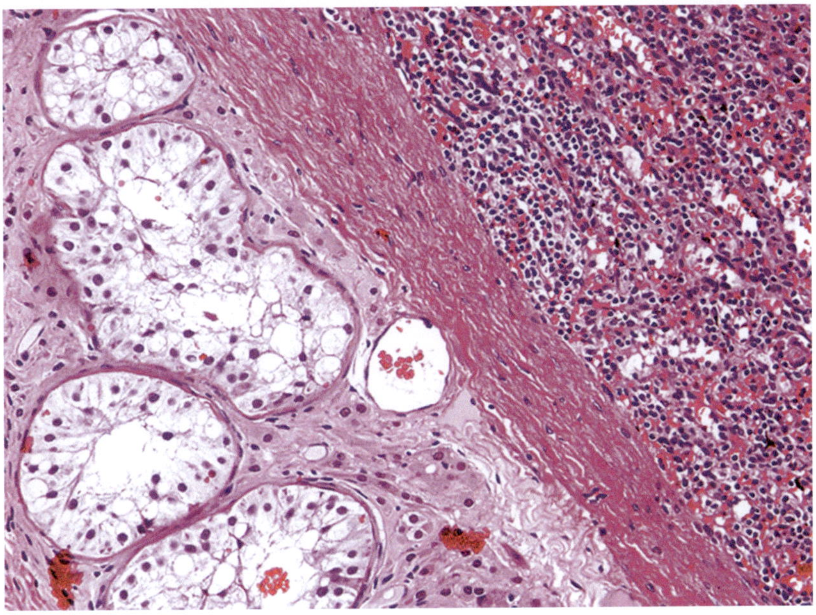

Fig. 36.6 Splenogonadal fusion. The splenic tissue is separated from the testicular parenchyma by a thin capsule. The seminiferous epithelium only consists of dysgenetic Sertoli cells

36.3 Hepatic Ectopia (Hepato-gonadal Fusion)

The presence of hepatic tissue joined to the superior testicular pole has been described in three patients, the first of them with right inguinal hernia [46], the second one with undescended testis [47], and the third one with right inguinal hernia and undescended testis [48]. In the first case, the hepatic tissue stood out as a reddish nodule which continued in a fibrous pedicle that rose from the scrotal pouch throughout the vaginal process, crossed the abdominal cavity, and ended in the porta hepatis. Histologically, this hepatic tissue appeared normal. In the second case, the testis was atrophied and was located in the abdominal cavity, while the hepatic tissue rose from the testis to the inferior-lateral aspect of the right lobe of the liver. In the third case, the hepatic tissue was present throughout the cord-like structure.

Heterotopic hepatic tissue has been observed in different organs and tissues, such as the gallbladder wall, umbilical cord, lung, splenic capsule, pancreas, adrenal gland, and retroperitoneum. The presence of hepatic parenchyma associated with the testis has been explained, like the occurrence of splenic tissue, on an embryological basis. When the testis initiates its descent, it is the bearer of mesenchymal cell clusters that develop the hepatic parenchyma. The knowledge of this and other ectopies should advise to perform a conservative surgery.

36.4 Orchidogastric Fusion

In orchidogastric fusion the testis remains firmly attached to the wall of the stomach. There is only one reported case of a newborn baby with a large gastroschisis defect and prolapsed large and small bowel. The left testis was attached to the anterior surface of the stomach. The vas deferens was normal and the vascular pedicle was short but allowing orchidopexia. Although the association between gastroschisis and undescended testicle is well known, the association of orchidogastric fusion and gastroschisis is unique. The author suggests that it is probably caused by an embryological defect coincident with the appearance of gastroschisis appearance where gut rotation is impaired rather than caused by secondary adherences between the stomach and the gonad by the exposition of both organs to amniotic fluid [49].

36.5 Renal Parenchyma Ectopia

The occurrence of ectopic nephrogenic blastema has been known for many years [50]. Ectopic renal tissue has been reported in the retroperitoneum [51], the sacrococcyx [52], or in the inguinal canal [53]. Renal blastema is frequently observed in fetal autopsies and has also been observed in some newborn babies (Fig. 36.7). This ectopic tissue has also been found associated with cryptorchidism in infants [54, 55]. The most common location of this ectopic tissue is the epididymis, the gubernaculum [56], and along the spermatic cord [57]. The size of these nephrogenic nodules may be large enough to be detected as a palpable mass, usually associated

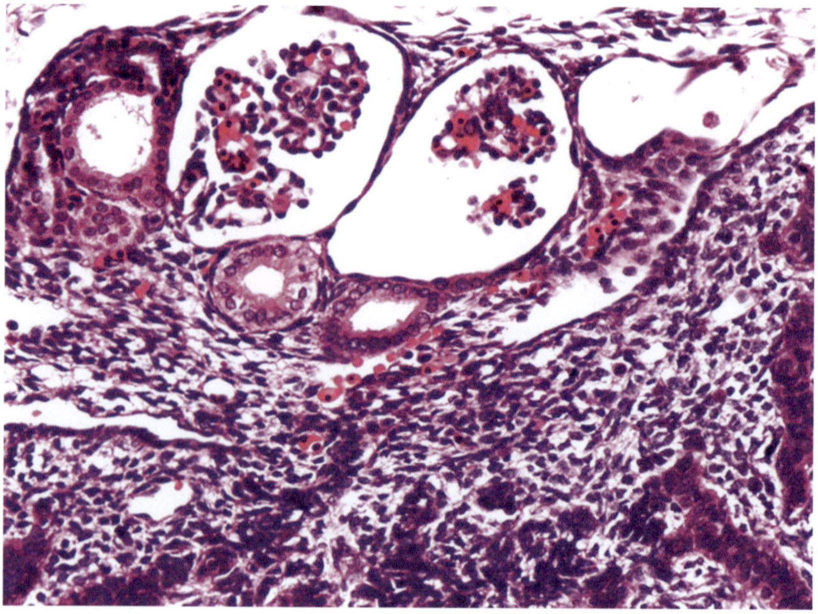

Fig. 36.7 Eight-week fetus autopsy. The mesonephros consisting of glomeruli and tubular structures is in contact with the cords of the rete testis

with congenital inguinal hernia. These nodules have been assumed to have originated in the mesonephros. Several Wilms' tumors described in the spermatic cord might have had their origin in this ectopic renal blastema [58, 59].

References

1. Dahl EV, Bahn RC. Aberrant adrenal cortical tissue near the testis in human infants. Am J Pathol. 1962;40:587–98.
2. Mares AJ, Shkolnick A, Sacks M, Fleuchtwanger M. Aberrant (ectopic) adrenocortical tissue along the spermatic cord. J Pediatr Surg. 1980;15:289–92.
3. Ozel SK, Kazez A, Akpolat N. Presence of ectopic adrenocortical tissues in inguinoscrotal region suggests an association with undescended testis. Pediatr Surg Int. 2007;23:171–5.
4. Beccia DJ, Krane RJ, Olsson CA. Clinical management of non-testicular intrascrotal tumors. J Urol. 1976;116:476–9.
5. Ketata S, Ketata H, Sahnoun A, FakhFakh H, Bahloul A, Mhiri MN. Ectopic adrenal cortex tissue: an incidental finding during inguinoscrotal operations in pediatric patients. Urol Int. 2008;81:316–9.
6. Wang XL, Dou JT, Gao JP, Zhong WW, Jin D, Hui L, Lu JM, Mu YM. Laparoscope resection of ectopic corticosteroid-secreting adrenal adenoma. Neuro Endocrinol Lett. 2012;33:265–7.
7. Nistal M, Paniagua R. Congenital anomalies of the testis and the epididymis. In: Testicular and epididymal pathology. New York: Thieme Stratton Inc; 1984. p. 74–5.
8. Czaplicki M, Bablok L, Kuzaka B, Janczewski Z. Heterotopic adrenal tissue. Int Urol Nephrol. 1985;17:177–81.
9. Mendez R, Tellado MG, Somoza I, Liras J, Sanchez-Abuin A, Pais E, Vela D. Ectopic adrenal tissue in the spermatic cord in pediatric patients: surgical implications. Int Braz J Urol. 2006;32:202–7.
10. Paner GP, Kristiansen G, McKenney JK, Amin MB. Rete testis-associated nodular steroid cell nests: description of putative pluripotential testicular hilus steroid cells. Am J Surg Pathol. 2011;35:505–11.
11. Zandanell E. Hyperplasie akzessorischer Nebennieren bei morbus Addison. Frankfurt Z Path. 1953;64: 100–19.
12. Rose EK, Enterline HT, Rhoads JE, Rose E. Adrenal cortical hyperfuntion in childhood. Report of a case with adrenocortical hyperplasia and testicular adrenal rests. Pediatrics. 1952;9:475–84.
13. Bostroem E. Demonstration eines Praparates von Verwachsung der Milz mit dem lenken Hoden. Gesellschaft deutscher Naturforscher und Aerzte, Verhandlungen der 56 Versammlung, Freiburg; 1883. p. 149.
14. Pommer G. Verwachsung die linken kryptorchischen Hodens und Nebenhodens mit der milz in einen Missegehurt mit zahlreichen Bildemsdefecten. Ber Naturw Med Ver Innsbruck. 1889;17-19:144–8.
15. Fernandez Atuan R, Burgues Prades P, Gonzalez Esgueda A, et al. Splenogonadal fusión: case report and review of literatura. J Pediatr Surg Case Rep. 2013;10:375–7.
16. Khairat AB, Ismail AM. Splenogonadal fusion: case presentation and literature review. J Pediatr Surg. 2005;40:1357–60.
17. Alivizatos G, Skolarikos A, Sopilidis O, Ferakis N, Chorti M. Splenogonadal fusion: report of a case and review of the literature. Int J Urol. 2005;12:90–2.
18. Halvorsen JF, Stray O. Splenogonadal fusion. Acta Paediatr Scand. 1978;67:379–81.
19. Bal K, Ermete M, Balcı U, Dinçel Ç. Splenogonadal fusion: a very rare congenital anomaly in the differential diagnosis of a testicular mass. Turk J Urol. 2014;40:62–4.
20. Velarde Ramos L, Sepulveda F, Silva E, Castillo OA. Discontinuous intrabdominal splenogonadal fusion with germ cell tumor. Excision with robotic assistance. Adult case report. Arch Esp Urol. 2012;65:762–5.
21. Kumar S, Jayant K, Agrawal S, Parmar KM, Singh SK. A rare case of continuous type splenogonadal fusion in a young male with primary infertility. Case Rep Urol. 2014;2014:796761.
22. Kaya C, Koca O, Karaman IM, Radmayr C. Splenogonadal fusion in a 13-year-old boy with contralateral displaced intra-abdominal testis. Urology. 2010;75:173–5.
23. Karaman MI, Gonzales Jr ET. Splenogonadal fusion: report of 2 cases and review of the literature. J Urol. 1996;155:309–11.
24. Sneath WA. Apparent third testicle consisting of a scrotal spleen. J Anat Physiol. 1913;47:340–3.
25. Shen XC, Du CJ, Chen JM, Zhang ZW, Qiu YQ. Splenogonadal fusion. Chin Med J (Engl). 2008;121:383–4.
26. Putschar W, Manion W. Splenic-gonadal fusion. Am J Pathol. 1956;32:15–33.
27. Knorr PA, Borden TA. Splenogonadal fusion. Urology. 1994;44:136–8.
28. Cortes D, Thorup JM, Visfeldt J. The pathogenesis of cryptorchidism and splenogonadal fusion: a new hypothesis. Br J Urol. 1996;77:285–90.
29. Ando S, Shimazui T, Hattori K, Yamamoto T, Kuriyagawa K, Akaza H. Splenogonadal fusion: case report and review of published works. Int J Urol. 2006;13:1539–41.
30. Duncan Jr WL, Barraza MA. Splenogonadal Fusion: a case report and review of literature. J Pediatr Surg. 2005;40:E5–7.
31. Carragher AM. One hundred years of splenogonadal fusion. Urology. 1990;35:471–5.
32. McPherson F, Frias JL, Spicer D, Opitz JM, Gilbert-Barness EF. Splenogonadal fusion-limb defect "syndrome" and associated malformations. Am J Med Genet A. 2003;120:518–22.

33. Le Roux PJ, Heddle RM. Splenogonadal fusion: is the accepted classification system accurate? BJU Int. 2000;85:114–5.
34. Celik A, Tiryaki S, Darcan S, Ergun O. Splenogonadal fusion-limb deformity syndrome: a rare but important cause of undescended testis. World J Pediatr. 2016;12:246–8.
35. Gouw ASH, Elema JD, Bink-Boelkens MTE, De Jongh HJ, Ten Kate LP. The spectrum of splenogonadal fusion. Case report and review of 84 reported cases. Eur J Pediatr. 1985;144:316–23.
36. Weiss L. The development of the primary vascular reticulum in the spleen of human fetuses (38 to 57 mm. crown-rump length). Am J Anat. 1973;136: 315–37.
37. Falkowski WS, Carter MF. Splenogonadal fusion associated with an anaplastic seminoma. J Urol. 1980;124:562–4.
38. Prada Arias M, Vazquez Castelo JL, Montero Sanchez M, Muguerza Vellibre R, Rodriguez Costa A. Supernumerary intrascrotal ectopic spleen: discontinuous splenogonadal fusion. An Pediatr (Barc). 2006;64:277–9.
39. Chen SL, Kao YL, Sun HS, Lin WL. Splenogonadal fusion. Formos Med Assoc. 2008;107:892–5.
40. Li YH. Preoperative detection of splenogonadal fusion by CT. Surg Radiol Anat. 2009;31:733–5.
41. Keyik B, Yanik B, Conkbayir I, Tuygun C, Kizilgoz V, Hekimoğlu B. Continuous-type splenogonadal fusion associated with an ipsilateral testicular atrophy: sonographic findings. J Clin Ultrasound. 2010;38:161–3.
42. Li WF, Luan MX, Ma Z, Chen YJ. Splenogonadal fusion: report of four cases and review of the literature. Exp Ther Med. 2013;6:816–8.
43. Bosnalı O, Cici İ, Moralıoğlu S, Cerrah-Celayir A. Continuous-type splenogonadal fusion: report of a rare case. Turk J Pediatr. 2014;56:680–3.
44. Alvarez Maestro M, López-Tello J, Domínguez Franjo P, Ríos González E, Martínez-Piñeiro L. Splenogonadal fusion. Report of a case and review of the literature. Actas Urol Esp. 2010;34:293–5.
45. Lopes RI, de Medeiros MT, Arap MA, Cocuzza M, Srougi M, Hallak J. Splenogonadal fusion and testicular cancer: case report and review of the literature. Einstein (Sao Paulo). 2012;10:92–5.
46. Ferro F, Lais A, Boldrini R, De Peppo F, Federici G, Bosman C. Hepatogonadal fusion. J Pediatr Surg. 1996;31:435–6.
47. Lund JM, Bouhadiba N, Sams V, Tsang T. Hepatotesticular fusion: an unusual case of undescended testes. BJU Int. 2001;88:439–40.
48. Fan R, Faught PR, Sun J, Meldrum KK. Hepatogonadal fusion. J Pediatr Surg. 2012;47(2):e5–6.
49. Muensterer OJ. Laparoscopic single-stage fowler-stephens orchidopexy in a case of orchidogastric fusion. Urology. 2011;78:687–8.
50. Meyer R. Nachnierenkanälchen mit Glomerulusanlage in der Leistengegend beim menschlichen Embryo: Ein Beitrag zur Adenomyomfrage. Virchows Arch Pathol Anat. 1911;204:94–105.
51. Goldberg J, Drut R. Ectopic immature renal tissue. Report of two cases. Pathol Res Pract. 1984;179: 115–23.
52. Posalaky Z, Drake RM, Mawk JR, Franciosi RA, Spencer BH, Athinarayanan PR, Baker TA, Viring N. Ectopic immature renal tissue over the dorsum of lumbar and sacral area in two infants. Pediatrics. 1982;69:336–9.
53. McDougall EM, Mikhael BR, Carpenter B. Ectopic renal tissue associated with an undescended testis: a case report. J Urol. 1986;135:1018–9.
54. Ducos R, Warrier RP, Mackenzie F, Evans B. Ectopic immature renal tissue in an infant with undescended testis. Am J Pediatr Hematol Oncol. 1986;8:264–6.
55. Yoshida K, Ohama K, Tsuchida K, Minato H, Kurumaya H. Embryonal renal remnant in the gubernaculum testis. Eur J Pediatr Surg. 1999;9: 186–8.
56. Shono T, Kai H, Suita S. Ectopic renal tissue in the gubernaculum associated with undescended testis. BJU Int. 2002;89:320–1.
57. Saito S, Higa L, Koyama Y, Hatano T, Hayakawa M, Osawa A, Toda T. Immature renal tissue in inguinal canal. J Urol. 1989;142:106–7.
58. Orlowky JP, Levin HS, Dyment PG. Intrascrotal Wilms` tumor developing in a heterotopic renal anlage of probable mesonephric origin. J Pediatr Surg. 1980;15:679–82.
59. Taylor WF, Myers M, Taylor WR. Extrarenal Wilms'tumour in an infant exposed to intrauterine phenitoin. Lancet. 1980;2:481–2.

37 Paratesticular Tumor-Like Acquired Lesions

Manuel Nistal, Pilar González-Peramato, and Álvaro Serrano

37.1 Meconium Periorchitis

The presence of meconium in the vaginal cavity is secondary to meconium peritonitis [1]. Less than 50 cases have been reported. The characteristic age of presentation are the first months of life, although this disorder has been reported also in a 5-year-old child [2].

Etiopathogenesis

Meconium reaches the scrotum through a patent vaginal process. In half of the cases, meconium peritonitis results from a perforation of the digestive tract with subsequent extrusion of meconium; in the other half, it is not possible to demonstrate the perforation [3]. Twenty percent of cases of meconium peritonitis are related to meconium inspissation secondary to cystic fibrosis [4, 5], and another 30 % are attributed to volvulus, intussusceptions, intestinal atresia, intestinal duplication, congenital bands, imperforate anus, Meckel diverticuli, or aganglionism of the colon.

Signs

Meconium vaginalitis occurs in the neonatal period as a hydrocele or acute scrotum [6]. A few weeks later, the scrotum acquires tumoral characteristics. Macroscopically yellowish nodules can be observed in the tunica vaginalis (meconium pearls) [2, 7]. Some cases of meconium periorchitis have been suspected during intrauterine routine ultrasound examination and confirmed after birth [8, 9].

Histology

Meconium produces a chemically aseptic inflammation in which macrophages predominate. Bile pigment can be shown in the cytoplasm of these cells. The study of scrotal fluid aspirates may help in the diagnosis if the meconium components (bile lipids, mucin salts, desquamated epithelial cells) are confirmed [10]. The natural evolution of meconium in the scrotum is toward spontaneous resolution [11]. In other cases the lesion evolves to fibrosis and dystrophic calcification [12] (Fig. 37.1).

Differential Diagnosis

Differential diagnosis is very easy when meconium periorchitis is associated with intraperitoneal calcifications, which happens in 50 % of patients [13]; a testicular or paratesticular tumor (rhabdomyosarcoma) must be ruled out in other cases [14]. Scrotal ultrasound and abdominal plain film are diagnostic [15].

Complications

Among the exceptional complications, necrosis of the scrotal wall with externalization of meconium and the testicle has been reported. The perforation could be secondary to ischemia caused by the pressure of the scrotal mass. This

M. Nistal et al., *Clues in the Diagnosis of Non-tumoral Testicular Pathology*, DOI 10.1007/978-3-319-49364-0_37

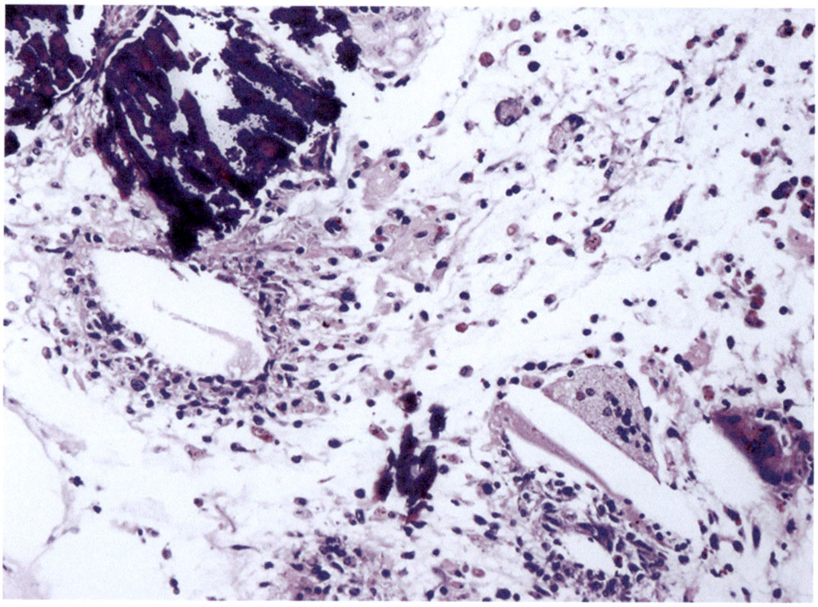

Fig. 37.1 Meconium periorchitis. The tunica vaginalis contains abundant pigmented macrophages, foreign body granulomas, and areas of dystrophic calcification

condition is known as testicular exstrophy [16, 17] or secondary scrotoschisis [18, 19].

37.2 Foreign Body Vaginalitis

Foreign bodies observed in the tunica vaginalis testis are varied; some are inert while others elicit a granulomatous reaction. Among the former there are various materials such as catheters from ventriculoperitoneal shunts, when they migrate from the abdominal cavity to the scrotum via the processus vaginalis [20, 21]. Among the latter there are granulomatous reactions produced by talc of gloves, vegetal fibers, and extravasation of parenteral nutrition solution [22].

Signs

They present clinically either with an acute scrotum simulating a testicular torsion or as a rapid onset hydrocele. This condition is more common in children [23–26] and on the right side, consequently with the distribution of inguinal hernias in children. A case of an adult in whom the foreign material perforated the scrotum [27] has been known. Sometimes the vaginal tunica is directly affected such as in scrotal operations; some other times it is indirectly affected, e.g., after interventions in the abdominal cavity, if a patent processus vaginalis exists. The interval between the operation and the detection of lesions is very variable (from 2 months to 45 years).

Histology

The most frequent granulomatous reactions are triggered by talc of gloves and vegetal fibers (lycopodium, talc, and starch). Histologically, the lesion is characteristic: a reaction of foreign body giant cells surrounding the material. In the case of talc, when polarized it shows double refractile crystals. Regarding glove-starch granuloma material, this is PAS positive and birefringent showing a Maltese cross image under polarization [28]. Scrotal granulomatous lesion due to plant fibers has been observed after jejunal perforation within an incarcerated inguinal hernia [29]. The size of these reactive processes can be so large that they result in a paratesticular mass [30].

37.3 Scrotal Lithiasis

Scrotal calculi are benign lesion consisting in the presence of one or more bodies moving freely inside a hydrocele. The prevalence with which it has been observed has been increasing as more and more ultrasound scans have been done – from

1.95 % of Tan et al. [31] in a study of 3435 patients evaluated retrospectively with radiology records to 9.6 % of Aslan et al. [32] using ultrasound. These figures are probably indicating that many calculi are not detected radiologically. The age of presentation varies from 4 months to 65 years. The incidence increases with age. In 50 % of the cases, the lesion is bilateral.

Signs
In some cases the diagnosis is made by the own patient on self-palpation of the testis; in other cases is a surgical or incidental finding in US examination of the scrotum. The ultrasound image is characteristic: a hyperechoic structure with posterior acoustic shadow that moves freely in the hydrocele [33]. In some cases the bodies may be attached to the wall [34]. They are observed in 13 % [35] to 56.8 % [31] of hydroceles. A very high incidence (81 % of hydroceles) has been observed in extreme mountain bikers [36]. Although considered a trivial finding, movements of the calculi secondary to daily life activities may repeatedly irritate the vaginal tunics and cause scrotal pain [32].

Histology
They are generally whitish, spherical bodies not exceeding 9 mm. They are constituted by connective tissue with areas of calcification and even ossification (Figs. 37.2 and 37.3). The calculi in hydroceles would originate by the deposition of calcium phosphates that crystallize the hydrocele's alkaline environment on a core of organic rests such as an infarcted testicular appendix, fibrin, red blood cells, sloughed mesothelial cells, and even parasites (filarial worms) [37].

37.4 Cholesterol Granuloma

Cholesterol granulomas occur associated with bleeding or tissue necrosis and can be observed in the vaginal cavity (hematocele), the epididymis (ischemic epididymitis) [38], and paratesticularly (hematomas) [39]. The most common clinical presentation mimics a testicular tumor.

Etiology
Hematocele causes are multiple. Some are local, like testicular trauma, torsion of the spermatic cord, or testicular appendages, or rupture of an underlying tumor. Other, less frequent, appear in patients with hematologic processes or when there is an increased tendency to mucous and serous bleeding. In children it has been reported in association with splenic rupture by a blunt abdominal trauma (communicant hematocele)

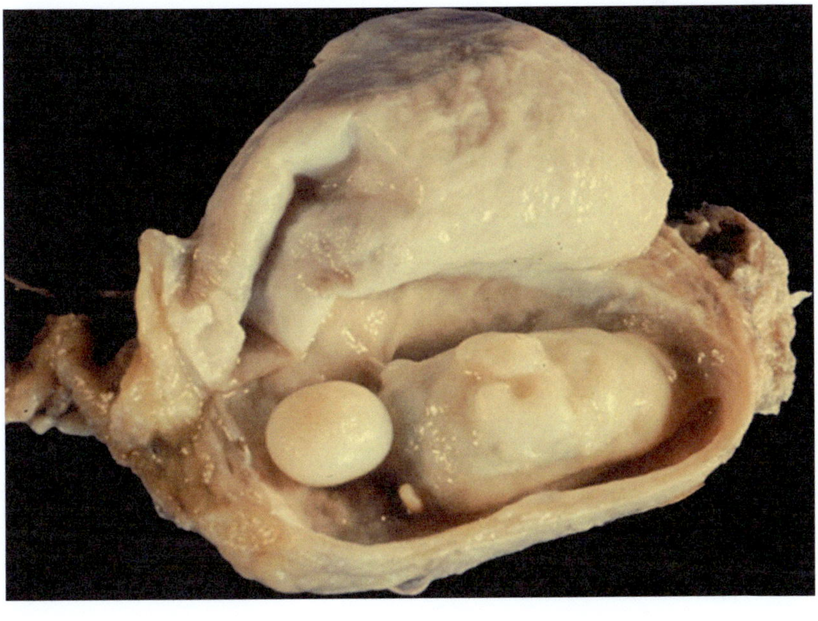

Fig. 37.2 Scrotal pearl. Whitish nodular formation in the tunica vaginalis of an elderly patient. The testis exhibits severe atrophy and the vaginal is markedly thickened

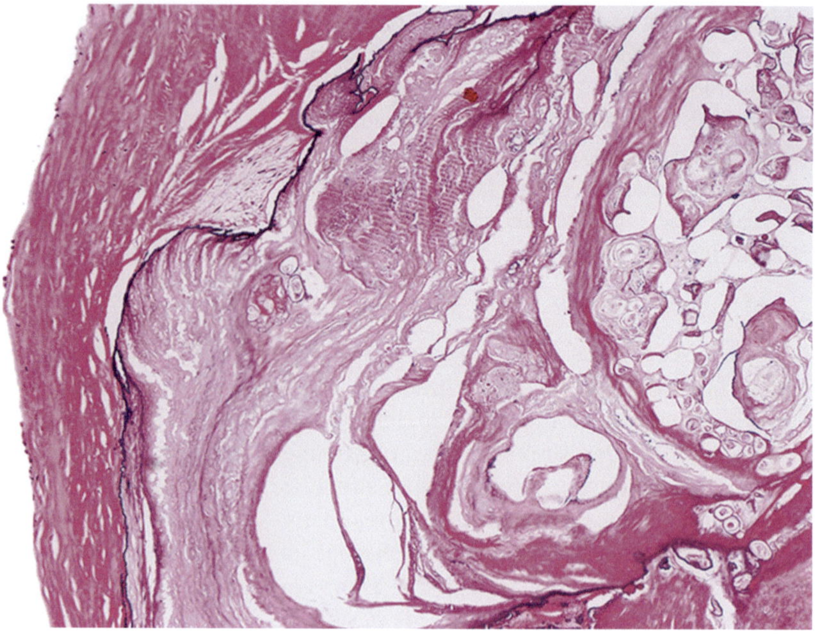

Fig. 37.3 Scrotal calculi. Free nodular formation in the vaginal cavity. It consists in connective tissue with laminated calcifications of eccentric arrangement

[40–42]. Most often the traumatic hematocele is due to a testicular rupture (80 %) [43] or ripping of the pampiniform plexus veins [44].

Diagnosis

Ultrasound [45] and computed tomography are very useful in diagnosing hematocele, but not in all cases they permit a differential diagnosis between a hematocele following a testicular blunt contusion with an intact tunica, which would not require surgery, and one secondary to testicular rupture in which the repair must be immediate to prevent ischemic necrosis or abscess formation [46]. MRI can aid a proper diagnosis [47].

Histology

In cases of short evolution, abundant fresh blood clots are observed upon opening of the tunica vaginalis. Afterward, the tunica vaginalis appears filled with a spongelike material in such a quantity that it can reach several times the testicular volume (Fig. 37.4). The material is preferably fibrin. In long-evolution hematoceles, the hematic material is partially or fully organized. It consists of a connective tissue with numerous neoformed vessels and macrophages with hemosiderin with a coating of fibrin toward the cavity. In the final stages, only a very thickened vaginal tunica with fibrosis and dystrophic calcification persists, in which bone metaplasia and cholesterol granulomas can be seen (Fig. 37.5). A complication of hematocele is testicular atrophy, but it does not occur in all cases [48]. Rare complications are rupture, infection, scrotal suppuration, and gangrene.

37.5 Vasitis Nodosa

Vasitis nodosa is a ductular proliferation that causes focal thickening of the vas deferens. It has received this name because it is reminiscent of the isthmic nodosa salpingitis. Most cases develop after a vasectomy, in other there is a history of trauma, and some are idiopathic. The most common symptoms are pain and tumor.

Benign ductular proliferation develops on or around the wall of the vas deferens. The ductular structures are formed by cuboidal cells and may have a central lumen. The cells have a pale cytoplasm and central nuclei and one nucleolus. Some of them are ciliated. The lesion shows nonspecific chronic inflammation and fibrosis. Perineural invasion [49] or benign vascular invasion is often

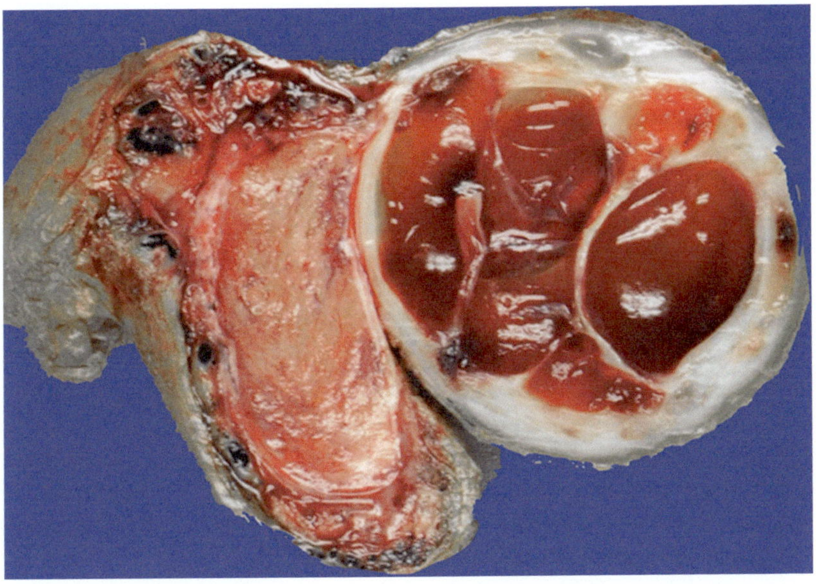

Fig. 37.4 Paratesticular hematoma. Well-defined ovoid formation with trabeculae inside that separate hematic material at different times of resorption. The tumor displaces and compresses the testis

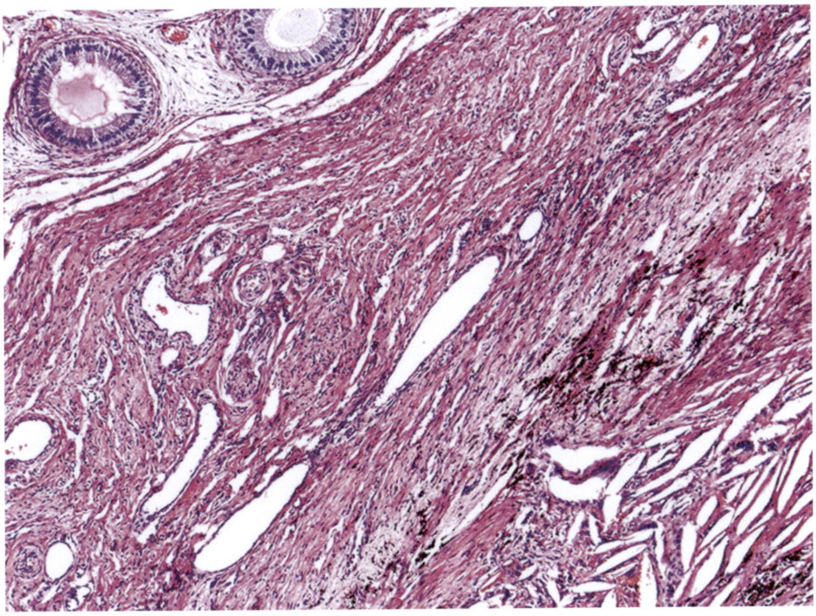

Fig. 37.5 Paratesticular hematoma. Cholesterol granulomas present in the wall of the previous figure hematoma. On top of the image, sections of epididymal ducts are recognized

observed [50]. The wall of the vas deferens may show muscle hyperplasia and perineural fibrosis, which could explain the pain experienced by some patients [51]. In 50 % of cases, there is a spermatic granuloma. A similar process can be observed in the epididymis (epididymitis nodosa) [52]. The differential diagnosis should include metastases of prostate adenocarcinoma [53].

37.6 Sperm Granulomas

This is a lesion characterized by a foreign body reaction to sperm extravasations. It appears in 42 % of vasectomized patients and 2.5 % of autopsies of adults [54]. Most cases are asymptomatic, but it is not uncommon to consult for localized pain in the head of the epididymis, spermatic cord, or testis [55].

The lesion consists of one or less frequently several nodes measuring up to four cm in diameter. Histology varies with time. At first, there is an extravasation of sperm that are rapidly engulfed by macrophages constituting a granuloma foreign body type. Late lesions are constituted by ceroid granulomas in which macrophages show abundant lipofuscins and fibrosis.

37.7 Endometriosis

Endometriosis has been reported in the bladder, prostate, seminal vesicles, retroperitoneum, lower abdominal wall, and paratesticular region. Endometriosis of the testes and paratesticular structures has been observed on the wall of a cyst in the epididymis [56], and cysts of the tunica vaginalis testis [57, 58], and in the spermatic cord [59]. Pain and a palpable mass are the most common clinical signs.

It is described as nodular or cystic formations consisting of glands with endometrial appearance. Most glands are dilated; the epithelium is cylindrical, and inside it there is an abundant eosinophilic granular, PAS-positive material. Stromal cells contain both ferric pigments and lipofuscins. The epithelium shows an endometrial phenotype that is positive for cytokeratin, vimentin, EMA, ER, and PR. The stromal cells express vimentin, estrogen and progesterone receptors, and CD10. Endometriosis, within its rarity, is more common in elderly patients with high estrogen levels secondary to estrogen therapy for prostate cancer. At least two patients lacked this background and were younger. There are two cytogenetic hypotheses not mutually exclusive – an origin in Müllerian remnants or an origin from metaplasia of the mesothelium.

37.8 Lipomembranous Fat Necrosis (LFN) of the Spermatic Cord

The LFN is a nonspecific reactive lesion of adipose tissue degeneration associated with impairment of the vascular supply to the adipose tissue. The term LFN was proposed by Poppiti in 1986 [60], although similar lesions had already been observed a decade before [61, 62], always in extragenital locations. The LFN of the spermatic cord was observed in three pubertal patients suffering from intravaginal spermatic cord torsion. They consulted for symptoms of pain, a mass in the groin, and absence of the testis in the scrotal sac [63] (Fig. 37.6).

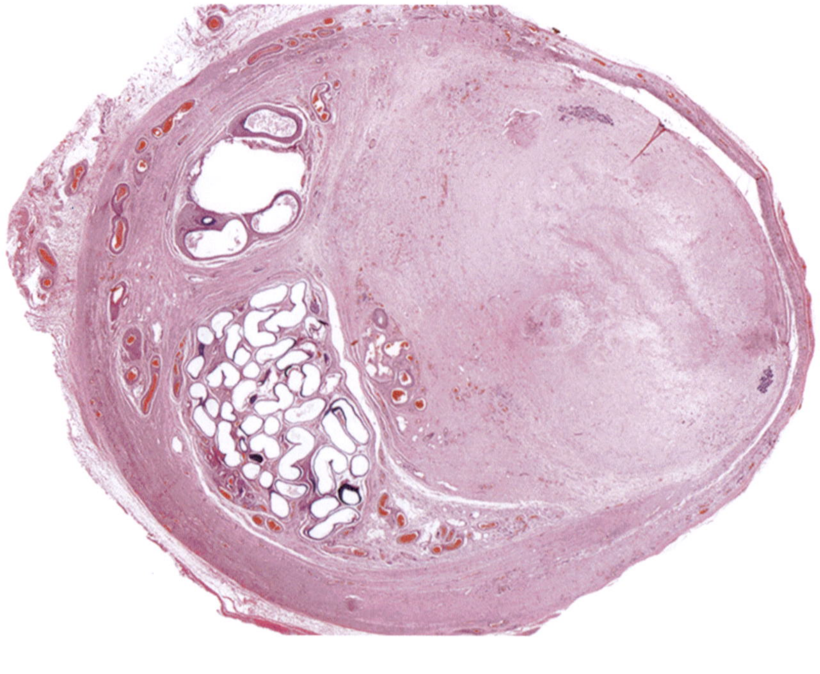

Fig. 37.6 Lipomembranous fat necrosis of the spermatic cord. Spermatic cord nodule in a patient who consulted for symptoms of pain, a mass in the groin, and absence of the testis in the scrotal sac

Histology

Light microscopy shows the silhouette of the seminiferous tubules with ischemic necrosis surrounded by granulation tissue. LFN is found in the epididymis and in the initial segment of the spermatic cord. The FLN is characterized by the occurrence of cystic cavities limited by eosinophilic, wavy outlined, refringent, hyaline membranes, which were stained with Sudan black, PAS (before and after diastase digestion) and orcein, and presented yellowish-green autofluorescence. Most of the degenerated fat cell remnants had been phagocytosed by multinucleated macrophages (Fig. 37.7). Foreign body granulomas surrounding necrotic areas are numerous. Histochemical tests suggested that the membranes seen in LFN were a lipopigment, which was probably the result of changes in the fragmented cell membranes of the degenerated fat cells. In all three cases, vascular thrombosis was confirmed. The fact that LFN has never been observed in torsions in newborn babies and infants is probably related to the absence of adipose tissue in this location at this age. Subsequently LFN evolves toward sclerosis in the cytoplasm of these cells, where both hemoglobin-derivate pigments and membrane fragments accumulate.

Differential Diagnosis

The diagnosis is usually easy; however, if the granulomatous pattern predominates and there are no clinical data, the differential diagnosis should be established with the following three processes: the presence of parasites or their eggs (filariae and schistosomes), sclerosing lipogranuloma, and granuloma secondary to material from a ruptured testicular prosthesis.

37.9 Pseudosarcomatous Periorchitis

This name describes the findings observed in two surgical specimens of adult patients with a recent history of testicular torsion. The lesion consisted of a crescent-shaped unencapsulated myofibroblastic proliferation surrounding necrotic seminiferous tubules. The cells were arranged in bundles and showed a focal storiform pattern. Among these cells, an infiltrate of neutrophils, lymphocytes, and histiocytes could be observed with variable intensity in different areas. Fusiform cells showed numerous mitoses, and the lesion in its whole looked like a malignant fibrohistiocytoma. The patients were well 2 and 3 years after orchiectomy without any treatment [64].

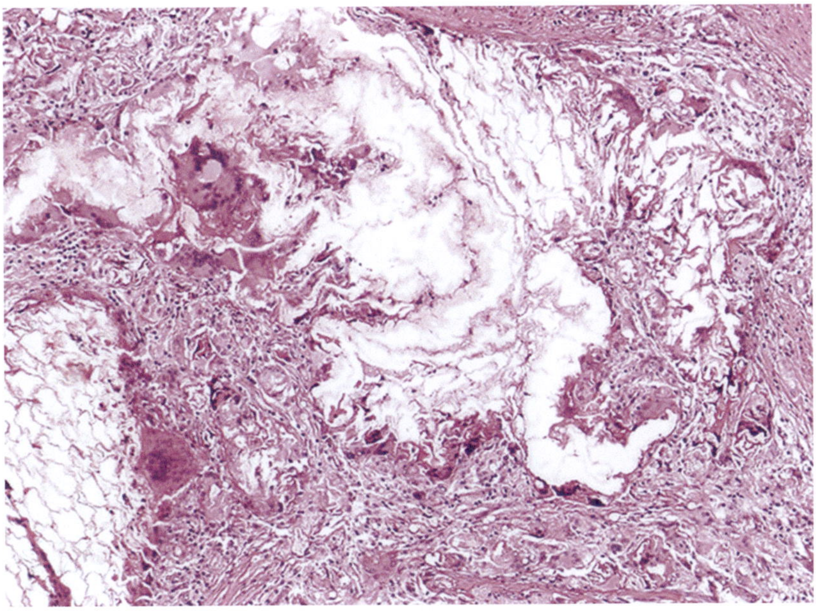

Fig. 37.7 Lipomembranous fat necrosis of the spermatic cord. Eosinophilic hyaline membranes of spiculated surface are surrounded by foreign body giant cells

37.10 Paratesticular Cyst

Mesothelial cysts, cyst-originated remains, Wolffian or Müllerian remnants, spermatoceles, epidermoid cysts (Fig. 37.8), and dermoid cysts, among others, have been described in paratesticular structures. Mesothelial cysts represent 53.8 % and originate from the cystic transformation of remains of the processus vaginalis [65]. Cord cysts can mimic hernia [66], a supernumerary testicle [67], or tumor [68, 69]. The twisting of epididymal cysts simulates a testicular torsion [70]. On the wall of cysts embryonic remains, albeit infrequently, different types of benign epithelial proliferations [71] and more rarely malignant ones [72] have been reported.

37.11 Fibrous Pseudotumor (Nodular and Diffuse Proliferation)

It refers to a chronic inflammatory process with a tendency to fibrosis, calcification, or ossification. It is known by a variety of names such as chronic periorchitis, reactive periorchitis, nodular fibrous periorchitis, fibromatous periorchitis, fibrous proliferation of the tunica, nonspecific paratesticular fibrosis, nodular fibrous pseudotumor, proliferative funiculitis, inflammatory pseudotumor, and fibroma, which are probably related to different macroscopic and histological aspects of this lesion throughout its evolution. It preferably affects testicular tunics, but it can also be located in the epididymis and the spermatic cord. It pres-

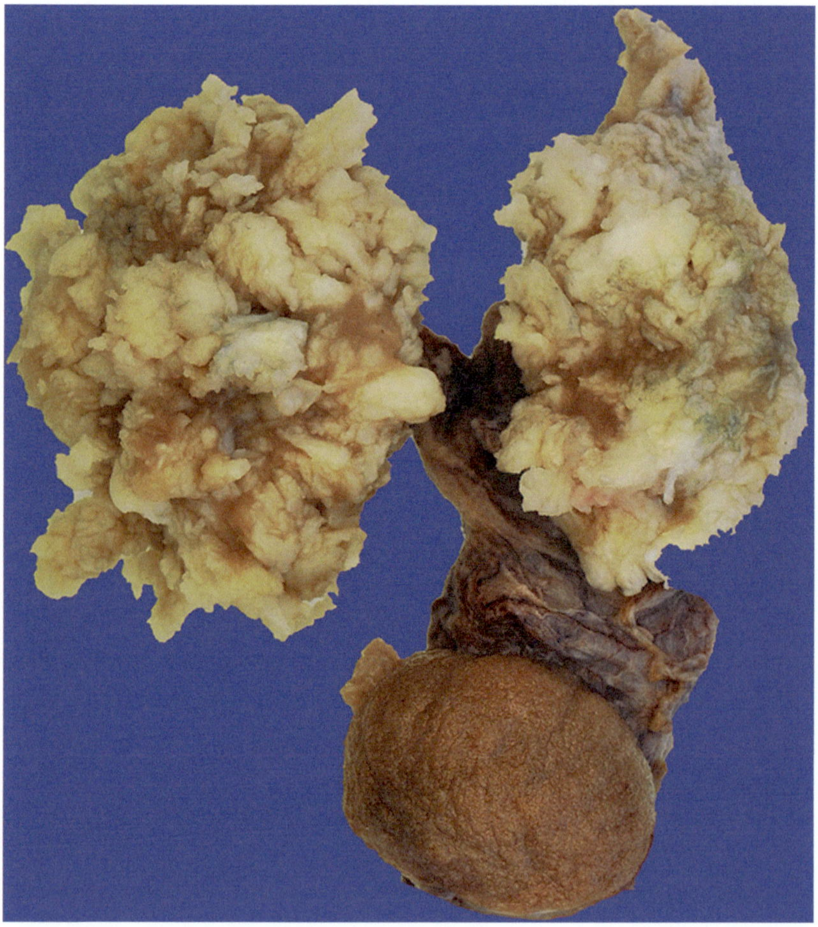

Fig. 37.8 Epidermoid cyst of the spermatic cord. Characteristic appearance of keratin masses after opening the cyst is shown

ents as single or multiple nodular lesions or as a diffuse lesion of the testicular tunics. It is more frequent in the third decade but it can occur at all ages. In many cases there is a history of orchio-epididymitis, trauma, or an inflamed hydrocele.

Histopathology
The initial lesions are formed by granulation tissue with chronic inflammation. The more evolved ones show a fibrous paucicellular connective tissue that is very hyalinized. Cell infiltrates may persist between collagen bundles and around vessel's plasma. The lesion may show calcification or ossification (Fig. 37.9). The differential diagnosis includes idiopathic fibromatosis, solitary fibrous tumor, neurofibroma, and leiomyoma.

Etiopathogenesis
Based on the histological similarity of fibrous pseudotumor to other conditions such as retroperitoneal fibrosis, sclerosing pancreatitis and cholangitis, Riedel's thyroiditis, and sclerosing sialadenitis, it is included in this growing list of IgG4-related diseases. Many cases meet most of the criteria required for the lesion to be considered an IgG4-related disease [73–78]: (a) presence of swelling or tumors that can affect one or more organs, (b) elevated serum IgG4 concentrations (>135 mg/dl), and (c) histopathological examination showing dense lymphoplasmacytic infiltrates, storiform-type fibrosis, obliterative phlebitis, and infiltration of IgG4-positive plasma cells (ratio of IgG4-positive/IgG-positive cells >40 % and >10 IgG4-positive plasma cells/HPF). The fibrosis and obliterative phlebitis are absent in some lesions that affect the lacrimal gland [79, 80]. The role of IgG4 in the disease is unknown.

37.12 Sclerosing Lipogranuloma

This is a reaction of the adipose tissue caused by trauma or exogenous lipid agents such as paraffin. In more than half of the cases, there is no precedent. Clinically, it is characterized by the development of a painless swelling. Most cases have been described in the scrotum, and only five were well-documented lipogranulomas of the spermatic cord [81–83]. It is a granulomatous lesion associated with a granulomatous foreign body reaction with infiltrates preferentially by lymphocytes and eosinophils and varying degrees of fibrosis around cystic spaces of varying sizes. Sudan black-positive remains of refracting membranes can be recognized inside the giant cells. The differential diagnosis includes infectious dis-

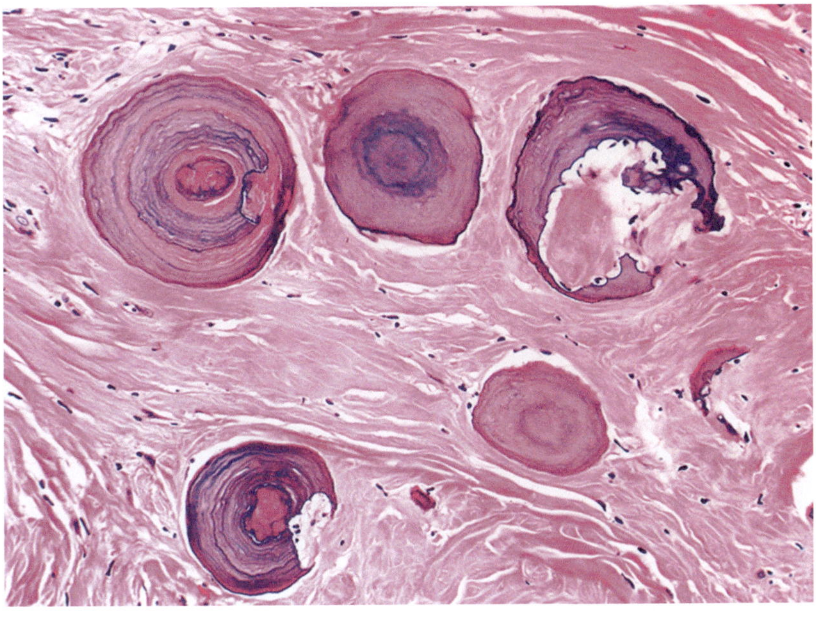

Fig. 37.9 Fibrous pseudotumor. Very collagenized connective tissue with scarce inflammatory cells shows numerous nodular calcifications of laminar architecture

eases that cause the granulomatous lesions and those caused by parasites.

37.13 Smooth Muscle Hamartomas (Smooth Muscle Hyperplasia)

This smooth muscle hyperplasia is seen in areas where it is usually abundant as in the tunica albuginea at the lower pole of the testis, in the tail of epididymis, and the wall of the vas deferens [84–87]. More than half of the cases have been reported in the epididymis. It presents as a mass of variable size up to 7 cm, simulating a malignancy on clinical examination. It is described at all ages, but its average age is 63 years [88].

Histologically it can take different growth patterns: periductal (around the vas deferens or the epididymis forming concentric layers), interstitial, in the connective tissue of the tail of the epididymis, and perivascular originating in the vessel walls. Mitoses and necrosis should be absent. A special form occurs in patients with androgen insensitivity syndrome in which the muscle tissue of the tunica continues with smooth muscle cell proliferation that simulates the uterine wall [89, 90]. In all cases the cells form irregularly arranged bundles (Fig.37.10). Between the bundles there is a loose stroma that may contain focal infiltrates of lymphoid cells, among which eosinophils stand out. In most cases there is no previous history of inflammation and only in three cases a history of inguinal hernia was reported [91].

The *etiology* of smooth muscle hyperplasia of the paratesticular structures is unknown, and since there are very few cases associated with a locally accompanying pathology, they are considered to be hamartomas. They are similar to their counterparts in other locations such as the gingival, palate, esophagus and pylorus, small intestine, large intestine, trachea, skin, and breast. The differential diagnosis includes leiomyomas and angioleiomyomas, and it is very important to highlight the periductal location of many paratesticular hamartomas along with the low cohesiveness of the bundles of smooth muscle cells. A peculiar cystic hamartoma constituted by a transformation of the rete testis, a proliferation of smooth muscle cells, and a wide myxoid stroma was reported in a 26-year-old patient [92].

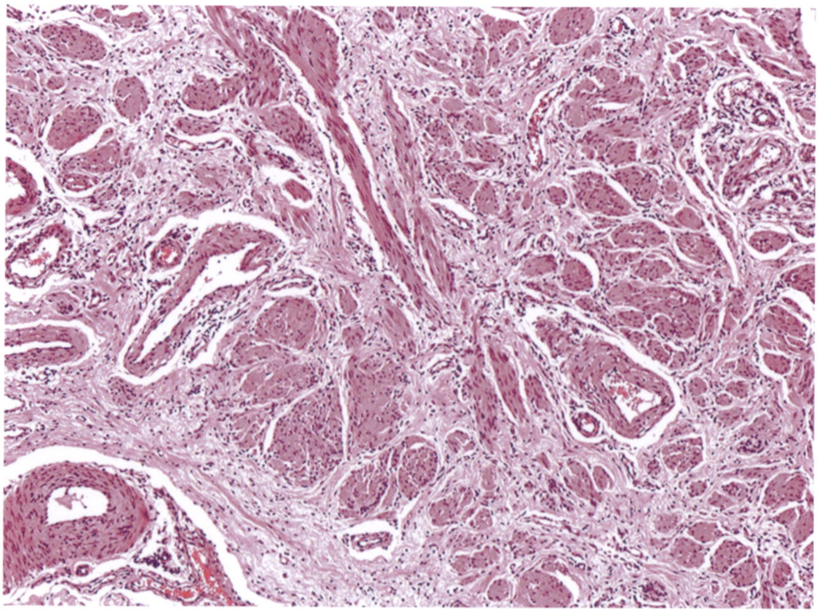

Fig. 37.10 Smooth muscle hamartoma of the cauda epididymis. Irregularly arranged bundles of smooth muscle cells separated by abundant connective tissue

References

1. Olnick HM, Hatcher MB. Meconium peritonitis. JAMA. 1953;152:582–3.
2. Kalra P, Radhakrishnan J. Meconium periorchitis. Urology. 2006;68:202.
3. Tibboel D, Gaillard JL, Molenaar JC. The importance of mesenteric vascular insufficiency in meconium peritonitis. Hum Pathol. 1986;17:411–6.
4. Drips RC. Meconium peritonitis with massive abdominal distention resulting in dystocia. Report of a case. Obstet Gynecol. 1966;27:335–7.
5. Berdon WE, Baker DH, Becker J, De Sanctis P. Scrotal masses in healed meconium peritonitis. N Engl J Med. 1967;277:585–7.
6. Stokes S 3rd, Flom S. Meconium filled hydrocele sacs as a cause of acute scrotum in a newborn. J Urol. 1997;158:1960–1.
7. Kesler SS, Glazier DB, Zaontz MR, Dean GE. Meconium pearls in the scrotum. J Urol. 2000;164:1350–1.
8. Regev RH, Markovich O, Arnon S, Bauer S, Dolfin T, Litmanovitz I. Meconium periorchitis: intrauterine diagnosis and neonatal outcome: case reports and review of the literature. J Perinatol. 2009;29:585–7.
9. Ochiai D, Omori S, Ikeda T, Yakubo K, Fukuiya T. A rare case of meconium periorchitis diagnosed in utero. Case Rep Obstet Gynecol. 2015;2015:606134.
10. Heydenrych JJ, Marcus PB. Meconium granulomas of the tunica vaginalis. J Urol. 1976;115:596–8.
11. Dehner LP, Scott D, Stocker JT. Meconium periorchitis: a clinico-pathologic study of four cases with a review of the literature. Hum Pathol. 1986;17:807–12.
12. Varkonyi l, Fliegel C, Rosslein R, Jenny P, Ohnacker H. Meconium periorchitis: case report and literature review. Eur J Pediatr Surg. 2000;10:404–7.
13. Bouhafs A, Bouvier R, Dodat H. Meconium periorchitis. Two case reports. Arch Pediatr. 2001;8:504–7.
14. Hegde D, Utture A. Meconium Periorchitis. Indian Pediatr. 2015;52:449.
15. Han K, Mata J, Zaontz MR. Meconium masquerading as a scrotal mass. Br J Urol. 1998;82:765–7.
16. Heyns CF. Exstrophy of the testis. J Urol. 1990;144:724–5.
17. Salle JLP, De Fraga JCS, Wojciechowski M, Antunes CRH. Congenital rupture of scrotum: an unusual complication of meconium peritonitis. J Urol. 1992;148:1242–3.
18. Chun K, St-Vil D. Scrotoschisis associated with contralateral meconium periorchitis. J Pediatr Surg. 1997;32:864–6.
19. Kojori F, DeMaria J. Scrotoschisis associated with meconium periorchitis. J Pediatr Urol. 2007;3:415–6.
20. Albala DM, Danaher JW, Huntsman WT. Ventriculoperitoneal shunt migration into the scrotum. Am Surg. 1989;55:685–8.
21. Karaosmanoglu D, Metin Y, Akata D, Haliloglu M. An unusual cause of hydrocele: malpositioned ventriculoperitoneal shunt in the scrotum. Ultrasound Med. 2008;27:159–60.
22. Krüse-Ruijter MF, Robben SG, Degraeuwe PL. Hydrocoele and periorchitis after extravasation of parenteral nutrition solution. Arch Dis Child Fetal Neonatal Ed. 2011;96:F359.
23. Oktem IS, Akdemir H, Koc K, Menku A, Tucer B, Selcuklu A, Turan C. Migration of abdominal catheter of ventriculoperitoneal shunt into the scrotum. Acta Neurochir. 1998;140:167–70.
24. Ozveren MF, Kazez A, Cetin H, Ziyal IM. Migration of the abdominal catheter of a ventriculoperitoneal shunt into the scrotum–case report. Neurol Med Chir (Tokyo). 1999;39:313–5.
25. Ward JF, Moquin RR, Maurer ST. Expanding the differential diagnosis of the acute scrotum: ventriculoperitoneal shunt herniation. Urology. 2001;58:281.
26. Kita D, Hayashi Y, Kinoshita M, Ohama K, Hamada J. Scrotal migration of the peritoneal catheter of a ventriculoperitoneal shunt in a 5-year-old male. Case report. Neurol Med Chir (Tokyo). 2010;50:1122–5.
27. Rehm A, Bannister CM, Victoratos G. Scrotal perforation by a ventriculoperitoneal shunt. Br J Neurosurg. 1997;11:443–4.
28. Miller RA, Kiviat MD, Graves J. Glove-starch granuloma in congenital hydrocele. Urology. 1974;3:610–1.
29. Martinez Alarcón M, Miranda Vallina C, Estefano BC. Inflamación crónica intraescrotal secundaria a cuerpos extraños libres en túnica vaginal. Arch Esp Urol. 1993;46:429–31.
30. Healey GB, McDonald DF. Talc granuloma presenting as a testicular mass. J Urol. 1977;118:122.
31. Tan S, Özcan MF, Karaoğlanoğlu M, Ipek A, Özcan AS, Arslan H. Prevalence of scrotal calculi and their relationship with pain. Diagn Interv Radiol. 2012;18:303–6.
32. Aslan A, Tan S, Yıldırım H, Dönmez U, Çam A, Gezer MC, Teber MA, Arslan H. Scrotal calculi in clinical practice and their role in scrotal pain: a prospective study. J Clin Ultrasound. 2015;43:406–11.
33. Dogra VS, Gottlieb RH, Oka M, Rubens DJ. Sonography of the scrotum. Radiology. 2003;227:18–36.
34. Valero Puerta JA, Medina Pérez M, Valpuesta Fernández I, Sánchez González M. Differential diagnosis of intrascrotal calcification: lithiasis attached to hydrocele wall. Arch Esp Urol. 2000;53:370–2.
35. Artas H, Orhan I. Scrotal calculi. J Ultrasound Med. 2007;26:1775–9.
36. Frauscher F, Klauser A, Stenzl A, Helweg G, Amort B, zur Nedden D. US findings in the scrotum of extreme mountain bikers. Radiology. 2001;219:427–31.
37. Hussein O, El Setouhy M, Ahmed ES, Kandil AM, Ramzy RM, Helmy H, Weil GJ. Duplex Doppler sonographic assessment of the effects of diethylcarbamazine and albendazole therapy on adult filarial worms and adjacent host tissues in Bancroftian filariasis. Am J Trop Med Hyg. 2004;71:471–7.
38. Nistal M, Mate A, Paniagua R. Granulomatous epididymal lesion of possible ischemic origin. Am J Surg Pathol. 1997;21:951–6.
39. Unal D, Kilic M, Oner S, Erkinuresin T, Demirbas M, Coban S, Aydos MM. Cholesterol granuloma of the

paratesticular tissue: a case report. Can Urol Assoc J. 2015;9(5–6):E390–2.
40. Skoog SJ, Belman AB. The communicating hematocele: an unusual presentation for blunt splenic trauma. J Urol. 1986;136:1092–3.
41. Shirvani AR, Ortenberg J. Communicating hematocele in children following splenic rupture: diagnosis and management. Urology. 2000;55:590.
42. Koumanidou C, Manopoulou E, Pantazis J, Dermentzoglou V, Georgoulis P, Vakaki M, Kakavakis K. Scrotal hematocele as an unusual presentation of blunt abdominal trauma in three male infants. J Clin Ultrasound. 2000;28:190–3.
43. Talic RF. Unilateral traumatic hematocele–an unusual presentation of bilateral testicular rupture. Scand J Urol Nephrol. 1999;33:131–2.
44. Vaccaro JA, Davis R, Belville WD, Kiesling VJ. Traumatic hematocele: association with rupture of the testicle. J Urol. 1986;136:1217–8.
45. Jeffrey RB, Laing FC, Hricak H, McAninch JW. Sonography of testicular trauma. AJR Am J Roentgenol. 1983;141:993–5.
46. Cass AS, Luxenberg M. Value of early operation in blunt testicular contusion with hematocele. J Urol. 1988;139:746–7.
47. Satake H, Inoue K, Sawada K, Shuin T. A case of traumatic rupture of the testis: usefulness of magnetic resonance imaging. Hinyokika Kiyo. 2001;47: 341–3.
48. Haddad FS, Manne RK, Nathan MH. The pathological, ultrasonographic and computerized tomographic characteristics of chronic hematocele. J Urol. 1988;139:594–5.
49. Balogh K, Travis WD. The frequency of perineural ductules in vasitis nodosa. Am J Clin Pathol. 1984;82:710–3.
50. Balogh K, Travis WD. Benign vascular invasion in vasitis nodosa. Am J Clin Pathol. 1985;83:426–30.
51. Hirschowitz L, Rode J, Guillebaud J, Bounds W, Moss E. Vasitis nodosa and associated clinical findings. J Clin Pathol. 1988;41:419–23.
52. Schned AR, Selikowitz SM. Epididymitis nodosa. An epididymal lesion analogous to vasitis nodosa. Arch Pathol Lab Med. 1986;110:61–4.
53. Warner JJ, Kirchner Jr FK, Wong SW, Dao AH. Vasitis nodosa presenting as a mass of the spermatic cord. J Urol. 1983;129:380–1.
54. Woodward PJ, Schwab CM, Sesterhenn IA. From the archives of the AFIP: extratesticular scrotal masses: radiologic–pathologic correlation. Radiographics. 2003;23:215–40.
55. Dunner PS, Lipsit ER, Nochomovitz LE. Epididymal sperm granuloma simulating a testicular neoplasm. J Clin Ultrasound. 1982;10:353–5.
56. Giannarini G, Scott CA, Moro U, Grossetti B, Pomara G, Selli C. Cystic endometriosis of the epididymis. Urology. 2006;68:203. e1-3
57. Zámečník M, Hošťáková D. Endometriosis in a mesothelial cyst of tunica vaginalis of the testis. Report of a case. Cesk Patol. 2013;49:134–6.
58. Fukunaga M. Paratesticular endometriosis in a man with a prolonged hormonal therapy for prostatic carcinoma. Pathol Res Pract. 2012;208:59–61.
59. Young RH, Scully RE. Testicular and paratesticular tumors and tumor-like lesions of ovarian common epithelial and müllerian types. A report of four cases and review of the literature. Am J Clin Pathol. 1986;86:146–52.
60. Poppiti Jr RJ, Margulies M, Cabello B, Rywlin A. Membranous fat necrosis. Am J Surg Pathol. 1986;10:62–9.
61. Hakola P. Lipomembranous polycystic osteodysplasia. Acta Psychiatr Scand Suppl. 1972;232:1–72.
62. Nasu T, Tsukahara Y, Terayama K. A lipid metabolic disease -"membranous lipodystrophy"- an autopsy case demostrating numerous peculiar membrane-structures composed of compound lipids in bone and bone marrow and various adipose tisues. Acta Pathol Jpn. 1973;23:539–58.
63. Nistal M, Gonzalez-Peramato P, Paniagua R. Lipomembranous fat necrosis in three cases of testicular torsion. Histopathology. 2001;38:443–7.
64. Nistal M, Paniagua R. Non-neoplastic diseases of the testis. In: Bostwick DG, Cheng L, editors. Urological surgical pathology. 3rd ed. Philadelphia: Saunders; 2014. p. 560–735.
65. Nistal M, Iniguez L, Paniagua R. Histological classification of spermatic cord cysts in relation to their histogenesis. Eur Urol. 1987;13:327–30.
66. Aslam MZ, Kheradmund F, Patel NS, Turner G, Cranston D. Dermoid cyst of the spermatic cord: a rare cause of benign inguinal lump. Can Urol Assoc J. 2009;3:E29–30.
67. Graif A, Gakhal M, Iacocca MV, Levy HM. Ruptured extratesticular epidermal inclusion cyst mimicking polyorchidism with torsion on sonography. Emerg Radiol. 2014;21:643–5.
68. Skorniakov MS, Ramírez AC, Delgado MS, Durán AC, Bernal CS. Spermatic cord dermoid cyst as paratesticular mass. Case report and bibliographic review. Arch Esp Urol. 2011;64:991–4.
69. Prada-Arias M, Ortiz-Rey JA, Fernández-Eire P, Montero-Sánchez M, Lema-Carril A, Segade-Andrade R. Dermoid cyst of the spermatic cord in children. J Pediatr Surg. 2010;45:2058–60.
70. Erikçi V, Hoşgör M, Yıldız M, Aksoy N, Okur Ö, Örnek Y, Demircan Y. Torsion of an epididymal cyst: a case report and review of the literature. Turk J Pediatr. 2013;55:659–61.
71. Nistal M, González-Peramato P, Serrano A, Vega-Perez M, De Miguel MP, Regadera J. Paratesticular cysts with benign epithelial proliferations of wolffian origin. Am J Clin Pathol. 2005;124:245–51.
72. Ulbright TM, Young RH. Primary mucinous tumors of the testis and paratestis: a report of nine cases. Am J Surg Pathol. 2003;27:1221–8.
73. Bösmüller H, von Weyhern CH, Adam P, Alibegovic V, Mikuz G, Fend F. Paratesticular fibrous pseudotumor–an IgG4-related disorder? Virchows Arch. 2011;458:109–13.

74. Hart PA, Moyer AM, Yi ES, Hogan MC, Pearson RK, Chari ST. IgG4-related paratesticular pseudotumor in a patient with autoimmune pancreatitis and retroperitoneal fibrosis: an extrapancreatic manifestation of IgG4-related disease. Hum Pathol. 2012;43: 2084–7.
75. Migita K, Miyashita T, Mizuno A, Jiuchi Y, Ito M, Matsuo M, Izumi Y, Takeoka A, Nishino A, Hayashi M. IgG4-related epididymo-orchitis associated with bladder cancer: possible involvement of BAFF/BAFF-R interaction in IgG4-related urogenital disease. Mod Rheumatol. 2014;24:188–94.
76. Dieckmann KP, Struss WJ, Frey U, Nahler-Wildenhain M. Paratesticular fibrous pseudotumor in young males presenting with histological features of IgG4-related disease: two case reports. J Med Case Reports. 2013;7:225.
77. de Buy Wenniger LM, Scheltema JM, Verheij J, Beuers U. Testicular inflammation as a new manifestation of IgG4-associated disease. Urology. 2013;82:e15–6.
78. Karashima T, Taniguchi Y, Shimamoto T, et al. IgG4-related disease of the paratestis in a patient with Wells syndrome: a case report. Diagn Pathol. 2014;9:225.
79. Umehara H. A new clinical entity: IgG4-related disease (IgG4-RD) discovered in the 21st century. Intern Med. 2012;51:821–2.
80. Deshpande V, Zen Y, Chan JK, et al. Consensus statement on the pathology of IgG4-related disease. Mod Pathol. 2012;25:1181–92.
81. Oertel YC, Johnson FB. Sclerosing lipogranuloma of male genitalia. Review of 23 cases. Arch Pathol Lab Med. 1977;101:321–6.
82. Maki A, Tajima M, Nakayama K, Matsushima M, Ando K, Atobe T. A case of primary lipogranuloma of the spermatic cord. Hinyokika Kiyo. 1984;30:371–4.
83. Marzouk E. Spontaneous localized lipogranuloma of the spermatic cord. Ital J Surg Sci. 1989;19:261–4.
84. Kikugawa T, Tanji N, Kurihara K, Shishido S, Mannami M. Smooth muscle hyperplasia of the epididymis: a case report. Pathology. 2003;35:454–5.
85. Yang DM, Kim HC, Lee HL, Kim GY. Sonographic findings of smooth muscle hyperplasia of the epididymis. J Ultrasound Med. 2009;28:963–5.
86. Sun X, Gong Y, Pins MR. Pathologic quiz case: a paratesticular mass in a 55-year-old man. Arch Pathol Lab Med. 2003;127:E111–2.
87. Blach O, Pollock A, Douglas D. Smooth muscle hyperplasia of the epididymis. J Surg Case Rep. 2011;2011:10.
88. Barton JH, Davis Jr CJ, Sesterhenn IA, Mostofi FK. Smooth muscle hyperplasia of the testicular adnexa clinically mimicking neoplasia: clinicopathologic study of sixteen cases. Am J Surg Pathol. 1999;23:903–9.
89. Krichen Makni S, Mnif Hachicha L, Ellouze S, Mnif M, Khabir A, Ketata H, Abid M, Sellami Boudawara T. Feminizing testicular syndrome with multiple hamartomas and bilateral paratesticular leiomyomas. Rev Med Interne. 2005;26: 980–3.
90. Goulis DG, Iliadou PK, Papanicolaou A, Georgiou I, Chatzikyriakidou A, Gerou S, Bondis IN, Papadimas I. R831X mutation of the androgen receptor gene in an adolescent with complete androgen insensitivity syndrome and bilateral testicular hamartomata. Hormones. 2006;5:200–4.
91. Nuciforo PG, Roncalli M. Pathologic quiz case: a scrotal sac mass incidentally discovered during autopsy. Arch Pathol Lab Med. 2003;127:239–40.
92. Fridman E, Skarda J, Ofek-Moravsky E, Cordoba M. Complex multilocular cystic lesion of rete testis, accompanied by smooth muscle hyperplasia, mimicking intratesticular Leydig cell neoplasm. Virchows Arch. 2005;447:768–71.

38 Intratesticular and Paratesticular Patterns of Mesonephric Remnants

Manuel Nistal, Pilar González-Peramato, and Álvaro Serrano

38.1 Structures Derived from Embryonic Remnants

The origin, structure, and pathology related to classic embryonic remnants are well known. The appendix of the testis (sessile hydatid of Morgagni) originates from the cephalic end of the Müllerian duct. Among the pathologies related to the hydatid, hydatid cystic transformation, torsion [1, 2], and tumoral degeneration [3, 4] stand out. The appendix of the epididymis (pediculate hydatid of Morgagni) is a remnant of the cephalic end of the Wolffian duct. Sometimes it may suffer a significant cystic transformation [5], torsion [6], and exceptionally a tumor [7]. Upper and lower aberrant ducts (Haller's organ) are mesonephric duct remnants located in the fissure between the testis and the epididymis [8]. Cystic transformation and torsion of the lower aberrant duct have been observed [9]. The paradidymis (Giraldés organ, Henles's paraepididymis, or innominate body), derives from the caudal mesonephric ducts. Torsion [10] and cystic transformation [11] of the paradidymis have also been reported, but not with the presence of other embryonic remains in the paratesticular structures or even in the testicle itself.

38.2 Histological Characteristics of the Mesonephric Remnants

Mesonephric remnants have been reported in virtually all parts of the male urogenital tract: kidney [12], renal pelvis [13], prostate [14, 15], prostatic urethra [16], and paratesticular structures [17]. One of the most surprising findings is the wide variety of histological patterns the embryonic remnants show. Often they are structures constituted by small acini/tubules lined by cuboidal or low columnar epithelium with or without colloid-like material inside, and less frequently as ductal formations reminiscent of efferent ducts, epididymis, or vas deferens due to its epithelium features (columnar or pseudostratified, sometimes ciliated), and condensed mesenchymal tissue around it. However, these remnants differ from the abovementioned normal ducts in that their lumen diameter is smaller (0.17 mm), in that such size does not increase with age, and in the absence of a true smooth muscle wall [18, 19].

The evidence of mesonephric remnants is completed by the immunohistochemical study that also allows to separate them from the

M. Nistal et al., *Clues in the Diagnosis of Non-tumoral Testicular Pathology*,
DOI 10.1007/978-3-319-49364-0_38

Müllerian remains. CD10 [20] is strongly positive in both the brush border of tubular formations reminiscent of the epididymis and vas deferens and the accompanying stroma, but it is negative in tubular and acinar structures. pP63 is expressed only in the basal cells of epithelia that resemble those of the epididymis and vas deferens. GATA3 and BCL2 react with the epididymis and vas deferens-like epithelium and some epithelia of acinar and glandular structures. PAX8 is strongly reactive in all epithelial structures.

38.3 Testicular and Paratesticular Mesonephric Remnants

Particularly interesting are the mesonephric remains that can be seen in the spermatic cord, the wall of hernial sacs, the testicular hydatid, the tunica vaginalis, and the testicle.

38.3.1 Mesonephric Remnants in the Spermatic Cord

In 28 % of the spermatic cords studied in autopsy of both adults and children, embryonic remnants have been observed. The material included a section proximal to the testicle, another one at a medium level, and the last one at a high level of the spermatic cord [21]. Most of it corresponded to mesonephric remnants. A variety of papillary and cystic benign lesions have been described in connection with these structures [4] (Fig. 38.1).

38.3.2 Mesonephric Remnants in Hernial Sacs

The incidence of glandular inclusions in the hernial sac walls of infants varies according to the series studied: 1.5 % [22], 2.6 % [19], 2.9 % [23], and 6 % [24] (Fig. 38.2). The highest peak is reached at the age of 4 months. The incidence reported in adults is remarkably lower, probably because the number of adult samples examined is much reduced. From 39 hernial sacs with epithelial inclusions studied by Cerili et al. in 2003 [20], nine corresponded to vas deferens-like, 13 to epididymis-like, and seven to Müllerian-like structures (Fig. 38.3).

38.3.3 Mesonephric Remnants in the Testicular Hydatid

The presence of tubular epididymis-like structures (aberrant epididymal tissue) in the testicular

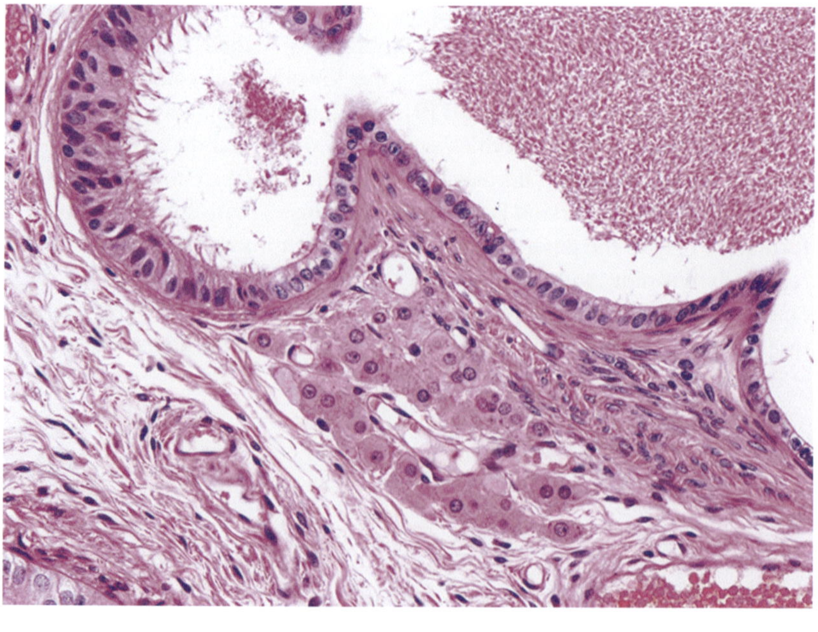

Fig. 38.1 Mesonephric remnants in the spermatic cord. The cystic formation has a lining which combines two areas. One area is reminiscent of the epididymal main duct epithelium because of its pseudostratified appearance and the presence of stereocilia. The other area shows cuboidal cells mimicking those of efferent ductules. In neighboring tissue a group of Leydig cells is shown

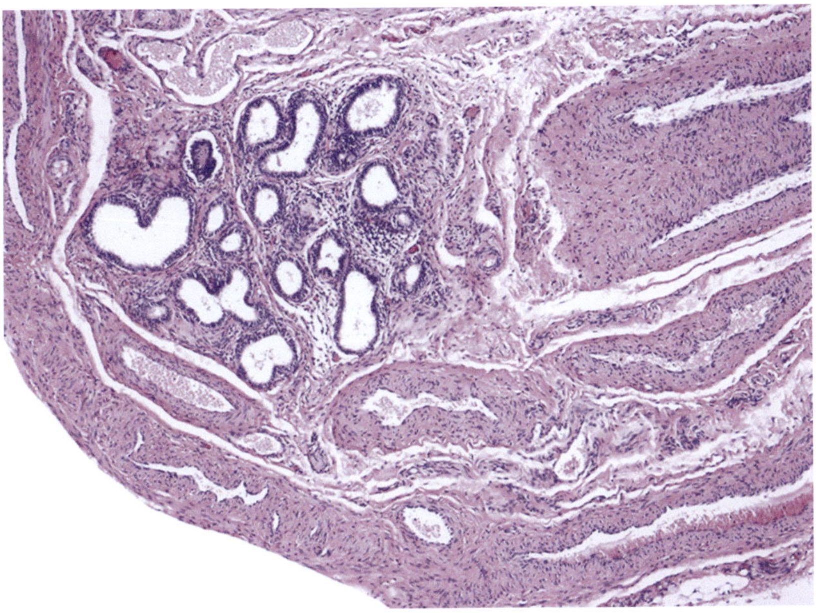

Fig. 38.2 Mesonephric remnants in the wall of a hernial sac. Group consisting in a dozen of glandular formations embedded in a dense stroma

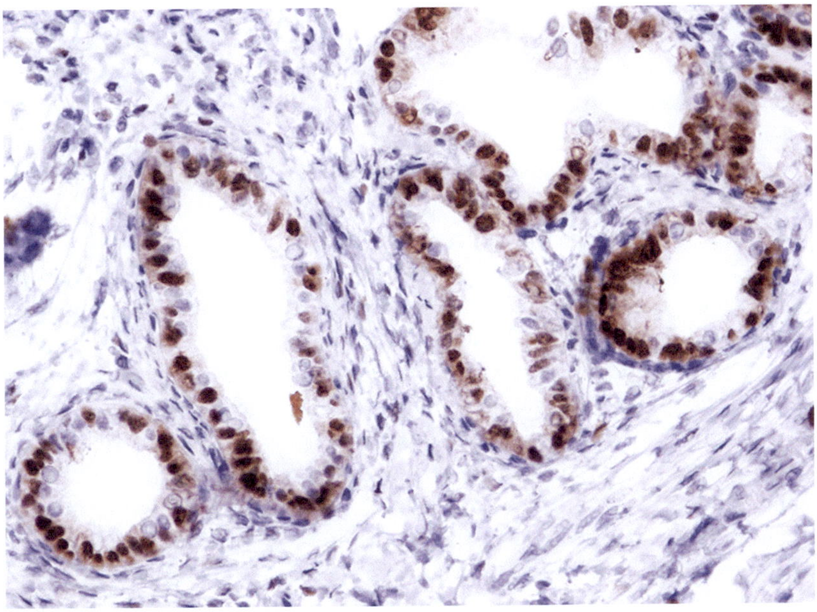

Fig. 38.3 Embryonal remnants in the wall of a hernia sac simulating efferent ducts. All epithelial cells have androgen receptor expression

hydatid is exceptional. It has been described in a 7-year-old boy with undescended testis found when the surgeon performed an orchidopexy and removed a pedunculated testicular appendage [25]. A second case has been observed in our department. The tubular formations in the first case were lying in loose stroma of the hydatid and showed no connection with the epithelial lining, but they formed cluster tubules with columnar epithelium surrounded by a layer of smooth muscle cells (Fig. 38.4). They showed no clear differentiation with efferent ductules or with the main duct of the epididymis, but they showed positivity with CD10 on the adluminal membrane, contrasting with the negativity of the epithelial lining of the hydatid. They could be considered immature epididymal structures. In the second case, to which the iconography in this chapter corresponds, the

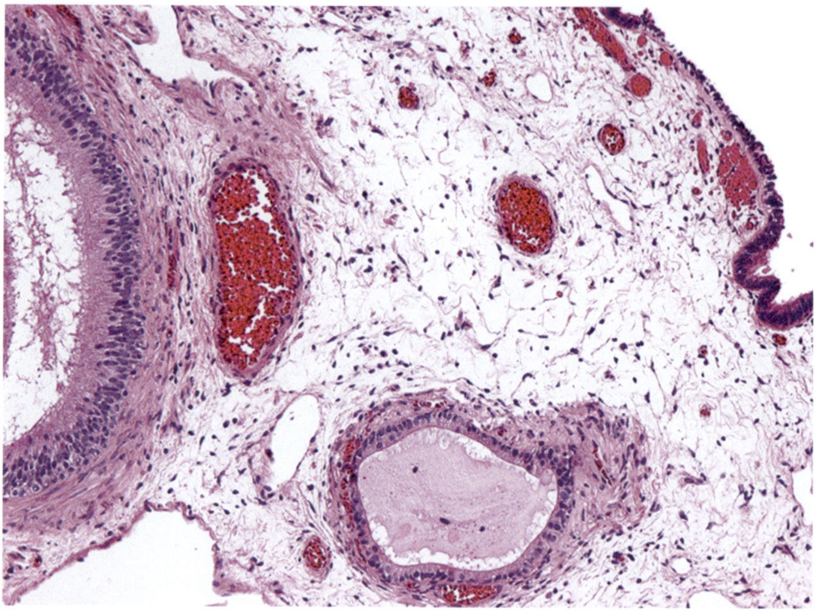

Fig. 38.4 Mesonephric remnants in the testicular hydatid. Two ducts lying in loose connective tissue of the hydatid are recognized. The largest one shows differentiation toward the main duct of the epididymis, and the smallest differentiates to efferent ductules

cluster of tubular formations had a pseudostratified epithelium with eosinophilic intranuclear inclusions, basal cells, and long stereocilia with intense adluminal positivity with CD10. An important layer of smooth muscle cells was arranged around the epithelial tubules. The structures were similar to the main duct of the epididymis. The explanation for the presence of mesonephric derivatives in a structure considered to be Müllerian is unknown. The very interesting and thorough work by Jacob and Barteczko in 2005 [26] on the embryological origin of the hydatid can shed some light on this matter. Other than hydatids of the testis and the epididymis, the authors describe a third type of hydatid, which could be found in the same locations as the previous ones, with a tubulus inside that is considered the remnant of a cystic mesonephric tubule.

38.3.4 Mesonephric Remains in the Tunica Vaginalis

Cysts of the tunica albuginea are sometimes mesothelial and sometimes originated in embryonic remnants. The epithelium of some cysts is similar to the epithelium of the efferent ductules, and so they can be considered of a mesonephric origin [27, 28].

38.3.5 Intratesticular Mesonephric Remnants

The presence of intratesticular structures resembling efferent ductules and also resembling the main duct of the epididymis was described by Nistal et al. in 2006 [29] in six patients in the course of a review of 1442 autopsies and 271 surgical specimens of adult men. The lesions were bilateral in five autopsy cases and unilateral in the surgical case. In six testes there were lesions affecting the testicular parenchyma next to the rete testis, in another four they affected the peripheral testicular parenchyma, and in one case they were both central and peripheral. The age of the patients ranged from 69 to 75 years. The iconography belongs to the study of a new case sent as consultation and was observed in a surgical specimen of a 67-year-old patient who was studied due to hypogonadism and showed a sonographic image suggestive of a testicular tumor.

Histopathology All of them had decreased testicular size. The cut showed multiple whitish areas of irregular contours alternating with testicular parenchyma. All patients had a small hydrocele. No macroscopic alterations were observed in the epididymis or the paratesticular structures. Histologically, most mesonephric remnants corresponded to epididymis-like structures, some were efferent-like, and only occasionally tubular or acinar formations were observed. The size of the tubular formations was highly variable; some were the same size as seminiferous tubules while others were cystically dilated up to 1 mm in diameter (Fig. 38.5). The contours of the longest formations were irregular with protrusions into the testicular parenchyma.

The epithelium of most tubes had basal cells, cylindrical cells with stereocilia, and eosinophilic inclusions in the nucleus as epididymal principal cells (Fig. 38.6). Cellular atypia or mitosis was not observed. In other patients the epithelium was cylindrical with ciliated cells similar to the efferent ductules. The interior of the tubular formations

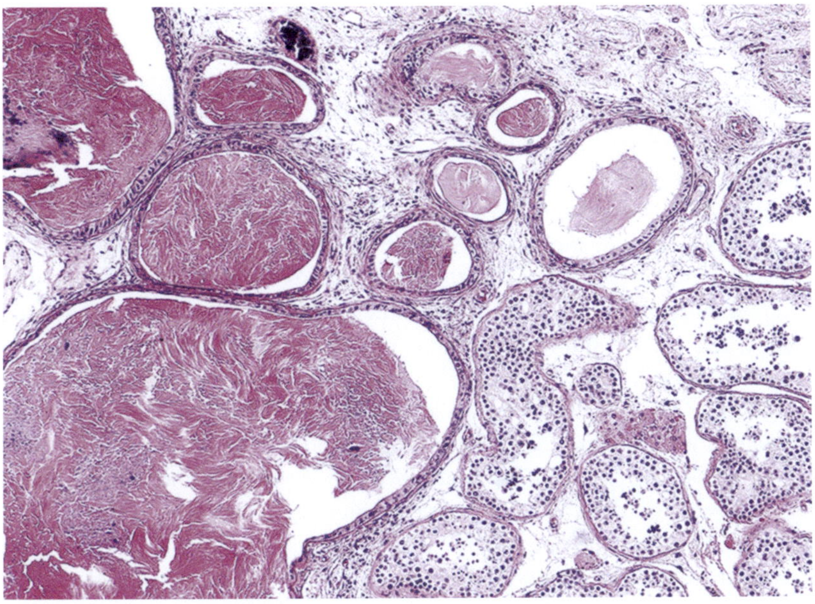

Fig. 38.5 Intratesticular mesonephric remnants. Numerous cystic formations of different sizes with eosinophilic content located among the seminiferous tubules

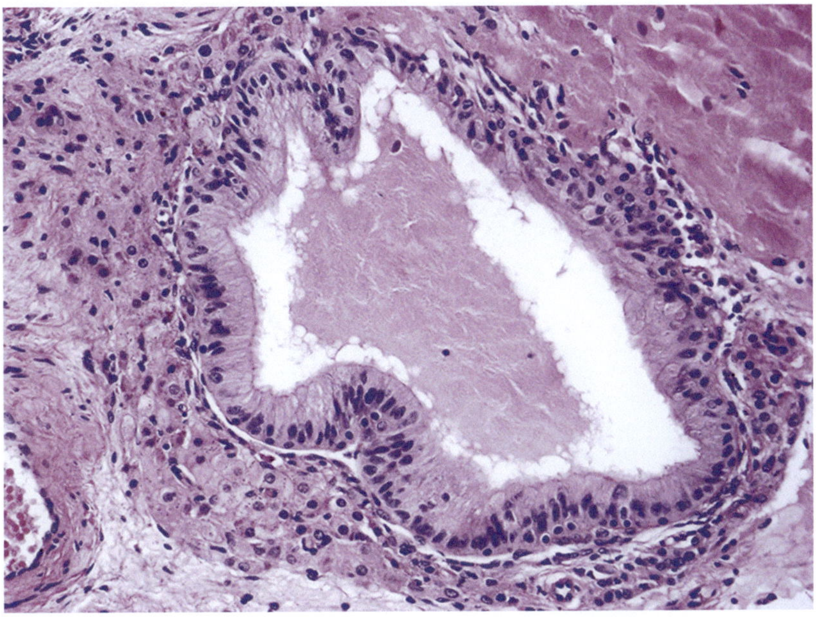

Fig. 38.6 Intratesticular mesonephric remnants. Ductal tubule lined by pseudostratified epithelium with stereocilia. It is partially surrounded by abundant Leydig cells

was occupied by an eosinophilic, granular, or fibrillar material, positive for PAS and Alcian Blue, with Liesegang rings. The thickness of the wall was variable, from a layer of smooth muscle cells around to more than half a dozen concentric layers of muscle cells.

The interstitium was expanded and extravasation of intratubular material could be observed, as well as a minimum lymphoid infiltrate and Leydig cell groups that were identified both in the interstitium and surrounding the epididymis-like structures. The microliths were frequent both inside the tubules and their walls and in the extravasation material (Fig. 38.7).

In three cases the testicular parenchyma showed completely hyalinized seminiferous tubules and in the rest of cases a mosaic of lesions including hyalinized tubules, dilated tubules, and tubules with marked atrophy of the seminiferous epithelium. Leydig cells were very scarce in four cases. All testes showed vascular lesions of arteriosclerosis.

The rete testis was atrophic in all cases. Two cases had lesions of intracavitary nodular proliferation, and four cases had microlithiasis. In five epididymides focal atrophy of efferent ductules was observed, and in two epididymides abundant microliths in the lumen were observed.

The immunohistochemical study of the tubular formations showed positivity in the basal cells for high-weight keratins and CK8,18,19 in most epithelial cells. Only the basal cells were p63 positive. Androgen receptor was expressed in most cylindrical cells of the efferent and epididymis-like structures. And intense adluminal CD10 positivity was observed in all kinds of tubular formations. Smooth muscle cells positive for smooth muscle actin were seen in the outer layer (Fig. 38.8).

The histological pattern of intratesticular Müllerian remnants is similar to the one described in other organs such as the kidney [30, 31] and prostate [32]. The predominance of the most differentiated efferent-like, epididymis-like structures against the tubular/alveolar pattern should be emphasized. In three cases the mesonephric remnants occupied more than half of the testicular parenchyma so the diagnosis of florid hyperplasia of the Müllerian remnants seems reasonable.

The differential diagnosis of intratesticular mesonephric remnants can be raised with teratomas and burned germ cell tumors. Teratomas appear on enlarged testicles, which do not occur in testicles with mesonephric remnants. Teratomas, including organoid teratomas, lack a

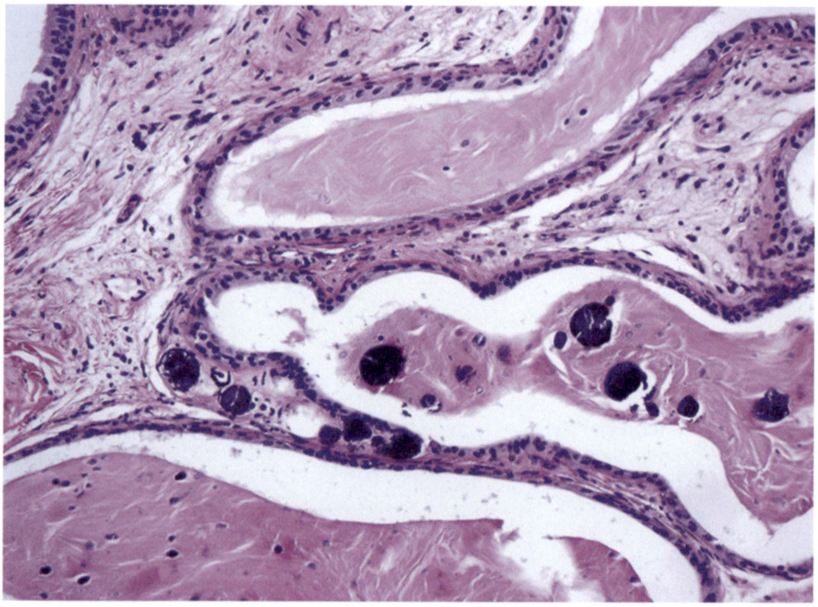

Fig. 38.7 Intratesticular mesonephric remnants. Eosinophilic material inside cystic formations shows several calcifications. These also are evident outside the tubules

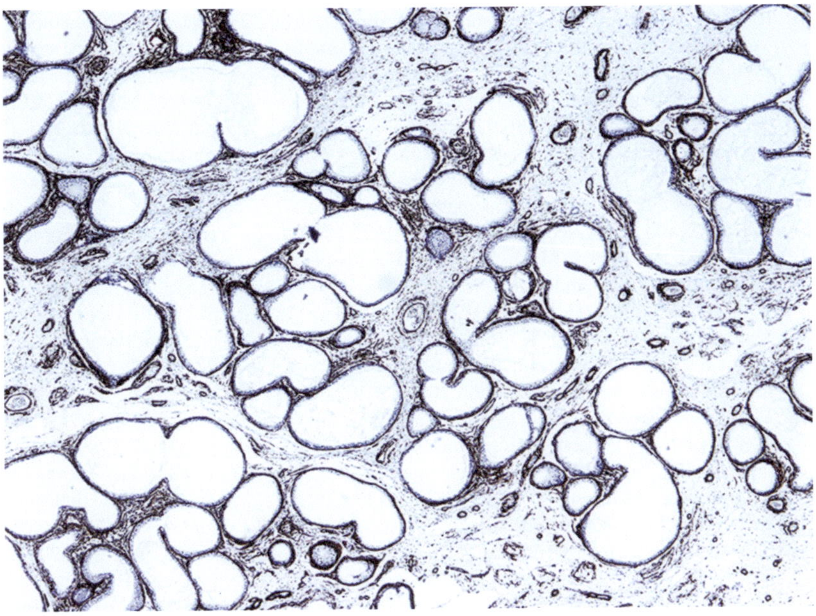

Fig. 38.8 Intratesticular mesonephric remnants. The wall of various formations shows an outer layer of smooth muscle cells as evidenced by immunostaining for smooth muscle actin

tubular development with a repetitive structure that reminds epididymal ducts. They have other mesodermal or ectodermal derivatives. And they are often accompanied by another germ cell tumor or germ cell neoplasia in situ. Burned out tumors are associated with normal or decreased in size testes and may contain some cysts and calcifications. However, they always show an area of scar fibrosis, the cysts contain keratin, the calcifications are amorphous, and there may be remains of another germ cell tumor and also intratubular germ cell neoplasia in situ.

The origin of the intratesticular mesonephric remnants could be found at a very early developmental abnormality of the gonad, when the mesonephros and the coelomic epithelium are practically in contact with one another. Mesonephric cells could be trapped between the nests of pre-Sertoli cells and germ cells before these constitute the testicular cords and produce AMH that determines the formation of the tunica and therefore the delimitation of the testicle. A second hypothesis for the epididymis metaplasia of Sertoli cell is suggested by the distribution of epididymal tubules among the seminiferous tubules whether they have spermatogenesis or not, but there is no data to support this hypothesis.

References

1. Nicolay L, Gitlin J, Palmer LS. Torsion of the appendix testis in an undescended testis: a case report. Can J Urol. 2013;20:6805–7.
2. Meher S, Rath S, Sharma R, Sasmal PK, Mishra TS. Torsion of a large appendix testis misdiagnosed as pyocele. Case Rep Urol. 2015;2015:430871.
3. Kernohan NM, Coutts AG, Best PV. Cystadenocarcinoma of the appendix testis. Histopathology. 1990;17:147–54.
4. Nistal M, González-Peramato P, Serrano A, Vega-Perez M, De Miguel MP, Regadera J. Paratesticular cysts with benign epithelial proliferations of wolffian origin. Am J Clin Pathol. 2005;124:245–51.
5. Kantarci F, Ozer H, Adaletli I, Mihmanli I. Cystic appendix epididymis: a sonomorphologic study. Surg Radiol Anat. 2005;27:557–61.
6. Remzi D, Erkan I, Yazicioglu A. Torsion of appendix epididymis. N Y State J Med. 1980;80:646–7.
7. Krukowski ZH, Auld CD. Torsion of the appendix epididymis in a maldescended testis. Br J Urol. 1983;55:244–5.
8. Wollin M, Marshall FF, Fink MP, Malhotra R, Diamond DA. Aberrant epididymal tissue: a significant clinical entity. J Urol. 1987;138:1247–50.
9. Virdi JS, Conway W, Kelly DG. Torsion of the vas aberrans. Br J Urol. 1990;66:435.
10. Orazi C, Fariello G, Malena S, Caterino S, Ferro F. Torsion of paradidymis or Giraldes´ organ: an uncommon cause of acute scrotum in pediatric age group. J Clin Ultrasound. 1989;17:598–601.
11. Schned AR, Seremetis GM, Rous SN. Paratesticular multicystic mass of wolffian, probably paradidymal, origin. Am J Clin Pathol. 1994;101:543–6.

12. Rizzardi C, Brollo A, Thomann B, Santirocco C, Melato M. Intra-abdominal ovarian-type mucinous cystadenoma associated with fallopian tube-like structure and aberrant epididymal tissue in a male patient. Hum Pathol. 2005;36:927–31.
13. Andersen CB, Horn T, Rasmussen F, Larsen S. Mesonephric remnants involving renal pelvis and prostatic urethra: a diagnostic problem towards adenocarcinoma. Scand J Urol Nephrol Suppl. 1994;157:119–22.
14. Bostwick DG, Qian J, Ma J, Muir TE. Mesonephric remnants of the prostate: incidence and histologic spectrum. Mod Pathol. 2003;16:630–5.
15. Yacoub M, Milin S, Irani J, Fromont G. Mesonephric remnant hyperplasia: an unusual benign mimicker of prostate cancer. Ann Diagn Pathol. 2009;13:402–4.
16. Malpica A, Ro JY, Troncoso P, Ordoñez NG, Amin MB, Ayala AG. Nephrogenic adenoma of the prostatic urethra involving the prostate gland: a clinicopathologic and immunohistochemical study of eight cases. Hum Pathol. 1994;25:390–5.
17. Saito S, Higa I, Koyama Y, Hatano T, Hayakawa M, Osawa A, Toda T. Immature renal tissue in inguinal canal. J Urol. 1989;142:106–7.
18. Gill B, Favale D, Kogan SJ, Bennett B, Reda E, Levitt SB. Significance of accessory ductal structures in hernia sacs. J Urol. 1992;148:697–8.
19. Gomez-Roman JJ, Mayorga M, Mira C, Buelta L, Fernandez F, Val-Bernal JF. Glandular inclusions in inguinal hernia sacs: a clinicopathological study of six cases. Pediatr Pathol. 1994;14:1043–9.
20. Cerilli LA, Sotelo-Avila C, Mills SE. Glandular inclusions in inguinal hernia sacs: morphologic and immunohistochemical distinction from epididymis and vas deferens. Am J Surg Pathol. 2003;27:469–76.
21. Nistal M, Iñiguez L, Paniagua R, Redondo E, Regadera J. Tubular embryonal remmants in the human spermatic cord. Urol Int. 1987;42:260–4.
22. Popek EJ. Embryonal remmants in inguinal hernia sacs. Hum Pathol. 1990;21:339–49.
23. Steigman CK, Sotelo-Avila C, Weber TR. The incidence of spermatic cord structures in inguinal hernia sacs from male children. Am J Surg Pathol. 1999;23:880–5.
24. Walker AN, Mills SE. Glandular inclusions in inguinal hernial sacs and spermatic cords: Müllerian-like remmants confused with functional reproductive structures. Am J Clin Pathol. 1984;82:85–9.
25. Val-Bernal JF, Val D, Garijo MF. Ectopic epididymal tissue in appendix testis. Virchows Arch. 2006;449:373–5.
26. Jacob M, Barteczko K. Contribution to the origin and development of the appendices of the testis and epididymis in humans. Anat Embryol (Berl). 2005;209:287–302.
27. Nistal M, Iñiguez L, Paniagua R. Cysts of the testicular parenchyma and tunica albuginea. Arch Pathol Lab Med. 1989;113:902–6.
28. Tanaka K, Kamidono S, Yoshimura K, Umezu K. Benign cystic lesion of the tunica albuginea: a case report. Hinyokika Kiyo. 2004;50:45–8.
29. Nistal M, García-Cabezas MA, Castello MC, De Miguel MP, Regadera J. Age-related epididymis-like intratesticular structures: benign lesions of Wolffian origin that can be misdiagnosed as testicular tumors. J Androl. 2006;27:79–85.
30. Ma XM, Liu HF, Wang LZ, Xia CY, Ge JH, Li YL, He J, Ye XD, Liu HM. Epididymal tissue in the dilated portion of a dysgenetic kidney with an ipsilateral seminal vesicle cyst and ectopic ureteral insertion. Asian J Androl. 2010;12:281–3.
31. Xiao GQ, Jerome JG, Wu G. Unilateral hypoplastic kidney and ureter associated with diverse mesonephric remnant hyperplasia. Am J Clin Exp Urol. 2015;3:107–11. eCollection 2015.
32. Chen YB, Fine SW, Epstein JI. Mesonephric remnant hyperplasia involving prostate and periprostatic tissue: findings at radical prostatectomy. Am J Surg Pathol. 2011;35:1054–61.

39 Testicular Changes in Elderly Men

Manuel Nistal, Pilar González-Peramato, and
Álvaro Serrano

39.1 Introduction

The testicular functions are both exocrine (spermatogenesis) and endocrine (androgen secretion), although there are large interindividual differences, and they slowly and progressively decline over the years [1]. It is a proven fact that the frequency of sexual dysfunction increases with age [2], and fertility decreases after 40 [3]. There is also a broad consensus that a significant loss of these functions occur between 65 and 70 years. To describe the gradual decline of male sexual function over the years, the terms "male climacteric" [4], "male menopause," or "andropause" [5] have been introduced. Today the terms "symptomatic" androgen deficiency in aging men (ADAM), "aging male syndrome," or even better "symptomatic" late-onset hypogonadism (LOH) [6, 7] are considered more appropriate.

The aging process affects both the structure and the function of the testes and in general of the whole male genital tract. The mechanisms involved in these changes may be of vascular, endocrine, and genetic type [8, 9]. Hormonal changes experienced by men with age, followed by testicular abnormalities, are successively exposed in this chapter. Finally, the mechanisms that are probably involved in their development are discussed.

39.2 Hormonal Changes with Age

The hypothalamic-pituitary-gonadal axis of older men experiences functional changes that lead to various changes in their hormone profiles. The hormonal profile and its configuration have no consistent and distinct patterns, since many factors such as inheritance [10], body mass index [11], smoking habit (plasma testosterone levels are higher in senior smokers than in nonsmokers) [12], or stress [13] are involved.

Testosterone levels decline with age from the third decade onward by 0.4–2 % per year [14]. Declining testosterone is more pronounced for the fraction of bioavailable free hormone, which may be due to increased levels and the binding capacity of sex hormone-binding protein (SHBP) [15–17]. The free testosterone level begins to decrease around 40, while the total testosterone remains relatively constant up to a very advanced age (80–90 years). Diseases, other comorbid conditions, and medications can exacerbate the decline.

LOH is a clinical and biochemical syndrome present in elderly patients and characterized by secondary symptoms of deficiency in serum testosterone levels. Hypogonadism is estimated to be present in 3.1–7.0 % of men between 30 and 69 years, and in 18.4 % of those over 70 years

M. Nistal et al., *Clues in the Diagnosis of Non-tumoral Testicular Pathology*,
DOI 10.1007/978-3-319-49364-0_39

[18]. The most frequent manifestations of the syndrome are low libido, erectile dysfunction, lower muscular mass and strength, increased body fat, decreased bone mineral density and osteoporosis, and decreased vitality and a depressed mood. The minimum criteria for the diagnosis of LOH are the presence of three sexual symptoms (decreased libido, morning erections, and erectile dysfunction) combined with a total testosterone level of less than 11 nmol/l and a free testosterone level of less than 220 pmol/l [19]. Hypogonadism may be primary and secondary. Secondary hypogonadism is six to seven times more common than primary and is associated more with obesity than with age, being particularly prevalent in middle-aged men. Primary hypogonadism is directly associated with age and comorbidity.

The existence of a *primary hypogonadism* is supported by a series of changes that occur in all testicular structures and specifically Leydig cells and Sertoli cells. Regarding Leydig cells, their number has been observed to decrease with age [20], the response to hCG stimulation is lowered [21], there is a decrease in steroid synthesis, and measurements of androgens in the spermatic vein yield low numbers [22]. Testosterone metabolites (estrogen, dihydrotestosterone) begin to gradually decline after 40 and have clearly descended over 80 [23]. The result is an increase in LH that in some men can reach up to 110 % compared to young individuals. In some cases this overstimulation would be sufficient to produce Leydig cell hypertrophy and maintain normal testosterone levels.

Target cells for FSH are the Sertoli cells. With age these cells show significant morphological changes that can justify increased FSH in senior patients [24]. Inhibin concentration decreases with age: at 40 years there are already detectable changes so it is likely that the Sertoli cells are affected even earlier than the Leydig cells [25, 26]. Serum FSH levels are negatively correlated to daily sperm production [20, 27].

Secondary hypogonadism is more common in the elderly with an associated pathology. Changes in the hypothalamic-pituitary axis occur with age that result secondarily in testicular damage. Nictameral variations in testosterone levels have been found to disappear [12, 28, 29]; the number of LH secretory pulses, both immunoreactive LH [29] and bioactive LH, decreases [30]; the frequency of the high-amplitude LH pulse decreases [31]; there is a failure in the ability to maintain normal testosterone levels in men with an adequate reserve of Leydig cells and gonadotropic cells [4]; and there is decreased or no response of LH to antiestrogens or antiopiates [32] and increased sensitivity of gonadotropic cells to the negative feedback of sex hormones [33]. The use of testosterone therapy in LOH seems to offer more benefits than contraindications [34] although the indication is preferential in primary hypogonadism [35].

39.3 Morphological Alterations of the Testes

The human testis undergoes involution with age. The lesions observed show great interindividual variation, but they may also be different in the testes of the same individual [36]. There is a significant decrease of testicular volume in elderly patients [37]. In our series testicular volume is decreased in 85 % of the individuals, and this decrease correlates with a decrease in the volume of the seminiferous tubules. The average weight of the testicle is lower in most cases, and this corresponds to a decrease of the testicular parenchyma [38]. The tunica albuginea undergoes changes in its thickness, structure, and weight. The thickness of the tunica can reach 900 microns [37, 39] compared to 400–450 microns of young adults, but this thickening only occurs when the vaginal tunica presents with reactive changes (Fig. 39.1). This increase probably depends more on the decreased testicular parenchyma than on the hypertrophy or hyperplasia of the elements that constitute it.

39.3.1 Seminiferous Tubules

Changes in length, diameter, number of diverticula, thickness of the lamina propria, decrease in

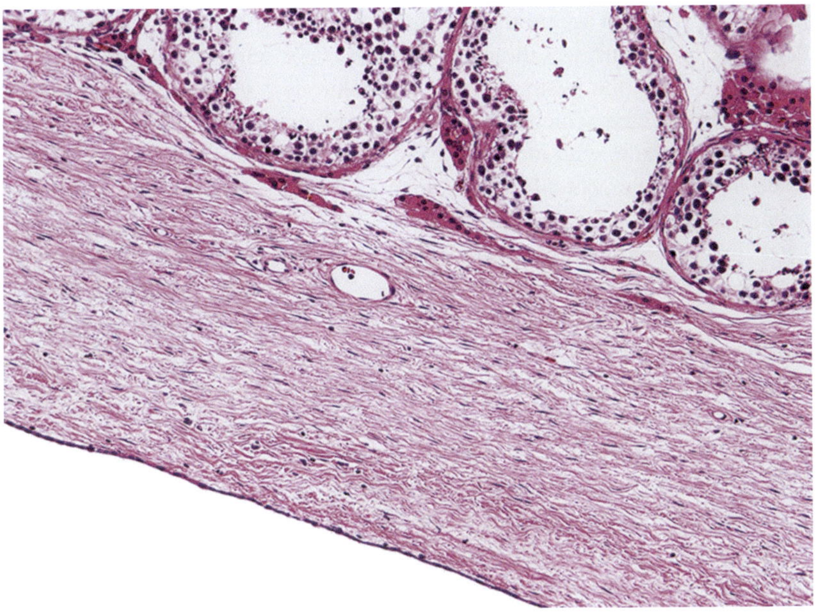

Fig. 39.1 Tunica albuginea undergoes loss of cellularity with increased collagen fibers. The seminiferous tubules show dilated lumen and preserved spermatogenesis

height of the seminiferous epithelium, and quantitative and qualitative alterations of germ cells have been described.

Tubular Length Shortening of the seminiferous tubules that occurs with age has been estimated at 25 %, probably being much higher in the seminiferous tubules that show a greater grade of atrophy of the seminiferous epithelium.

Tubular Diameter The tubular diameter always depends on two facts: the height of the seminiferous epithelium and the breadth of the tubular lumen. In most senior patients, there is a significant atrophy of the seminiferous epithelium, and although the tubular lumen is generally increased, the tubular diameter is often reduced. But the amplitude of the lumen may be equally important in some cases in which the seminiferous tubules can reach more than 300 microns in diameter. The most interesting fact is that the tubular diameter does not decrease regularly throughout the testicle, but appears in a patchy pattern in the testicle varying from one to another lobule [40].

Diverticula In elderly patients the number of diverticula is increased, and this is a consistent finding in all testes studied in patients over 70 years of age. Their number and size is greater in those with obstructive disease of the spermatic ducts [41].

Tubular Wall The normal thickness of the lamina propria of the seminiferous tubules is five microns in young adults. In older men this structure undergoes a progressive thickening parallel to a decrease in the height of the seminiferous epithelium. More than 55 % of men over 65 have a lamina propria more than ten microns thick. Another important event that occurs with age is the changes experienced by the peritubular cells and specifically the myoid cells. A dedifferentiation process has been observed in which those cells adopt the appearance of fibroblasts [41].

Seminiferous Epithelium Huge differences in the degree of development of the seminiferous epithelium from one to another individual, between the testicles, and even in some lobules as compared to others within the same testicle have been observed in senior patients. They range from patients with a normal spermatogenesis to those showing varying degrees of hypospermatogenesis, generally associated with spermatocyte sloughing and tubular ectasia. Common findings are the presence of one or more groups of hyalinized seminiferous tubules between preserved seminiferous tubules. The degree of involvement of the germline is also not uniform within the testis. Some seminiferous tubules are detected, which in serial studies belong to the same lobule, with identical lesions as compared to each other, but different from those of the seminiferous tubules of neighboring lobules. All cells in the seminiferous epithelium undergo changes with age.

Sertoli Cells Sertoli cells suffer changes both in the number and in morphology and function upon aging [42]. The Sertoli cell population is estimated to be 500 million per testicle between the ages of 20 and 48, a number that drops to approximately 300 million per testis in men aged 50–85 years [43]. This reduction is not evident in the transverse tubular sections that maintain a stable number of Sertoli cells; it is only explicable by the marked shortening of the length of the seminiferous tubule [44].

Many Sertoli cells undergo morphological changes. It is estimated that 50 % show typical adult Sertoli cell characteristics, 30 % show an abundant accumulation of lipids, 8 % show intense cytoplasmic vacuolization, 4 % are multinucleated, and 7 % are dedifferentiated [45]. Lipid accumulation is a gradual process that starts at age 15 and intensifies in patients older than 70 years [46]. In the young adult lipids, they are located in the basal cell cytoplasm [47]. Another characteristic feature of old age is supranuclear location.

Cytoplasmic vacuolization is another fact that is accentuated with age. Vacuoles are preferably located at the apical pole. They are surrounded by a membrane that retains the adjacent cytoplasm specializations that are common between Sertoli cells and germ cells (spermatocytes and spermatids), which represent extracellular spaces that would have been occupied by germ cells.

When aging, Sertoli cells tend to form syncytia. In senior men, bi- and trinucleated cells are frequent [46, 48]. Their number is higher in the tubules containing Sertoli cells only [49]. These cells probably arise by a cytoplasmic fusion mechanism. The Sertoli cells of the tubules have low or no spermatogenesis and show increased vimentin filaments and reexpression of keratin filaments [50].

Germ Cells If even in young men there is a potential loss of spermatogenesis that has been estimated between 36 and 45 % [51, 52], in elderly patients these figures soar. The low rate of cell proliferation, the high number of abnormal cells, and frequent phenomena of apoptosis [53] are inscribed among the causes of low spermatogenesis in the elderly. Cell loss occurs mostly during meiosis and increases with the withdrawal or lowering of testosterone levels and gonadotropins [54, 55].

Spermatogonia Aging forces spermatogonia to undergo changes in number, morphology, and distribution. The number of Ap and Ad types of spermatogonia decreases with age. Ap spermatogonia begin to disappear by 50 and Ad by 60 [56]. At the same time, there is an increase in the number of multinucleated spermatogonia [57] (Fig. 39.2). The same cell can contain nuclei with characteristic Ad and Ap spermatogonia [58]. These cells slough into the tubular lumen or else they degenerate [59]. Spermatogonia with large nuclei (greater than eight microns in nuclear size), probably diploid cells, are very common in old age. Giant spermatogonia or hypertrophic spermatogonia (larger nuclear size, nine to ten microns) also increase with age [60, 61]. These are probably formed by DNA cell replication that is not followed by cell division [62]. Dislocated spermatogonia also increase with age – they can be seen forming several layers in 75 % of patients over 65 years [63].

Spermatocytes A decrease in the number of first-order spermatocytes, a tendency to binucleation, and meiosis alterations are noticed with age. This decrease would be secondary to a poor number of spermatogonia, to a defect in the early stages of meiosis, or to early sloughing in patients with obstruction of the spermatic pathway [56]. First-order spermatocytes are frequently multinucleated

[57, 59, 64–66]. Even though occasionally observed in young men with and without another pathology, the number of megalospermatocytes rises in 64 % of men over 65 [63] (Fig. 39.3). Megalospermatocytes are shifted to the adluminal compartment where some disintegrate and are phagocytosed by Sertoli cells, and others are released to the lumen.

Young Spermatids With age, a decrease of young spermatids and an increase of multinucleated forms are observed. Multinucleated spermatids increase in parallel with age [66]. About 10 % of men over 60 years with some kind of germline lesion present with bi- and trinucleate spermatogonia compared to 1.4 % of young adults [57]. The number of nuclei that can be observed in the

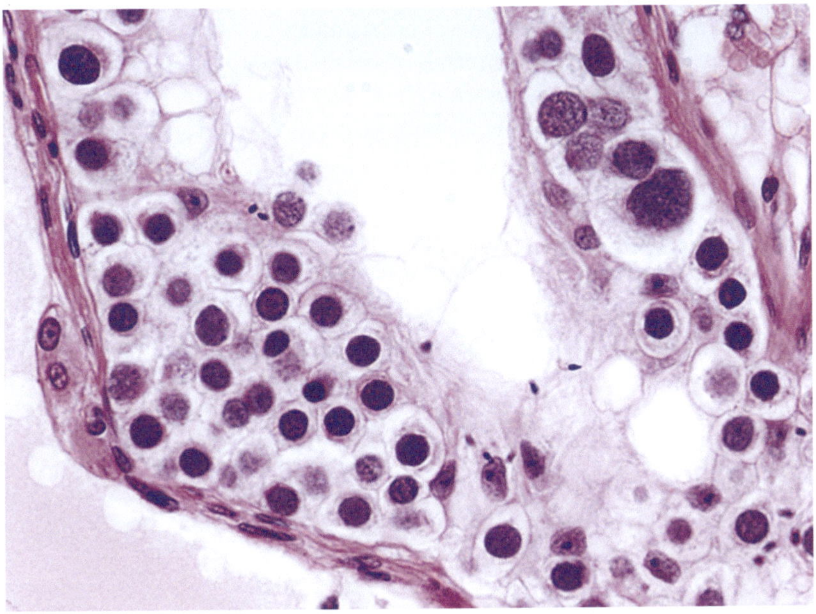

Fig. 39.2 Most spermatogonia are Ad type. A cell clone consisting in more than a dozen Ad spermatogonia is shown. Hypertrophic and multinucleated spermatogonia can also be observed in this tubule

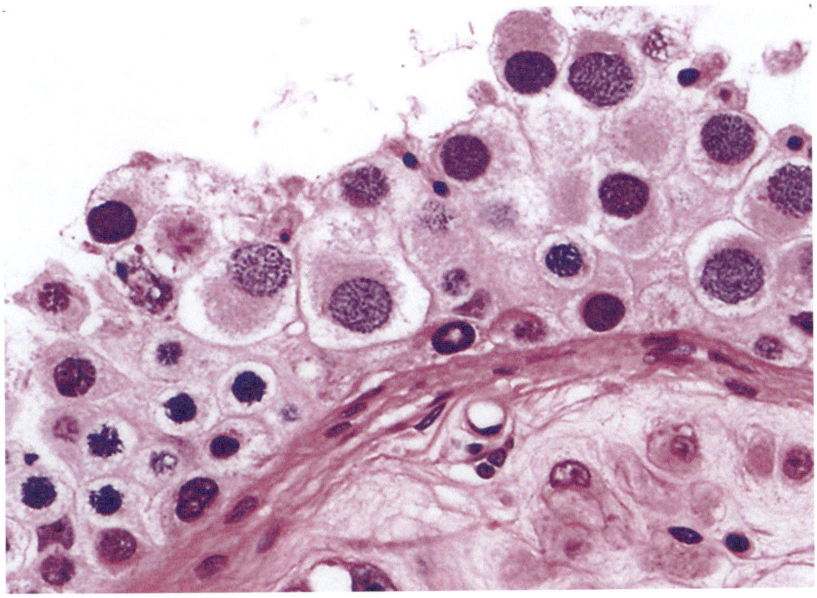

Fig. 39.3 The seminiferous epithelium with decreased height shows abundant megalospermatocytes and scarce spermatids

cytoplasm is highly variable – cells with as many as 86 nuclei have been reported [64].

Adult Spermatids There is a gradual reduction in number with age. If in testicular biopsies of men between 20 and 40 years 90 % of the seminiferous tubules contain adult spermatids, the numbers are reduced to 50 % in individuals aged between 40 and 60 years and to 10 % if they are older than 80 [67]. Apart from the decrease in the number of adult spermatids with age, the most important fact is the increase in deformed spermatids. Spermatids with two nuclei are often observed [68], as well as spermatids with elongated nuclei with postacrosomal strangulation [57].

39.3.2 Interstitium

Leydig Cells It is estimated that the normal number of Leydig cells is 1.2 accumulations by tubular section. A decrease in the number of Leydig cells is usually observed with aging. The testes of men over 60 years contain about half the number of Leydig cells in 20-year-old men. It has also been observed that age brings about not only a decrease of their number but also the volume of cytoplasm and the nuclear volume [20]. The decrease in the number of Leydig cells is not linked to an increase in other cell types, so it suggests that these cells degenerate [69].

We have observed the following changes with age in our material [57]:

(a) The number of Leydig cells is better preserved in individuals with intact spermatogenesis.
(b) When there is an important tubular atrophy, especially in cases of diffuse tubular hyalinization, there is an apparent increase in the number of Leydig cells.
(c) With age a tendency to form clumps occurs.

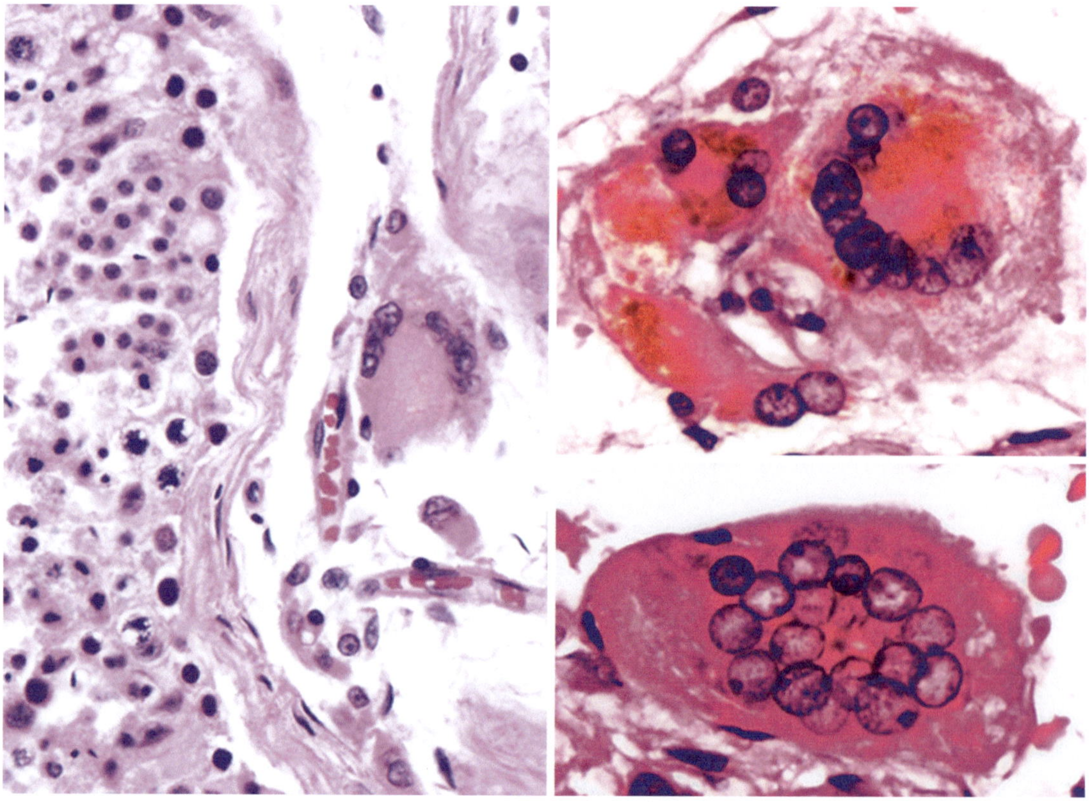

Fig. 39.4 Different types of multinucleated Leydig cells (Langhans type and Touton type) in an elderly patient

(d) In any case when the number of Leydig cells is expressed by the seminiferous tubule, including hyalinized tubes, the number of Leydig cells is higher than normal.
(e) Leydig cells often have involutive signs such as nuclear pyknosis, cytoplasmic shrinkage, and increased lipofuscins. Sometimes an excessive accumulation of lipids or intense cytokeratin immunoexpression is observed.

The most common ultrastructural changes in Leydig cells with age are an increase in the number of Reinke crystals and paracrystalline structures [70]; involutional changes in structures related to steroidogenesis (endoplasmic reticulum, mitochondria, etc.) [71]; increase of lipids, lipofuscins, and residual bodies [72]; and the appearance of multinucleated cells (Fig. 39.4). The same changes are expressed by extraparenchymal Leydig cells [73]. These morphological features are the expression of profound changes in the physiology of the Leydig cells. Multiple defects have been identified in the steroidogenic pathway of aged Leydig cells, reduction of LH-stimulated cAMP production, the cholesterol transport inducing protein steroidogenesis, acute regulatory protein (STAR) and the outer mitochondrial membrane cholesterol-binding translocator protein, and downstream steroidogenic enzymes of the mitochondria and smooth endoplasmic reticulum [74–76].

Stromal Giant Cells They are a normal finding in the testes of elderly patients and their number increases with age [77]. They are not related to the degree of tubular atrophy. These cells derive from CD34 positive fibroblasts.

Vascular Disorders The testicular blood flow decreases with age [78]. The testicular artery, which normally follows a straight course along the spermatic cord, forms loops along its trajectory. Doppler measurements of blood flow in the testicular artery have shown increased vascular resistance in the testes of men between 51 and 80 years, as compared to those under 40 [79]. The centripetal and centrifugal arteries of the testicular parenchyma undergo spiraling that may be secondary to a decreased testicular volume [80].

Vascular lesions can be found in most of the testes of patients of an advanced age [66] (Fig. 39.5). Hyperplasia of the muscular layer of the arteries, sclerosis of the medium layer, fibrosis of the intima of arterioles, arteriolar hyalinosis [81], or regression of the peritubular capillary network [82] have been reported.

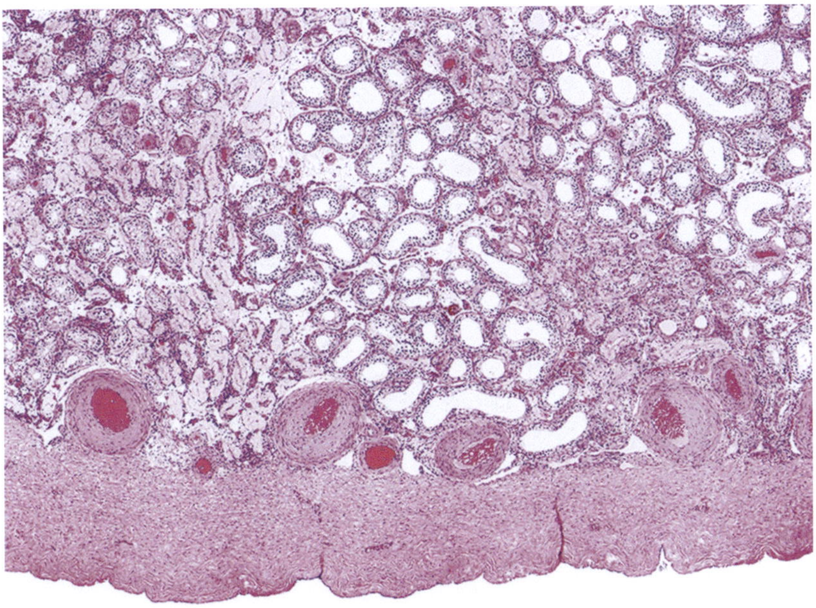

Fig. 39.5 Testis with marked atherosclerosis of the vascular tunic vessels. Atrophic lobules side by side to others with mild tubular ectasia

Another frequent finding in adults is varicocele. The incidence in young adults is estimated at 16 % and in the infertile population at 40 %. These percentages increase in old age. Many young patients with varicocele often show abnormalities in the semen analysis, hormone levels in serum, and testicular histology in both the ipsilateral testis and the contralateral one. The testes show two types of lesions, some of them are a diffuse sloughing of germ cells with more advanced maturity, and some are focal with the presence of multiple patchy lesions as well as more severe spermatogenesis lesions.

39.4 Mechanisms of Testicular Lesions

There are multiple potential mechanisms involved in the decline of testicular functions with age: genetic, environmental, hormonal, vascular (Fig. 39.6), obstruction of the spermatic ducts. In many cases, the lesions caused by these agents associate others lesions that depend directly on the specific condition the individual may be suffering from, so the identification of the damage caused by the two types of lesions is very difficult.

A good starting point to approach the etiology of these lesions is to classify them in two groups: diffuse alterations and focal abnormalities. Genetic, environmental, and hormonal causes naturally produce diffuse changes since all the parenchyma is exposed to the same noxa. Secondary injuries to vascular pathology and obstruction of the spermatic ducts will preferably be focal.

Explanation of most of the observed changes has been attempted by considering the testicle an exclusively endocrine gland, but this would not justify the most frequently encountered findings, the focal nature of some lesions, or the variability of lesions in the other testicle. In other words, not enough attention has been paid to the fact that the testicle is also an exocrine gland, and as such, an obstruction of the spermatic ducts can lead to serious damage to the structures that drain through them (Fig. 39.7).

Two populations of patients of similar age, one group formed by 100 orchiectomy specimens from patients without any other pathology but untreated prostate cancer, and a second group comprising the testes and spermatic ducts of 100 autopsies of men older than 65 who had died from causes not directly related to a testicular pathology, were compared in our department.

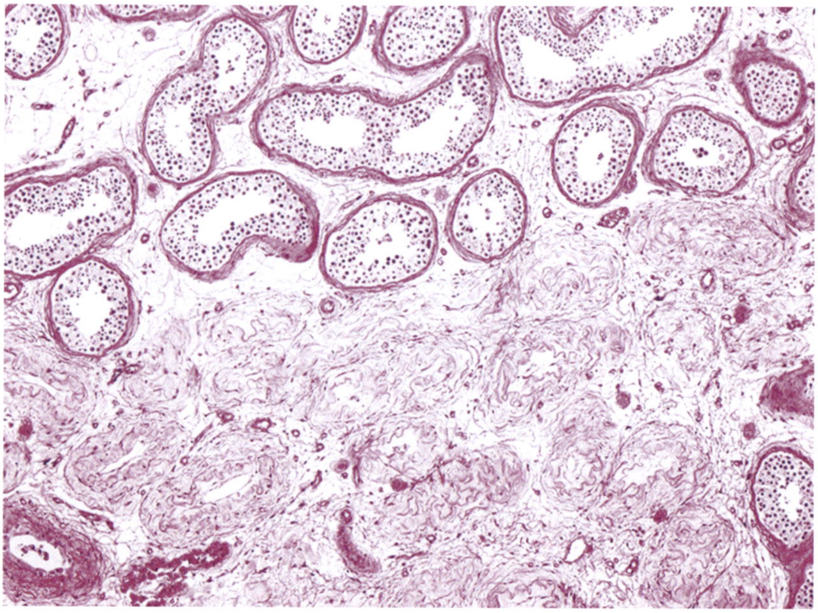

Fig. 39.6 Tubular hyalinization caused by ischemic mechanism. Silhouettes of hyalinized tubules nor Leydig cells in the interstitium are hardly recognized. The neighbor lobule has a partially preserved spermatogenesis

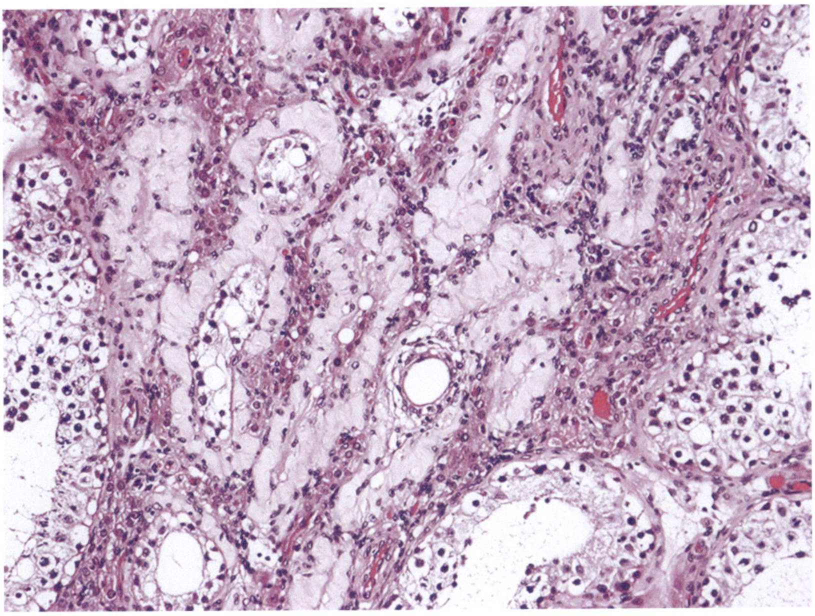

Fig. 39.7 Atrophy of seminiferous tubules of a testicular lobule caused by obstructive mechanism. Small cystic dilations within some hyalinized tubules associated with an apparent increase in Leydig cells in the interstitium

The orchiectomy specimens showed normal spermatogenesis in 6 % of the cases, diffuse spermatogenesis changes in 94 %, and focal lesions associated with diffuse lesions in 78 %. The quantitative study of the seminiferous epithelium in the testes with diffuse lesions specified the following diagnoses in decreasing order of frequency: hypospermatogenesis associated with spermatocyte sloughing, pure hypospermatogenesis, and maturation arrest in spermatogonia. About half of these lesions were accompanied by tubular ectasia (tubular lumen larger than the height of the seminiferous epithelium). It is noteworthy that the most common etiology of hypospermatogenesis associated with spermatocyte sloughing is obstruction of spermatic ducts.

Normal spermatogenesis was observed in the autopsy material in only 2 % of the cases, diffuse lesions of spermatogenesis in 98 %, and focal lesions associated with diffuse lesions in 68 %. Most diffuse lesions were associated with hypospermatogenesis associated with first-order spermatocyte sloughing, followed by incomplete maturation in spermatogonia, Sertoli cell-only and diffuse tubular hyalinization. The presence of more serious lesions in this material is consistent with the pathology the patients were suffering from and with the treatment they had received. After histological serialization of several cases of both the biopsy and the autopsy material, it was evident that each focal lesion corresponded to a common pathology of the seminiferous tubules of the same lobule, and the lesions characteristic of these tubules were of an obstructive nature and superimposable to those observed when the efferent duct ligation [83] or vasectomy [84] occurred.

By studying the first part of the spermatic pathway, i.e., the rete testis in the autopsy material, the following lesions were identified: diffuse cystic transformation (72 %), focal cystic transformation (20 %), and rete testis atrophy (8 %) (Fig. 39.8). Cases of regular and diffuse cystic transformation of the rete testis corresponded to epididymis having focal or diffuse atrophy at a head level or efferent duct ectasia. The most common cause was a hormone deficiency in some cases, and a lesion in the upper epididymal artery in other cases [79]. When transformation of the rete testis was focal and irregular, we often observed dilated veins with a hyalinized wall in the testicular mediastinum, typical lesions of varicose veins that compressed the cavities of the rete testis, thus justifying the post-obstructive lobular atrophy.

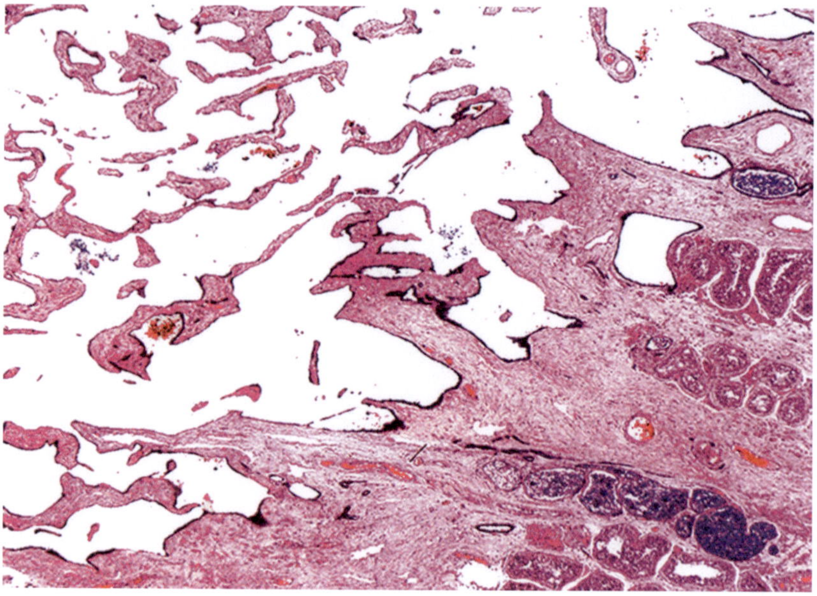

Fig. 39.8 Simple ectasia of the rete testis. Both mediastinal and septal rete testes are expanded

In summary, the testis undergoes aging of all its structures. Testicular changes may be aggravated by the coexistence of a vascular, arterial, or venous disease, which directly or indirectly causes a blockage of the first part of the spermatic ducts.

References

1. Kaufman JM, Vermeulen A. Declining gonadal function in elderly men. Baillières Clin Endocrinol Metab. 1997;11:289–309.
2. Rowland DL, Greenleaf WJ, Dorfman LJ, Davidson JM. Aging and sexual function in men. Arch Sex Behav. 1993;22:545–57.
3. Tserotas K, Merino G. Adropause and the aging male. Arch Androl. 1998;40:87–93.
4. Vermeulen A. The male climaterium. Ann Med. 1993;25:531–4.
5. Mastrogiacomo I, Feghali G, Foresta C, Ruzza G. Andropause: incidence and pathogenesis. Arch Androl. 1982;9:293–6.
6. Araujo AB, O'Donnell AB, Brambilla DJ, Simpson WB, Longcope C, Matsumoto AM, McKinlay JB. Prevalence and incidence of androgen deficiency in middle-aged and older men: estimates from the Massachusetts male aging study. J Clin Endocrinol Metab. 2004;89:5920–6.
7. Yeap BB, Almeida OP, Hyde Z, Norman PE, Chubb SA, Jamrozik K, Flicker L. In men older than 70 years, total testosterone remains stable while free testosterone declines with age. The health in men study. Eur J Endocrinol. 2007;156:585–94.
8. Everit AV, Meites J. Aging and antiaging effects of hormones. J Gerontol. 1989;44:B139–47.
9. Vijg J, Papaconstantinou J. Aging and longevity genes: strategies for identifying DNA sequences controlling life span. J Gerontol. 1990;45:B179–82.
10. Meikle AV, Stanish WM, Taylor N, Edwards CQ, Bishop CT. Familial effects on plasma sex steroid content in man: testosterone, estradiol and sex hormone- binding globulin. Metabolism. 1982;31:6–9.
11. Cameron JL, Weltzin TE, McConaha C, Helmreich DL, Kaye WH. Slowing of pulsatile luteinizing hormone secretion in men after forty-eight hours of fasting. J Clin Endocrinol Metab. 1991;73:35–41.
12. Deslypere JP, Vermeulen A. Leydig cell function in normal men: effect of age, life-style, residence, diet, and activity. J Clin Endocrinol Metab. 1984;59:955–62.
13. Vermeulen A. Androgens in the aging male. J Clin Endocrinol Metab. 1991;73:221–4.
14. Wu FC, Tajar A, Pye SR, Silman AJ, Finn JD, O'Neill TW, Bartfai G, Casanueva F, Forti G, Giwercman A, Huhtaniemi IT, Kula K, Punab M, Boonen S, Vanderschueren D, European Male Aging Study Group. Hypothalamic-pituitary-testicular axis disruptions in older men are differentially linked to age and modifiable risk factors: the European male aging study. J Clin Endocrinol Metab. 2008;93: 2737–45.
15. Gray A, Feldman HA, McKinlay JB, Longcope C. Age, disease and changing sex hormone levels in middle-aged men: results of the Massachusetts male aging study. J Clin Endocrinol Metab. 1991;73:1016–25.
16. Mass D, Jochen A, Lalande B. Age-related changes in male gonadal function. Implications for therapy. Drugs Aging. 1997;11:45–60.

17. Ahn HS, Park CM, Lee SW. The clinical relevance of sex hormone levels and sexual activity in the ageing male. BJU Int. 2002;89:526–30.
18. Araujo AB, Esche GR, Kupelian V, O'Donnell AB, Travison TG, Williams RE, Clark RV, McKinlay JB. Prevalence of symptomatic androgen deficiency in men. J Clin Endocrinol Metab. 2007;92:4241–7.
19. Tajar A, Huhtaniemi IT, O'Neill TW, Finn JD, Pye SR, Lee DM, Bartfai G, Boonen S, Casanueva FF, Forti G, Giwercman A, Han TS, Kula K, Labrie F, Lean ME, Pendleton N, Punab M, Vanderschueren D, Wu FC. EMAS Group. Characteristics of androgen deficiency in late-onset hypogonadism: results from the European Male Aging Study (EMAS). J Clin Endocrinol Metab. 2012;97:1508–16.
20. Neaves WB, Johnson L, Porter JC, Parker Jr CR, Petty CS. Leydig cell numbers, daily sperm serum production and gonadotrophin levels in aging men. J Clin Endocrinol Metabol. 1984;59:756–63.
21. Nankin HR. Fertility in aging men. Maturitas. 1985;7:259–65.
22. Pirke KM, Sintermann R, Vogt HJ. Testosterone and testosterone precursors in the spermatic vein and in the testicular tissue of old men. Reduced oxygen supply may explain the relative increase of testicular progesterone and 17alpha hidroxy-progesterone content and prediction in old age. Gerontology. 1980;26:221–30.
23. Ravaglia G, Forti P, Maloli F, Scali RC, Boschi F, Pratelli L, Pizzoferrato A, Gasbarrini G. Hormonal changes in male subjects over-ninety. Boll Soc Ital Biol Sper. 1995;71:133–9.
24. Davidson JM, Chen JJ, Crapo L, Gray JD, Greenleaf WJ, Catania JA. Hormonal changes and sexual function in aging men. J Clin Endocrinol Metab. 1983;57:71–7.
25. Veldhuis JD, Urban RJ, Dufau ML. Differential responses of biologically active luteinizing hormone secretion in older versus young men to interruption of androgen negative feedback. J Clin Endocrinol Metab. 1994;79:1763–70.
26. Mahmoud AM, Goemaere S, De Bacquer D, Comhaire FH, Kaufman JM. Serum inhibin B levels in community-dwelling elderly men. Clin Endocrinol (Oxf). 2000;53:141–7.
27. Johnson L, Grumbles JS, Bagheri A, Petty CS. Increased germ cell degeneration during postprophase of meiosis is related to increased serum folliclestimulationg hormone concentrations and reduced daily sperm production in aged men. Biol Reprod. 1990;42:281–7.
28. Bremner WJ, Vitiello MV, Prinz PN. Loss of circadian rhythmicity in blood testosterone levels with aging in normal men. J Clin Endocrinol Metab. 1983;56:1278–81.
29. Deslypere JP, Kaufman JM, Vermeulen T, Vogelaers D, Vandalen JL, Vermeulen A. Influence of age on pulsatile luteinizing hormone release and responsiveness of the gonadotrophs to sex hormone feedback in men. J Clin Endocrinol Metab. 1987;64:68–73.
30. Urban RJ, Veldhuis JD, Blizzard RM, Dufau ML. Attenuated release of biologically active luteinizing hormone in healthy aging men. J Clin Invest. 1988;81:1020–9.
31. Vermeulen A, Kaufmann JM. Ageing of the hypothalamo-pituitary-testicular axis in men. Horm Res. 1995;43:25–8.
32. Coiro V, Passeri M, Volpi R, Marchesi M, Bertoni P, Fagnoni F, Schianchi L, Bianconi L, Marcato A, Chiodera P. Different effects of aging on the opioids mechanisms controlling gonadotropin and cortisol secretion in man. Horm Res. 1989;32:119–23.
33. Winters SJ, Sherins RJ, Troen P. The gonadotropin-suppressive activity of androgen is increased in elderly men. Metabolism. 1984;33:1052–9.
34. Saad F, Yassin A, Haider A, Doros G, Gooren L. Elderly men over 65 years of age with late-onset hypogonadism benefit as much from testosterone treatment as do younger men. Korean J Urol. 2015;56:310–7.
35. Dean J, Maggi M, de Boer BJ, Hellstrom W, Khera M, Kim ED, McCullough A, Wu F, Zitzmann M. Diagnosing secondary hypogonadism: important consequences for fertility and reversibility. BJU Int. 2016;117:552–4.
36. Sibert L, Lacarrière E, Safsaf A, Rives N. [Aging of the human testis]. (Article in French). Presse Med. 2014;43:171–7.
37. Arenas MI, Bethencourt FR, Fraile B, Paniagua R. Immunocytochemical and qualitative study of the tunica albunigea testis in young and ageing men. Histochem Cell Biol. 1997;107:469–77.
38. Gosden RG, Richardson DW, Brown N, Davidson DW. Structrue and gametogenic potencial of seminierfous tubules in ageing mice. J Reprod Fertil. 1982;64:127–33.
39. Nistal M, Paniagua R. Non-neoplastic diseases of the testis. In: Bostwick DG, Cheng L, editors. Urological surgical pathology. 3rd ed. Philadelphia: Saunders; 2014. p. 560–735.
40. Meacham RB, Murray MJ. Reproductive function in the aging male. Urol Clin North Am. 1994;21:549–56.
41. Nistal M, Santamaría L, Regadera J, Paniagua R. Diverticula of human seminiferous tubules in the normal and pathologic testis. J Androl. 1988;9:55–61.
42. Arenas MI, Bethencourt FR, de Miguel MP, Fraile B, Romo E, Paniagua R. Immunocytochemical and quantitative study of actin, desmin and vimentin in the peritubular cells of the testes of elderly men. J Reprod Fertil. 1997;110:183–93.
43. Harbitz TB. Morphometric studies of the Sertoli cells in elderly men with special reference to the histology of the prostate. An analysis in an autopsy series. Acta Pathol Microbiol Scand. 1973;81:703–14.
44. Johnson L, Zane RS, Petty CS, Neaves WB. Quantification of the human Sertoli cell population: its distribution, relation to germ cell numbers, and age-related decline. Biol Reprod. 1984;31:785–95.
45. Paniagua R, Nistal M, Amat P, Rodriguez MC, Martin A. Seminiferous tubule involution in elderly men. Biol Reprod. 1987;36:939–47.

46. Paniagua R, Amat P, Nistal M, Martin A. Ultrastructural changes in Sertoli cells in ageing humans. Int J Androl. 1985;8:295–312.
47. Lynch KM, Scott WW. The lipid content of the Leydig cell and Sertoli cell in the human testis as related to age, benign hypertrophy and prostatic cancer. J Urol. 1950;64:767–671.
48. Holstein AF, Roosen.Runge EC. Sertoli cells during senescence. In: Illustrated pathology of human spermatogenesis. Berlin: Grosse; 1988. p. 230–4.
49. Schulze W, Schulze C. Multinucleate Sertoli cells in aged human testis. Cell Tissue Res. 1981;217:259–66.
50. De Miguel MP, Bethencourt FR, Arenas MI, Fraile B, Paniagua R. Intermediate filaments in the Sertoli cells of the ageing human testis. Virchows Arch. 1997;431:131–8.
51. Barr AB, Moore DJ, Paulsen CA. Germinal cell loss during human spermatogenesis. J Reprod Fertil. 1971;25:75–80.
52. Johnson L. Efficiency of spermatogenesis. Microsc Res Tech. 1995;32:385–422.
53. Brinkworth MH, Weinbauer GF, Bergmann M, Nieschlag E. Apoptosis as a mechanism of germ cell loss in elderly men. Int J Androl. 1997;20:222–8.
54. Brinkworth MH, Weinbauer GF, Schlatt S, Nieschlag E. Identification of male germ cells undergoing apoptosis in adult rats. J Reprod Fertil. 1995;105:25–33.
55. Sinha Hikim AP, Rajavashisth TB, Sinha Hikim I, Lue Y, Bonavera JJ, Leung A, Wang C, Swerdloff RS. Significance of apoptosis in the temporal and stage-specific loss of germ cells in the adult rat after gonadotropin deprivation. Biol Reprod. 1997;57:1193–201.
56. Nistal M, Codesal J, Paniagua R, Santamaria L. Decrease in the number of human Ap and Ad spermatogonia and in the Ap/Ad ratio with advancing age. New data on the spermatogonial stem cell. J Androl. 1987;8:64–8.
57. Paniagua R, Martín A, Nistal M, Amat P. Testicular involution in elderly men: comparison of histologic quantitative studies with hormone patterns. Fertil Steril. 1987;47:671–9.
58. Miething A. Multinuclearity of germ cells in the senescent human testis originates from a process of cell-cell fusion. J Submicrosc Cytol Pathol. 1995;27:105–13.
59. Paniagua R, Nistal M, Saez FJ, Fraile B. Ultrastructure of the aging human testis. J Electron Microsc Tech. 1991;19:241–60.
60. Holstein A. Morphological evidence for the involution of spermatogenesis during senescence. In: Holstein A, Voigt K, Grasslin D, editors. Reproductive biology and medicine. Berlin: Diesbach Verlag; 1989. p. 66–77.
61. Codesal J, Nistal M, Queizan A, Carretero JL, De Vega RM, Perez A, Paniagua R. Number and DNA content of hypertrophic spermatogonia in normal and cryptorchid human testes. Arch Androl. 1992;29:157–62.
62. Schulze W. Normal and abnormal spermatogonia in the human tetis. Fortsch Androl. 1991;7:33–45.
63. Holstein AF, Bustos-Obregon E, Hartmann M. Dislocated type-A spermatogonia in human seminiferous tubules. Cell Tissue Res. 1984;236:35–40.
64. Holstein AF, Eckmann C. Multinucleated spermatocytes and spermatids in human seminiferous tubules. Andrologia. 1986;18:5–16.
65. Miething A. Multinucleated spermatocytes in the aging human testis: formation, morphology, and degenerative fate. Andrologia. 1993;25:317–23.
66. Nistal M, Codesal J, Paniagua R. Multinucleate spermatids in aging human testes. Arch Androl. 1986;16:125–9.
67. Sasano N, Ichijo S. Vascular patterns of the human testis with special reference to its senile changes. Tohoku J Exp Med. 1969;99:269–80.
68. Merino G, Carranza-Lira S. Semen characteristics, endocrine profiles, and testicular biopsies of infertile men of different ages. Arch Androl. 1995;35: 219–24.
69. Neaves WB, Johnson L, Petty CS. Age-related change in numbers of other interstitial cells in testes of adult men: evidence of the fate of Leydig cell lost with increasing age. Biol Reprod. 1985;33:259–69.
70. Kaler LW, Neaves WB. Attrition of the human Leydig cell population with advancing age. Anat Rec. 1978;192:513–8.
71. Paniagua R, Amat P, Nistal M, Martín A. Ultrastructure of Leydig cells in human ageing testes. J Anat. 1986;146:173–83.
72. Holstein AF, Roosen-Runge EC, Schirren C. Leydig cells during senescence. In: Illustrated pathology of human spermatogenesis. Berlin: Grossse Verlag; 1988. p. 237–8.
73. Regadera J, Cobo P, Martinez-Garcia F, Nistal M, Paniagua R. Testosterone immunoexpression in human Leydig cells of the tunica albuginea testis and spermatic cord. A quantitative study in normal foetues, young adults elderly men and patients with cryptorchidism. Andrologia. 1993;25:115–22.
74. Luo L, Chen H, Zirkin BR. Temporal relationships among testosterone production steroidogenic acute regulatory protein (StAR), and P450 side-chain cleavage enzyme (P450scc) during Leydig cell aging. J Androl. 2005;26:25–31.
75. Culty M, Luo L, Yao ZX, Chen H, Papadopoulos V, Zirkin BR. Cholesterol transport, peripheral benzodiazepine receptor, and steroidogenesis in aging Leydig cells. J Androl. 2002;23:439–47.
76. Beattie MC, Adekola L, Papadopoulos V, Chen H, Zirkin BR. Leydig cell aging and hypogonadism. Exp Gerontol. 2015;68:87–91.
77. Coyne JD, Dervan PA. Multinucleated stromal giant cells of testis. Histopathology. 1997;31:381–3.
78. Suoranta H. Changes in small blood vessels of the adult human testis in relation to age and to some pathological conditions. Virchows Arch A Pathol Pathol Anat. 1971;352:165–81.
79. Wielgos M, Bablok L, Fracki S, Marianowski L. Doppler flowmetry measurements in testicular artery of aging men. Ginekol Pol. 1998;69:537–40.
80. Regadera J, Nistal M, Paniagua R. Testis, epididymis and spermatic cord in elderly men: correlation of angi-

ographic and histologic studies with systemic arteriosclerosis. Arch Pathol Lab Med. 1985;109:663–7.

81. Hatakeyama S, Segoku K, Takayama S. Histological and submicroscopic studies on arteriolar hialinosis of the human testis. Bull Tokyo Med Dent Univ. 1966;13:511–30.
82. Takizawa T, Hatakeyama S. Age-associated changes in microvasculature of human adult testis. Acta Pathol Jpn. 1978;28:541–5.
83. Johnson AL, Howards SS. Intratubular hydrostatic pressure in testis and epididymis before and after vasectomy. Am J Physiol. 1975;228:556–64.
84. Flickinger CJ, Howards SS, Carey PO, Spell DR, Kendrick SJ, Caloras D, Gallien TN, Herr JC. Testicular alterations are linked to the presence of elevated antisperm antibodies in Sprague-Dawley rats after vasectomy and vasovasostomy. J Urol. 1988;140:627–31.

40 Treatment-Related Testicular Changes

Manuel Nistal, Pilar González-Peramato, and Álvaro Serrano

40.1 Introduction

The number of people diagnosed with cancer is rising steadily. In Europe, an estimated 3.5 million cancers were diagnosed in 2012 [1]. Nowadays, the improvements achieved in diagnosis and therapy in oncology as surgery, radiotherapy, and chemotherapy have led to relatively high rates of remission and long-term survival. Also, improving survival rates for many cancers – some 1–2 % per annum – and 5-year relative survival for all cancers combined now exceeding 50 % have led to greater focus addressing the side effects and toxicities of treatments [2]. These trends mean that there are increasing numbers of "cancer survivors" in the population. About 49 % of these cancer survivors are male [3]. Early detection and improved cancer treatment protocols in the past 20 years have led to a dramatic increase in the number of men surviving cancer at a young age. A diagnosis of cancer is a life crisis for any person. Younger persons face the additional potential loss of their reproductive function and the opportunity to have children. Studies show that more than 50 % of young male survivors will desire paternity after treatment, including 75 % of those who were childless at the time of diagnosis [4]. But despite the continuous improvement of cancer treatment protocols, an altered testicular function and infertility are frequently the major adverse effects of oncologic treatments.

Testicular cancer, Hodgkin's disease, and leukemia are the most frequent male malignancies during the reproductive years. Acute lymphoblastic leukemia (ALL) is the most common type of cancer in childhood, representing about one-third of all cancers in children younger than 15. Other frequent cancers in children are Wilms' tumor, non-Hodgkin's lymphoma, germ cell tumors, Ewing's tumor, osteosarcoma, soft tissue sarcomas, retinoblastoma, and brain tumors [5].

Additionally, chemotherapy also is often used for noncancerous conditions such as autoimmune diseases like systemic lupus erythematosus (SLE) and hematological diseases. Also, treatments with estrogens and antiandrogenic hormones used in prostate cancer patients with gender dysphoria (GD) changing from male to female as a prerequisite for sex reassignment surgery cause testicular lesions.

40.2 Testicular Function and Cancer Treatments

Sexual dysfunction is found in 25–50 % of patients who are treated for cancer [6]. It is particularly important as 5 % of cancers occur in patients under 35 years of age, and approximately 1 in every 600 children will develop cancer before 15. Today, nearly 85 % of tumors in children and young men can be successfully treated [7, 8], and up to 80 % of these patients

M. Nistal et al., *Clues in the Diagnosis of Non-tumoral Testicular Pathology*, DOI 10.1007/978-3-319-49364-0_40

can now be cured [9]. In 2010, estimates pointed to one in every 250 young adults between 20 and 29 years as having survived pediatric cancer [10, 11].

Gonadal damage in men treated for cancer can result from either systemic chemotherapy or radiation therapy involving the spinal or pelvic area. This damage may involve both the germ cells and the somatic cells of the testis (Sertoli and Leydig cells). The testis has been shown to be highly susceptible to the toxic effects of cancer therapy at all stages of life [12]. Although earlier studies suggested that germ cells of younger males were less vulnerable to the toxic effects of chemotherapy compared to older boys and young adults, recent studies have failed to support this contention [13, 14]. Low-dose chemo- and/or radiotherapy can deplete progenitor type A pale spermatogonia and differentiating B spermatogonia in both the pubertal and adult testis, while less sensitive spermatogonial stem cells (which in adults are most likely a subpopulation of the quiescent A dark spermatogonia) survive, and spermatocytes and spermatids continue their maturation and spermiation and are finally released from the testis as spermatozoa [15]. If the damage is severe (e.g., as a result of high-dose treatment), all the spermatogonial stem cells undergo apoptosis, or alternatively the damaged Sertoli cells are unable to support the spermatogonial stem cells. This may lead to complete depletion of the pool of spermatogonial stem cells and seminiferous tubules leading to a Sertoli cell-only (SCO) pattern [16], making the patient permanently infertile. Testicular biopsies show that these SCO tubules frequently have Sertoli cells of the involuting type with lobulated nuclei with very irregular outlines, coarse chromatin granules, and inconspicuous nucleoli. These seminiferous tubules have central lumina, decreased diameters, and variable thickening of the basement membrane. Elastic fibers are present in normal or diminished amounts. Lengthy cancer chemotherapy combined with radiation therapy invariably causes hyalinization [17].

The main risk factors concerning fertility in child cancer survivors are the age at the time of the treatment, chemotherapy using alkylating agents, and irradiation of the reproductive organs or the hypothalamus/pituitary. In testicular cancer patients, it has also been suggested that in individuals with certain genotypes of LH receptor (LHR) and 5alpha-reductase II (SRD5A2), might be more vulnerable to these treatments [18].

In addition, gonadal dysfunction and reduced male fertility may also be associated with specific malignancies, even prior to treatment, as the disease itself may contribute to male gonadal dysfunction, particularly in testicular germ cell tumors (TGCTs), Hodgkin's disease [19], and leukemia. Patients with TGCT bear the highest risk of having poor semen quality before cancer treatment [20]. The association of TGCT and impaired spermatogenesis is well known, and both are included in the testicular dysgenesis syndrome. Up to 34–44 % of patients with Hodgkin's disease, assessed before and after treatment, have azoospermia or oligospermia [21, 22], and overall impaired spermatogenesis is seen in about 50–70 % of patients [23, 24]. This impairment seems to occur with other malignancies as well, although perhaps not to the same extent. Delayed maturation in spermatogenesis has been found in prepubertal patients prior to treatment of solid mesenchymal tumors [25]. The mechanisms of this dysfunction are poorly understood but they are likely multifactorial. The proposed mechanisms include primary germ cell deficiency, systemic release of cytokines by tumor cells injurious to both the seminiferous tubules and the Leydig cells, alterations of the immune system, and alteration of the hypothalamo-hypophyseal axis [26, 27]. In addition to the disease itself, other nonspecific conditions commonly observed at disease presentation (e.g., fever, anorexia, and pain) or later (stress, malnutrition) can impair semen quality. These findings on semen quality prior to treatment have been investigated only in adult patients, since similar studies on prepubertal boys cannot be performed [28].

The three main options for cancer treatment are surgery, radiotherapy, and chemotherapy.

40.2.1 Surgery

Any surgery involving the gonads or reproductive organs may impair fertility. Radical unilateral orchiectomy remains the standard treatment for testicular tumors. Decreased sperm concentration is seen in most men after unilateral orchiectomy for testicular cancer, and 10 % of patients with preoperative normal sperm counts will become azoospermic [29]. There is some recovery after 1 year [30]. Some authors recommend offering semen cryopreservation before unilateral orchiectomy [31].

Partial orchiectomy has become a favored option as a method to preserve hormonal and sperm cell production in carefully selected patients with bilateral testicular tumors or a unilateral tumor in a solitary testis. In these cases strict instructions should be followed to avoid tumor relapse or metastasis.

Retroperitoneal surgery may injure the adjacent sympathetic ganglia of the hypogastric plexus which are responsible for semen emission and ejaculation. Modifications of surgical techniques of retroperitoneal lymph node dissection (RPLND) have reduced the incidence of loss of anterograde ejaculation from 90 % in the late 70s and early 80s to nearly 0 % as today, since virtually all patients treated with nerve-sparing RPLND have a preserved ejaculatory function [32, 33].

40.2.2 Radiation Therapy

The testicular parenchyma is one of the most radiosensitive tissues of the body. Very low doses of radiation cause significant function impairment both in spermatogenesis and hormonal regulation of the testes. Radiation-induced gonadal damage is most often encountered following direct testicular irradiation, as what occurs in the management of testicular relapse of leukemia, or following total body irradiation as what happens prior to bone marrow transplantation. Fertility and endocrinological disturbances including both early and delayed puberty may also occur following cranial radiation [34]. In most patients treated with I^{131} for thyroid cancer, treatment-induced permanent infertility is not a concern [35], although fertility decreases briefly at the beginning of the treatment [36]. Also, recent evidence shows that prostate brachytherapy has a minimum or even no effect on spermatogenesis as the dose received by the testes from I^{125} brachytherapy of the prostate is close to 0.18 Gy [37].

The degree and persistence of gonadal damage depend on the total dose, the patient's age, the field of treatment, and the fractionation schedule [38]. Temporary azoospermia among testicular cancer patients has been reported following 0.2–0.6 Gy [38]. No significant effects on FSH levels or sperm counts are seen at doses below 0.2 Gy, but transient dose-dependent changes between 0.2 and 0.7 Gy, which all returned to normal within 12–24 months, have been reported in Hodgkin's lymphoma patients [39]. Fractionated radiation dosing, although the most common form of radiotherapy, is more harmful to sperm than the bioequivalent single-dose radiotherapy. The testes are more sensitive to fractioned treatment as the time available for repair is reduced. The repeated hits first activate and then hit the reserve stem cells. A fractionated total dose of 1.2 Gy is found to be a threshold dose after which permanent testicular damage is possible [40, 41].

The *germ cells* are the most radiosensitive testicular cells in men of all ages [42]. The more immature the cells, the more radiosensitive they are. Late spermatogonia (Ap and B) are more radiosensitive than early (Ad) spermatogonia. Ap and B spermatogonia are destroyed with doses as low as 0.1–1.2 Gy, while B spermatogonia tolerate doses higher than 4 Gy. Doses of 2–3 Gy result in overt damage to spermatocytes, which lead to a reduction in spermatid numbers. At doses of 4–6 Gy, the numbers of spermatozoa are significantly decreased, and this implies damage to spermatids. Prolonged azoospermia should be expected at 2.5 Gy total doses [43]. Doses of more than 4 Gy can cause irreversible damage to spermatogenesis [44], whereas doses higher than 6 Gy produce a SCO pattern (Fig. 40.1). Testicular irradiation (16–18 Gy) therapy as used to treat germ cell neoplasia in situ is associated with a high rate of permanent sterility [20].

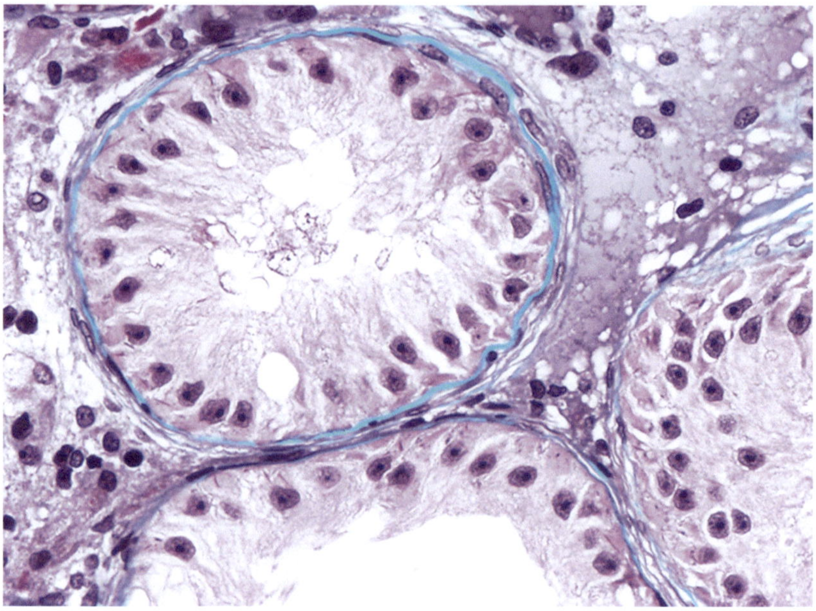

Fig. 40.1 A 25-year-old patient that underwent radiation therapy in childhood by retroperitoneal tumor. Sertoli cell-only pattern with complete disappearance of germ cells when he consulted by infertility

Leydig cells are less radiosensitive than the germ cells, and their biochemical abnormalities are usually mild. Leydig cell damage is shown to be dose dependent and inversely related to the age at treatment. Leydig cells' function is usually preserved up to 20 Gy in prepubertal boys and 30 Gy in sexually mature men; this fact explains that progression through puberty with normal testosterone levels is common and that many patients get to develop secondary sexual characteristics despite the severe impairment of spermatogenesis [45]. However, since a raised plasma concentration of LH has been observed, subclinical injury to Leydig cell occurs even at these levels of radiation. In children with acute lymphoblastic leukemia involving the testis, radiotherapy with doses of 20–25 Gy, either alone or combined with chemotherapy, causes irreversible damage of the seminiferous tubules and Leydig cells. These patients develop azoospermia and hypogonadotropic hypogonadism with low serum testosterone levels [17].

Sertoli cells tolerate up to 60 Gy, although they show ultrastructural alterations after low doses of radiation [17, 28].

Even with optimal protection, the contralateral testis absorbs 0.2–1.4 Gy when the opposite testis is irradiated [46] or in adjuvant therapy for rectal cancer [47].

High doses of radiation therapy, as those used for treatment of testicular leukemia, frequently cause tubular hyalinization. In addition, radiation induces dense interstitial fibrosis and loss of peritubular cells, thus obscuring the borders between the interstitium and the tubules (Fig. 40.2). This makes the tubules difficult to see in hematoxylin- and eosin-stained sections. Leydig cells are atrophic and decreased in numbers. Ischemia secondary to radiation-induced vascular injury also contributes to hyalinization [17].

Recovery of Spermatogenesis Spermatogenesis is generally restored 1–2 years after treatment, but it may be incomplete or need more years in some patients. Recovery of spermatogenesis takes place from surviving stem cells (type A spermatogonia) and depends on the radiation dose. Complete recovery takes place within 9–18 months following radiation with 1 Gy or less, 30 months for 2–3 Gy, and 5 years or more for doses of 4 Gy and above [44].

Cranial Irradiation While not harming the gonads directly, fertility can be impaired by disruption of the hypothalamic-pituitary-gonadal axis. Cranial irradiation (CRI) is responsible for the development of secondary gonadal failure in some long-term survivors, but, as a whole, overt

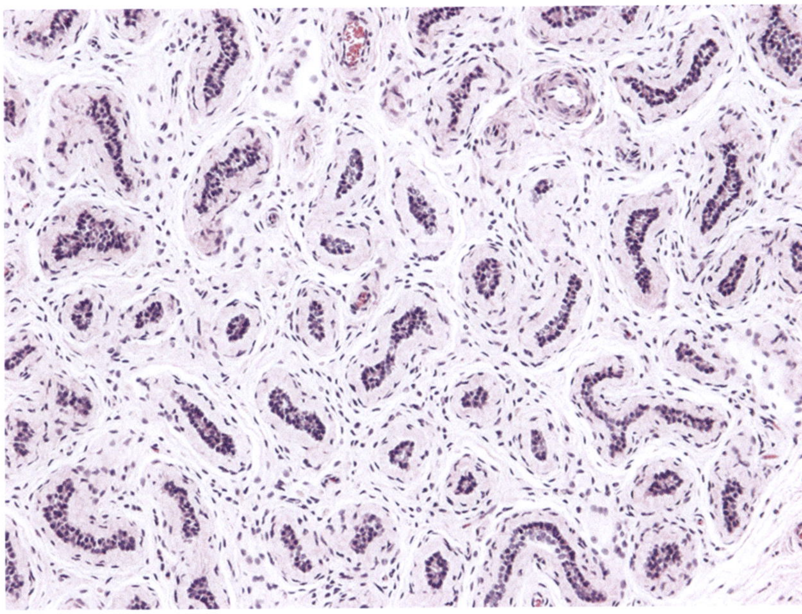

Fig. 40.2 A 12-year-old patient treated for acute lymphoblastic leukemia. Severe atrophy of both seminiferous tubules and Leydig cells. Seminiferous tubules show complete disappearance of germ cells and thickened tubular wall

gonadotropin deficiency is rare and mainly related to high radiation doses (35–45 Gy) that are used in the treatment of brain tumors [41]. The clinical sequelae of gonadotropin deficiency exhibit a broad spectrum of severity: from subclinical abnormalities detectable only by the GnRH test to a significant reduction in circulating sex hormone levels, delayed puberty [28], and infertility [48].

40.2.3 Chemotherapy

Numerous chemotherapeutic agents have been identified as being gonadotoxic because they target rapidly proliferating cells, killing not only differentiating spermatogonia but also the stem cells themselves. In addition, stem spermatogonia that do survive fail to further differentiate, and this causes permanent infertility. Leydig cells are more resistant than germ cells due to their lower turnover rate (Fig. 40.3). Leydig cell dysfunction after chemotherapy is dose dependent and usually limited to elevated LH concentrations with normal or low normal testosterone levels, and thus the secondary sexual characteristics develop normally. Less frequently patients show hypogonadism. Leydig cells can also be secondarily affected by damage of the germ cell epithelium and reduction of the testicular volume causing alterations in the paracrine control of Leydig cells.

Chemotherapy has a profound negative effect on spermatogenesis by different mechanisms: causing chromosomal aberrations (platinum antineoplastic agents and topoisomerase inhibitors), maturation arrest by inhibiting microtubule polymerization (vinca alkaloids), mutagenic effect in all stages of spermatogenesis (alkylating agents), and impaired spermatozoa motility. Taxanes inhibit microtubule function, thereby inhibiting the cell division process. Additionally, taxanes induce the reduction of inhibin B and reciprocal elevation of follicle-stimulating hormone, which are associated with significant gonadal damage [49].

The nature and the extent of chemotherapy on gonadal toxicity depend on several factors: type of drug, cumulative doses, treatment duration, combinations used, patient's age, patient's pretreatment gonadal status, and individual sensitivity [50, 51]. Most of the chemotherapy regimens are multi-agent, and thus the relative contribution of each individual drug is difficult to determine.

Type of Drug and Dosage The alkylating drugs are the most gonadotoxic cytostatics [43]. Testicular toxicity of alkylating agents on childhood

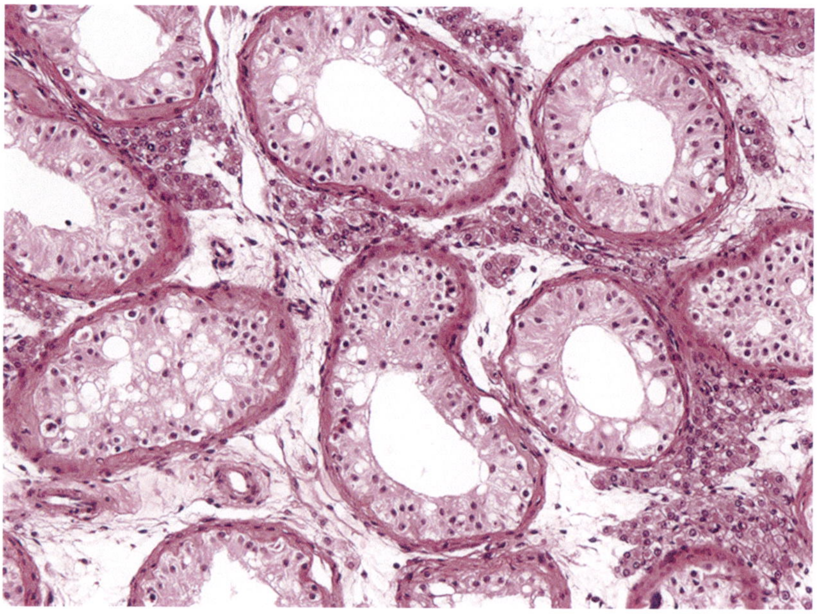

Fig. 40.3 A 50-year-old patient treated for bladder carcinoma. Seminiferous epithelium consists only of isolated germ cells and Sertoli cells showing marked vacuolization. Leydig cells are better preserved

lymphoma survivors is dose dependent and not correlated to diagnosis, age, or pubertal status at diagnosis [52]. In children, cyclophosphamide reduces the seminiferous tubular diameter and the germ cell numbers; nuclei in the residual spermatogonia are enlarged. Puberty may progress, even during treatment. In adults, cyclophosphamide and isophosphamide caused permanent azoospermia in 80–90 % of cases, most commonly in patients with a pretreatment testis volume lower than 13 ml or a low sperm count with high FSH (>10 IU/l). In adults cyclophosphamide destroys the seminiferous epithelium, induces a SCO pattern, and increases FSH serum concentration [53]. Alkylating agents may also induce reversion to a dedifferentiated Sertoli cell with immature phenotype (reexpression of cytokeratins 18) [54]. These agents also impair Leydig cell function and cause low testosterone levels, normal or elevated LH serum levels, and an exaggerated response of LH to GnRH administration [55] (Figs. 40.4 and 40.5).

Fludarabine, used for the treatment of chronic lymphocytic leukemia, produces testicular damage with diminished ejaculate volume, oligozoospermia, increased FSH and LH serum levels, and decreased testosterone levels. DNA in spermatozoa is markedly abnormal, an effect that persists for several months [56].

Cisplatin-based regimens are at present the main chemotherapeutic agent in oncological protocols for testicular tumors. Cisplatin affects the cellular DNA and its effects are dose related. It causes azoospermia when the dosage is high (400–600 mg/m^2) [57]. If not azoospermic prior to treatment, there is a medium chance (defined as 65 % at 3 years and 80 % at 4 years) of recovery to at least oligospermia after up to four cisplatin-based cycles [58]. In addition, cisplatin has a synergic interaction with the spermiotoxicity of radiotherapy.

There are little systematically achieved data for newer drugs such as taxanes, oxaliplatin, irinotecan, monoclonal antibodies, and tyrosine kinase inhibitors. Inhibin-B was slightly reduced after treatment with oxaliplatin [59]. Experimental studies in prepubertal mice have shown that irinotecan metabolite SN38 induces a marked dose-dependent sensitivity in the testicular germ cells [60]. Imatinib mesylate (a tyrosine kinase inhibitor) used in the treatment of chronic myeloid leukemia causes severe oligozoospermia [61].

Combination of Drugs The impact of chemotherapy used in the treatment of Hodgkin's disease has been widely reported. The MOPP (mustine, vincristine, procarbazine, and prednisolone) regi-

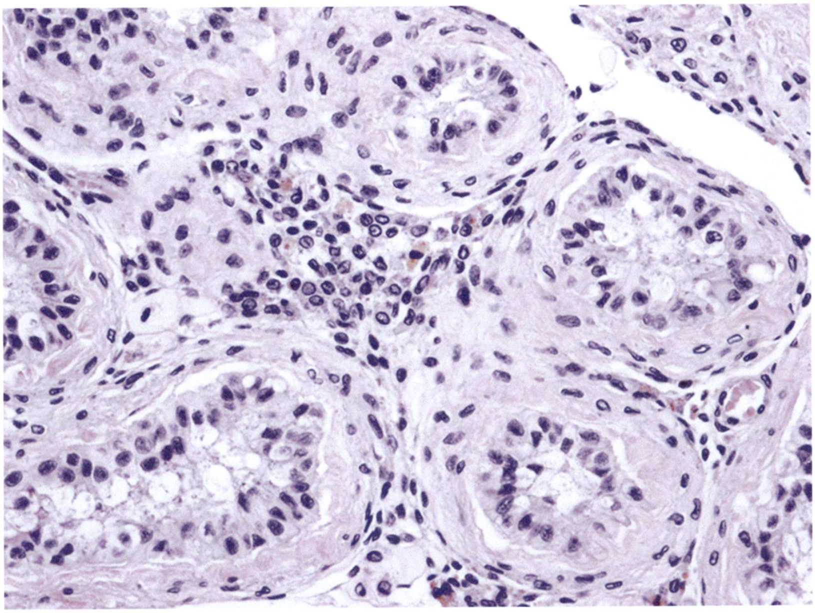

Fig. 40.4 Testicular parenchyma of a patient treated with busulfan showing severe decrease in tubular diameter, Sertoli cell-only pattern with dedifferentiated Sertoli cell and Leydig cell atrophy

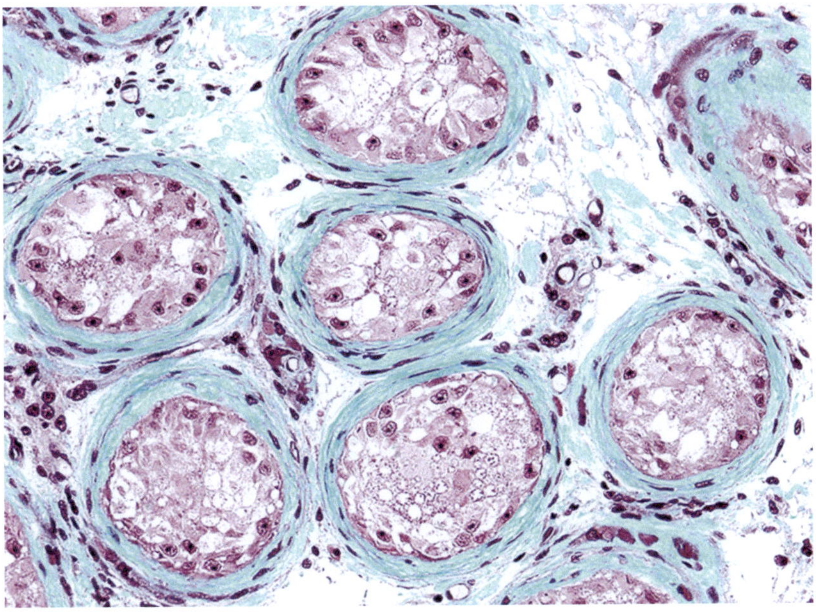

Fig. 40.5 Patient treated for nephroblastoma in childhood. Seminiferous tubules with low number of adult Sertoli cells as the only lining cells

men, which was commonly used in the past, leads to permanent sterility in most (97 %) male patients and raises LH concentrations, suggesting Leydig cell impairment. Patients treated with the COPP (cyclophosphamide, vincristine, procarbazine, and prednisone) protocol do not recover spermatogenesis even if the cyclophosphamide dose does not exceed 4800 mg/m2. After treatment with the ABVD (Adriamycin, bleomycin, vinblastine, and dacarbazine) regimen, the first nonalkylating agent combination, which is commonly used today, azo- or oligospermia was induced in 54 % of patients [62] with a posttreatment sperm recovery rate of 90 % within 1–5 years of treatment [63]. The alternating use of MOPP and ABVD regimens causes testicular dysfunction in

87 % of patients, but 40 % retrieve spermatogenesis [64]. Chemotherapy regimens used for the treatment of non-Hodgkin's lymphoma are generally less gonadotropic than those used for Hodgkin's disease.

Patients with TGCT who received chemotherapy with BEP (bleomycin, etoposide, and cisplatin) regimens become azoospermic 7–8 weeks after starting treatment. When the total doses reach 600 mg/m2, infertility is irreversible; at lower dosages, fertility may be recovered over a period of approximately 2 (50 % of patients) to 5 (80 %) years [65] although a high percentage of spermatozoa with DNA abnormalities will persist [66].

Age The prepubertal testis is very vulnerable to cytotoxic therapy, probably because of the steady turnover of early germ cells that undergo spontaneous degeneration before the haploid stage is reached, which is essential for normal adult function [67].

Pretreatment gonadal status of the patient has previously been commented.

Additionally, besides impairment of sperm production and Leydig cell dysfunction, concerns have been raised about the possible mutagenic effect of chemotherapy on sperm resulting in transmissible genetic damage. However, no clear evidences have been reported in humans [51].

Therefore, fertility preservation requires careful selection of less gonadotoxic therapeutic regimens. Cryopreservation of semen has become a standard practice and should be offered to all men before undergoing potential sterilizing therapy. Advances in assisted reproductive techniques have increased the chance of successful pregnancy using cryopreserved spermatozoa [51]. However, there are limitations to this method of preserving fertility, as it is not an option for prepubertal patients or patients with impaired spermatogenesis prior to treatments. Cryopreservation of immature testicular tissue or isolated germ cells from prepubescent males in order to achieve restoration of fertility following treatment, either by germ cell transplantation or by in vitro maturation of the germ cells harvested, remains experimental [25, 28, 68, 69]. Research in the field of spermatogenic stem cells may lead to improved treatment options such as autotransplant of stem cells for repopulation of the testes after cancer treatment [49]. In 12 % of men, no sperm could be banked as a result of the absence of spermatozoa or the very low numbers of nonmotile spermatozoa.

40.2.4 Potential for Fertility Following Cancer Treatment in Childhood

The prevention of sterility in survivors of cancer in childhood and youth is a major reproductive challenge for the coming decades. Due to the broad variety of gonadotoxic effects of chemotherapy or radiation therapy on the testes, it is often difficult to predict whether a child undergoing cancer treatment will subsequently have impaired fertility as an adult. Besides, in the prepubertal age, there is no sensitive marker of gonadal function that allows early prediction of gonadal damage. Great interest is currently placed on plasma inhibin B [14, 28, 70] or inhibin B to FSH [71] as a potential marker of gonadotoxicity in this age group as it is in adults. The risk of subfertility can be categorized according to drugs, the type of malignancy, and the associated treatment and is shown in Table 40.1.

40.3 Estrogen and Antiandrogen Therapy

Estrogen treatments in adult humans have been used mainly in two types of patients: patients with prostate cancer and patients with gender dysphoria (GD) changing from male to female in whom cross-sex hormone treatment is a prerequisite for sex reassignment surgery.

Patients with prostate cancer treated with estrogens have shown some similarities with hypogonadism such as reduced spermatogenesis, SCO seminiferous tubules, or spermatogonia-only-containing tubules, reduced Leydig cell numbers, and sclerosed tubules [72].

Patients with Gender Dysphoria Changing from Male to Female Testicular lesions have been studied in bilateral orchiectomy specimens after definitive surgical treatment. Estrogen exposure during adulthood not merely causes atrophy but exerts true dedifferentiation of adult human Sertoli cells [73], including immaturity immunophenotype such as reexpression of anti-Müllerian

Table 40.1 Risk of gonadal subfertility due to cytotoxic drugs and current treatments for disease

High risk	Medium risk	Low risk	Limited data
Drugs			
Alkylating drugs Cyclophosphamide Isofosfamide Busulfan Melphalan Chlorambucil Chlormethine Procarbazine	Platinum analogs Cisplatin Carboplatin Doxorubicin BEP ABVD	Plant derivatives Vincristine Vinblastine Antibiotics Bleomycin Dactinomycin Antimetabolites Methotrexate Mercaptopurine 5-Fluoruracil	Taxanes Oxaliplatin Irinotecan Tyrosine kinase inhibitors Monoclonal antibodies
Disease/treatment			
Total body irradiation Localized radiotherapy: pelvic/testicular Chemotherapy conditioning for bone marrow transplant Hodgkin's disease: alkylating agent-based therapy Soft tissue sarcoma: metastatic	Acute myeloblastic leukemia Hepatoblastoma Osteosarcoma Ewing's sarcoma Soft tissue sarcoma Neuroblastoma Non-Hodgkin's lymphoma Hodgkin's disease: "alternating therapy" Brain tumor: craniospinal radiotherapy Cranial irradiation >24 Gy	Acute lymphoblastic leukemia Wilms' tumor Soft tissue sarcoma: stage 1 TGCT (gonadal preservation and no radiotherapy) Retinoblastoma Brain tumor (surgery only) Cranial irradiation <24 Gy	

Adapted from Brydoy (2007) and Broughman (2003)

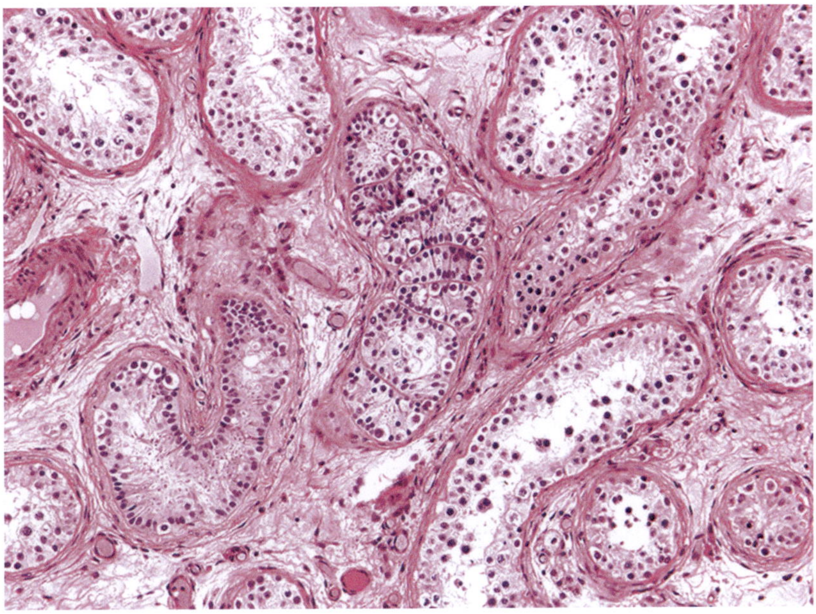

Fig. 40.6 Patient with gender dysphoria changing from male to female. Testicular parenchyma showing complete, although quantitatively abnormal, spermatogenesis with numbers of spermatocytes and spermatids lower than expected. Note a group of hypoplastic tubules in the center of the figure

hormone, D2-40, and inhibin bodies [74]. Nistal el al. found that based on the seminiferous epithelium pattern of the greatest part of the testicular parenchyma, patients can be classified in three subgroups: (1) patients with complete, although quantitatively abnormal spermatogenesis showing numbers of spermatocytes and spermatids lower than expected (Fig. 40.6); (2) patients with mostly pubertal-like seminiferous tubules (the most frequent pattern); and (3) patients with mostly infantile seminiferous tubules. In the majority of cases (72 %), spermatogenesis was considered pubertal-like, with seminiferous tubules containing Sertoli cells and spermatogonia only, or spermatogonia and primary spermatocytes, as the only germ cells. Spermatogonial

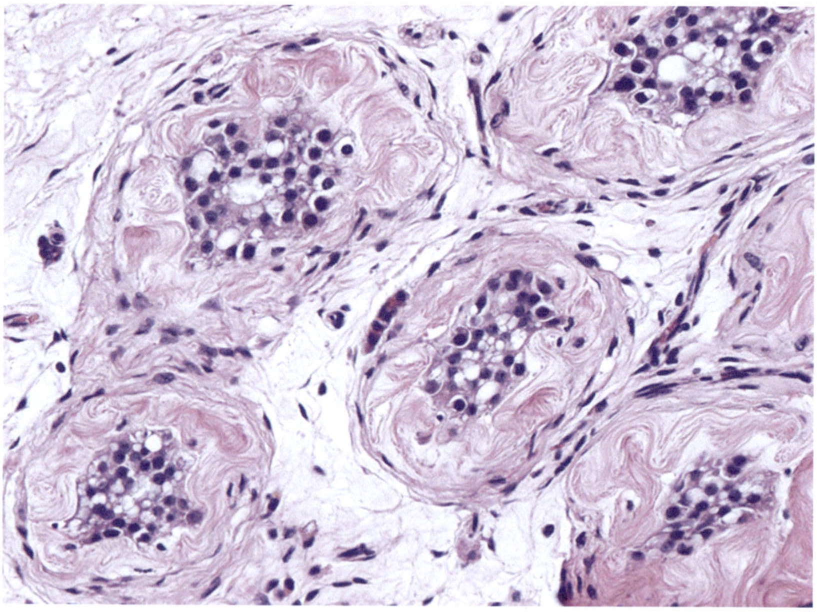

Fig. 40.7 Patient with gender dysphoria changing from male to female. Spermatogonial numbers is reduced; Sertoli cell nuclei are rounded instead of indented as in adults, and the tubular wall is thickened. Leydig cell numbers are lower than normal

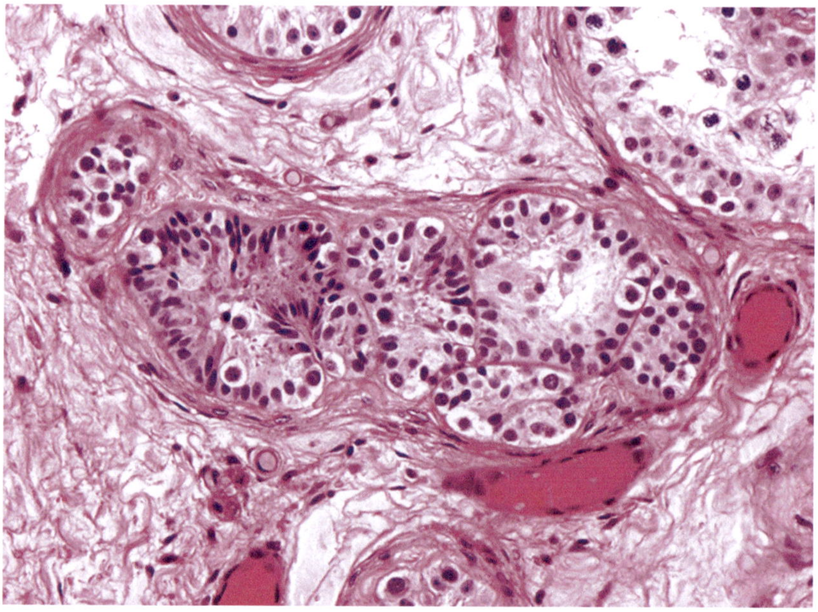

Fig. 40.8 Patient with gender dysphoria changing from male to female. Hypoplastic involuting tubules with dedifferentiated Sertoli cells (round or even ovoid SC nuclei, no lumen) grouped in involuting seminiferous cords, showing intratubular wall protrusions

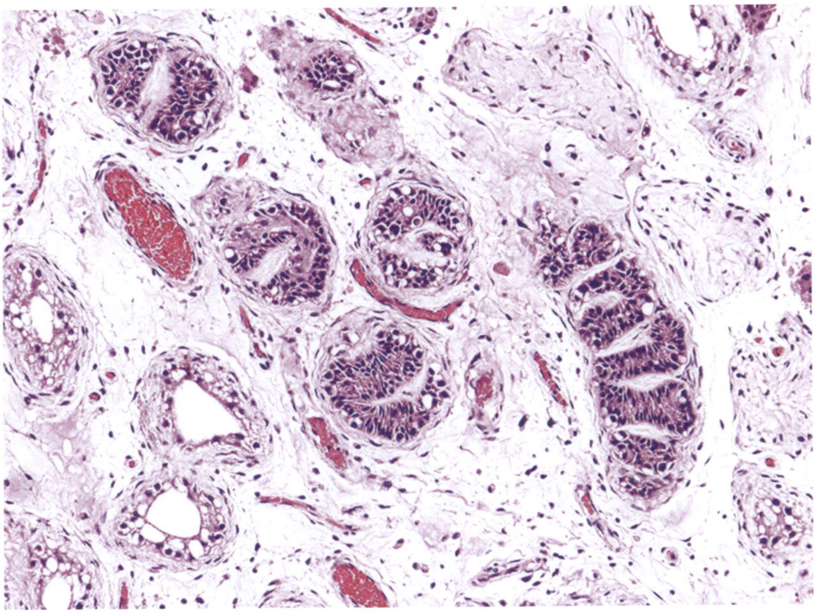

Fig. 40.9 Patient with gender dysphoria changing from male to female. Involuting zones showing several involuting tubules with pubertal pattern. The neighbor seminiferous tubules show severe atrophy

numbers were highly variable; Sertoli cell nuclei were rounded instead of indented as in adults, and the tubular wall was thickened (Fig. 40.7).

A progression in the involution and the extent of the lesions was observed related to increasing estrogen dosage intake. Lesions progressed from involuting tubules to involuting zones showing several involuting tubules with pubertal pattern (triangular-shaped SC nuclei, germ cells' presence, tubular lumen) together with Sertoli cell-only involuting tubules (round or even ovoid SC nuclei, no germ cells, no lumen) even in adjacent zones of the same seminiferous tubule. The wall of these tubules was highly thickened. These lesions progressed to even more extended areas, where most tubules were grouped in involuting seminiferous cords, showing intratubular wall protrusions and frequently containing multinucleated spermatogonia (Figs. 40.8 and 40.9). Leydig cell numbers are more frequently lower than normal although they can also be higher or normal [74]. Other studies found seminiferous cords containing only Sertoli cells and spermatogonia as the only germ cells [73, 75], or 48 % of patients with spermatogenesis [76] probably related to differences in the dosage of estrogens and antiandrogen hormones received.

References

1. Ferlay J, Steliarova-Foucher E, Lortet-Tieulent J, Rosso S, Coebergh JW, Comber H, Forman D, Bray F. Cancer incidence and mortality patterns in Europe: estimates for 40 countries in 2012. Eur J Cancer. 2013;49:1374–403.
2. Verdecchia A, Guzzinati S, Francisci S, De Angelis R, Bray F, Allemani C, Tavilla A, Santaquilani M, Sant M. EUROCARE Working Group: Survival trends in European cancer patients diagnosed from 1988 to 1999. Eur J Cancer. 2009(45):1042–66.
3. Sharp L, Deady S, Gallagher P, Molcho M, Pearce A, Alforque Thomas A, Timmons A, Comber H. The magnitude and characteristics of the population of cancer survivors: using population-based estimates of cancer prevalence to inform service planning for survivorship care. BMC Cancer. 2014;14:767.
4. Schover LR, Brey K, Lichtin A, Lipshultz LI, Jeha S. Knowledge and experience regarding cancer, infertility, and sperm banking in younger male survivors. J Clin Oncol. 2002;20:1880–9.
5. Nistal M, Paniagua R, Gonzalez-Peramato P, Reyes-Múgica M. Chapter 23.- Testicular pathology secondary to physical and chemical injury. Pediatr Dev Pathol. 2016. [Epub ahead of print].
6. Arai Y, Kawakita M, Okada Y, Yoshida O. Sexuality and fertility in long-term survivors of testicular cancer. J Clin Oncol. 1997;15:1444–8.
7. Aslam I, Fishel S, Moore H, Dowell K, Thornton S. Fertility preservation of boys undergoing anti-cancer therapy: a review of the existing situation and prospects for the future. Hum Reprod. 2000;15:2154–9.

8. Schrader M, Heicappel R, Muller M, Straub B, Miller K. Impact of chemotherapy on male fertility. Onkologie. 2001;24:326–30.
9. Brenner H, Steliarova-Foucher E, Arndt V. Up-to-date monitoring of childhood cancer long-term survival in Europe: methodology and application to all forms of cancer combined. Ann Oncol. 2007;18:1561–8.
10. Bleyer WA. The impact of childhood cancer on the United States and the world. CA Cancer J Clin. 1990;40:355–67.
11. Blatt J. Pregnancy outcome in long-term survivors of childhood cancer. Med Pediatr Oncol. 1999;33:29–33.
12. Jahnukainen K, Ehmcke J, Hou M, Schlatt S. Testicular function and fertility preservation in male cancer patients. Best Pract Res Clin Endocrinol Metab. 2011;25:287–302.
13. Kenney LB, Laufer MR, Grant FK, Grier H, Diller L. High risk of infertility and long term gonadal damage in males treated with high dose cyclophosphamide for sarcoma during childhood. Cancer. 2001;91:613–21.
14. van Casteren NJ, van der Linden GH, Hakvoort-Cammel FG, Hählen K, Dohle GR, van den Heuvel-Eibrink MM. Effect of childhood cancer treatment on fertility markers in adult male long-term survivors. Pediatr Blood Cancer. 2009;52:108–12.
15. van Alphen MM, van de Kant HJ, de Rooij DG. Depletion of the spermatogonia from the seminiferous epithelium of the rhesus monkey after X irradiation. Radiat Res. 1988;113:473–86.
16. de Rooij DG, van de Kant HJ, Dol R, Wagemaker G, van Buul PP, van Duijn-Goedhart A, de Jong FH, Broerse JJ. Long-term effects of irradiation before adulthood on reproductive function in the male rhesus monkey. Biol Reprod. 2002;66:486–94.
17. Nistal M, Paniagua R, González-Peramato P. Non-neoplastic diseases of the testis. Chapter 12. In: Bostwick DG, Chen L, editors. Urologic surgical pathology. Philadelphia: Mosby/Elsevier; 2014. p. 560–735.
18. Aschim EL, Oldenburg J, Kristiansen W, Giwercman A, Witczak O, Fosså SD, Haugen TB. Genetic variations associated with the effect of testicular cancer treatment on gonadal hormones. Hum Reprod. 2014;29:2844–51.
19. Caponecchia L, Cimino G, Sacchetto R, Fiori C, Sebastianelli A, Salacone P, Marcucci I, Tomassini S, Rago R. Do malignant diseases affect semen quality? Sperm parameters of men with cancers. Andrologia. 2016;48:333–40.
20. Dohle GR. Male infertility in cancer patients: review of the literature. Int J Urol. 2010;17:327–31.
21. Viviani S, Ragni G, Santoro A, Perotti L, Caccamo E, Negretti E, Valagussa P, Bonadonna G. Testicular dysfunction in Hodgkin's disease before and after treatment. Eur J Cancer. 1991;27:1389–92.
22. Lass A, Akagbosu F, Abusheikha N, Hassouneh M, Blayney M, Avery S, Brinsden P. A programme of semen cryopreservation for patients with malignant disease in a tertiary infertility centre: lessons from 8 years' experience. Hum Reprod. 1998;13:3256–61.
23. Rueffer U, Breuer K, Josting A, Lathan B, Sieber M, Manzke O, Grotenhermen FJ, Tesch H, Bredenfeld H, Koch P, Nisters-Backes H, Wolf J, Engert A, Diehl V. Male gonadal dysfunction in patients with Hodgkin's disease prior to treatment. Ann Oncol. 2001;12:1307–11.
24. Fitoussi, Eghbali H, Tchen N, JP B, Soubeyran P, Hoerni B. Semen analysis and cryoconservation before treatment in Hodgkin's disease. Ann Oncol. 2000;11:679–84.
25. Pietzak 3rd EJ, Tasian GE, Tasian SK, Brinster RL, Carlson C, Ginsberg JP, Kolon TF. Histology of testicular biopsies obtained for experimental fertility preservation protocol in boys with cancer. J Urol. 2015;194:1420–4.
26. Costabile RA, Spevak M. Cancer and male factor infertility. Oncology (Williston Park). 1998;12:557–70.
27. Agarwal A, Allamaneni SS. Disruption of spermatogenesis by the cancer disease process. J Natl Cancer Inst Monogr. 2005;34:9–12.
28. Brougham MF, Kelnar CJ, Sharpe RM, Wallace WH. Male fertility following childhood cancer: current concepts and future therapies. Asian J Androl. 2003;5:325–37.
29. Petersen PM, Skakkebæk NE, Rørth M, Giwercman A. Semen quality and reproductive hormones before and after orchiectomy in men with testicular cancer. J Urol. 1999;161:822–6.
30. Jacobsen KD, Theodorsen L, Fossa SD. Spermatogenesis after unilateral orchiectomy for testicular cancer in patients following surveillance policy. J Urol. 2001;165:93–6.
31. Brydøy M, Fosså SD, Dahl O, Bjøro T. Gonadal dysfunction and fertility problems in cancer survivors. Acta Oncol. 2007;46:480–9.
32. Donohue JP, Thornhill JA, Foster RS, Rowland RG, Bihrle R. Retroperitoneal lymphadenectomy for clinical stage A testis cancer (1965 to 1989): Modifications of technique and impact on ejaculation. J Urol. 1993;149:237–43.
33. Jacobsen KD, Ous S, Wæhre H, Trasti H, Stenwig AE, Lien HH, Lien HH, Aass N, Fosså SD. Ejaculation in testicular cancer patients after postchemotherapy retroperitoneal lymph node dissection. Br J Cancer. 1999;80:249–55.
34. Gleeson HK, Shalet SM. The impact of cancer therapy on the endocrine system in survivors of childhood brain tumours. Endocr Relat Cancer. 2004;11:589–602.
35. Bal C, Kumar A, Tripathi M, Chandrashekar N, Phom H, Murali NR, Chandra P, Pant GS. High-dose radioiodine treatment for differentiated thyroid carcinoma is not associated with change in female fertility or any genetic risk to the offspring. Int J Radiat Oncol Biol Phys. 2005;63:449–55.
36. Esfahani AF, Eftekhari M, Zenooz N, Saghari M. Gonadal function in patients with differentiated

thyroid cancer treated with (131)I. Hell J Nucl Med. 2004;7:52–5.
37. Khaksar SJ, Laing RW, Langley SE. Fertility after prostate brachytherapy. BJU Int. 2005;96:915.
38. Hansen PV, Trykker H, Svennekjær IL, Hvolby J. Long-term recovery of spermatogenesis after radiotherapy in patients with testicular cancer. Radiother Oncol. 1990;18:117–25.
39. Kinsella TJ, Trivette G, Rowland J, Sorace R, Miller R, Fraass B, Steinberg SM, Glatstein E, Sherins RJ. Long-term follow-up of testicular function following radiation therapy for early-stage Hodgkin's disease. J Clin Oncol. 1989;7:718–24.
40. Ash P. The influence of radiation on fertility in man. Br J Radiol. 1980;53:271–8.
41. Centola GM, Keller JW, Henzler M, Rubin P. Effect of low-dose testicular irradiation on sperm count and fertility in patients with testicular seminoma. J Androl. 1994;15:608–13.
42. Lambrot R, Coffigny H, Pairault C, Lécureuil C, Frydman R, Habert R, Rouiller-Fabre V. High radiosensitivity of germ cells in human male fetus. J Clin Endocrinol Metab. 2007;92:2632–9.
43. Lee SJ, Schover LR, Partridge AH, Patrizio P, Wallace WH, Hagerty K, Beck LN, Brennan LV, Oktay K. American society of clinical oncology recommendations on fertility preservation in cancer patients. J Clin Oncol. 2006;24:2917–31.
44. Howell SJ, Shalet SM. Spermatogenesis after cancer treatment: damage and recovery. J Natl Cancer Inst Monogr. 2005;34:12–7.
45. Shalet SM, Didi M, Ogilvy-Stuart AL, Schulga J, Donaldson MD. Growth and endocrine function after bone marrow transplantation. Clin Endocrinol (Oxf). 1995;42:333–9.
46. Hahn EW, Feingold SM, Simpson L, Batata M. Recovery from aspermia induced by low-dose radiation in seminoma patients. Cancer. 1982;50:337–40.
47. Piroth MD, Hensley F, Wannenmacher M, Zierhut D. Male gonadal dose in adjuvant 3-d-pelvic irradiation after anterior resection of rectal cancer: influence to fertility. Strahlenther Onkol. 2003;179:754–9. [in German].
48. Edgar AB, Morris EM, Kelnar CJ, Wallace WH. Long-term follow-up of survivors of childhood cancer. Endocr Dev. 2009;15:159–80.
49. Polland A, Berookhim BM. Fertility concerns in men with genitourinary malignancies: treatment dilemmas, fertility options, and medicolegal considerations. Urol Oncol. 2016;34:399–406. pii: S1078-439(16)30058-8.
50. Arnon J, Meirow D, Lewis-Roness H, Ornoy A. Genetic and teratogenic effects of cancer treatments on gametes and embryos. Hum Reprod Update. 2001;7:394–403.
51. Howell SJ, Shalet SM. Testicular function following chemotherapy. Hum Reprod Update. 2001;7:363–9.
52. Servitzoglou M, De Vathaire F, Oberlin O, Patte C, Thomas-Teinturier C. Dose-effect relationship of Alkylating agents on testicular function in male survivors of childhood lymphoma. Pediatr Hematol Oncol. 2015;32:613–23.
53. Müller J, Hertz H, Skakkebaek NE. Development of the seminiferous epithelium during and after treatment for acute lymphoblastic leukemia in childhood. Horm Res. 1988;30:115–20.
54. Bar-Shira Maymon B, Yogev L, Marks A, Hauser R, Botchan A, Yavetz H. Sertoli cell inactivation by cytotoxic damage to the human testis after cancer chemotherapy. Fertil Steril. 2004;81:1391–4.
55. Friedman NM, Plymate SR. Leydig cell dysfunction and gynaecomastia in adult males treated with alkylating agents. Clin Endocrinol (Oxf). 1980;12: 553–6.
56. Chatterjee R, Haines GA, Perera DM, Goldstone A, Morris ID. Testicular and sperm DNA damage after treatment with fludarabine for chronic lymphocytic leukaemia. Hum Reprod. 2000;15:762–6.
57. Colpi GM, Contalbi GF, Nerva F, Sagone P, Piediferro G. Testicular function following chemo-radiotherapy. Eur J Obstet Gynecol Reprod Biol. 2004;113(Suppl. 1):S2–6.
58. Lampe H, Horwich A, Norman A, Nicholls J, Dearnaley DP. Fertility after chemotherapy for testicular germ cell cancers. J Clin Oncol. 1997;15:239–45.
59. Levi M, Shalgi R, Brenner B, Perl G, Purim O, Amit L, Stemmer SM, Ben-Aharon I. The impact of oxaliplatin on the gonads: from bedside to the bench. Mol Hum Reprod. 2015;21:885–93.
60. Lopes F, Smith R, Nash S, Mitchell RT, Spears N. Irinotecan metabolite SN38 results in germ cell loss in the testis but not in the ovary of prepubertal mice. Mol Hum Reprod. 2016;22:745–55. pii: gaw051. [Epub ahead of print].
61. Mariani S, Basciani S, Fabbri A, Agati L, Ulisse S, Lubrano C, Spera G, Gnessi L. Severe oligozoospermia in a young man with chronic myeloid leukemia on long-term treatment with imatinib started before puberty. Fertil Steril. 2011;95:1120. e15–17.
62. Viviani S, Santoro A, Ragni G, Bonfante V, Bestetti O, Bonadonna G. Gonadal toxicity after combination chemotherapy for Hodgkin's disease. Comparative results of MOPP vs ABVD. Eur J Cancer Clin Oncol. 1985;21:601–5.
63. Fosså SD, Magelssen H. Fertility and reproduction after chemotherapy of adult cancer patients: malignant lymphoma and testicular cancer. Ann Oncol. 2004;15:259–65.
64. van den Berg H, Furstner F, van den Bos C, Behrendt H. Decreasing the number of MOPP courses reduces gonadal damage in survivors of childhood Hodgkin disease. Pediatr Blood Cancer. 2004;42:210–5.
65. Delbes G, Hales BF, Robaire B. Effects of the chemotherapy cocktail used to treat testicular cancer on sperm chromatin integrity. J Androl. 2007;28:241–9.
66. Spermon JR, Ramos L, Wetzels AM, Sweep CG, Braat DD, Kiemeney LA, Witjes JA. Sperm integrity pre- and postchemotherapy in men with testicular germ cell cancer. Hum Reprod. 2006;21:1781–6.

67. Muller J, Skakkebaek NE. Quantification of germ cells and seminiferous tubules by stereological examination of testicles from 50 boys who suffered from sudden death. Int J Androl. 1983;6:143–56.
68. Agarwal A, Said TM. Implications of systemic malignancies on human fertility. Reprod Biomed Online. 2004;9:673–9.
69. Bahadur G, Chatterjee R, Ralph D. Testicular tissue cryopreservation in boys. Ethical and legal issues: case report. Hum Reprod. 2000;15:1416–20.
70. Cicognani A, Cacciari E, Pasini A, Burnelli R, De Iasio R, Pirazzoli P, Paolucci G. Low serum inhibin B levels as a marker of testicular damage after treatment for a childhood malignancy. Eur J Pediatr. 2000;159:103–7.
71. Bordallo MA, Guimarães MM, Pessoa CH, Carriço MK, Dimetz T, Gazolla HM, Dobbin J, Castilho IA. Decreased serum inhibin B/FSH ratio as a marker of Sertoli cell function in male survivors after chemotherapy in childhood and adolescence. J Pediatr Endocrinol Metab. 2004;17:879–87.
72. Oshima H, Sarada T, Ochiai OK, Tamoaki B. Effects of synthetic estrogen upon steroid bioconversation in vitro in testis of patients with prostatic cancer. Invest Urol. 1974;12:43–9.
73. Schulze C. Response of the human testis to long-term estrogen treatment: morphology of Sertoli cells, Leydig cells and spermatogonial stem cells. Cell Tissue Res. 1988;251:31–43.
74. Nistal M, Gonzalez-Peramato P, De Miguel MP. Sertoli cell dedifferentiation in human cryptorchidism and gender reassignment shows similarities between fetal environmental and adult medical treatment estrogen and antiandrogen exposure. Reprod Toxicol. 2013;42:172–9.
75. Sapino A, Pagani A, Godano A, Bussolati G. Effects of estrogens on the testis of transsexuals: a pathological and immunocytochemical study. Virchows Arch A Pathol Anat Histopathol. 1987;411:409–14.
76. Schneider F, Neuhaus N, Wistuba J, Zitzmann M, Heß J, Mahler D, van Ahlen H, Schlatt S, Kliesch S. Testicular functions and clinical characterization of patients with Gender Dysphoria (GD) undergoing Sex Reassignment Surgery (SRS). J Sex Med. 2015;12:2190–200.

MIX
Papier aus verantwortungsvollen Quellen
Paper from responsible sources
FSC® C105338

If you have any concerns about our products,
you can contact us on
ProductSafety@springernature.com

In case Publisher is established outside the EU,
the EU authorized representative is:
Springer Nature Customer Service Center GmbH
Europaplatz 3, 69115 Heidelberg, Germany

Printed by Libri Plureos GmbH
in Hamburg, Germany